AUDIOLOGY REVIEW

Preparing for the Praxis
and Comprehensive Examinations

Editor-in-Chief for Audiology
Brad A. Stach, PhD

AUDIOLOGY REVIEW

Preparing for the Praxis and Comprehensive Examinations

Jeremy J. Donai, AuD, PhD
Katharine Fitzharris, AuD, MS, PhD, CCC-A

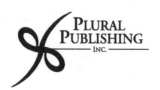

PLURAL
PUBLISHING
INC.

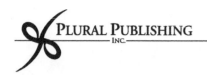

9177 Aero Drive, Suite B
San Diego, CA 92123

email: information@pluralpublishing.com
website: https://www.pluralpublishing.com

Typeset in 12/14 Adobe Garamond by Flanagan's Publishing Services, Inc.
Printed in the United States of America by Integrated Books International
27 26 25 24   2 3 4 5

Library of Congress Cataloging-in-Publication Data

Katharine, author, editor.
Title: Audiology review : preparing for the praxis and comprehensive
    examinations Names: Donai, Jeremy J. (Jeremy James), author, editor. | Fitzharris,
/ Jeremy J. Donai, Katharine Fitzharris.
Description: San Diego, CA : Plural Publishing, Inc., 2024. | Includes
    bibliographical references.
Identifiers: LCCN 2023042392 (print) | LCCN 2023042393 (ebook) | ISBN
    9781635505528 (paperback) | ISBN 1635505526 (paperback) | ISBN
    9781635504415 (ebook)
Subjects: MESH: Audiology | Study Guide
Classification: LCC RF290 .D66 2024 (print) | LCC RF290 (ebook) | NLM WV
    18.2 | DDC 617.8--dc23/eng/20231214
LC record available at https://lccn.loc.gov/2023042392
LC ebook record available at https://lccn.loc.gov/2023042393

Contents

Chapter 3. Acoustics, Psychoacoustics, and Instrumentation   87
Jenna Cramer, Katharine Fitzharris, and Jeremy J. Donai

Chapter 4. Communication Across the Lifespan: Typical vs. Disordered   135
Angela Van Sickle and Brittany Hall

Section III. Assessment and Differential Diagnosis

Section IV. Prevention, Identification, and Treatment

Chapter 8. Screening and Hearing Conservation   377
Leigh Ann Reel

Chapter 9. Treatment: Topics in Amplification   417
Emily Jo Venskytis and Melanie Lutz

Section V. Research and Professional Topics

Preface

*A*udiology Review: Preparing for the Praxis and Comprehensive Examinations* is intended to serve as a review guide for audiologists and audiology students preparing for formal assessments such as Praxis and comprehensive examinations. The material from this text serves as a comprehensive resource for instructors teaching courses (such as capstone courses) designed to review audiology content and prepare students for various types of evaluations. The text is also designed to be a centralized resource for practicing audiologists and those who are required to take the Praxis exam. Over 13 chapters, topics related to audiology basics, diagnostics, treatment, research, and professional issues are reviewed. Section I begins with a description of test question types, then discusses strategies to select an answer, and finally discusses techniques to utilize when taking the Praxis. Section II covers the fundamentals of audiology: auditory and vestibular anatomy, physiology, and disorders; psychoacoustics, principles of sound, and audiometric instrumentation; as well as information regarding the development of speech and language in individuals with typical and atypical hearing. Section III further discusses audiological diagnostic techniques for adult and pediatric patients, vestibular testing and interpretation, and differential diagnosis of auditory and vestibular disorders. Section IV is a review of the screening and identification methods for hearing and balance disorders; industrial audiology; and treatment practices for amplification, implantable devices, as well as audiological counseling, and documentation. Section V concludes the handbook with a review of research, information on evidence-based practice, and professional topics in audiology. Together, this handbook covers information presented during graduate-level education to prepare the reader to approach milestone assessments with confidence. There are practice questions at the end of each chapter, as well as additional materials available on the PluralPlus companion website, including a practice exam and integrated cases with questions.

Acknowledgments

We thank our former professors for challenging and inspiring us to strive for excellence in our respective careers. We would also like to thank all of the contributors, reviewers, and students who assisted in the development of the text. Specifically, Texas Tech University Health Sciences Center AuD student Ashley Reynard played a significant role in the development and editing of various components of the text.

Contributors

Jamie M. Bogle, AuD, PhD
Assistant Professor and Division Chair
Mayo Clinical Arizona
Division of Audiology
Scottsdale, Arizona

Jackie L. Clark, BS, MS, PhD
Clinical Professor of Audiology
University of Texas at Dallas
Dallas, Texas

Trey A. Cline, AuD, CCC-A
Doctor of Audiology
Department of Otolaryngology-Head and Neck
    Surgery
University of Kentucky
Lexington, Kentucky

Jenna Cramer, AuD, CCC-A
Instructor
Texas Tech University Health Sciences Center
Lubbock, Texas

Jeremy J. Donai, AuD, PhD
AuD Program Director
Associate Professor
Texas Tech University Health Sciences Center
Lubbock, Texas

Katharine Fitzharris, AuD, MS, PhD
Associate Clinical Professor
Wichita State University
Wichita, Kansas

Laura N. Galloway, AuD, CCC-A
Assistant Professor
Department of Otolaryngology-Head and Neck
    Surgery and Communication Disorders
University of Louisville
School of Medicine
Louisville, Kentucky

Karah Gottschalk, AuD, PhD, CCC-A
Research Audiologist
James H. Quillen VA Medical Center
Mountain Home, Tennessee

Tori J. S. Gustafson, AuD
Associate Professor
Department of Speech, Language, and Hearing
    Sciences
Texas Tech University Health Sciences Center
Lubbock, Texas

Brittany Hall, MS, CCC-SLP, LSLS Cert. AVT
Assistant Professor and Program Director
Department of Speech, Language and Hearing
    Sciences
Texas Tech University Health Sciences Center
Lubbock, Texas

Candace Bourland Hicks, PhD, CCC-A
Professor and Chair
Department of Speech, Language, and Hearing
    Sciences
Texas Tech University Health Sciences Center
Lubbock, Texas

Melanie Lutz, AuD, CCC-A
Audiologist
UPMC Children's Hospital of Pittsburgh
Pittsburgh, Pennsylvania

Alex Meibos, AuD, PhD, CCC-A
Assistant Professor
School of Speech-Language Pathology and
    Audiology
The University of Akron
Northeast Ohio AuD Consortium
Akron, Ohio

Kay T. Payne, PhD, CCC-SLP (Retired)
Professor Emeritus
ASHA Honors
Washington, DC

Leigh Ann Reel, AuD, PhD, CCC-A
Associate Professor
Department of Speech, Language, and Hearing
  Sciences
Texas Tech University Health Sciences Center
Lubbock, Texas

Angela Van Sickle, PhD, CCC-SLP
Assistant Professor
Department of Speech, Language, and Hearing
  Sciences
Texas Tech University Health Sciences Center
Lubbock, Texas

Emily Jo Venskytis, AuD, ABAC, CCC-A
Director of Clinical Education
Assistant Professor
MGH Institute of Health Professions
Boston, Massachusetts

C. Renee Zimmerman, AuD, CCC-A
Assistant Professor and Audiology Clinical
  Coordinator
Department of Speech, Language, and Hearing
  Sciences
Texas Tech University Health Sciences Center
Lubbock, Texas

Reviewers

Plural Publishing and the editors would like to thank the following reviewers for taking the time to provide their valuable feedback during the manuscript development process. Additional anonymous feedback was provided by other expert reviewers.

Tricia Dabrowski, AuD
Director of Clinical Education
Associate Professor
A.T. Still University
Mesa, Arizona

Richard W. Danielson, PhD, CPS-A, Colonel (U.S. Army)
Retired
Houston, Texas

Diana C. Emanuel, PhD, CCC-A
Professor
Towson University
Towson, Maryland

Karah Gottschalk, AuD, PhD
Research Audiologist
James H. Quillen VA Medical Center
Mountain Home, Tennessee

Julie Hazelbaker, PhD
Clinical Assistant Professor
The Ohio State University
Columbus, Ohio

Kristen Janky, AuD, PhD
Director: Balance and Vestibular Research Lab
Boys Town National Research Hospital
Omaha, Nebraska

Kenneth Morse, AuD, PhD
Assistant Professor
West Virginia University
Morgantown, West Virginia

Leigh Ann Reel, AuD, PhD
Associate Professor
Texas Tech University Health Sciences Center
Lubbock, Texas

Sherry Sancibrian, MS, CCC-SLP, BCS-CL
ASHA Fellow
Grover E. Murray Professor
Program Director—Speech-Language Pathology
Texas Tech University Health Sciences Center
Lubbock, Texas

Gail M. Whitelaw, PhD, MHA
Clinical Associate Professor
Clinic Director
The Ohio State University
Columbus, Ohio

Section I

Test-Taking Strategies and What to Expect

Chapter 1

Test-Taking Strategies

Kay T. Payne

Introduction

Perhaps you have observed that you perform better on some types of exams and not quite as well on others. For example, despite all effort devoted to study, you score high on classroom exams but not standardized tests such as the Praxis. The reason for this difference is that, rather than mere passive verbatim recall of course knowledge, Praxis questions require active use of logic, cognitive processes, critical thinking, and application of academic knowledge. This is often the case for comprehensive examinations required by academic training programs, and as such, the information from this chapter should be helpful on those types of exams. For example, note the difference between the following questions.

In acoustic reflex decay testing, an abnormal decay occurs when the amplitude of the reflex decreases
A. At least one fourth of the initial amplitude
B. At least one half of the initial amplitude
C. Within the first 2 seconds
D. Within the first 5 seconds

An adult patient free of dexterity issues has normal hearing through 750 Hz with a steeply sloping, moderate-to-severe sensorineural hearing loss. Which of the following is most likely to be an appropriate hearing aid fitting?
A. Full shell with small vent
B. BTE with open dome
C. BTE with full shell mold and small vent
D. CIC with medium vent

In addition to the active reasoning skills required to interpret and answer the questions on the Praxis, the time-limited, multiple-choice format requires the examinee to have a planned approach and procedure for advancing through the exam, as well as proven strategies to optimize performance. This chapter will discuss (1) reasoning skills for understanding the question and selecting the answer, (2) guessing strategies, and (3) a recommended test-taking procedure for successful performance on the Audiology Praxis. Demonstrative Praxis-type questions with explanations will be presented, as well as additional questions for practicing the strategies.

For the sample questions above, the first question, known as verbatim recall, is typical of classroom exams wherein you need only recall the answer. Naturally, if you recognize the answer, nothing further is required. For the first question, you should immediately recognize the correct answer as (B). In acoustic reflex decay testing, a signal is presented for 10 seconds, and abnormal decay is observed when the amplitude decreases more than half of the initial amplitude.

By contrast, the second question, which is typical of the Praxis, requires you to be actively engaged in specific cognitive processes and to use professional judgment in selecting the correct answer. For the second question, utilizing your inherent mental processes, you should reason that since hearing in the low frequencies is normal, it is important that the hearing aid provide less amplification for low frequencies than for high frequencies and account for the occlusion effect. A BTE hearing aid with an open dome is the best means for amplifying the high-frequency region and minimizing occlusion by allowing a maximum amount of low-frequency information to escape the ear canal with the open dome. Therefore, (B) is the correct answer.

Known as reasoning skills, several cognitive processes required for Praxis-type questions will be discussed in this chapter. The cognitive processes and logic are demonstrated in the explanations to the correct answers. It is important to know that reasoning skills are not a general approach to taking the Praxis, but conscious processes to be executed for tackling questions that you must methodically think through or make an intelligent guess.

None of the processes are new skills to be learned, nor do they require you to memorize them. Rather, they are inherent and easy operations to be mindful of and apply when you encounter tough questions. As you will see, the reasoning skills are often tied to a typical question format, but not exclusively. Indeed, you can elect to use any reasoning skill with any type of question if it assists in selecting the answer. While reasoning skills are required for most questions on the Praxis, some are useful for understanding the question, while others are to be applied when selecting the intended answer. In fact, you will find that you often use reasoning skills for both the question and the answer.

Understanding the Question

Focusing

Focusing requires conscious awareness of what the question is really asking, that is, what the specific points of information in the question stem imply and what information is relevant to the answer. The question stem may appear as a wordy, narrative clinical scenario from which you must extrapolate the facts and intuit their relevant implication. The major demand of focusing is the ability to summarize wordy questions into concise statements. As a demonstration, note the two versions of the next question.

Version 1

In an investigation of infants' ability to discriminate auditory stimuli, the investigator presents pure-tone signals at various frequencies and dB levels to 30 infants between the ages of 3 and 6 months and observes changes in the rate of their sucking reflex response. The investigator observes an increased rate of sucking correlated with increments of increases in dB level but not frequency. For this investigation, the sucking response is the. . . .

Version 2

In an investigation of infants' discrimination of auditory stimuli, the investigator presents stimulus sounds and observes changes in the rate of sucking reflex responses. For this investigation, the sucking response is the . . .

Now, consider the answer options.

A. Intervening variable

B. Dependent variable

C. Independent variable

D. Control variable

Perhaps a result of test anxiety, or other reason, some examinees fail to translate Version 1 into the more precise Version 2 or recognize that the question is not concerned with the experimental procedures or the outcomes, but the identification of one of the variables. The correct answer is (B). In an experimental study, the dependent variable is the response or change that the investigator measures after applying a stimulus to elicit a response.

Abstracting

This type of question presents information or evidence for the examinee to interpret the meaning of data, extrapolate relationships among variables, and draw appropriate conclusions. Abstracting also requires making clinical judgments, knowledge of and application of diagnostic and treatment principles, and reading tables, charts, graphs, spectrograms, tympanograms, and audiograms. Specifically, abstracting requires the following operations: deriving meaning from charts and graphic displays; identifying relationships among variables presented visually; deriving implications of test results, statements, or conditions; generalizing data or information to novel conditions; and applying principles or rules to novel situations. The following question presented verbally is typical of questions requiring abstracting.

A patient has a conductive hearing loss accompanied by absent middle ear muscle reflexes (ipsilateral and contralateral), delayed waves I, III, and V on the auditory brainstem response, and excellent word recognition scores at 40 dB SL. This result is suggestive of:

A. Cochlear dysfunction

B. Temporal lobe lesion

C. Middle ear dysfunction

D. VIIIth cranial nerve disorder

For this question, the examinee must utilize abstracting to piece together the symptoms described in the question and mentally formulate a diagnosis. The correct answer is (C) since the diagnostic profile suggests middle ear dysfunction (conductive loss, absent reflexes, delayed ABR waves, and preserved word recognition at 40 dB SL).

Ethics and Values

For the Praxis, examinees are frequently required to make ethical clinical decisions based upon professional values and appropriate clinical procedures. These may be reflected in both the question and the answer options. Typical values questions include law abidance, fairness and equity, protecting patient rights, professional decorum, referrals/cooperation with other professionals, objectivity, and the scientific method. It is extremely important to read the ASHA Code of Ethics. Such ethics questions are quite easy, but the points in the Code of Ethics are sufficiently specific that it can be difficult to select the answer without having read the document. The following is an example of a question that reflects ethics and professional values.

An audiologist completes an evaluation due to a complaint of recent hearing loss in one ear. Results of the evaluation reveal a moderate-to-severe, flat sensorineural hearing loss in the right ear and normal hearing in the left ear. The word recognition scores for recorded, full-list NU-6 in quiet at 40 dB SL is 24% in the right ear and 100% in the left ear. Which of the following is the audiologist's appropriate next step?

A. Recommend a Contralateral Routing of Signal (CROS) amplification system

B. Refer the patient for a comprehensive auditory processing disorder (APE) evaluation

C. Refer the patient to a physician

D. Refer the patient for magnetic resonance imaging (MRI)

According to the ethical and professional values of the profession, any recent onset of hearing loss and significant, unexplained, asymmetry between right and left ear requires medical evaluation. Thus, the patient should be referred to a physician for diagnosis, so (C) is correct.

Another type of ethics and values question requires the examinee to recognize and assume the mind-set of the question writer. In the classroom, students adapt to the instructor's style and what the instructor deems as important. Either consciously or subconsciously, students learn to predict what will be on an exam. However, for the Praxis, one should not assume that the emphasis or camp of thought presented in his or her training applies universally or that the same textbooks are used overall. Thus, predicting the examiner is a useful skill that involves selecting the universal or most socially acceptable response. This is supremely important for professionals who have been away from academic study for a prolonged time and may have developed a personal slant, approach, or belief. It is necessary to recognize these and set them aside for the Praxis and select the textbook answer or the most highly professional option.

Negative Stem Questions

Best practices for test question writing recommend against negative stem questions, but they are nevertheless used quite often. Negative stem questions often contain the words *not*, *least*, or *except* or negative prefixes in the terminology. These questions sometimes pose a problem because they require a temporary cognitive shift that demands keen concentration. The best strategy for negative stem questions is known as the true/false strategy, which will be detailed further in a subsequent section. For the true/false strategy, as you read each option, physically (or mentally if the test is online) mark options that are true with **T** and those that are false with **F**. This will provide an immediate visual indication of the correct answer. Then select the option that is consistent with the question stem as it is stated.

An additional strategy is to write the negative word on scratch paper as a reminder of its significance, then select the answer option that is most incompatible with or unlike the others. The following is an example.

Which of the following is the most commonly accepted reason for not using pure tones during soundfield testing?

A. Responses to pure-tone stimuli are less reliable.

B. Pure-tone stimuli are more prone to create standing waves during soundfield testing.

C. Responses to pure-tone stimuli in soundfield are too difficult to hear for most patient populations.

D. Pure-tone stimuli cannot be accurately calibrated for soundfield testing.

After mentally emphasizing the negative word *not*, you must rule out the faulty answer options. Using the true/false method, your decisions in selecting the answer should be visibly rendered as indicated below. This method clearly displays the correct answer as (B) since it is the only one that is true.

A. *F*

B. *T*

C. *F*

D. *F*

Key Words

Key words are superlatives, quantity/quality words, adjectives, or adverbs within the question or answer option that are crucial to selecting the correct answer or eliminating incorrect answers. Some key words provide valuable clues to the correct answer due to their semantic similarity or dissimilarity. The list below contains typical key words for Praxis questions.

- *Best* signals that the answer options include two or more plausible options.
- *Most* and *least* signify a hierarchy among the answer options.
- *Primary* signifies first in sequence, priority, or immediacy.
- *Major, main* signify a hierarchy of importance.
- *Preferred* signifies a value judgment.

Consider the following question that contains a typical and important key phrase.

A long-time hearing aid user is fit with a new set of hearing aids. What is the most likely indicator of good acceptance by the patient of the new technology?

A. New hearing aid processing strategy matches previous aids

B. Client Oriented Scale of Improvement (COSI) goals as described by the patient

C. Improved wireless connectivity features of the new hearing aids

D. Patient's declaration of high motivation to wear new amplification

The key phrase *most likely* signals that several options are plausible, hence it will be necessary to prioritize the statements according to their impact. Option (D) is correct since the patient will successfully adjust to a hearing aid when she or he feels motivated to accept it as an alternative for better communication.

Selecting the Answer

Some Praxis-type questions require reasoning skills to be used when choosing among the answer options. For this type of question, the examinee must select the single best answer. Always remember that the best answer is the textbook response rather than the examinee's personal opinion or experience. Like skills that assist in understanding the question, reasoning skills applied to the answer options are not a test-taking approach applied to every question, but cognitive operations for use only when you are uncertain, or if you do not immediately recognize the answer. The skills presented in this section are familiar operations that you already perform in daily life. However, it is important to recognize that they are required for Praxis-type questions and to practice these skills to be able to apply them automatically and instinctively while taking the Praxis.

Critiquing

While it may be said that all questions involve critiquing the answer options, this reasoning process deserves special mention. In critiquing, after reading the question, each answer option is critiqued individually before deciding upon the answer. Typically, the answer options are lengthy or wordy. Elements of critiquing involve several cognitive processes, including determining the relevance of the statement, determining and evaluating the negative attributes, identifying the worst answer, and applying the process of elimination. Critiquing questions often requires a relative amount of academic knowledge, as reflected in the following example.

An audiologist has completed an evaluation of an adult client. After providing informational counseling, which of the following would not be an expected outcome of the counseling session?

A. The client will understand the degree of hearing loss.

B. The client will share feelings about hearing loss and its effect on their life.

C. The client will know about assistive listening technologies.

D. The client will be knowledgeable of aural rehabilitation options.

As you focus on the question, do not overlook the key phrase *informational counseling*, or the negative stem format. Then, as you critique each option as to whether it is an outcome of informational counseling, the correct answer is (B). Sharing of feelings would not be an expected outcome of informational counseling.

Comparing

Like questions where critiquing is required, some questions require conscious, active comparison of the answer options. Here, the stem appears to be a verbatim recall question. However, selecting the correct answer requires more than mere recognition or recall. Comparison questions require the examinee to discriminate between the options and evaluate quality, degree, impact, or relevance as it relates to the information presented in the question. As an example, the next question requires comparing the answer options.

A 40-year-old female experienced trauma to the head during a motor vehicle accident approximately 2 months ago. She was hospitalized for a week after suffering a concussion and lacerations to her head and scalp. Upon discharge from the hospital, she is reporting brief (15–20 second) episodes of vertigo when going from a sitting to a supine position and when rolling over in bed. The case history should lead the audiologist to suspect which of the following?

A. Central vestibular dysfunction

B. Temporal bone fracture

C. Benign paroxysmal positional vertigo (BPPV)

D. Ossicular disarticulation

This question demonstrates how focusing on the question stem, together with comparing and critiquing the answer options, can lead to the correct answer. The main concerns of the question are the brief symptoms of vertigo when moving from sitting to a supine position and/or rolling over in bed. Together with this information, the examinee must then compare each option for its relevance to the question and assess its potential contribution to the symptoms. Option (C) is correct because head trauma can lead to BBPV.

Classifying

Questions that require classification are typically theoretical and abstract. The question stem may be brief and contain little or no information, while it is the answer options that are wordy and contain the necessary facts. Classification involves discriminating the subtle differences among the options, distinguishing their quality and quantity aspects, and prioritizing and placing them in hierarchical relationships. The question might require selecting the worst answer or the one that is not consistent with the others. The question stem often contains key words *best*, *least*, *primary*, *preferred*, *major*, or *main*. Several answer options may be plausible, but there is one single best answer. The following question demonstrates classifying.

A typically developing middle-school age child who is performing at grade level is referred for further evaluation after failing a school hearing screening. Although she reports no difficulties with her hearing, the audiologist finds hearing loss after a complete audiological workup. Which of the following hearing losses is most likely to go unnoticed?

A. Bilateral moderate sloping to severe sensorineural hearing loss

B. Precipitously sloping to moderately severe sensorineural hearing loss

C. Bilateral moderate conductive hearing loss

D. Bilateral mild to severe mixed hearing loss

After classifying the options to select the condition most likely to be unperceived, (B) is correct. A sharply sloping bilateral sensorineural hearing loss most likely affects only high frequencies, and children with this type of hearing loss may be able to function relatively normally in most situations. Thus, the hearing loss could be unperceived.

Creating

Praxis-type questions frequently present course material differently than the way it was introduced in the classroom. Typically, Praxis questions present a clinical case scenario that requires knowledge of facts or principles to be transformed into a plan of action. Hence, these questions call for active imagination through generating novel thoughts or innovative ideas, or generating a realistic situation from a theoretical notion. Creativity questions may require you to select a course of action and make a diagnosis, prognosis, or recommendation for treatment as in the following example.

While recording the auditory brainstem response (ABR), how can an audiologist effectively delineate between true ABR waveforms and a cochlear microphonic?

A. Increasing the click rate

B. Using supraural earphones to eliminate artifact

C. Lowering stimulus intensity

D. Reversing the polarity of the stimulus

Creativity questions often resemble those requiring critiquing, classifying, or comparing. Indeed, these skills can be used in conjunction or in lieu of creating. The nuance of difference is that in creativity questions, the clinical case scenario is unique, and the answer represents a novel, imaginative thought. For this question, (D) is correct. The cochlear microphonic response can create "noise" that makes it difficult to interpret the ABR waves, such as in auditory neuropathy spectrum disorder (ANSD). The polarity of the cochlear microphonic response, but not that of the ABR, varies with that of the stimulus, so by reversing (e.g., going from rarefaction to condensation) the polarity of the clicks used as stimuli, the cochlear microphonic response will be canceled out and a true ABR can be visualized.

Fusing

Fusing is the inverse of classifying. However, the fusion question may not necessarily contain key words such as *most* or *best*. The question usually contains little information, while much information is contained in the answer options. One or more options might need to be eliminated initially. Fusion questions require finding commonalities among the answer options and identifying the ultimate option that encompasses the others, hence fusing the options. The correct answer is the one that is the most complete. In these questions, several options are fitting or true. The correct answer is the one that is most inclusive or most general in scope, while the others are too limited and specific. The following is an example:

Self-advocacy in the realm of adult aural rehabilitation includes listener training wherein the patient is taught to:

A. Ask the talker to slow down their rate of speech

B. Inform the speaker of the listener's hearing loss

C. Employ a variety of techniques to elicit additional responses from the speaker

D. Employ acoustic information to detect the speaker's message

The correct answer can be selected by fusing the three plausible options into a single broad statement that encompasses their separate ideas. The overall objective of self-advocacy training is to facilitate listening skills using multiple phrases directed at the speaker to gain additional information (e.g., repetition, clearer speech) as represented by (C).

Grouping

Grouping is the inverse of elimination because various options are ruled in rather than ruled out. Thus, grouping involves finding commonalities among the options and selecting all that satisfy the specifications of the question. As such, the true/false strategy described previously is supremely helpful. Presented in several different formats, grouping questions are verbatim recall questions. The question stem often contains key words such as *except*, *not*, and *only*. Among the answer options, a single option stands out from the others (e.g., apples, oranges, grapefruit, cabbage). Some utilize the Roman numeral format, which identifies a combination of items listed in Roman numeral style as in the following example.

The elements necessary for sound to be created are

    I. Energy source
    II. Compression
    III. Transmitting medium
    IV. Vibrator

A. I, II, and IV

B. I, III, and IV

C. I and III only

D. II and III only

The correct answer is (B). The examinee must recognize that the three necessary elements for sound are I, III, and IV and (B) is the only option that contains all three. Another quick and efficient method of selecting the answer is to eliminate any option (i.e., (A) and (D)) that contains the incorrect element, II. Also eliminate any option (i.e., (C)) that does **not** contain one of the required elements, IV. The following grouping question is presented in a different format.

In a hearing conservation program, a significant threshold shift from baseline audiogram warrants further counseling regarding the use of ear protection. The standard threshold shift is

A. 10 dB at 2000, 3000, and 4000 Hz

B. 20 dB at 2000, 3000, and 4000 Hz

C. 10 dB at 500, 1000, 2000, 3000, and 4000 Hz

D. 10 dB at 1000, 2000, 3000, and 6000 Hz

The Occupational Safety and Health Administration (OSHA) Standard Threshold Shift (STS) is defined as a notable change in the hearing ability in one or both ears of an average of 10 dB or more at three frequencies of 2000, 3000, and 4000 Hz. As you group these three frequencies, eliminate any option that contains more than three frequencies, (C) and (D), and with your academic knowledge, choose between (A) and (B). The correct answer is (A).

Cluing

For the Praxis, clues may be intentional or unintentional hints you can detect by consciously matching concepts, words, or semantic styles in the question stem that signal the correct answer. With practice, examinees can develop the skill of recognizing clues through focusing, attending to detail, and making a conscious effort to find a clue. The following example contains a clue that may or may not be obvious to you.

A 64-year-old patient with a unilateral, flat, moderate mixed hearing loss was fit with a single invisible-in-the-canal hearing aid. She reports having trouble tracking the talker when in a group of colleagues or friends. The patient's complaint is most likely linked to which of the following?

A. Disrupted outer ear resonance

B. Poor processing of interaural timing cues

C. Differences in sound quality between ears

D. Diminished frequency selectivity

Using cluing, you should recognize the correct answer as (B). The patient's reported problem implies difficulty in using spatial cues for sound localization, which the patient described as "*tracking the talker.*" Interaural timing differences are important for spatial listening; notice the similarity of concepts in the words *spatial* and *tracking*. You should expect few questions with obvious clues on the Praxis. However, the skill of cluing may be useful for intelligent guessing, as well as for changing to the correct answer when you recheck the exam.

Guessing

The Praxis test makers encourage guessing since it is likely to increase your score, although you should not plan for guessing to be your general approach. Rather, guessing should always be used to assist in selecting the correct answer when you experience uncertainty or difficulty in making your final answer selection. There are two types of guesses: random guess and intelligent guess. This section will distinguish the two and make suggestions for when each should be employed.

If you know nothing about the question content, the rule is simple: Make a random guess. A multiple-choice question is always a game of chance. Since Praxis questions contain four answer options, even a random guess has a 25% chance of being correct. Intelligent guessing will increase this to a greater probability. So, the best guessing strategy is to avoid random guessing since it has the least probability of being correct. Intelligent guessing is an essential skill for multiple-choice exams. Several effective strategies can be useful for intelligent guessing on questions for which you have partial knowledge.

Elimination

Of course, if you know the answer, guessing as a strategy is unnecessary. But most Praxis questions are not the verbatim recall type wherein the answer is automatic or immediately recognized. The reasoning skills discussed above performed on the answer options enable you to rule in options that are likely to be correct. Conversely, the process of elimination rules out untenable options to narrow the possibilities, thereby increasing the probability of a correct intelligent guess. The following are strategies that can be useful for eliminating incorrect options.

- *True/False Strategy.* The true/false strategy was demonstrated previously as a quick method for answering negative stem and grouping questions. Recall that this strategy required marking each option with **T** if it is true and **F** if it is false. The true/false strategy should always be used to help eliminate incorrect answers. This variation requires you to first use your scratch paper to write down the letter options A, B, C, D. Then, as you read through each option on the computer screen, make a **T** beside an option if it is acceptable and an **F** beside all other options to be eliminated. This will allow visual tracking of your decisions, so you won't need to reread each option. Finally, in deciding upon your answer, select the one that is marked with **T**.

- *Avoid Extremes.* Avoiding semantic extremes in the wording of the answer options is an age-old strategy used widely. The presence of negative words in the options (e.g., *no, nothing, not, never,* and *none*) as well as extremes such as *never, always, only,* and *completely* is a signal to avoid that option. Other extreme words contain negative prefixes such as *unimportant, impossible,* and *unlikely.* Avoiding extremes can also entail eliminating the lowest and highest values in a numerical sequence, as well as avoiding (A) and (D) in making a random guess.

- *Avoid Both Opposites.* Akin to avoiding extremes, avoiding both opposites is a useful strategy for intelligent guessing. Be warned, however, that this strategy is not absolute. Using inherent knowledge together with this strategy is always advisable.

- *Avoid Absurd Answers.* Absurd answers are not difficult to recognize, especially if they cause you to chuckle or are unscientific or unethical. It is wise to first eliminate the absurd option then choose among the remaining options.

- *Beware Negative Statements.* Except in rare cases, answer options presented as negative statements are almost always a clue that they should be eliminated.

- *Distrust Unfamiliar Terminology.* When you encounter an answer option you do not recognize, there is a good probability that it is not correct. An example might be a totally unfamiliar word, syndrome, or condition. Yet, there is a proclivity for examinees under stress to select that unknown option. However, this tendency should be avoided.

Taking the Praxis

General Procedure

This general process for taking the Praxis will discuss mental and psychological preparation and behaviors for successful performance. The following is a recommended approach to taking the Praxis.

- Assume an active, rather than passive, approach to each question. The answers will not be readily apparent. Put your mind to work to figure out the answer.

- Take each question at face value. Don't overthink the question by trying to find subtleties, tricks, or hidden meanings.

- Establish a quick yet comfortable pace as you move through each question. Because guessing is recommended, answer every question, guessing if you must.

- When you encounter a question that you know nothing about, take a random guess. Some examinees prefer to use the same letter for every guess. This strategy is as good as any.

- If you think you know the answer but do not immediately find it among the options, use elimination. If you can, eliminate all but two and use intelligent guessing. Flag these questions to return to when you complete the exam.

- If you know the material within the question, flag it if:

  □ You have a memory block.

  □ The question takes more time than it should.

  □ You do not grasp the meaning.

  □ The question appears to be ambiguous.

  □ The implication of a chart, graph, or audiogram is not apparent.

  □ You disagree with the answer options.

- If there is time remaining when you complete the exam, return to the questions you flagged. Do not start at the beginning and attempt to redo the entire exam in sequence.

- If there is time remaining after you return to the questions you flagged, check the exam from the beginning checking for errors. But do not change the answer unless it is clearly an error.

Combatting Test Anxiety

Test anxiety is that unsettling, unpleasant, discomforting feeling experienced in anticipation of or during an exam. Some examinees respond to test anxiety as a positive force, resulting in enhanced performance. However, extremely elevated levels of anxiety can cause distress, confusion, fear, physical malaise, and worry, resulting in ineffective coping strategies that diminish performance. The following are tips to combat test anxiety.

- *Distrust myths heard about the Praxis.* Read all the information about the test from the American Speech-Language-Hearing Association (ASHA) and Educational Testing Service (ETS).

- *Don't focus on past failure.* Adopt an attitude of confidence.

- *Don't trust the reports of others.* Each individual experiences the Praxis differently.

- *Avoid toxic people.* Avoid negative, test-anxious acquaintances.

- *Begin preparation well in advance.* Being prepared will boost confidence and ease anxiety.

- *Visit the student counseling center.* Professionals can provide useful coping strategies.

- *Don't cram.* Relax the night before. Get your usual hours of sleep.

- *Do warm-up exercises before the exam.* Do puzzles or word games unrelated to audiology.

- *Avoid drugs and other stimulants.* These may dull knowledge and induce fatigue during the exam.

- *Write down mnemonic devices and memory joggers on scratch paper.* Do this in the first minute to help combat memory blocks and thus ease anxiety.

- *Take brief relaxation breaks.* To refresh your brain cells.

- *Use anxiety to your advantage.* The adrenaline boost from a little anxiety can be beneficial to performance.

As a final thought, confidence is the antithesis of test anxiety. Indeed, the more you can utilize these and other strategies to bolster confidence, the less you will experience debilitating test anxiety.

Pacing Yourself

For the Praxis, you have 150 minutes to complete 120 questions. The main goal is to complete the exam with time to recheck questions you guessed and flagged for review. Thus, it is important to set your pace early so that you do not worry whether you will finish or rush to finish at the end. The following is a recommended strategy to set your pace.

- Establish a rapid, yet comfortable and efficient pace for the first several questions. Your pace must be comfortable to ensure accuracy. DO NOT speed read the questions.

- After 15 minutes, check the number of questions completed. You should have completed at least 20 questions. (To ensure completion with time to recheck, as a rule of thumb, the number of questions completed should be slightly more than the minutes lapsed.)

- If you have not reached 20 questions, don't panic. Hasten your speed for short verbatim recall questions, avoiding the temptation to speed read. Remember that random guessing on unknown questions will save time.

- Continue working until 30 minutes have lapsed. You should have completed at least 40 questions.

If you have answered 40 questions at this point, your pace is on target for completion. If you have not reached 40 questions, determine the reason. You may still be able to complete the exam. However, you must alter your behavior, or risk not being able to return to the flagged questions. The following timing strategies assist in setting a healthy pace.

Preview Strategy

The preview strategy is useful with a particular question format. The preview strategy is recommended only when the question stem is lengthy, but the answer options are composed of one-word or single-line phrases. It is a practice for saving time with lengthy questions that have one-word or short phrases as options. This strategy is useful because it allows a quick preview of the options. The strategy is exercised as follows:

- Take a quick glance at the question, noting whether the question stem is lengthy. Also notice whether the answer options are one word or short phrases.

- If the answer options are lengthy, answer the question as usual.

- If the answer options are one word or short phrases, scan the options. If none are familiar, make a random guess and select any answer immediately.

- If the answers are familiar, glance at them quickly to gain a sense of the question topic.

- Return to the question and read it thoroughly.

- As you reread the options, if you recognize the correct answer, select it without reviewing the other options and move to the next question.

- If you need to reread all the options, use elimination or reasoning skills to select the best answer.

Single-Letter Strategy

If you run out of time, there is an effective strategy for guessing on questions you have not reached. This is done to gain a few additional points. The single-letter strategy is effective **only** when you have not completed the exam and have several questions remaining. This strategy requires that you continue working until the final minute. In the final minute, choose any letter and mark the same letter for all remaining questions, that is, mark all the options with (A), for example. It does not matter which letter you choose, (A), (B), (C), or (D), as long as you mark every question with that same letter.

For this strategy to be effective, it is important to avoid randomly selecting different options for each question because this will not lead to scoring additional points. As a demonstration of this principle, consider, for example, that you have 15 questions remaining. There is a good probability that (B) is the answer for two or three of those questions. Marking all questions with (B) ensures that you will get those two or three questions correct. Note that this single-letter strategy is effective **only** for a group of final unanswered questions. The strategy is not particularly useful when you must make a random guess on individual questions.

Practice Questions

Complete the practice questions as if you were taking the actual Praxis. Allow no more than 10 minutes and note whether you finish or if you require more time. If you know the information, mark your answer, and proceed to the next question. If you must think through the question or guess, decide on the answer using the test-taking strategies described in this chapter.

1. A 48-year-old male has been referred for an audiological evaluation by his physician. The patient is experiencing hearing loss with vertigo and nystagmus. Medical history indicates that he has recently experienced head trauma resulting in a longitudinal fracture of the temporal bone. Which of the following would be the expected audiological finding?

   A. Cochlear hearing loss

   B. Retrocochlear hearing loss

   C. Conductive hearing loss

   D. Mixed hearing loss

2. Which of the following individuals is the most appropriate candidate for a cochlear implant?

   A. A 50-year-old woman who has tinnitus

   B. A 3-year-old boy who has acquired a profound bilateral hearing loss following a case of meningitis

   C. A 6-year-old girl who has moderate sensorineural hearing loss due to viral infection

   D. A 45-year-old woman who has been diagnosed with Meniere's disease

3. The pure-tone audiogram of a 38-year-old female diagnosed with bilateral otosclerosis exhibits a 40 dB air-bone gap. Which of the following will probably reflect the acoustic immittance results?

    A. Type C tympanogram; low static compliance; absent acoustic reflexes

    B. Type As tympanogram; low static compliance; present acoustic reflexes

    C. Type As tympanogram; low static compliance; absent acoustic reflexes

    D. Type B tympanogram; normal static compliance; elevated acoustic reflexes

4. A patient has come to an ASHA-certified audiologist for a hearing aid fitting. In counseling regarding appropriate expectations, which of the following statements by the audiologist to the patient is not in accordance with the ASHA Code of Ethics?

    A. "You will hear some sounds that you have not heard before."

    B. "Your voice may sound different."

    C. "Using your hearing aid guarantees that your hearing will return to normal."

    D. "It may still be difficult to hear people talking in another room."

5. In the battery of immittance tests, which of the following is most likely to be affected by the cognitive effects of aging?

    I. Tympanometry

    II. Static admittance values

    III. Acoustic reflex thresholds

    IV. Acoustic reflex decay tests

    A. I, II, and IV

    B. III and IV

    C. All are affected

    D. None are affected

6. Otoacoustic emissions (OAE) testing has been found to be most successful in identifying which of the following types of lesions?

    A. Cochlear

    B. Retrocochlear

    C. VIIIth nerve

    D. Temporal lobe

7. The typical immittance pattern for a left-sided facial paralysis where a VIIth cranial nerve lesion is located medial to the stapedial muscle will include which of the following when measured from the left ear?

    A. Normal tympanogram, normal static compliance, absent acoustic reflexes

    B. Normal tympanogram, normal static compliance, normal acoustic reflexes

    C. Abnormal tympanogram, abnormal static compliance, absent acoustic reflexes

    D. Normal tympanogram, normal static compliance, elevated acoustic reflexes

8. Sudden hearing loss can result from all of the following except
   A. Viral labyrinthitis
   B. Vascular occlusion
   C. Genetic disposition
   D. Ototoxic drug ingestion

9. A 47-year-old man is referred for auditory brainstem response (ABR) testing. The referral indicates that he is suspected of having a bilateral functional hearing loss. Medical history indicates that a new medication has been prescribed. Which of the following is a likely observation of ABR testing?
   A. All waves will be delayed
   B. Delayed wave I–V interpeak latency
   C. A single wave (V) will be identified
   D. Results will not be affected by medication

10. A patient is referred to an ASHA certified and licensed audiologist for central auditory processing disorder (CAPD) testing. The audiologist has never administered a CAPD test. According to the ASHA Code of Ethics, which of the following should be the appropriate action?
    A. Refer the patient to another audiologist with experience in CAPD testing.
    B. Delegate the testing to an assistant and provide supervision.
    C. Refuse to schedule the patient.
    D. Administer the CAPD test and request consultation from an experienced audiologist.

Answers

After completing the practice questions, check the accuracy of your answers. For incorrect answers, use the answer explanations for knowledge of the question content as well as the recommended reasoning skill, which is bolded.

1. (C) **Creating**. Use your creativity to anticipate the impact of a longitudinal temporal bone fracture on the hearing process. Longitudinal fracture to the temporal bone will result in ossicular and tympanic membrane injury, thus disrupting sound transmission to the cochlea, producing a conductive hearing loss.

2. (B) **Comparing**. The key word *most* in the question stem renders this a comparison question. A cochlear implant will restore nerve conduction in the cochlea for an individual with a permanent sensorineural hearing loss. Compare the effect on hearing of each of the conditions listed in the options. (B) is the option that would result in a permanent sensorineural hearing loss.

3. (C) **Creating/Grouping**. In otosclerosis, stapes fixation often reduces the mobility of the middle ear system, leading to limited tympanic membrane mobility (Type As). Using creativity, conclude that immittance results will reflect a Type As tympanogram with low static immittance

and absent acoustic reflexes. Using this knowledge together with grouping, eliminate options (A), (B), and (D).

4. (C) **Values/Critiquing**. Critique each option using your academic knowledge and sense of professional values. Ethically, as well as in accordance with the ASHA Code of Ethics, an audiologist must not guarantee the results of a treatment or procedure. Therefore, (C) is correct.

5. (D) **Grouping/Critiquing**. Using the true/false strategy, each of the Roman numeral options is deemed as false, revealing (D) as the correct answer. Since the immittance test battery is composed of physiological measurements, cognitive symptoms of aging will not affect the test results.

6. (A) **Verbatim Recall**. OAE is successful in identifying lesions within the cochlea that affect outer hair cell function.

7. (A) **Grouping/Elimination**. Marking each with **T** or **F**, use the true/false strategy for each of the three elements of option (A); then mark the same in all the other options. When measured from the left ear, a VIIth cranial nerve lesion before the stapedial muscle point of innervation will prevent reflex action, resulting in absent acoustic reflexes, which is marked as **T**, so (B) and (D) should be eliminated. Finally, (C) should also be eliminated since tympanogram and static compliance measurements will be normal.

8. (D) **Negative Stem/Critiquing**. Use the true/false strategy as you critique each option, marking it as **T** or **F**. Ototoxic drug ingestion results in gradual onset of hearing loss, so (D) should be marked **F** since it is false, thereby identifying (D) as the correct answer.

9. (D) **Creating**. Using the specific information in the question, creativity should be used to anticipate the ABR test results. The ABR test provides information on the ability of the peripheral auditory system to transmit information to the auditory nerve and beyond. As such, it does not assess the patient's hearing, and thus the results will not be affected by the patient's medication.

10. (A) **Values**. Using the values of the profession, as well as knowledge of the ASHA Code of Ethics, the only acceptable action is (A). An audiologist must be able to competently provide clinical services or refer the patient to another audiologist to ensure that competent service is provided.

Acknowledgment

The author acknowledges the contributions of editors Jeremy Donai and Katharine Fitzharris in the production of this chapter.

Section II

Foundational Knowledge

Chapter 2

Anatomy, Physiology, and Relevant Pathologies

Jackie L. Clark and Katharine Fitzharris

Auditory System

A broad and deep knowledge base regarding the anatomy and physiology of the auditory system is a necessary asset for the delivery of comprehensive hearing services both in clinical and research domains in audiology. This chapter provides descriptions, tables, and figures for the following classical anatomical terms of orientations as well as anatomy and physiology according to the classic division of the auditory system: outer ear, middle ear, inner ear, central auditory, and vestibular systems. It also includes common pathologies associated with each system and an overview of genetics and embryology.

Anatomical Terms of Orientation

It is important to possess a deep understanding regarding the orientation (both visually and in text) of each anatomical structure according to proximity and possible interactions between auditory and nonauditory structures. Each anatomical orientation is identified in-situ according to axis (or plane) of position when referring to each anatomical structure as if the subject were in a standing position with palms, feet, and head facing in a forward position.

As seen in Figure 2–1, each orientation is referenced accordingly:

- Sagittal/Longitudinal Plane: body being divided (medially) into left and right (lateral) sections with proximal being positioned near a reference point and distal being away from a reference point
- Transverse/Axial Plane: body being divided into upper (superior) and lower (inferior) sections
- Coronal/Frontal Plane: body being divided into front (anterior or ventral) and back (posterior or dorsal) sections

Regardless of body position, a structure within the body can also be described relative to another body structure. For example, the in-situ human cochlea would be distal from the cortex and anterior to the vestibule. Conversely, the left tympanic membrane would be lateral to the human cochlea and proximal to the malleus.

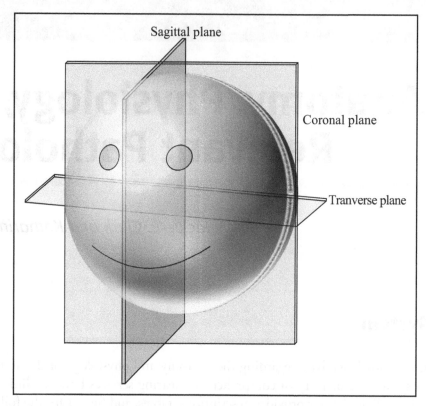

FIGURE 2–1. Classic anatomic orientation for humans.

Typical Anatomy of the Auditory Mechanism

Despite the minute size of the auditory system in total, due to its complexity, scientists will continue to discover new aspects about its anatomy and physiology. The auditory system will be described in four classic sections with basic anatomic and physiologic functions.

- The classic anatomical divisions and their appropriate labels for the major components of the auditory system are seen in Figure 2–2 and described in Table 2–1. Figure 2–2 provides a view of the anatomical structure of the hearing mechanism's peripheral system, while Table 2–1 lists the function of those (and other) major structures of the peripheral and central auditory system (hearing mechanism).

An important task of the peripheral hearing mechanism (comprising the outer ear, middle ear, cochlea/inner ear, and auditory nerve) is to convert minute, but rapid, pressure variations in the air (initiated by vibrating objects in and about the environment) into neural impulses. These will ultimately facilitate a transfer of the information to the central system while preserving the acoustic characteristics of sound for identification and discrimination. Peripheral hearing mechanisms and their function within the auditory sensory system are displayed in Table 2–2. Each anatomical section manages important transduction of energy to varying degrees from mechanical to hydrodynamic to electroacoustic action of activity. Depending upon the frequency, intensity, distance, and mode of transmission of sound, there are instances in which pathology or anatomical abnormalities may (or may not) yield a small to dramatic loss of acoustic energy transmission, resulting in significant disruption in communication abilities.

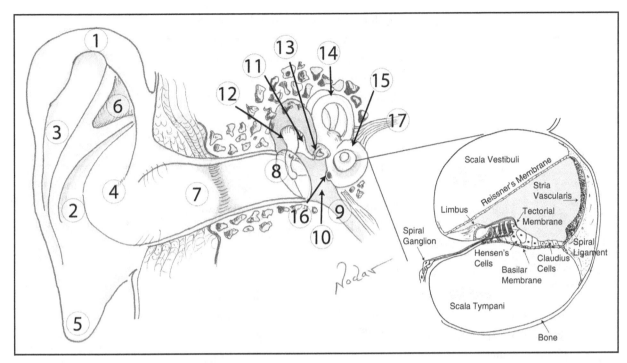

FIGURE 2–2. Main structures of the outer, middle, and inner ear with a cochlear cross section. Key: 1: helix; 2: antihelix; 3: scaphoid fossa; 4: concha; 5: lobe; 6: triangular fossa; 7: external auditory canal; 8: tympanic membrane; 9: Eustachian tube; 10: middle ear space; 11: incus; 12: malleus; 13: stapes; 14: superior semicircular canal; 15: bony cochlea; 16: round window; 17: CN VIII. *Source:* From *The Auditory System: Anatomy, Physiology, and Clinical Correlates, Second Edition* (pp. 1–487) by Musiek, F. E., & Baran, J. A. Copyright © 2020 Plural Publishing, Inc. All rights reserved.

TABLE 2–1. Auditory System

AUDITORY SENSORY SYSTEM: HEARING MECHANISM	
PERIPHERAL SYSTEM	**CENTRAL SYSTEM**
• Outer Ear	• Cochlear Nucleus
• Middle Ear	• Superior Olivary Complex
• Cochlea	• Lateral Lemniscus
• Auditory Nerve	• Inferior Colliculus
	• Medial Geniculate Body
	• Auditory Cortex
	• Association Areas

Outer Ear

Of the two major features within the outer ear (i.e., pinna/auricle and external auditory canal/meatus), the typical human pinna is the largest and most visible auditory structure, which facilitates entry of air-conducted sound into the hearing mechanism (see Figure 2–2).

TABLE 2–2. Peripheral Anatomy and Physiology of the Hearing Mechanism

AREA	OUTER EAR	MIDDLE EAR	COCHLEA	NEURAL
FUNCTION	Sound Localization & Directing Sound	Impedance Matching	Convert Mechanical to Electrical Signal	Translate Electrical Signals
ENERGY TYPE	Acoustic	Mechanical	Hydraulic & Electrochemical	Electrochemical
ANATOMY	• Pinna • Tragus • Helix • Antihelix • Triangular Fossa • Scaphoid Fossa • Concha • Lobe • External Auditory Canal	• Tympanic Membrane • Pars Tensa • Pars Flaccida • Incus • Malleus • Stapes • Eustachian Tube	• Cochlea/Otic Capsule • Round Window • Oval Window • Spiral Ganglion • Reissner's Membrane • Basilar Membrane • Scala Tympani • Scala Vestibuli • Scala Media • Tectorial Membrane	• Auditory/ Vestibulocochlear (CN VIII) Nerve • Facial (CN VII) Nerve

■ The outer ear is important for sound localization and directing sound into the system. Such sound can occur in isolation or multiplicity within varying levels and angles in a listener's environment. The pinna is responsible for an approximate 10 dB "boost" (gain) in an auditory signal around 5000 Hz (Shaw, 1974).

■ Any pathology, absence, or malformation of the outer ear may result in some loss of hearing acuity in the mid-to-high frequencies (2000–5000 Hz). It is believed that the convolutions seen in the outer ear—the helix, antihelix, triangular fossa, and scaphoid fossa—work as a funnel directing acoustic signals into the external auditory meatus/canal (EAM/EAC). Physically, the EAC is oriented lateral to the tympanic membrane (TM).

The pinna is attached to the head (specifically, the temporal bone) at a 15° to 30° angle at the following points:

■ Zygomatic arch anteriorly

■ Mastoid process posteriorly

■ External auditory canal medially

It comprises yellow fibrous cartilage, vestigial musculature, and ligaments and is covered by perichondrium and squamous epithelium. Note that it is common for individuals to develop squamous cell carcinoma on the pinna; this is often treated with surgical removal of the affected area, which distorts the shape of the pinna.

On the left pinna, starting superiorly and working clockwise (anterior–inferior–posterior), major landmarks of the pinna include:

■ Helix; triangular fossa, crura of the antihelix, concha cymba; crus of the helix; supertragic notch, concha cavum, tragus, intertragal notch, antitragus, lobule, antihelix, Darwin's tubercle (not present on every pinna), scaphoid fossa

The superior pinna is innervated by the auriculotemporal nerve (a portion of the CN V, the trigeminal nerve); the concha is supplied by CN VII (facial), CN IX (glossopharyngeal), and CN X (vagus). The lobe and inferior/posterior portion of the pinna is served by the greater auricular nerve (C2 and C3).

- There is some debate about the exact innervation patterns of the pinna, but the previously mentioned nerves are commonly accepted. With regards to vasculature, the pinna receives its blood supply from the external carotid artery, specifically from two branches: the superficial temporal artery (STA) and the posterior auricular artery (PAA).

- The epithelial layer of the pinna is continuous within the EAC. This cartilaginous and bony tube (typically closed at one end with a resonance of ¼ wavelength frequency) is approximately 1 inch long in adults and about 6 to 8 mm in diameter; in children, it is straighter and shorter. In adults, it provides an approximate 12 dB "boost" (gain) around 3000 Hz.

- The EAC is tortuous (S-shaped) and comes to its narrowest point at the osseocartilaginous juncture, or isthmus. The outer one third to one half of the EAC is cartilaginous (i.e., mobile), while the inner one half to two thirds is bony. The cartilaginous portion, in most humans, runs anterior and superior from the tragus to the first bend, then runs posterior and superior from the first bend to the isthmus; note that these turns are helpful in protecting the TM from damage and also play a role in altering acoustic properties of a signal. The osseous portion of the EAC runs inferior and anterior, ending at the TM. The entire structure is housed within the tympanic portion of the temporal bone.

 Q & A

Question: Why is it important for audiologists to be familiar with EAC anatomy?

Answer: Typically, one of the first clinical procedures conducted during an audiological appointment is otoscopy, which is done to visualize the anatomical orientation of the EAC prior to inserting probes, earphones, or otoblocks. During otoscopy, one will pull upward and back (for the adult patient) on the superior posterior edge of the pinna in order to straighten the cartilaginous portion of the EAC to better view the TM. Knowing the landscape of the EAC helps with choosing the appropriately sized probe and insert earphone. It is equally important to know where each bend of the EAC occurs to achieve a deep placement of an otoblock for production-ready earmold investments.

The osseous and cartilaginous portions of the EAC vary in terms of their anatomical elements. At the entry of the EAC, where cerumen is produced, is the cartilaginous portion containing squamous epithelia (~0.5–1 mm thick), hair follicles (pointing outward to provide obstruction and protection), vasculature, subcutaneous fat, as well as sebaceous and ceruminous glands. Cerumen is made of a mix of minerals, lipids, and protein-free amino acids and has protective functions:

- It maintains a pH balance of ~6.1, which creates a toxic environment for most insects.
- It is slightly antifungal and antibacterial.
- It keeps the ear canal lubricated.

Further beyond the cartilaginous portion resides the bony portion of the canal, which has a thinner layer of squamous epithelium (~0.02–0.1 mm) and vasculature.

AUDIOLOGY NUGGET

Cerumen is secreted at the base of the hair cells (HCs) in the cartilaginous EAC. The different types of cerumen are determined by age, genetics, and race. It is determined by a single gene variant, which creates cerumen along the spectrum of dry, crumbly/flaky, gray to tan in color to wet, sticky, yellow-brown to dark brown in color. If there is a blockage of typical epithelial migration exiting the EAC or an overproduction of cerumen in the canal, an occlusion of the EAC can create a conductive hearing loss (CHL). Note that the longer the cerumen remains in the EAC, the drier and more difficult extraction becomes. Audiologists, depending upon state licensure laws, can practice cerumen management. Several techniques to remove impacted cerumen blockage include mechanical (using instruments such as curettes and forceps), lavage (forcing warmed water —sometimes mixed with alcohol, mineral oil, and hydrogen peroxide to flush the cerumen out of the EAC), and microsuctioning. Different ages and types of cerumen require specific removal techniques. It is important to recall the contraindications to cerumen management procedures: If the patient is on blood thinners or has diabetes, undesirable medical side effects may occur. If the cerumen is too deep or if the audiologist is uncomfortable proceeding, a referral to an ENT or other specialty physician is necessary.

Disorders of the Outer Ear

While not exhaustive, Appendix 2–A lists a variety of pathologies, conditions, malformations, or absence of any mechanism within the outer ear. However, outer ear disorders are often treatable (if specialized services are available) and hearing loss may be resolved if treated quickly without chronicity of the etiology in the future.

Middle Ear

By the very resistive anatomical nature of the middle ear mechanisms, not all airborne sound molecules traveling from the peripheral outer ear mechanism will be transformed into mechanical energy within the middle ear space. Fortunately, the impedance matching mechanisms found in the middle ear are critical to make up for the power loss of sound traveling through absorbent human tissue blanketing the cartilaginous pinna and EAC. It is important to recall that impedance is defined as the resistance to the flow of energy.

- One border of the middle ear is the TM, which is the commencement of a series of actions through the connectiveness of the ossicular chain (malleus, incus, and stapes) that results in amplifying acoustic signals via mechanical energy (ossicular chain shown in Figure 2–2).
- The TM is surrounded by an annular ligament that attaches to the temporal bone (tympanic sulcus) and is thought to comprise three to five layers, depending upon the school of thought,

from lateral to medial: the epithelial layer, fibrous layer (radial, circular, radial), and mucosal layer. The pars flaccida (or Shrapnell's membrane) is the superior portion while the pars tensa makes up the majority of the TM.

■ Otoscopic inspections allow visualization of the cone of light typically seen with a normal TM, which appears gray to pearly white, and connects to the manubrium of the malleus that is bisected from the superior to midportion, ending in the umbo. Typically, the cone of light will point to the side that matches the ear being observed (i.e., if the cone of light and umbo are pointing right, it is the right ear; if they are pointing left, it is the left ear).

 Q & A

Question: Describe the changes in modes of vibration of the stapes according to sound intensities.

Answer: As the ossicular joints (malleoincudal and incudostapedial) pivot, the footplate of the stapes will rotate side-to-side with moderate-intensity signals and rock front to back with high-intensity signals. The TM also changes its vibratory patterns depending on frequency and intensity of the acoustic signal. The stapes does not act like a piston, but has rather more complex movement patterns concomitant with the intensity of the incoming signal.

There are three primary ratios (impedance matching mechanisms) responsible for dealing with the impedance mismatch:

1. Area ratio: also known colloquially as the high-heel principle (think walking in flat shoes on a soft surface versus stiletto heels—the latter sinks in a soft surface), the area of the TM is about 17 times the area of the stapes footplate. When the same force is applied to a smaller area, there is a dramatic increase in pressure; this gives the area ratio a value of 17:1.

2. Ossicular lever ratio: there is a lever formed by the manubrium of the malleus and the long process of the incus. These ossicles are tightly bonded at their articulation point, causing them to move as a unit, thereby resulting in a gain of approximately 1.3:1.

3. Curved membrane ratio: also known as the buckling effect, there are two layers of TM tissue vibrating around the fulcrum (malleus). As a result of the curvature, there is greater movement of the curved membranes and less movement of the manubrium, which can increase the force on the manubrium to move with a gain from this ratio of approximately 2:1.

When combined, these three ratios create a force that is 46 times greater at the stapes footplate than at the TM and translates into approximately 33 dB SPL of gain. Without the middle ear mechanism, there would be a loss of 33 dB SPL of the acoustic signal reaching the oval window.

The middle ear anatomy is described below and shown in Figure 2–2, which is much like a six-sided box with the ossicles suspended in the center with the following landmarks.

1. Lateral wall: TM
2. Medial wall: oval window, round window, promontory (covered by branches of CN IX), semi-canal of the tensor tympani, bony eminence of the facial nerve, lateral semicircular canal

AUDIOLOGY NUGGET

When there are concerns regarding middle ear function negatively contributing to hearing, it is possible to monitor middle ear status over a long period of time through immittance testing. Not only is there value in documenting any changes in the outer ear canal volume but also the amount of flexibility (or specific periods of limited mobility) at the TM from infancy and through the lifespan (from infancy through geriatric ages). For example, it is expected that infants to young children will experience more otitis media than older children and adults. When coupled with the pure-tone and speech audiometry, any information yielded about the middle ear system through immittance measures can be used to confirm the type (i.e., conductive [CHL], mixed [MHL], or sensorineural [SNHL]) of hearing loss.

3. Inferior wall (floor): jugular vein (inferior to the inferior wall)

4. Superior wall (roof): tegmen tympani (tegmental wall/roof), the thin petrous part of the temporal bone, separating intracranial compartment and middle ear

5. Anterior wall: Eustachian/auditory tube and carotid canal, as well as the chorda tympani exit

6. Posterior wall: aditus ad antrum, pyramid of the stapedius canal, bony eminence of the chorda tympani (entrance), fossa incudus

Vascularization of the middle ear is via the internal carotid artery (which occasionally may be a cause of pulsatile tinnitus), external carotid, and sometimes subclavian arteries. For specific branches of these arteries, see Musiek and Baran (2020). Venous drainage occurs via the jugular bulb and sigmoid sinus. The middle ear is innervated by CN IX. Although the chorda tympani branch of CN VII travels through the middle ear space, it carries taste and pain fibers from the tongue and face and does not provide sensory innervation.

KNOWLEDGE CHECKPOINT

The Eustachian tube passively opens during natural middle ear pressure changes and actively opens from tensor palatini muscle contraction that elevate the soft palate, at which point the epiglottis will fold down. Pressure within the Eustachian tube will occur when middle ear pressure exceeds the nasopharyngeal pressure, thus forcing the Eustachian tube to open. When air and gasses exit the ear through the Eustachian tube, pressure is then reduced. Though significantly small, the Eustachian tube can become problematic and influential in proliferation of pathologies (such as otitis media, necrotizing otitis media, cholesteatoma) when chronically closed due to thick phlegm plugging the tube secondary to allergies, upper respiratory infections, dramatic/excessive weight loss, or chronic acid reflux disorder.

Disorders of the Middle Ear

Disorders of the middle ear mechanism are shown in Appendix 2–B. Much like disorders of the outer ear, most disorders of the middle ear **if** attended to early may be medically managed and result in transient CHL. However, when these disorders are ignored or co-occur with disorders of the inner ear, mixed losses can occur. Most often the TM is implicated in disorders of the middle ear. Consequently, completing inspection and otoscopy of the outer ear provides insight into possible etiologies that create hearing loss. Immittance testing (discussed in more detail in Chapters 5 and 6) can also provide useful information regarding the status of the middle ear system.

Auditory Inner Ear Structure and Function

The primary function of the cochlea (seen in Figure 2–2) is to convert the acoustic signal into electrical energy that can be utilized by the auditory/cochlear portion of the vestibulocochlear nerve (CN VIII). Mechanisms found at the junction of the stapes and cochlea (the oval window) are the last waystations critical for translating the mechanical energy to hydrodynamic energy to electrical energy. Between the vibrations of the TM to the movement of the stapes in the oval window, frequency and intensity information is preserved for processing within the cochlea via hydrodynamic and electrical events.

Temporal Bone Anatomy

Auditory and vestibular structures are housed within the temporal bone, which is located on the lateral position of the skull. There are four major portions of the temporal bone:

1. Tympanic: contains the osseous EAM and tympanic sulcus
2. Mastoid: point of attachment for several muscles; contains mastoid air cells and tympanic ad antrum
3. Squamous: thin and fairly smooth portion that contains the zygomatic process
4. Petrous: houses the middle and inner ear; canals for nerves and vasculature

Cochlear Anatomy

Located in the petrous portion of the temporal bone is the bony inner ear, which contains the cochlea, vestibule, and semicircular canals. The human cochlea, shown as a cross section in the right side of Figure 2–2, comprises ~2¾ spiraling turns in its membranous form. At its core of the turns is the modiolus, where the spiral ganglia nerve fibers merge to form CN VIII as the fibers exit the inner ear. In addition to the nerve fibers, the modiolus also contains blood vessels for vascular support of each cochlea.

- Each turn can be further divided into three sections or scalae: the scala vestibuli (top; articulates with the oval window), scala media (middle; also known as the cochlear duct), and scala tympani (bottom; articulates with the round window). These three scalae contain cochlear fluids: perilymph (high in sodium, low in potassium; similar to cerebral spinal fluid) in the vestibuli and tympani and endolymph (high in potassium and low in sodium) in the media. There are two fluid systems within the cochlea: cochlear aqueduct (containing perilymph) and the vestibular aqueduct (containing endolymph). The scala tympani and vestibuli meet at the apex of the cochlea at an area called the helicotrema. The scala vestibuli and media are divided by Reissner's (vestibular) membrane while the scala media and tympani are divided by the basilar membrane.

- Basilar membrane
  - □ Contains organ of Corti (see below)
  - □ Supported medially by the spiral lamina (where spiral ganglion nerve fibers pass through to the modiolus) and laterally by the spiral ligament
  - □ Wider (more mass) at apex than at the base (however, note that the cochlear shell is wider at the base of the cochlea than at the apex)
  - □ Stiffer and thicker at base than at apex
  - □ Tonotopically organized: high frequencies at base, low frequencies at apex

The organ of Corti runs the length of the scala media and is the true sensory organ of the inner ear. Here, hydrodynamic forces are translated into electrochemical energy and sent to the auditory nerve fibers. There are numerous cells and components to the organ of Corti, but arguably the most important are the inner and outer hair cells (IHCs and OHCs, respectively), the tops of which are embedded in the reticular lamina and contain stereocilia.

- Outer hair cells (OHCs)
  - □ Supported by Deiter's cells; distal from the modiolus
  - □ Three to five rows
  - □ Cylindrical-shaped
  - □ ~12,000 per cochlea
  - □ Resting charge of −70 mV; K+ channels
  - □ Taller/longer and double the mass at cochlear apex than at base
  - □ Contain contractile proteins for active cochlear mechanism
  - □ Few afferent connections (one afferent nerve fiber to many OHCs); Type II fibers (unmyelinated)
  - □ Many efferent connections (myelinated)
  - □ Stereocilia
    - 50–150 per OHC
    - Embedded in tectorial membrane
    - W-shaped
    - Connected by tip-links and cross-links
    - Shorn by movement of the tectorial membrane
- Inner hair cells (IHCs)
  - □ Tightly supported by supporting cells (stronger HCs); proximal to modiolus
  - □ One row
  - □ Flask-shaped
  - □ 3,500 per ear

☐ Resting charge of –40 mV; K+ and Na+ channels

☐ Majority (90%–95%) of afferent connections (many afferent nerve fibers to one IHC); Type I fibers (myelinated)

☐ Few efferent connections (unmyelinated)

☐ Stereocilia

- 50–75 per IHC

- Curved line

- Longer at apex than base

- Connected by tip-links and cross-links

- Moved by endolymph

While fine structure is beyond the scope of this text, grossly the cochlea is supplied with blood from the labyrinthine artery, which branches off either the basilar artery or the anterior inferior cerebellar artery (AICA) traveling along the brainstem. The cochlea is innervated by CN VIII.

 Q & A

Question: The macromechanics of the basilar membrane can be seen as two distinct mechanical actions. What are those two specific types of actions?

Answer:

Passive mechanics—membrane mechanics are powered purely by simple sound propagation and affected by the mechanical properties of the material that the sound is passing through. The basal portion of the basilar membrane is stiffness limited, whereas the apical portion is mass limited. Both stiffness and mass will affect the acoustic wave in varying degrees.

Active mechanics—refers to vibrations that are powered by additional energy. With the assistance of OHC activity, a mechanical energy is injected into a passive (traveling) wave. The basilar membrane moves up and down, and a sheer force is created at the apical end of the OHCs between the tectorial membrane and stereocilia. This action is often referred to as the cochlear amplifier.

Both the stereocilia and tectorial membrane are the most compromised structures within the organ of Corti.

- Stereocilia and HCs physically interact with the tectorial membrane and are considered mechanoelectric organelles found within the organ of Corti. Through its very nature, the hydromechanical action (initiated by sound waves along the basilar membrane) will be converted into a mechanical form of energy from the stereocilia tips of the OHCs and IHCs that are either embedded or touching/tapping the tectorial membrane. Next, the electrical transduction of energy will aid in modulating a neurotransmitter release (glutamate) at the base of the HCs. Each component of the chain reaction is sensitive to and selectively responds to frequency and intensity of the external signal received in the auditory system.

■ The tectorial membrane is one continuous gelatinous structure that runs from the base to the apex of the organ of Corti. The tips of each of the thousands of longer stereocilia erupt out of the cuticular plate of the HCs and will attach to the underside of the tectorial membrane. Alternatively, thousands of shorter stereocilia erupt out of the cuticular plate of HCs and rest on the underside of (without attaching to) the tectorial membrane.

AUDIOLOGY NUGGET

High-frequency hearing loss due to chronic exposure to excessive levels of noise is most often reported and considered a significant public health problem. Though it is not possible to obtain a visualization of the gross to fine cochlear structure from conception through the lifespan of humans, there is some validity in postulating, from the growing knowledge base about the cochlear anatomy and physiology, about cause and effect of chronic and excessive sound assaults on the hearing mechanism. Consider the anatomy of the cochlea: High-frequency processing has been shown to occur maximally at the basal end of the cochlea. Coincidentally, the mechanical and hydrodynamic activity could be considered at their maxima at the oval window, where the stapes articulates and creates the hydrodynamic energy within the membranous cochlea. It would be reasonable to believe an unusually intense influx of power would result in an intense hydro-dynamic force. Next, consider individuals who work in a noisy environment without wearing hearing protection. What frequencies would likely be negatively impacted initially in this scenario? When considering the tonotopic organization of the human auditory system, the high frequencies would most likely be nega-tively impacted from the environment. It is currently impossible to definitively identify and precisely quantify cause and effect of high-frequency hearing loss as a consequence to the intense hydrodynamics generated at the oval window.

Cochlear Mechanics

As mentioned earlier, when the mechanical/vibratory compression action occurs as a consequence of the stapes footplate vibrating into the oval window, there will be a reciprocal/vibratory energy expansion at the round window, which can be visualized as a traveling wave into the cochlea, as discovered by Georg von Békésy. Such dynamic reciprocal action of expansion and compression at the two separately articu-lating membranous round and oval windows is the beginning of the cochlear transduction of energy.

■ While Reissner's membrane moves down (or up, depending on the phase of the signal) along the cochlea, the basilar membrane also moves; the area of movement is dictated by the mass and stiffness gradient, which contributes to tonotopic organization.

■ In condensation/compression phases, the TM moves inwardly, pushing the stapes into the oval window, which forces downward motion of the basilar membrane; this action is inhibitory. Conversely, for rarefaction stimuli, the TM and stapes footplate move outward, and the basilar membrane moves upward, leading to excitatory actions.

■ When considering HC movement, condensing stimuli move the HCs toward the stria vascularis (lateral wall), which shears the stereocilia toward the modiolus (medial); this creates hyperpolarization of the HCs and the release of gamma-aminobutyric acid (GABA). In rarefaction phases, the HCs move toward the modiolus and the stereocilia deflect toward the stria vascularis, opening the mechanically gated channels and depolarizing the cell, releasing glutamate (an excitatory neurotransmitter) into the intercellular space.

AUDIOLOGY NUGGET

While an AuD student at NSU, Tara Collela introduced acronyms regarding the physiology of rarefaction and condensation stimuli: DERP: depolarize, excitatory, rarefaction, positive auditory effect; CHIN: condensation, hyperpolarizing, inhibition/inward movement, negative auditory effect.

Acoustic signals that generate traveling waves are complex—any given acoustic stimuli can create several traveling waves that simultaneously generate excitatory responses in multiple areas of the basilar membrane. The oscillation rate (speed) of the stapes' movement dictates frequency while the amount of displacement dictates intensity, but fine tuning is controlled by the metabolic function, neural tuning curves, and nonlinearity in the cochlea.

- Metabolic function: unfortunately, von Békésy's experiments were conducted on cadavers with no metabolic function, and his proposed traveling wave cannot adequately or definitively explain the fine tuning and nonlinear actions of the cochlea.
  - Without metabolic function, von Békésy was unable to witness the effects of the cochlear amplifier, which provides gain to low-level sound inputs and is in effect for acoustic stimuli around or below 40 dB SPL.
    - The cochlear amplifier stimulates motor proteins (namely, prestin) of the OHC to shorten or lengthen, effectively enhancing the flow of endolymph across the IHC stereocilia.
    - For more intense sounds (i.e., >40 dB), the cochlear amplifier is not necessary.
- Tuning curves: neural tuning curves can depict the preferential frequency of HCs as well as the frequency range to which a given HC will respond.
  - The tips of the curves are representative of frequencies eliciting a response at the lowest intensity presented.
- Cochlear nonlinearity: at greater intensities, larger portions of the basilar membrane (and more HCs) are stimulated despite the stapes' relatively linear movement.
  - Large areas of the basilar membrane are excited with greater intensities, which were observed by von Békésy.
    - Due to the cochlear amplifier, smaller areas of the basilar membrane can react to acoustic stimuli at lower intensities and lead to more discrete tuning (allowing for improved frequency selectivity as discussed in Chapter 3).

In addition to cochlear mechanics, it is important to understand the cochlear chemical makeup. It is the interaction between both sodium (Na+) rich and potassium (K+) rich molecules that facilitates the electrical charges within the cochlear "battery." Depending upon the cochlear regions, there are relative differences in nutrients, fluids, and ionic charges: 0 mV in perilymph, +80 mV in endolymph, –70 mV in OHCs, and –45 mV in IHCs (Carlson, 1986; Musiek & Baran, 2020), providing nutrients to inner ear structures.

- K+ enters the HCs via channels on the stereocilia and is then expelled under the reticular lamina.

- Electrical synapses move K+ into fluid surrounding HCs, then through the basilar membrane into the scala tympani.

- K+ is picked up by fibrocytes of the spiral ligament, which leads to the stria vascularis.
  □ K+ moves through basal cells, then intermediate cells, through marginal cells, and back into the endolymph of the scala media.
  □ Sodium (Na+) is also transported through the stria vascularis but is removed from entering the endolymph (for the most part).
  □ Genetic mutations such as Connexin 26 can disrupt the gap junctions between the basal and intermediate cells, preventing K+ transport, leading to damage to or destruction of the organ of Corti (Musiek & Baran, 2020).

Theories of Frequency Encoding

Within microseconds of acoustic signals entering the ear canal, the cochlea is able to process the signal: first as sound pressure waves (that are simultaneously processed according to signal frequency and intensity) and next synapse within the efferent and afferent nerves of the inner and/or outer hair cells to immediately begin the sequential neural impulses to enable synapsing at the auditory nerve. These unique sequential synapses, secondary to auditory stimulation, continue delivery via neural input to the central auditory system. As such, the auditory nerve fiber is discriminately stimulated by various frequencies within a wide range of intensities.

- Characteristic Frequency: the frequency at which the lowest amount of sound intensity elicits a neural response (threshold) within specific nerve fibers. There are other frequencies that a nerve fiber will respond to, but not to the same low intensity as the characteristic frequency (CF). It is possible to map the specific CF of each nerve fiber within the cochlea to identify sharp or broad tuning curves. Most of the evidence with frequency coding of the auditory nerve has clearly indicated that the basal portion of the human cochlea (i.e., the point proximal to the oval window and middle ear) encodes the high frequencies. Conversely, when neural signals ascend from the cochlea to the apical aspect of the human cochlea, it is presumed that low frequencies are encoded.

- Temporal Coding: related to the firing rate and phase-locking ability of the auditory nerve. It is conceivable that both coding processes work simultaneously and parallel to each other, which results in more accuracy of frequency coding. Conversely, temporal frequency coding is still not well understood.

- Intensity Coding: the auditory nerve fibers are dependent upon generated spontaneous firing rates (SFRs) as well as the number of neurons activated by stimulus frequencies and intensities.
  □ Firing rates can be described as low, medium, or high. Those neurons with high SFRs are most sensitive to responding to low-intensity signals, whereas those with low SFRs are most sensitive to firing to higher intensities.

- □ It is presumed that the dichotomy of coding mechanisms is the neural correlates of perceived loudness, which allow listeners to effectively process and perceive a wide range of intensities.

- □ Neurons with low SFRs usually have a wider dynamic range and those with high SFRs have a smaller dynamic range in terms of the intensities they are capable of encoding. Together, these two fiber types are thought to account for the significant dynamic range for intensity among human listeners.

Disorders of the Inner Ear

There are a variety of disorders and malformations that can occur at the level of the cochlea, ranging from part or a complete absence of the cochlea resulting from naturally or medically induced teratogens or genetic traits. Appendix 2–C provides a summary of inner ear disorders typically attributed to SNHL in which both bone-conduction and air-conduction thresholds would be abnormal and within 10 dB of each other.

- ■ There may be occasions in which a patient presents with no attributable physical manifestation or etiology but has been identified with SNHL. Unfortunately (for the curious), such a lack of etiology may remain mysterious with unsubstantiated assumptions about the existence of an unknown genetic trait link or abnormal embryonic or preembryonic formation but due to lack of scientific evidence cannot be attributed to the hearing loss.

- ■ More recent translational research and clinical outcomes have provided evidence about cochlear HCs and the active processes of the cochlea being negatively impacted with potential permanence from ototoxic agents (described below), intense acoustic sounds, viruses, bacteria, teratogens during embryologic development, and genetic traits.

  - □ Ototoxic drugs fall into many classes: antibiotics (e.g., aminoglycosides [gentamicin, kanamycin, amikacin, neomycin], amphotericin B, bacitracin, chloramphenicol, macrolides, nystatin, polymyxin B); chemotherapy drugs (platinum compounds such as cisplatin, carboplatin, vincristine); nonsteroidal anti-inflammatory drugs (NSAIDs; ibuprofen, indomethacin, paracetamol, phenylbutazone, salicylates); and other (antimalarials [quinine], loop diuretics [Lasix]). Note that several of these drugs are also vestibulotoxic (gentamicin, streptomycin, tobramycin, chemotherapy agents).

  - □ Other toxic agents include asphyxiants (carbon monoxide), heavy metals (mercury, lead), and solvents (benzalkonium chloride, polyethylene glycol, propylene glycol, styrene, toluene, xylene). Ethyl benzene, styrene, trichloroethylene, and toluene are all vestibulotoxic.

Central Auditory Nervous System: Auditory Nerve to Cortex

Type I and Type II nerve fibers within the cochlea will ultimately become bundled and exit through the habenula perforata of the osseous spiral lamina, into the modiolus, and onward to the internal auditory meatus of the temporal bone. At that point, they are bundled as spiral ganglion and will ascend to the brainstem as the vestibulocochlear nerve (CN VIII; the first auditory bottleneck). As inferred with the name of the cranial nerve, they remain dedicated to either vestibular or auditory input that ascends from the cochlea through the subcortical strata to the auditory cortex. For reference, Table 2–3 includes the 12 human cranial nerves. Importantly, the tonotopic organization that begins in the cochlea is maintained throughout the central auditory nervous system (CANS).

TABLE 2–3. Human Cranial Nerves

CRANIAL NERVES NUMBER/NAMES		TYPE	FUNCTION
I	Olfactory	Sensory	Olfaction (smell)
II	Optic	Sensory	Vision
III	Oculomotor	Motor	Eyelid and eyeball muscles
IV	Trochlear	Motor	Eyeball movement
V	Trigeminal	Mixed	Sensory: facial sensation Motor: chewing muscles
VI	Abducens	Motor	Eyeball movement
VII	Facial	Mixed	Sensory: taste Motor: facial muscles and salivary glands
VIII	Vestibulocochlear	Sensory	Hearing, vestibular, and balance
IX	Glossopharyngeal	Mixed	Sensory: taste Motor: swallowing
X	Vagus	Mixed	Sensory: taste in the epiglottis, EAC, visceral sensation, larynx Motor: parasympathetic nervous system (PNS)
XI	Accessory	Motor	Swallowing; moving head and shoulder
XII	Hypoglossal	Motor	Tongue muscles

Anatomically and physiologically, CN VIII, the outermost fibers, represent the high-frequency information while the innermost fibers are the low frequencies. Cranial nerves VII and VIII travel in the internal acoustic meatus, divided into four quadrants, twisting as the nerves course toward the brainstem. The cochlear portion of CN VIII is located in the anterior-inferior section as shown in Figure 2–3. A simple way to recall the course of each nerve is 7-Up, Coke down, meaning that CN VII is anterior-superior and the cochlear portion of CN VIII is anterior-inferior. The vestibular portions of CN VIII (superior and inferior) are located posteriorly and are self-explanatory.

The ascending tract (CSLIMA, as defined below) is as follows and shown in Figure 2–4:

- Cochlear nucleus (C): the first obligatory synapse of the CANS
  - Located bilaterally through the cerebellopontine angle in the pontomedullary junction, inferior to the fourth ventricle and located below the cerebellar peduncle
  - Divided into anteroventral, posteroventral, and dorsal sections (AVCN, PVCN, and DCN, respectively)
  - CN VIII enters via the root entry zone, then its fibers synapse throughout the cochlear nucleus

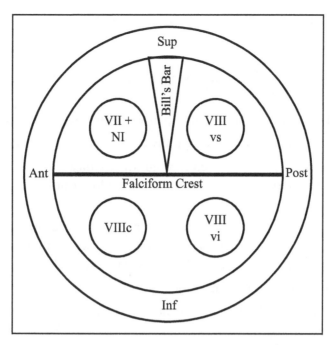

FIGURE 2–3. Figure of the left internal auditory meatus. Key: Ant: anterior; Sup: superior; Post: posterior; Inf: inferior; VII + NI: facial nerve and nervous intermedius; VIII vs: superior vestibular branch of vestibulocochlear nerve; VIII vi: inferior vestibular branch of vestibulocochlear nerve; VIIIc: auditory (cochlear) branch of vestibulocochlear nerve.

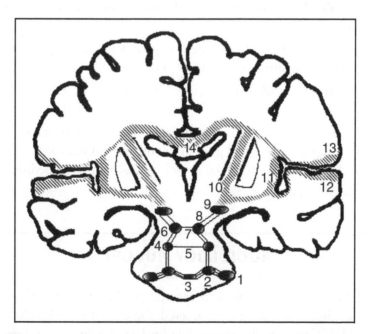

FIGURE 2–4. Coronal slice of the brainstem and brain illustrating the CANS. Key: 1: cochlear nucleus; 2: superior olivary complex; 3: trapezoid body; 4: nuclei of the lateral lemniscus; 5: commissure of Probst; 6: inferior colliculus; 7: commissure of inferior colliculus; 8: brachium of inferior colliculus; 9: medial geniculate body; 10: internal capsule; 11: insula; 12: Heschl's gyrus; 13: inferior central gyri of the parietal lobe; 14: corpus callosum. *Source:* From *The Auditory System: Anatomy, Physiology, and Clinical Correlates, Second Edition* (pp. 1–487) by Musiek, F. E., & Baran, J. A. Copyright © 2020 Plural Publishing, Inc. All rights reserved.

- □ 55+ different cell types with unique coding patterns for spectral and intensity information from CN VIII
  - Different cell types project via different pathways within and outside of the cochlear nucleus
  - Octopus cells themselves are tonotopically organized (Oertel et al., 2000)
- □ The acoustic startle reflex is mediated through the cochlear nucleus, which then goes through the pontine reticular formation, the medial longitudinal fasciculus, and then to spinal cord neurons
  - This reflex, used in very early newborn hearing screening techniques, occurred after a loud sound was played. If the infant startled, the hearing screening was judged "Pass." Note: Use of the startle reflex is not considered best practice for hearing screening purposes.
- □ Location site of auditory brainstem implants
- ■ Superior olivary complex (S/SOC): the cochlear nuclei project to the bilateral SOC
  - □ Located in the caudal pons
  - □ Grossly divided into the lateral and medial SOC (LSO and MSO), but also includes periolivary nuclei and the nuclei of the trapezoid body
    - Trapezoid body contains the largest synapses in the human body—the calyces of Held
  - □ First level of bilateral auditory important, which is important for localization
    - MSO: responsible for encoding the low-frequency interaural timing/phase differences (ITD/IPDs)
    - LSO: responsible for encoding the high-frequency interaural intensity/level differences (IID/ILD); this is relevant to the head shadow effect
  - □ Plays major role in the middle ear muscle reflex (MEMR) or acoustic reflex (AR), which is a bilateral response
    - Acoustic information enters the outer, middle, and inner ear, travels up CN VIII to the cochlear nucleus, then the signal goes to the bilateral SOC, to the bilateral facial nerve nuclei (FNN), down CN VII (facial nerve) to the bilateral stapedius muscles
    - See Figure 5–7 for the reflex arc

 AUDIOLOGY NUGGET

The MEMR is an important tool in the audiologist's toolbox. There are four conditions in which the testing is completed; these are named for the ear receiving the stimulus. These conditions are right ipsilateral (stimulus and recording in the right ear), right contralateral (stimulus in the right ear, recording in the left ear), left ipsilateral (stimulus and recording in the left ear), and left contralateral (stimulus in the left ear, recording in the right ear). Depending on the pattern of test result, different pathologies can be indicated. See Chapter 5 for common patterns of results. For more information, see D. Emanuel's Acoustic Reflex Threshold (ART) Patterns: An Interpretation Guide for Students and Supervisors at https://www.audiologyonline.com/articles/acoustic-reflex-threshold-art-patterns-875

- Lateral lemniscus (L/LL): a large, nonobligatory fiber tract along the CANS
  - Located within the pons
  - Contains two nuclei: ventral (VNLL) and dorsal (DNLL)
    - Bilateral dorsal nuclei communicate with each other via commissure of Probst
    - VNLL has many cells sensitive to ITDs
    - DNLL has many cells sensitive to ILDs and responsive to binaural input
  - Receive bilateral and ipsilateral input from cochlear nuclei and SOC, then project to the ipsilateral inferior colliculus
- Inferior colliculus (I/IC): essentially an obligatory synapse in the CANS; this is an important relay point within the CANS as signals travel to the thalamus
  - Visible on the dorsal surface of the midbrain
  - Endpoint for the acoustic chiasm
    - Formed with ipsilateral low-frequency fibers and contralateral high-frequency fibers from the LSO
  - Comprising several nuclei, projecting mainly ipsilaterally through the brachium to the thalamus
  - First area with time duration–sensitive neurons, which are important for gap detection
- Medial geniculate body of the thalamus (M/MGB): located in the central part of the brain, the MGB projects off of the posterior end of the thalamus
  - The MGB is further divided into the ventral (MGV), dorsal (MGD), and medial (MGM) sections
    - All three sections output to areas of the auditory cortex
  - Important waystation in the nonclassical auditory pathway as well
    - MGM projects directly to the amygdala, prefrontal cortex, and nucleus accumbens, among others
    - Responsible for emotional responses to auditory stimuli
  - A lesioned thalamus does not automatically include auditory areas, but the MGB is responsible for frequency discrimination, localization, the conditioned fear response, and rapid ordering of acoustic elements
- Auditory cortex (A): located on the superior temporal plane of the temporal lobe, located in the Sylvian fissure
  - Also called Heschl's gyrus, the auditory cortex has been traditionally thought of being divided into primary, secondary, and tertiary areas; more recently, these are termed the core, belt, and parabelt, which radiate from a center source (core)
  - Posterior to the auditory cortex is the planum temporale, superior to which is the supramarginal gyrus and posterior to that is the angular gyrus
    - These areas integrate sensory information and are important for activities such as reading
  - Deep to the Sylvian fissure, one will find the insular cortex (or insula or Island of Reil); this is involved in cognitive, emotional, and sensory processes

□ The auditory cortex completes advanced processing of auditory stimuli and, by many interconnections to the remainder of the cortex, is responsible for speech understanding

□ The auditory cortex is asymmetrical in most humans, with the left being larger, which is thought to be the basis for language dominance

The processing of auditory signals does not cease at the auditory cortex. There are many surrounding association areas and tracts (e.g., corpus callosum, cerebellum, insula) where auditory signals are represented and transmitted, but these are beyond the scope of this chapter. Additionally, auditory signals are not only processed in an afferent (ascending) manner, but there are efferent (descending) tracts as well. For more information on these points, the reader is directed to Musiek and Baran (2020).

Vasculature of the Central Auditory Nervous System

Ascending from the neck are the vertebral arteries deep to the external carotid arteries. The latter join together in the brainstem to form a basilar artery, which then leads into the circle of Willis. The vertebrobasilar system is responsible for blood supply to the cochlear nucleus, SOC, IC, LL, and corpus callosum. The circle of Willis supplies the internal and external capsules and thalamus. The internal carotid branches into the middle cerebral artery (MCA), which supplies the temporal lobe, primary auditory cortices, and insula.

Disorders of the CANS

Some disorders of the central auditory system are displayed in Appendix 2–D. These will present with SNHL. Central disorders can present with abnormal MEMRs, rollover, asymmetrical hearing losses, or sometimes normal hearing sensitivity due to the types and places of lesions, as well as the type of stimuli presented (e.g., a person may effectively perceive tones but not words). Much like inner ear disorders, there are no otoscopic findings that provide insight into possible etiologies of central disorders.

Vestibular System

The vestibular system is one of three systems (visual, proprioceptive, and vestibular) responsible for maintaining normal posture, balance, and orientation. It reaches mature size by 17 to 19 weeks' gestation and functions to transduce forces associated with head acceleration and gravity into awareness of head and body in space and produce motor reflexes for postural and ocular stability. The following is an overview of the structure and function of the vestibular system. Additional details are provided in Chapter 7.

Peripheral Vestibular System

The peripheral vestibular system grossly is divided into two sections within the bony and membranous labyrinths: the semicircular canals and the vestibule. The vestibular apparatus is located posterior to the cochlea in the petrous portion of the temporal bone (Jacobson et al., 2021). This is shown in Figure 2–5.

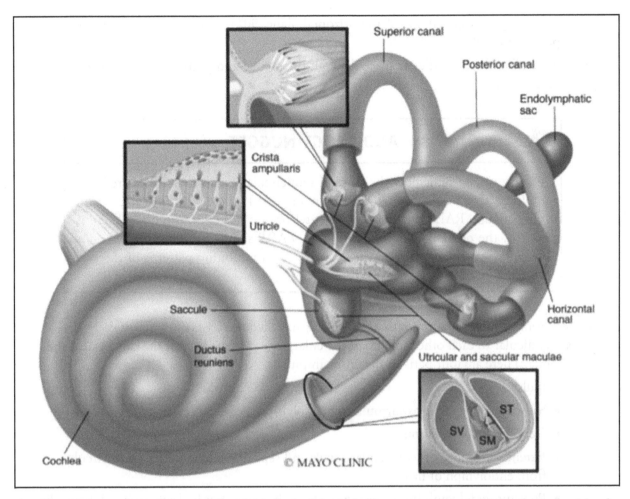

FIGURE 2–5. Anatomy of the peripheral vestibular labyrinth. The structures include the three semicircular canals (horizontal/lateral, superior/anterior, and posterior) and two otolith organs (utricle and saccule). Semicircular canal sensory epithelium contains the crista ampullaris and the otolith organs contain maculae for the otolith organs. *Source:* From Lane JI, Witte RJ, Bolster B, Bernstein MA, Johnson K & Morris J. *AJNR Am J Neuroradiol.* 2008 Sep;29(8):1436–1440; used with permission of Mayo Foundation for Medical Education and Research, all rights reserved.

■ Endolymph fills the membranous labyrinth, created by the stria vascularis (continuous with the scala media) and transmitted to the vestibular system by the ductus reuniens of Hensen.

■ Perilymph fills the space between the membranous and bony labyrinths, providing cushioning between the two. It is supplied from the subarachnoid space via the perilymphatic duct.

Semicircular Canals

■ Detect angular motion

■ Three on each side: work as antagonistic pairs

    1. Anterior/superior: 45° to frontal plane (angled forward); 90° to posterior canal

    2. Posterior: 45° to frontal plane (angled backward)

3. Horizontal/lateral: 20° to 30° to horizontal plane; 90° to anterior/superior and posterior canals

■ Canal extends into middle ear space through the medial and posterior walls (Furman & Lempert, 2016)

AUDIOLOGY NUGGET

An easy way to remember the pairs of semicircular canals that are excited and inhibited together is through the acronyms RALP and LARP (not live-action role-playing). RALP stands for right anterior, left posterior, meaning if one is excited, the other is inhibited. Similarly, LARP stands for left anterior, right posterior, which correlates to the excitation and inhibition patterns of the two semicircular canals.

■ Each semicircular canal contains a sensory organ called the crista ampullaris; these sit perpendicular to each other and are in the enlargement at the base of the canal called the ampulla. There are four parts to the crista ampullaris:

1. Cupula
   - Same specific gravity as surrounding endolymph
   - Gelatinous composition
   - Extends to "roof" of semicircular canals and separates endolymph of semicircular canals from endolymph of utricle
   - Prevents endolymph from moving freely in the canal, but is elastic so it will bend slightly in either direction

2. Type I and Type II HCs
   - Resting charge of −40 mV
   - Stereocilia contain tiplinks
   - Calcium (Ca+) and potassium (K+) channels
   - Type I more responsive within a small area of sensory epithelium
     o Flask-shaped
     o Crest of crista ampullaris and striola of macula
     o Calyx (calyces; large synapses that look like the calyx flower) to afferents
   - Type II react to stronger stimuli over entire sensory epithelium
     o Cylindrical
     o Small bouton afferents
     o Efferents synapse directly to cells

3. 20 to 100 stereocilia and one kinocilium (longest stereocilia) on surface of HCs
   - Project through crista and embedded in cupula

- Arranged in "haystacks" as opposed to stereocilia of the IHCs and OHCs
- Second law of Ewald (1882)—see Chapter 7 for a review of the laws of Ewald

4. Afferent nerve endings projecting to the vestibular nuclei in the brainstem

 KNOWLEDGE CHECKPOINT

If a person turns their head to the left, endolymph will flow to the right in both lateral canals. This will be excitatory (utricopetal) in the left semicircular canals and inhibitory (utricofugal) in the right semicircular canals. The utricle is located anterior to the semicircular canals, so if the endolymph is moving forward, it will deflect the cupula forward, or toward the utricle. On the other hand, if the endolymph is moving backward, it will deflect the cupula backward, or away from the utricle.

- Physics of the semicircular canals
  - Friction, viscosity, mass, and acceleration determine fluid lag and angle of displacement
    - Greater mass means that there needs to be a greater force/acceleration to move the fluid and/or cupula
  - Increase of cupula stiffness or increase of endolymph viscosity: lower canal sensitivity and shorter postrotary sensations
  - Increase of absolute endolymph mass: higher canal sensitivity and longer postrotary sensations
  - Change of endolymph specific mass compared to that of the cupula: sensitivity of the canals for gravity and linear accelerations is induced

Vestibule

- Detect linear motion (up/down, front/back, head tilt, gravity)
- Two organs on each side
  1. Utricle
     - Oriented horizontally
     - Superior to the saccule, anterior to the semicircular canals
  2. Saccule
     - Oriented vertically
     - Inferior to the utricle
- Each organ contains a macula
  - Utricular macula detects linear horizontal acceleration and is not sensitive to constant velocities
  - Saccular macula detects linear vertical acceleration and is not sensitive to constant velocities

- □ The macula is similar to cupula (or tectorial membrane of the cochlea), but does not extend to the roof of the vestibule; instead, it has otoliths/otoconia that sit on top of the maculae
- □ Otoliths provide a weightbearing system (utricle and saccule are also referred to as otolithic organs)
  - Calcium carbonate crystals
  - Sit on top of gelatinous material of macula
  - Gravity causes displacement, which causes deflection of hair cells
- □ There is an imaginary center line of the utricular and saccular maculae called the striola
  - Utricular striola: Hair cells have short stereocilia, polarized toward center
  - Saccular striola: Hair cells have long stereocilia, polarized away from center (Furman & Lempert, 2016)

AUDIOLOGY NUGGET

An easy way to remember the motions detected by the otolithic organs is as follows: When writing an "S" for saccule, your pen moves from top to bottom. This correlates with the vertical acceleration detected by the saccular maculae. When writing a "U" for utricle, your pen moves from left to right. This corresponds to the horizontal acceleration detected by the utricular maculae.

Otolithic Organ Function

- Head accelerates
  - □ Lower part of utricular or saccular (basement) membrane immediately follows
  - □ Otoconia lag behind, deflecting stereocilia toward or away from kinocilium
  - □ Hair cells de- or hyperpolarize (depending on direction of deflection)
- Head decelerates to stopping
  - □ Basement membrane decelerates to stopping
  - □ Otoconia remain in motion, deflecting the stereocilia in the opposite direction
  - □ Hair cells de- or hyperpolarize (depending on direction of deflection)

Peripheral Vestibular Vasculature

The peripheral vestibular system is first supplied by the AICA (or sometimes the basilar artery), which then branches to the labyrinthine artery. This divides into the anterior vestibular artery and the common cochlear artery, which then branches into the posterior vestibular artery. The anterior vestibular artery supplies blood to the utricle, ampullae of the lateral and anterior semicircular canals, and some to the saccule. The posterior vestibular artery supplies blood to other areas: the inferior saccule and the ampulla of the posterior semicircular canal (Jacobson et al., 2021).

Cranial Nerve VIII: Vestibular Portion

The vestibular portion of CN VIII comprises approximately 15,000 bipolar neurons; their cell bodies make up Scarpa's ganglion. These first-order neurons will synapse with vestibular nuclei in the brainstem, which are located on the floor of the fourth ventricle after traveling through the posterior portion of the internal auditory canal. The nerve is divided into two branches: inferior and superior. The inferior vestibular nerve carries input from the saccule and posterior semicircular canal. The superior vestibular nerve carries input from the horizontal and anterior semicircular canals, as well as the utricle and some of the saccule. Figure 2–3 shows the orientation of the vestibular portion of CN VIII in the internal acoustic meatus.

Central Vestibular System

In the central vestibular system, there are four primary vestibular nuclei located in the dorsal medulla and pons (Furman & Lempert, 2016). Note that no primary afferents cross midline, unlike in the auditory system.

1. Superior—receives primary inputs from the vestibular end organs (semicircular canals) and commissural fibers from the contralateral superior vestibular nucleus

2. Inferior—receives inputs from the vestibular end organs (saccule), cerebellum, and contralateral vestibular nuclei

3. Medial—receives main input from vestibular end organs (semicircular canals), reticular formation, contralateral medial vestibular nucleus, cerebellum, and spinal cord

   - Sends efferent signals to the CN III (oculomotor) and VI (abducens) via the medial longitudinal fasciculus (MLF)

4. Lateral—receives main input from the utricle, cerebellum, and spinal cord as well as some fibers from the frontal and parietal cortices

   The central vestibular system is responsible for communicating with the central visual and proprioceptive systems to make motor controls based on the head's movement in space (Furman & Lempert, 2016). There are three main outputs from the vestibular nuclei:

1. CN III and VI—two main routes
   - MLF: direct pathway good for quick communication
   - Reticular formation: maintains spontaneous activity, is the integration circuit for many sensory systems, and is responsible for compensatory eye movements
2. Spinal cord—via the reticulospinal or vestibulospinal pathways
3. Cerebellum—via the vestibulocerebellar pathway through the cerebellar peduncle

   There are four main reflexes that follow the abovementioned pathways:

1. Vestibulo-ocular reflex (VOR)
2. Vestibulo-spinal reflex (VSR)
3. Vestibulo-collic reflex (VCR)
4. Cervico-ocular reflex (COR)

Vestibulo-Ocular Reflex (VOR)

Under normal circumstances, the visual and vestibular systems act synchronously to keep a target image steadily focused on the fovea (back portion) of the eye, referred to as the foveal reflex. However, head movements can be very fast while the "recording" of the foveal images can be slow. This would create blurred/unfocused images to be perceived. The visual system alone cannot keep a target image focused during movement, which is where the vestibular system plays a role.

- Compensatory eye movements (nystagmus) are initiated by stimulus exciting the vestibular end organs, which then triggers a response in the VOR arc

- Eye movements can be conjugate (both eyes moving in the same direction) or vergent (eyes moving in opposite directions)

- Nystagmus—defined as involuntary eye movements with clearly defined slow and fast components; it is normal to have nystagmus in some cases, but pathological in others

  □ The slow component (tracking/pursuit) is the compensatory movement while the fast component is generated by the central nervous system

  □ The direction of the fast component (saccade) defines the nystagmus (i.e., right-beating nystagmus is when the fast phase is to the right)

    • When the head is turning to the left, the slow phase of nystagmus will be to the right as the eyes try to keep the visual target centered on the fovea. When this is no longer possible, the eyes will snap back to center, moving quickly to the left. This is the fast phase of nystagmus, which is left-beating in this case. If the head is turning to the right, the individual will experience right-beating nystagmus.

  □ Nystagmus normally occurs when the head is rotating, can be visually evoked (watching a passing picket fence), under caloric stimulation (differing temperatures of water or air being forced into the outer ear), or when gaze is focused at the extreme lateral (i.e., endpoint nystagmus)

  □ It is pathological when these eye movements occur spontaneously, result from changes in head position, or result from changes in gaze position

 AUDIOLOGY NUGGET

When a patient undergoes vestibular evaluation, pathological and normal nystagmus is being recorded. Under caloric testing, cool and/or warm stimuli (sometimes the testing is completed monothermally, sometimes bithermally, and in some cases, ice water is used) are applied to each ear and the resultant nystagmus is evaluated for direction and strength. To remember the direction in which the nystagmus should occur, the acronym COWS is used; this stands for cold-opposite, warm-same, meaning that cold stimuli should result in nystagmus beating toward the contralateral ear and warm stimuli should result in nystagmus beating toward the ipsilateral ear. Caloric results are compared to normative values as well as between ears to determine if a "weakness" or reduced degree of nystagmus is produced in a certain testing condition, which can be indicative of peripheral vestibular pathology.

        □   Table 2–4 provides additional details about types of nystagmus (Jacobson et al., 2021)

    ■   For the VOR arc to be complete, extraocular muscles are included. These work in antagonistic pairs, similar to the semicircular canals. The muscles and their innervations are shown in Table 2–5.

    ■   The VOR is a three-neuron arc: vestibular afferents project to the vestibular nuclei, which go to the ocular nuclei, which go to the extraocular muscles

        □   For example, if the head is turning left, the left horizontal semicircular canal is excited, which sends excitatory signals to the medial vestibular nuclei, to the ipsilateral abducens nucleus, which then goes to the ipsilateral (left eye) medial rectus via the medial longitudinal fasciculus and oculomotor nucleus as well as directly to the contralateral (right eye) lateral rectus. Inhibitory signals from the right horizontal semicircular canals go to the vestibular nuclei, then ipsilateral abducens to the contralateral (left eye) lateral rectus); it also sends projections to the ipsilateral MLF, oculomotor nucleus, and ipsilateral (right eye) medial rectus. These steps are shown in Figure 2–6.

TABLE 2–4. Types of Nystagmus

NYSTAGMUS TYPE	INDUCED	SPONTANEOUS	NORMAL	ABNORMAL	NOTES
Postrotary	X		X		
Optokinetic	X		X		
Caloric	X		X		
Galvanic	X		X		
Endpoint	X		X		
Gaze	X		X		
Positional	X			X	
Hallpike	X			X	
Fistula	X			X	
Vestibular type		X		X	Fast and slow phase; can be suppressed with fixation; horizontal
Ocular type		X		X	Seen in blindness and miners
Central type		X		X	Irregular fast and slow phases; oblique, vertical; cannot be suppressed with fixation

TABLE 2–5. Extraocular Muscles

MUSCLE	INNERVATION	MOVEMENT	EXCITATORY INPUT	INHIBITORY INPUT
Medial rectus	CN III	Adduction	Ipsilateral horizontal SCC	Contralateral horizontal SCC
Lateral rectus	CN VI	Abduction	Contralateral horizontal SCC	Ipsilateral horizontal SCC
Superior rectus	CN III	Elevation	Ipsilateral anterior SCC	Contralateral posterior SCC
Inferior rectus	CN III	Depression	Contralateral posterior SCC	Ipsilateral anterior SCC
Superior oblique	CN IV	Extorsion	Ipsilateral posterior SCC	Contralateral anterior SCC
Inferior oblique	CN III	Intorsion	Contralateral anterior SCC	Ipsilateral posterior SCC

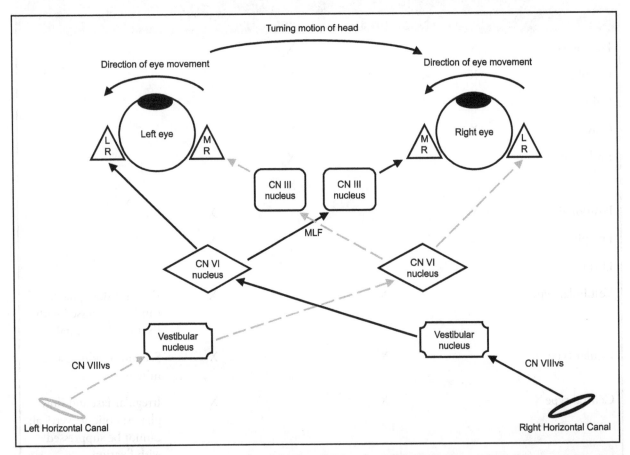

FIGURE 2–6. VOR pathway of right head turn. Black solid lines indicate excitatory signaling; gray dashed lines indicate inhibitory signaling. Key: LR: lateral rectus; MR: medial rectus; MLF: medial longitudinal fasciculus, CN VIIIvs: superior vestibular portion of the vestibulocochlear nerve.

The VOR can be evaluated clinically via ocular vestibular evoked myogenic potentials (oVEMP), calorics, or video head impulse testing (vHIT; Jacobson et al., 2021). See Chapter 7 for additional details of these tests.

Vestibulospinal Reflex (VSR)

The VSR is responsible for maintaining head and body posture (general control of posture) during daily activities (Jacobson et al., 2021). It serves to stabilize the head relative to inertial space by generating a command to move the head in the opposite direction of the existing head-in-space velocity and consists of a three-neuron arc:

1. Vestibular afferents
   - The lateral VSR comes from afferents stemming from the posterior semicircular canal and utricle while the medial VSR comes from afferents of the saccule and horizontal and superior semicircular canals (in fact, a bit from everywhere). The reticulospinal VSR has afferents from the entire peripheral vestibular system.
2. Vestibular nuclei
3. (Cervical) spinal cord

The VSR is clinically evaluated with posturography, specifically the sensory organization test (SOT).

Vestibulocollic Reflex (VCR)

The VCR maintains head position and horizontal gaze relative to gravity. This reflex is evaluated via cervical VEMPs (cVEMP).

Cervico-Ocular Reflex (COR)

The COR is responsible for eye movements in relation to head or torso movements. It is thought to come into play when there are disturbances in VOR function. There are no clinical tests designed to specifically examine the COR (Jacobson et al., 2021).

Higher-Order Vestibular Processing

This section provides a brief overview of the central vestibular system. For more detailed information, see Chapter 7. Five main areas of the cerebellum receive vestibular input:

1. Lobules I to V of anterior lobe—proprioceptive (neck) and vestibular signals for VSR
2. Deep cerebellar nuclei—communication point and tract for VSR
3. Lobules VI to VII (oculomotor vermis of posterior lobe)—visual-vestibular processing
4. Lobes IX and X (nodulus and central vulva)—inertial motion processing
5. Central paraflocculus and flocculus—compensatory eye movements (Furman & Lempert, 2016)

From the cerebellum (and vestibular nuclei), projections run through the thalamus to the cortex, primarily to the temporal and parietal lobes. Most areas of the thalamus and cortex receive and integrate input from the visual, vestibular, and somatosensory systems. The parietoinsular vestibular cortex (PIVC) is critical for shaping perception of self-movement, spatial orientation, and body representation. The dorsal medial superior temporal cortex (MSTd) plays a role processing optic flow information (smooth pursuit) and heading direction. Projections to the cortex also go to the frontal eye field as well as Brodmann's areas 2, 3, and 7 (Furman & Lempert, 2016).

AUDIOLOGY NUGGET

Throughout a vestibular assessment, the peripheral and central vestibular systems are subject to evaluation. Specific patterns of results are indicative of specific pathologies. However, the patient's history and symptoms are equally, if not sometimes more, important. Appendix 2–E displays common pathologies and their associated symptomology. Differential diagnostic procedures and results are discussed in Chapter 7.

Disorders of the Vestibular System

Obtaining a detailed case history for patients undergoing vestibular evaluation is paramount. Vestibular disorders will vary in description and time course of symptoms, provoking factors, and symptoms related to auditory and other domains. Unfortunately, "dizziness" does not mean the same thing for every patient, so further questioning is required. For example, true vertigo is the sensation of movement, either of the individual or their surroundings, when no movement is occurring. Unsteadiness is what precedes falls, or the sensation that one is going to fall. "Dizziness" is the catch-all term for every other sensation associated with feelings of disorientation, imbalance, lightheadedness, or unsteadiness.

- Symptoms can differ between peripheral and central vestibular pathologies. For example, peripheral origins of vertigo will often be accompanied by severe nausea/vomiting, mild imbalance, mild oscillopsia (unstable vision), and hearing loss and will generally recover with treatment or be compensated for with time. Central disorders rarely include hearing loss, but do have severe imbalance and oscillopsia (unstable vision with movement), as well as neurological symptoms and some nausea and vomiting (not to the extent of peripheral disorders). Compensation for central disorders is usually quite slow.

- The goal of a vestibular evaluation is to determine the site of lesion and plan the best course of rehabilitation. The following provides a brief overview of selected disorders; for an exhaustive list of disorders with associated history and site of lesion, see Appendix 2–E. Chapter 7 also describes the differential diagnoses of vestibular disorders.

Genetics

While a number of causes for hearing loss are documented within the general population, there is speculation that as much as 60% of hearing loss occurring in babies is simply due to genetic traits inherited through transmission by their parents (Korver et al., 2017). Some genetic traits are easily traced through mendelian inheritance (autosomal dominant, autosomal recessive, X-linked recessive, and X-linked dominant). In brief, an individual's inheritance of traits is controlled by only a single gene with two alleles. One of the alleles may have genetic dominance over the other. Unfortunately, there are many occasions when a baby or child is identified with hearing loss that may have a specific genetic trait, but genetic testing is not pursued since none of the family members are known to have hearing loss associated with a genetic trait (i.e., autosomal recessive).

Some of the challenges arise from the vast ranges of hearing loss, especially in onset and degree occurring coupled with variability of genetic traits. Such differences in penetrance of traits may result in delayed identification for any genetic traits that upon closer investigation might be found in other family members. Many syndromes involve chromosomal abnormalities that could result in first-trimester miscarriages because of specific gene(s) shared and transmitted through the family lineage. Nearly 20 years ago, there were more than 300 documented forms of syndromic hearing loss that had distinctive features clinically recognized (Morton & Nance, 2006). In fact, there were specific genes associated with hearing loss, such as Connexin 26, impacting the vestibular apparatus and multiple aspects of the hearing mechanism throughout the cochlea, including stereocilia of the fine structure within the cochlea. Further, there are genetic traits attributed to multifactorial inheritance that are influenced by the environment. Though not substantiated, there have been proposed examples of multifactorial traits impacting hearing loss during embryogenesis that can result in other conditions such as neural tube defects, Type 1 insulin-dependent diabetes, cleft lip with or without cleft palate, presbycusis, otitis media, and so on. Genetic disorders and syndromes associated with hearing loss are shown in Appendix 2–F.

Major Embryological Developments

The gestational period is divided into three main stages: preembryonic (fertilization to 3 weeks), embryonic (4–8 weeks), and fetal (9 weeks to birth). A summary of the development of the auditory and vestibular systems is depicted in Table 2–6.

In Utero Development

Syngamy: Preembryonic Stage

At the time of syngamy (fertilization), gametes are formed from the female egg (ovum) and male sperm, each contributing 22 chromosomes and 1 sex chromosomes (46 total) forming a zygote (fertilized egg) (Northern & Downs, 2014), thereby resulting in a fusion of one (or more) "embryo" (Greek term: "to swell"). Embryogenesis is an important process in which an embryo is formed by a collection of cells undergoing mitosis and myosis, resulting in an accelerated growth of cells. By about the third day postfertilization, the zygote (i.e., blastocyst) has three main elements:

- Embryoblast: inner layer of cells that forms the embryo
- A fluid-filled sac connected to the embryoblast
- Rudimentary placenta: a thin layer of cells surrounding the first two components

The blastocyst implants into the uterine lining about a week after fertilization and it will either be unsuccessful and result in spontaneous abortion or more firmly implanted by the second week of gestation. When successful implantation occurs, gastrulation is the next critical embryogenesis stage in which the embryonic disk develops from the embryoblast and contains three (germ cell) layers of tissue divided into ectoderm, mesoderm, and endoderm, which lead to the development of the organs and tissues of the fetus (Figure 2–7). The ectoderm is most relevant for the auditory and vestibular systems

TABLE 2–6. Embryological Development of the Ear

GESTATIONAL WEEK	EXTERNAL EAR	MIDDLE EAR	INNER EAR
3		Development of tubotympanic recess	Otic placode and pit
4	Thickening of tissue begins		Otocyst forms Division of cochlear and vestibular portions
5	External auditory meatus begins to form		
6	Six auricular hillocks are present Begin formation of cartilage		Presence of utricle and saccule Semicircular canals begin formation
7	Pinnae move dorsally and laterally		Sensory cells in utricle and saccule Presence of one cochlear turn
8	Outer 1/3 of external auditory canal formed (cartilaginous)	Cartilaginous malleus and incus Lower half of tympanic cavity	Sensory cells in semicircular canals Ductus reuniens present
9		Membranous layers of TM present	
11			Innervation by CN VIII Completed cochlear turns
12			Cochlear sensory cells Ossification of otic capsule Completed membranous labyrinth
15		Stapes formed (cartilaginous)	
16		Beginning of ossification of malleus and incus	
18		Beginning of ossification of stapes	
20	Adult-shaped pinna (not size)		Adult-size inner ear
21		TM exposed due to meatal plug disintegration	

TABLE 2–6. *continued*

GESTATIONAL WEEK	EXTERNAL EAR	MIDDLE EAR	INNER EAR
30	Maturation of external auditory canal (until 7 years)	Aeration of epitympanum	
32		Malleus and incus ossified	
34		Development of mastoid air cells	
35		Aeration of aditus ad antrum	
37		Change in tympanic membrane position (until 2 years) Aeration of epitympanum Stapes continues development until adulthood;	

Source: Adapted from *Hearing in Children, Sixth Edition* (pp. 1–720) by Northern, J. L., & Downs, M. P. Copyright © 2014 Plural Publishing, Inc. All rights reserved.

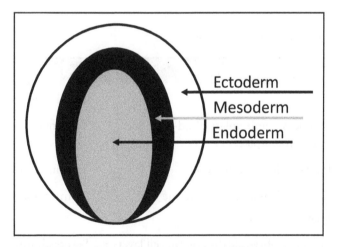

FIGURE 2–7. The three primary germ cell layers present during the third week of gestation: the endoderm in gray, mesoderm in black, and ectoderm in white.

as it gives rise to the inner ear, sensory epithelia, epidermis, and central nervous system. However, the epithelial lining of the Eustachian tube and middle ear cavity are from the endoderm (Northern & Downs, 2014).

At about the 14th to 17th day postfertilization, the process of neurulation ensues, in which the neural tube, brain, and spinal cord begin to develop. The notochord (primitive nervous system;

develops into the axial skeleton) develops during this period of gestation (Northern & Downs, 2014). Ultimately, the ectoderm further develops a thickened layer of cells, which becomes the neural plate, folding into a neural groove that then become neural folds. At or about the fourth week of gestation, the neural tube is closed, giving rise to the central nervous system. An overview of the preembryonic and embryonic stages is displayed in Tables 2–7 and 2–8 (Northern & Downs, 2014).

Embryonic Stage

Appearance of the embryo becoming more recognizable human shape occurs around the end of Week 4. There are several small structures that develop and move dorsolaterally from the neck region eventually much closer to the final placement near the lower mandible/jaw. The external auditory meatus is formed from the pharyngeal/branchial groove, which is the counterpart of the pharyngeal pouch on the endodermal side. Four pairs each of pharyngeal (branchial) arches and pharyngeal pouches are present, which are destined to evolve into bone, cartilage, muscles, nerves, glands, and connective tissue of the head and neck:

1. Pharyngeal/Branchial Arch 1 (mandibular arch)—becomes malleus, incus, upper (maxilla) and lower (mandible) jaws, as well as other aspects of the face, muscles of mastication, tensor tympani, tensor veli palatini; tympanic membrane will arise from the ectoderm and mesoderm; innervated by CN V (trigeminal)

2. Pharyngeal/Branchial Arch 2 (hyoid arch)—becomes stapes, part of the malleus and incus, stapedius, stapedial artery, parts of the hyoid, styloid process, and muscles of facial expression; innervated by CN VII (facial)

TABLE 2–7. Preembryonic Development

TIME	MAJOR DEVELOPMENTS	RESULTS OF INTERRUPTION
Fertilization	Zygote	Termination
Day 3	Blastocyst: embryolast; fluid-filled sac; rudimentary placenta	Termination
Days 6–7	Implants into uterine wall	Termination
Week 2	Firm implantation into uterine wall Bilayer embryonic disk	Termination
Week 3	Trilayer embryonic disk (germ cell layers): ectoderm, mesoderm, endoderm Notochord Neural plate/groove/folds from ectoderm Primitive cardiovascular system	Severe abnormalities of spinal cord and brain
Week 4	Fully closed neural tube Early development of the inner ear Heart begins to beat with primitive blood	Severe abnormalities of spinal cord and brain

Source: Adapted from *Hearing in Children, Sixth Edition* (pp. 1–720) by Northern, J. L., & Downs, M. P. Copyright © 2014 Plural Publishing, Inc. All rights reserved.

3. Pharyngeal/Branchial Arch 3—becomes parts of the hyoid, common and proximal internal carotid arteries, stylopharyngeus; innervated by CN XI (glossopharyngeal)

4. Pharyngeal/Branchial Arch 4—becomes muscles of the soft palate, larynx, and pharynx, cartilages of the larynx; innervated by CN X (vagus; superior laryngeal branch)

Other structures are present during the fourth week as well:

■ Otic pit—develops into the inner ear
  □ Forming the otocyst, which folds, deepens, and elongates to become the vestibular and cochlear structures (accomplished Weeks 5–11)
  □ Cochlear turns develop through Week 16
  □ Membranous and bony labyrinths become fully developed by Week 20 (marking anatomic and mechanical structure is in place, but neuroelectrical system and outer hearing mechanisms are not yet primed to establish functional hearing)

TABLE 2–8. Embryonic Development

TIME	MAJOR DEVELOPMENTS	RESULTS OF INTERRUPTION
Week 4	4 pharyngeal arches Otic pits Lens placodes Limb buds Organ systems	
Week 5	Enlarged head secondary to increased brain size Facial features Limb differentiation Organ systems	Termination or severe congenital abnormalities in multiple organ systems Ventricular septal defect Tracheoesophageal fistula
Week 6	Auricular hillocks Limb definition Growing head size Organ systems	
Week 7	Limb definition Gonadal development Growing head size Organ systems	
Week 8	Distinctive limbs and facial features, including pinna and external auditory canals All major organ systems at least in primitive state	

□ Cochlear bony and membranous structures are at full size by Week 34; developing base to apex (i.e., high frequencies first)

■ Lens placode—develops in the eye

■ Limb buds—develop into the arms and legs

In the fifth week, facial features become more distinct, as do the limbs. Due to increased brain size, the head also becomes larger. Auricular hillocks (which fuse and become the external ear) emerge during the sixth week, and the first branchial groove will deepen to become the external auditory canal. Limbs further differentiate as the head grows larger. These developments continue into the seventh and eighth weeks; at the end of the eighth week, the embryo has an identifiably human-like appearance with a large head, distinctive limbs, and facial features. Throughout the embryonic stage, major organ systems appear and are differentiated, including the central nervous system (neural tube), peripheral nervous system (neural crest), cardiovascular system, respiratory system (laryngotracheal tube), urinary system, and the fore-, mid- (forming the umbilical cord), and hindgut. A summary of the development during the embryonic stage is shown in Table 2–8.

Fetal Stage

With the onset of organ systems formation marking the embryonic stage, the fetal stage is marked by great growth and maturation (Northern & Downs, 2014).

■ Weeks 9–16: The body and limbs of the fetus grow so that their relative sizes approximate a newborn's. The external ears (recognizable pinnae) migrate to the final newborn position.

■ Weeks 17–20: Fetal skin tissue begins to approximate that of a newborn, hair grows, and fetal movements continue to increase. The external auditory canal is blocked with a meatal plug (which becomes the epithelial layer of the tympanic membrane) until the 21st week of gestation.

■ Week 21: External auditory canal becomes filled with mesenchymal tissue and amniotic fluid.

■ Weeks 22–25: Weight gain significantly increases and alveoli develop in the fetal lungs.

■ Weeks 26–29: Full development of hair and the beginning of subcutaneous fat.

The respiratory system reaches maturity in the last 9 to 10 weeks of development; weight and subcutaneous fat increases are noted as well. Aside from overall typical physical development, there are many ways typical auditory development can be significantly slowed, disrupted, or ceased by pharmacologic or natural teratogens creating any degree or type of hearing loss. Some are included in Table 2–9 (Northern & Downs, 2014).

Postnatal Development

Postnatally, typically the auditory and vestibular systems continue to develop.

■ Pinna: develops to adult size by 9 years of age

■ EAC: infant (0.5 cm) grows to about 2.2 cm into adulthood

■ Eustachian tube: elongates and changes orientation (from more horizontal to more angled) during childhood

TABLE 2–9. Developmental Disorders and Syndromes

DEVELOPMENTAL STAGE	DISORDER/ SYNDROME	AFFECTED AREAS	HEARING LOSS TYPE	ETIOLOGY
Week 4	First arch syndrome	Microtia, atresia, ossicles/ middle ear, maxilla, mandible, palate, eyes	Conductive	Cellular migration disruption
	Treacher Collins syndrome	Microtia, atresia, middle & inner ear, eyelids, underdeveloped zygomatic bone	Conductive, mixed, sensorineural	
	Pierre Robin sequence	Outer ear, small lower jaw, palate	Conductive	
Weeks 4–10		CNS, PNS, organ systems, limbs	Sensorineural	Teratogens, e.g., CMV, TORCH infections, rubella virus
Weeks 7–8	Mondini aplasia	Cochlea	Sensorineural	Genetic, syndromes, teratogens (e.g., CMV)

Note: CMV: cytomegalovirus; TORCH: toxoplasmosis, other bacterial or viral infection (e.g., syphilis), rubella, CMV, herpes simplex virus.

Source: Adapted from *Hearing in Children, Sixth Edition* (pp. 1–720) by Northern, J. L., & Downs, M. P. Copyright © 2014 Plural Publishing, Inc. All rights reserved.

     □ This is important because younger children can be prone to middle ear infections secondary to Eustachian tube dysfunction from a more horizontal orientation, resulting in pathological fluid buildup within the middle ear space.

- Cochlea: development (e.g., tuning curve sharpening, especially at the apex) continues until age 8

- CN VIII: myelination continues through the first several months of infancy (up to 6 months to full maturation)

- Auditory brainstem: pons and midbrain continue to grow until the ages of 8 and 6 years, respectively; myelination in the auditory brainstem is typically complete by approximately 1 year of age

- Auditory cortex: fully developed at about 20 years of age due to the caudal-to-rostral maturation of the central nervous system

Other aspects of the brain, such as the corpus callosum, also have a protracted maturation course (Musiek & Baran, 2020).

AUDIOLOGY NUGGET

The infant EAC creates some interesting clinical effects related to diagnostic testing and the fitting of amplification. Their canal is less stiff and has a smaller volume than adults (0.4–1.0 cm^3 vs. 0.6–1.5 cm^3, respectively), which directly affects resonant properties. Otoacoustic emissions (OAEs) may have a greater range of amplitudes in infants than in older patients because of the potentially increased intensity resulting from a smaller resonating cavity. It is important to be mindful of the physics of sound waveforms and the linear interaction of waveforms unpredictably resulting in constructive or destructive interference within the external auditory canal. Consequently, when undertaking hearing aid fittings with infants and children with personal amplification systems, programming modifications would account for the increased or decreased sound intensity delivered to the TM (depending upon EAC shape, length, width, and also frequency of the stimulus). When completing verification measures, clinicians can somewhat account for such differences by measuring real ear to coupler differences (RECD) or utilizing appropriately sized couplers to appropriately match the actual hearing aid output delivered within the ear canal of infants and children. In addition, this smaller chamber can ultimately result in a higher resonant frequency. Ultimately, these differences can lead to more variability in OAE amplitudes, especially in the higher frequencies, as well as an increase in high-frequency amplification. Finally, it is also imperative that clinicians are mindful of the canal size differences when inserting materials (specula, inserts, probe tips) prior to testing so that the TM is not punctured (Musiek & Baran, 2020).

Lifetime Changes of the Auditory and Vestibular Systems

Auditory System

With age, the peripheral auditory system is subject to degradation, especially the OHCs. The middle ear can also be subject to aging, such as arthritic changes and the formation of sclerotic tissues. The pinna and EAC become less elastic, with the pinna lengthening with age. From infancy through young adulthood, the CANS is largely in a plasticity and development mode. Once adulthood is achieved, there is considerable evidence in various animal species that age-related changes occur within the CANS structures. The few studies with humans about CANS changes have implicated a reduction in density of nuclei of the anatomical structural lateral lemniscus, inferior colliculus, superior temporal gyrus, superior temporal gyrus, and lobe (e.g., Ferraro & Minckler, 1977; Thompson et al., 2003). Though the changes were seen in humans with advancing ages, there is also unpredictable variability in degree of anatomical changes as well as ages of the adult humans.

- A variety of studies on the aging central auditory system have demonstrated an expected deterioration of CANS function resulting from the natural aging process: reduced myelination at the corpus collosum (Musiek & Weihing, 2011); loss of vascular density that leaves fewer viable vessels (Kalaria, 1996); atrophy of vessels along with reduced metabolism, resulting in reduced optimal neural function (Clinkard et al., 2013); reduction of cerebral spinal fluid and blood circulation in the brain (Kalaria, 2010); and physiological consequences of reduced blood supply (Thore et al., 2007). With all of these changes, it is expected that auditory processing abilities become altered with advanced aging in adults.

Vestibular System

The vestibular system is fully formed at birth, developed by the 12th to 14th week of gestation and adult-like by the 24th week of gestation (Jacobson et al., 2021). Like the auditory system, the vestibular organs arise from the otic placode and begin development in the third to fourth week of gestation: Disruptive events occurring in this time period can have catastrophic results on the vestibular system. By Week 5, the utricle is formed, and the saccule is formed by Week 9. The sensory epithelium is differentiated between the maculae, cristae, and cochlea in Weeks 8 through 10. Hair cells are fully formed by Weeks 12 to 15 and reach adult-like structure by Weeks 20 to 23. The peripheral system may be developed at birth, but the integration of information and processing of vestibular information is not completely developed until adolescence/early teenage years. Childhood years yield significant changes and maturation in the various postural and motoric responses to vestibular input, including alterations in the VOR (Jacobson et al., 2021).

- With advancing age, there are several factors that result in an increased incidence of dizziness, vertigo, imbalance, and falls (e.g., polypharmacy, disordered vision or proprioception, neuromuscular changes, and medical comorbidities). One of these is the changes that occur in the vestibular system, both peripheral and central.

- In the peripheral vestibular system (semicircular canals and otolithic organs), sensory cells degenerate with age, which leads to degradation of the nerve fibers in the vestibular portion of cranial nerve VIII. The number of otoconia has been observed to decrease with age.

- Alterations have been noted in the connectivity of the central vestibular system as well. On the positive side, vestibular rehabilitation may decrease the fall risk in older adults.

Recommended Readings

Babu, S., Schutt, C. A., & Bojrab, D. I. (Eds.). (2019). *Diagnosis and treatment of vestibular disorders.* Springer. https://doi.org/10.1007/978-3-319-978 58-1

Casale, J., Browne, T., Murray, I, & Gupta, G. (2022, May 8). Physiology, vestibular system. https://www .ncbi.nlm.nih.gov/books/NBK532978.

Jahn, A. F., & Santos-Sacchi, J. (2001). *Physiology of the ear* (2nd ed.). Singular-Thomson Learning.

Katz, J. (2014). *Handbook of clinical audiology* (7th ed.). Lippincott Williams & Wilkins.

Seikel, J. A., Drumright, D., & Seikel, P. (2004). *Essentials of anatomy & physiology of communication disorders.* Thomson Delmar Learning.

References

Carlson, N. R. (1986). Audition, vestibular senses, somatosenses, gustatory, and olfaction. In *Physiology of audition* (3rd ed.). Allyn & Bacon.

Clinkard, D., Amoodi, H., Kandasamy, T., Grewal, A. S., Chen, S., Quian, W., . . . Lin, V. Y. W. (2013). Changes in the cochlear vasculature and vascular endothelial growth factor and its receptors in the aging c57 mouse cochlea. *International Scholarly Research Notices: Otolaryngology, 2013*, 430625. https://doi.org/10.1155/2013/430625

Ewald, J. R. (1882). *Physiologische Untersuchungen uber das Endorgan des Nervus Octavus.* Bergmann.

Ferraro, J. A., & Minckler, J. (1977). The human lateral lemniscus and its nuclei. The human auditory pathways: A quantitative study. *Brain and Language, 4*, 277–294.

Furman, J., & Lempert, T. (Eds.). (2016). *Neuro-otology: Handbook of clinical neurology* (Vol. 137). Elsevier.

Jacobson, G. P., Shepard, N. T., Barin, K., Burkard, R. F., Janky, K., & McCaslin, D. L. (2021). *Balance function assessment and management* (3rd ed.). Plural Publishing.

Kalaria, R. M. (1996). Cerebral vessels in ageing and Alzheimer's disease. *Pharmacology & Therapeutics, 72*, 193–214.

Kalaria, R. M. (2010). Vascular basis for brain degeneration: Faltering controls and risk factors for dementia. *Nutrition Reviews, 68*(Suppl. 2), S74–S87.

Korver, A. M., Smith, R. J., Van Camp, G., Schleiss, M. R., Bitner-Glindzicz, M. A., Lustig, L. R., . . . Boudewyns, A. N. (2017). Congenital hearing loss. *Nature Reviews. Disease Primers, 3*, 16094. https://doi.org/10.1038/nrdp.2016.94

Morton, C. J., & Nance, W. E. (2006). Newborn hearing screening—A silent revolution. *New England Journal of Medicine, 354*, 2151–2165. https://doi.org/10.1056/NEJMra050700

Musiek, F. E., & Baran, J. A. (2020). Normal development, auditory plasticity, and aging effects. In *The auditory system: Anatomy, physiology, and clinical correlates* (2nd ed.). Plural Publishing.

Musiek, F. E., & Weihing, J. (2011). Perspectives on dichotic listening and the corpus callosum. *Brain and Cognition, 76*, 225–232.

Northern, J. L., & Downs, M. P. (2014). Early development. In *Hearing in children* (6th ed., pp. 51–109). Plural Publishing.

Oertel, D., Bal, R., Gardner, S. M., Smith, P. H., & Joris, P. X. (2000). Detection of synchrony in the activity of auditory nerve fibers by octopus cells of the mammalian cochlear nucleus. *Proceedings of the National Academy of Sciences, 97*(22), 11773–11779.

Shaw, E. A. (1974). Transformation of sound pressure level from the free field to the eardrum in the horizontal plane. *The Journal of the Acoustical Society of America, 56*(6), 1848–1861.

Thompson, P. M., Narr, K. L., Blanton, R. E., & Toga, A. W. (2003). Mapping structural alterations of the corpuscallosum during brain development and degeneration. In E. Zaidel & M. Iacoboni (Eds.), *The parallel brain: The cognitive neuroscience of the corpus callosum* (pp. 93–130). MIT Press.

Thore, C. R., Anstrom, J. A., Moody, D. M., Challa, V. R., Marion, M. C., & Brown, W. R. (2007). Morphometric analysis of arteriolar tortuosity in human cerebral white matter of preterm, young, and aged subjects. *Journal of Neuropathology and Experimental Neurology, 66*(5), 337–345.

Practice Questions

1. A patient is being evaluated for an osseointegrated device due to microtia, atretic ear canals, and abnormal middle ear structures. The audiologist also notices craniofacial abnormalities (e.g., eyes slant downward with a notch in the lower eyelid, small jaw and mouth) often seen in Treacher Collins syndrome. Which pharyngeal arch is most likely implicated in this patient?

   a. 1

   b. 2

   c. 3

   d. 4

Explanation: Treacher Collins syndrome is a first arch syndrome; the first brachial arch is responsible for the feature changes of the face and aspects of the ear, especially external and middle ears. Since this patient was being evaluated for an osseointegrated device, a conductive component can be safely assumed to be present, so a is the correct answer.

2. At what gestational age is the cochlea fully developed?

   a. 6 weeks

   b. 12 weeks

   c. 18 weeks

   d. 24 weeks

Explanation: The cochlea begins to develop at approximately 7 weeks (one cochlear turn). At 11 weeks, the cochlear turns are completed, and the following week, cochlear sensory cells are present. The cochlea reaches adult size (i.e., full development) by 20 weeks. Thus, the best answer is d (24 weeks).

3. Which of the following is considered a fine structure mechanism within the auditory system:

   a. Malleus

   b. Modiolus

   c. Tectorial membrane

   d. Reissner's membrane

Explanation: The fine structure refers to the cochlea mechanisms responsible for the conversion of energy from mechanical to electrochemical. The malleus continues the mechanical transfer of energy from the tympanic membrane to the stapes. Modiolus is simply part of the cochlear osseous structure and does not contribute to the transfer of energy. In this instance, the ONLY structure involved in conversion of energy from hydrodynamic to electrical is the tectorial membrane, which is where the hair cells of the stereocilia are embedded . Thus, c is the correct answer.

4. What region of the basilar membrane will vibrate maximally for 100 Hz tone?

   a. Apical/apex

   b. Basal/base

   c. Mid-basal/base

   d. None of the above

Explanation: The basilar membrane is tonotopically organized and is less stiff and compliant at the apex/apical portion, vibrating best with low-frequency signals. Despite not having specific information about the age or frequency response of the cochlea, a is the best answer as the apical/apex portion of the cochlear membrane because it vibrates best in the low frequency similar to 100 Hz.

5. The auditory system serves as a transducer of sensory information. Where does this transduction take place?
   a. Sound entering the external auditory meatus after being funneled by the pinna
   b. Fluid filling the middle ear space due to Eustachian tube dysfunction
   c. Stimulation of hair cells on the basilar membrane in response to sound
   d. The ear canal changing an auditory event into an electrical signal

Explanation: Transduction refers to the conversion of energy from mechanoreceptive as initiated at the cochlear hair cells of the stereocilia contacting or embedded into the tectorial membrane and anchored at the basilar membrane within the organ of Corti to become an equivalent electrical waveform. In this question, the best answer is c, which will ultimately result in a conversion of energy from mechanical to electrical, which allows delivery of the signal to the sensory system.

6. The definition of "matching" relatively low-resistant airborne signals to a mechanism that is highly resistant to airborne signals would be relevant for the following term (choose one that is most appropriate):
   a. Impairment matching
   b. Impedance matching
   c. Incident matching
   d. Impediment matching

Explanation: The major function of the middle ear is to match very low-resistance airborne sounds to the highly resistant fluid contained in the inner ear. This is completed through the mechanical action of the ossicular chain in the middle ear. The best answer for this question is b, which transfers energy from sound traveling in the middle ear through the three major dynamic mechanisms (malleus, incus, and stapes) that through their unified actions ensure very little loss of energy as sound travels into the oval window.

7. One of the structures found within the organ of Corti is:
   a. Reissner's membrane
   b. Malleus
   c. Pars flaccida
   d. Reticular lamina

Explanation: The listing of possible answers contains mechanisms that range from the tympanic membrane, middle ear, and the larger cochlea. Not only by deductive reasoning through elimination, the stiff reticular lamina/membrane extends from the outer hair cells to the Hensen's cells—all reside within the organ of Corti so the correct answer is d.

8. What is an important characteristic of the outer hair cells?

   a. Connected to all Type I spiral ganglia

   b. Responsible for cochlear amplification

   c. Structurally the strongest hair cell

   d. Significant afferent connections

Explanation: The outer hair cells remain stiff when displaced, but the stiffness varies with potential discharges. They also possess contractile proteins and are populated with more stereocilia at the base than the apex. Though outer hair cells have very few afferent connections, they have the most efferent connections. Their electromotile abilities create the cochlear amplifier so that responses to low-level stimuli are enhanced. Responses a, c, and d are characteristics of the inner hair cells, but this question pertains to outer hair cells. Therefore, the best answer would be b.

9. Choose the most appropriate choice of term that would fit the following definition: the frequency at which the lowest amount of energy is needed to stimulate the neural response.

   a. Cochlear amplifier

   b. Low frequency

   c. Characteristic frequency

   d. Compound action potential

Explanation: The key terms to guide the reader are lowest amount of energy and stimulate the neural response. Low frequency is neither a relevant nor a logical response. Inarguably, the cochlear amplifier and compound action potential are important in the transduction of energy, but they do not relate to creating more or less energy to trigger the neural response. Therefore, the only logical and relevant term used for energy use at the neural level is characteristic frequency or c.

10. Which of the following is the reason that the frequency/telephone theory is unable to explain all of frequency encoding abilities displayed by the auditory system?

    a. Neural refractory period

    b. Neural restoration period

    c. Not all neurons fire at the same place in a cycle

    d. Neural fine tuning is greater than what would be expected

Explanation: Though it only lasts a few milliseconds, the neural refractory period can potentially impact the temporal coding of acoustic stimuli by auditory neurons; due to this, the higher frequencies cannot be adequately encoded by the frequency/telephone theory alone. The volley principle involves different neurons firing at the same place in alternating cycles and the place theory is driven by the traveling wave, which has been shown to have broader areas of excitation than are psychophysically measured. Thus, the best answer is a.

Appendix Key

ABR: auditory brainstem response; ANSD: auditory neuropathy spectrum disorder; Audio: audiometry; BPPV: benign paroxysmal positional vertigo; CHARGE: coloboma, heart defects, atresia choanae (also known as choanal atresia), growth retardation, genital abnormalities, and ear abnormalities; CHL: conductive hearing loss; CULLP: congenital unilateral lower lip palsy; ET: Eustachian tube; HL: hearing loss; MEMR: middle ear muscle reflexes (acoustic reflexes); MHL: mixed hearing loss; OAEs: otoacoustic emissions; SCC: semicircular canals; SNHL: sensorineural hearing loss; TM: tympanic membrane; Tymps: tympanometry; VNG: vestibulonystagmography; WNL: within normal limits.

Appendix 2–A

Outer Ear Disorders

DISORDER	ETIOLOGY AND PATHOLOGY	SYMPTOMS	DIFFERENTIAL DIAGNOSIS
Atresia	Congenital malformation of the external auditory canal due to interrupted development of the outer ear Type A—meatal atresia Type B—partial atresia Type C—total atresia Type D—hypopneumatic atresia	Visible abnormalities (often in conjunction with microtia and other craniofacial abnormalities) Speech and language delays Possible inflammation, otalgia, and/or otorrhea	Otoscopy: Abnormal EAC Tymps: Small ECV MEMR: Conductive pattern Audio: CHL OAEs: Reduced to absent
Cerumen impaction	Cerumen that has been prevented from naturally exiting out of EAC	Otalgia/discomfort/ itchiness Hearing loss	Otoscopy: partially or fully occluding cerumen Tymps: Type B with small ECV MEMR: Conductive pattern Audio: CHL (can be mixed) OAEs: Reduced to absent
Exostoses	Broad, round, bony growths that occur in the osseous portion of the EAC	Primarily asymptomatic Hearing loss if large enough Otalgia Cerumen impaction Otitis externa	Case Hx: report of exposure to cold temperatures (e.g., swimming, diving) Otoscopy: Abnormal broad round growths deep in canal Tymps: Type A MEMR: Consistent with audio Audio: Possible CHL OAEs: Consistent with audio

continues

APPENDIX 2–A. *continued*

DISORDER	ETIOLOGY AND PATHOLOGY	SYMPTOMS	DIFFERENTIAL DIAGNOSIS
Foreign bodies	Insects, small toys, earrings/earring backs, beads, etc. either placed or volitionally entered into EAC	Otalgia/discomfort Audible movement Tactile perception	Otoscopy: Abnormal Tymps: Depends on if the foreign body perforated the TM; possibly Type A, possibly Type B with small or large ear canal volume MEMR: Consistent with audio and tymps Audio: Possible CHL OAEs: Consistent with audio
Furunculosis	Raised, reddish lesions at the base of hair follicles on the outer EAC	Otalgia	Otoscopy: Abnormal Tymps: Type A MEMR: WNL Audio: Normal hearing OAEs: WNL
Herpes zoster oticus (shingles)	Lesions/blisters on the pinna as a result of chicken pox virus; swelling on side of face	Otalgia Facial weakness/paralysis Erythema Hearing loss	Otoscopy: Abnormal Tymps: Type A MEMR: Possibly elevated Audio: SNHL OAEs: Consistent with audio
Microtia	Small or misshapen pinna (e.g., peanut) Anotia—complete absence of pinna	Visible abnormalities (often co-occurs with other anomalies such as atresia and craniofacial abnormalities)	Otoscopy: Abnormal pinna Tymps: Depends on comorbidities; microtia in isolation would yield type A tymps MEMR: Depends on comorbidities; microtia in isolation would yield normal MEMR Audio: Depends on comorbidities; microtia in isolation would yield normal hearing OAEs: Consistent with audio

DISORDER	ETIOLOGY AND PATHOLOGY	SYMPTOMS	DIFFERENTIAL DIAGNOSIS
Osteoma	Pedunculated benign tumors in the osseous portion of the EAC	Primarily asymptomatic Hearing loss if large enough Otalgia Vertigo Cerumen impaction Otitis externa	Otoscopy: Abnormal growths with narrow base Tymps: Type A MEMR: Consistent with audio, possible conductive pattern Audio: Normal hearing, possible CHL OAEs: Consistent with audio
Otitis externa	Infection of the outer ear (ear canal and/or pinna) caused by bacteria or fungus Can progress to necrotizing	Otalgia Otorrhea Possible fever	Otoscopy: Abnormal Tymps: Type A (dependent on EAC edema) MEMR: WNL, possible conductive pattern (dependent on EAC edema) Audio: Normal hearing, possible CHL (dependent on EAC edema) OAEs: Consistent with audio
Perichondritis	Infection of pinna resulting typically from trauma	Otalgia Erythema Edema	Otoscopy: Reddened, swollen pinna with normal EAC Tymps: Type A MEMR: WNL Audio: Normal hearing OAEs: Consistent with audio

Appendix 2–B

Middle Ear Disorders

DISORDER	ETIOLOGY AND PATHOLOGY	SYMPTOMS	DIFFERENTIAL DIAGNOSIS
Cholesteatoma	Overproduction of keratin from squamous cell epithelium within the middle ear, most often in the epitympanum Can be caused by chronic inflammation and infection of the middle ear (acquired) or related to embryonic epithelial cell nests Most often unilateral	Chronic middle ear issues Aural fullness Otalgia Smelly otorrhea Numbness or muscle weakness of affected side Hearing loss Dizziness	Otoscopy: White mass behind TM; debris in EAC Tymps: Type Ad or B MEMR: Conductive pattern Audio: Unilateral CHL or MHL with normal speech OAEs: Reduced to absent VNG: ordered if dizzy
Disarticulation of the ossicular chain	Continuity of the ossicles becomes disrupted, most often at the incudostapedial joint Possibly related to congenital abnormalities, ear infections, or trauma	Primarily asymptomatic Hearing loss	Otoscopy: WNL Tymps: Type Ad MEMR: Absent contralaterally Audio: CHL (can be mixed) OAEs: Absent
Eustachian tube dysfunction	ET fails to open or becomes chronically closed, which prevents the middle ear from ventilating Creates excess negative pressure, which can lead to other middle ear disorders	Aural fullness Possible sinus issues Possible hearing loss and tinnitus on affected side Autophony Difficulty popping ears	Otoscopy: WNL or retraction Tymps: Type C MEMR: Conductive pattern ETF: No/minimal change in peak pressure for Valsalva or Toynbee Audio: Low-frequency CHL OAEs: Reduced to absent

DISORDER	ETIOLOGY AND PATHOLOGY	SYMPTOMS	DIFFERENTIAL DIAGNOSIS
Glomus tumor (paraganglioma)	Jugulare or tympanicum Arise from paraganglion cells in jugular bulb or adjacent to Arnold's or Jacobson's nerve	Pulsatile tinnitus Aural fullness Otalgia Facial nerve weakness Hoarse voice & dysphagia Vertigo	Otoscopy: Red mass behind TM; Brown's sign Tymps: Match heartbeat (can see with decay protocol) MEMR: Consistent with audio Audio: Unilateral CHL or MHL OAEs: Absent unilateral VNG: Order if dizzy
Otitis media	Inflammation of the middle ear creates effusion behind the TM, which can develop bacterial infection Can be acute, serous, chronic, recurrent Primarily caused by ET dysfunction	Otalgia Otorrhea Aural fullness Possible history of recent respiratory infection Possible facial nerve palsy (rare) Pulling ears (child)	Otoscopy: Cloudy, bubbles, redness, inflammation; landmarks not visible Tymps: Type B MEMR: Conductive pattern Audio: Low-frequency or flat CHL with normal speech scores (at elevated presentation levels) OAEs: Absent
Otosclerosis	Metabolic alteration of temporal bone in the otic capsule—stapes footplate becomes mineralized around oval window, causing stapes fixation	Autophony Difficulty hearing when chewing Possible tinnitus Trouble in background noise Hearing loss Related to hormone changes; women in 30s/40s, after giving birth	Otoscopy: Schwartze's sign (TM appears reddish) Tymps: Type A or As MEMR: Upward deflection Tuning Fork: Weber (to CHL), Rinne (CHL-louder on mastoid) Audio: Carhart's notch (CHL with SNHL at 2 kHz), can progress into flat MHL OAEs: Consistent with audio
Perforation	Perforation in the pars flaccida or pars tensa of TM Related to trauma, infections, or surgery	Otalgia Hearing loss Possible history of head trauma Possible blood or drainage in EAC	Otoscopy: Visible hole in TM Tymps: Type B with large ECV MEMR: Conductive pattern Audio: Unilateral low-frequency CHL OAEs: Absent unilateral

continues

APPENDIX 2–B. *continued*

DISORDER	ETIOLOGY AND PATHOLOGY	SYMPTOMS	DIFFERENTIAL DIAGNOSIS
Temporal bone trauma (otic capsule sparing)	Result of blunt force, penetrating, compressing, or barotrauma Otic capsule (i.e., cochlea and SCC) remains intact	Otalgia Bloody otorrhea Loss of consciousness Possible facial nerve issues	Otoscopy: Hematoma, debris or blood in EAC, hemotympanum or CSF behind TM Tymps: Depend on damage (Ad, As, B) Audio: Unilateral CHL OAEs: Absent unilateral VNG: Possible comorbid BPPV
Tympanosclerosis	White calcified plaques on TM	Primarily asymptomatic	Otoscopy: Abnormal; white areas of TM Tymps: Type A or As Audio: Typically normal hearing; can have CHL OAEs: Consistent with audio

Appendix 2–C

Inner Ear Disorders

DISORDER	ETIOLOGY AND PATHOLOGY	SYMPTOMS	DIFFERENTIAL DIAGNOSIS
Autoimmune inner ear disorder	Caused by body's immune response directed at inner ear	Progressive Aural fullness Fluctuating tinnitus Gradual vertigo Typically treated as ear infection Common in middle-aged women	Otoscopy: WNL Tymps: Type A MEMR: Consistent with audio Audio: Fluctuating or progressive SNHL OAEs: Consistent with audio Dx by exclusion
Diabetes mellitus	Elevated blood glucose levels and altered lipids and proteins cause vascular changes that impact the stria vascularis and other cochlear anatomy and auditory nervous system	Gradual progressive symptoms Postural instability due to neuropathy Hearing loss	Otoscopy: WNL Tymps: Type A MEMR: Consistent with audio Audio: Bilateral high-frequency SNHL OAEs: Consistent with audio
Enlarged vestibular aqueduct syndrome	Vestibular aqueduct within the temporal bone is abnormally large Age of onset: Typically diagnosed around age 3–4	Possible history of head trauma Delayed motor milestones General imbalance Poor coordination Head tilting with vomiting	Otoscopy: WNL Tymps: Type A MEMR: Consistent with audio Audio: Fluctuating and progressive HL with low-frequency air-bone gap OAEs: Absent VNG: See Chapter 7
Hidden hearing loss	Abnormalities in the inner hair cells or ribbon synapses of the cochlea due to exposure to noise, but present with normal hearing	History of noise exposure Hearing loss Difficulty with speech in noise and background noise	Otoscopy: WNL Tymps: Type A MEMR: Elevated to absent Audio: Normal hearing OAEs: Absent ABR: Missing/reduced wave I ECochG: Abnormal SP/AP

continues

APPENDIX 2–C. *continued*

DISORDER	ETIOLOGY AND PATHOLOGY	SYMPTOMS	DIFFERENTIAL DIAGNOSIS
Meniere's disease	Excess endolymph fluid pressure, overproduction, or underabsorption	Roaring tinnitus Aural fullness Episodes of vertigo Fluctuating hearing loss that worsens during episodes	Otoscopy: WNL Tymps: Type A MEMR: Consistent with audio Audio: Unilateral low-frequency SNHL (progresses to bilateral) with poor word recognition OAEs: Consistent with audio VNG: See Chapter 7
Meningitis	Inflammation of the meninges of the brain and spinal cord (due to primarily bacterial or viral infection) enter the inner ear	Fever Stiff neck Persistent headache Nausea and vomiting Symptoms occur 3–7 days following exposure	Otoscopy: WNL Tymps: Type A MEMR: Consistent with audio Audio: Bilateral SNHL Ossificans VNG: Possibly abnormal
Noise-induced hearing loss	Excessive stimulation to the inner ear causes damage to hair cells and auditory nerve fibers Related to exposure to impulse noise (acoustic trauma) or gradual noise, causing temporary or permanent threshold shifts	History of noise exposure Hearing loss High-frequency constant tinnitus Possible aural fullness with threshold shift	Otoscopy: WNL Tymps: Type A MEMR: Consistent with audio Audio: SNHL with poorer thresholds 3–6 kHz (noise notch) OAEs: Consistent with audio
Ototoxicity	Toxic effect of the inner ear—degeneration of cochlear hair cells and auditory nerve and possible alteration to fluid in the organ of Corti	History of ototoxic medications or exposure to ototoxic chemical Hearing loss Tinnitus General dizziness Oscillopsia Atypical gate	Otoscopy: WNL Tymps: Type A MEMR: Consistent with audio Audio: Bilateral progressive high-frequency SNHL; poor word recognition VNG: See Chapter 7

DISORDER	ETIOLOGY AND PATHOLOGY	SYMPTOMS	DIFFERENTIAL DIAGNOSIS
Perilymphatic fistula	Perilymph leaks from the oval or round window, which alters the pressure differences between the scalae in the cochlea Causes are related to head trauma, barotrauma, and activities that produce straining	Episodic vertigo (during strain) Aural fullness Tinnitus Nausea Possible history of head trauma Ocular tilt	Otoscopy: WNL Tymps: Type A with reports of dizziness or presence of nystagmus MEMR: Consistent with audio Audio: Fluctuating flat or sloping SNHL OAEs: Consistent with audio Fistula test: Nystagmus during pressure changes (Hennebert's sign) VNG: See Chapter 7
Presbycusis	Decrease of auditory function (in the peripheral and central auditory system) due to aging	Gradual symptoms Hearing loss Tinnitus Poor speech understanding (especially in noise) Older age	Otoscopy: WNL Tymps: Type A MEMR: Consistent with audio Audio: Bilateral high-frequency SNHL with decreased word recognition, poor speech in noise performance Hyperacusis
Sudden SNHL	Acute onset, idiopathic hearing loss	Sudden decrease in hearing Unilateral tinnitus Aural fullness Trouble in background noise Possible dizziness and imbalance	Otoscopy: WNL Tymps: Type A MEMR: Consistent with audio Audio: SNHL with poor word recognition especially in noise OAEs: Consistent with audio ABR: WNL (rule out tumor) VNG: Possible unilateral peripheral findings

continues

APPENDIX 2–C. *continued*

DISORDER	ETIOLOGY AND PATHOLOGY	SYMPTOMS	DIFFERENTIAL DIAGNOSIS
Superior semicircular canal dehiscence	Bony covering of the superior semicircular canal thins or falls open, creating a fistula at times	Autophony Tinnitus Hyperacusis Aural fullness Distorted sensation of sounds Chronic imbalance Possible history of recent head trauma Tullio's (vertigo and/ or nystagmus to loud sounds)	Otoscopy: WNL Tymps: Type A MEMR: WNL Audio: Enhanced bone thresholds (esp. at 250 Hz) OAEs: WNL VNG: See Chapter 7
Temporal bone fracture (otic capsule disrupting)	Fracture of the otic capsule extends into the cochlea and/or vestibule, which can disrupt the membranous labyrinth and damage auditory nerve fibers	Raccoon eyes Hearing loss Vertigo Facial nerve paralysis Possible history of trauma	Otoscopy: Hemotympanum Tymps: Dependent on fracture MEMR: Consistent with audio Audio: SNHL OAEs: Consistent with audio

Appendix 2–D

Retrocochlear Disorders (Auditory Nerve and Central Auditory Nervous System)

DISORDER	ETIOLOGY	SYMPTOMS	DIFFERENTIAL DIAGNOSIS
Auditory neuropathy spectrum disorder	Impaired function of the auditory nerve	Adult: Hearing loss Difficulty with speech in noise Child: Abnormal birth history Delay of speech milestones	Otoscopy: WNL Tymps: Type A MEMR: Absent Audio: Varies from normal hearing to profound SNHL OAEs: Present (can progress to absent) ABR: Absent or highly abnormal with CM only
Labyrinthitis	Viral inflammation of CN VIII	Possible recent viral infection Vertigo Unilateral hearing loss Tinnitus Imbalance Nausea	Otoscopy: WNL Tymps: Type A MEMR: Consistent with audio Audio: Unilateral SNHL OAEs: Consistent with audio VNG: See Chapter 7
Multiple sclerosis	Autoimmune disease that causes demyelination	Numbness of extremities Neural shock during neck movement Tremors Loss of vision/double vision Speech and swallowing difficulties Vertigo Ataxia	Otoscopy: WNL Tymps: Type A MEMR: Consistent with audio Audio: Asymmetric high-frequency SNHL OAEs: Consistent with audio ABR: Possibly abnormal; abnormal morphological breakdown/latency prolongations with high rates VNG: See Chapter 7

continues

APPENDIX 2–D. *continued*

DISORDER	ETIOLOGY	SYMPTOMS	DIFFERENTIAL DIAGNOSIS
Vestibular schwannoma	Benign tumor of the vestibular branch (primarily) of CN VIII originating from Schwann cells (wrap around the neurons that conduct signal) Commonly resulting from Neurofibromatosis Type 2	Gradual changes Unilateral tinnitus Progressive unsteadiness and vertigo Nausea Possible facial weakness Possible headaches Aural fullness Difficulty on the phone	Otoscopy: WNL Tymps: Type A MEMR: Retrocochlear pattern Reflex Decay: Positive Audio: Unilateral SNHL with positive rollover OAEs: Consistent with audio ABR: Prolonged wave V VNG: See Chapter 7

Appendix 2–E

Vestibular Pathologies

DIAGNOSIS	VESTIBULAR SYMPTOMS	DURATION	NUMBER OF ATTACKS	PROVOCATION	AUDITORY SYMPTOMS	ASSOCIATED SYMPTOMS	LESION SITE
Anxiety	Nondescriptive; vague	Constant or episodic	Multiple or constant	Stress	None	Agoraphobia; instability/swaying	Central
Benign paroxysmal positional vertigo (BPPV)	Sudden onset vertigo	30–60 seconds	Multiple	Moving head in certain directions; lying down; rolling over in bed	None	Nausea; vomiting	Semicircular canal/s (posterior most often)
Benign paroxysmal vertigo of childhood (BPVC)	Episodic vertigo	Minutes to hours	Multiple	Stress, fatigue, motion intolerance	None	Aura, phono, or photophobia; nausea; vomiting; changes in vision; anxiety	Semicircular canal/s
Cerebellar ataxia with neuropathy and bilateral vestibular areflexia syndrome (CANVAS)	Unsteadiness/ imbalance with standing and walking	Constant with standing and walking	Multiple or constant	None	None	Swallowing difficulties; peripheral neuropathy	Vestibular labyrinth; cerebellum; peripheral nervous system
Concussion/ traumatic brain injury	Unsteadiness; dizziness; rotational/ rocking vertigo	Constant or episodic	Multiple or constant	Position changes; visual stimuli	Aural fullness, otalgia; tinnitus	Headache; cognitive changes; mood disorders; sleep disorders	Likely diffuse central

continues

DIAGNOSIS	VESTIBULAR SYMPTOMS	DURATION	NUMBER OF ATTACKS	PROVOCATION	AUDITORY SYMPTOMS	ASSOCIATED SYMPTOMS	LESION SITE
Enlarged vestibular aqueduct (EVA)/ large vestibular aqueduct syndrome (LVAS)	True vertigo; feelings of unsteadiness/ imbalance	Minutes to hours	Multiple	Positional; head trauma; pressure change; loud sounds	Hearing loss (sensorineural or mixed; usually bilateral) around 3–4 years old; false conductive component in low frequencies; hearing loss can fluctuate, be stable, or progress	Delayed motor development; difficulty climbing stairs, riding a bike, moving in the dark; often seen as clumsy	Labyrinth
Herpes zoster oticus (Ramsay Hunt syndrome)	True vertigo				Unilateral tinnitus; unilateral hearing loss; hyperacusis	Preceded by intense ear pain and blisters in and around the tongue, face, mouth, and ear; can be accompanied by facial paralysis; nausea; vomiting	CN VIII and VII; CPA
Labyrinthitis	True vertigo	30 minutes to hours (possibly longer)	Single	Sometimes preceded by illness	Sudden unilateral sensorineural hearing loss; unilateral tinnitus	Possible oscillopsia	Auditory and vestibular labyrinth
Mal de debarquement syndrome	Persistent rocking (no imbalance or rotational vertigo)	Constant (over days to months; relieved when in motion)	Constant	Preceded by prolonged travel	None	None	Unknown

DIAGNOSIS	VESTIBULAR SYMPTOMS	DURATION	NUMBER OF ATTACKS	PROVOCATION	AUDITORY SYMPTOMS	ASSOCIATED SYMPTOMS	LESION SITE
Ménière's disease	Episodic vertigo occurring before hearing loss	Minutes to hours	Multiple (must have at least two episodes for diagnosis)	Changes in atmospheric pressure or weather; diet; not necessarily accompanied by an aura/knowing attack is imminent	Low-frequency fluctuating hearing loss; low pitch/roaring tinnitus; aural fullness	Burnout after several years (no more dizziness; hearing loss remains); drop attacks	Labyrinth
Migraine/vestibular migraine	Episodic vertigo	1 minute to several days	Multiple	Headaches (not necessarily), light, sound, certain positions; visual stimuli	Many report ear pain, fullness	Aura, phono-, or photophobia; sensitivity to smells; head pain does not necessarily accompany dizziness	Thought to be labyrinth and vestibular nuclei; include other areas of the midbrain and brainstem
Nonorganic/physiologically inconsistent	Vague case history; inconsistent timeline and description	Variable	Variable	Variable	Variable	Variable	None
Orthostatic hypotension/dysautonomia	True vertigo, lightheadedness, unsteadiness	A few seconds	Multiple	Standing up quickly; changes in body posture; may be taking antihypertensive medication	None	Blurred vision; fatigue; nausea; palpitations; headache; weakness	Central

continues

DIAGNOSIS	VESTIBULAR SYMPTOMS	DURATION	NUMBER OF ATTACKS	PROVOCATION	AUDITORY SYMPTOMS	ASSOCIATED SYMPTOMS	LESION SITE
Perilymph fistula	Dizziness; imbalance/ unsteadiness; vertigo	Seconds to minutes	Multiple	Pressure changes	Hearing loss; tinnitus	Preceded by barotrauma, head trauma, middle ear surgery (stapedectomy), Valsalva maneuver; nausea; vomiting	Labyrinth
Persistent postural-perceptual dizziness	Dizziness; unsteadiness	Constant for days (>3 months)	Constant/ multiple	Motion; upright posture; moving/ complex visual stimuli	None	Preceded by acute/ episodic vestibular syndromes, neurologic, psychological, or other illnesses	None
Superior semicircular canal dehiscence (SSCD)	Episodic vertigo following loud sounds	Lasts as long as the sound (30–60 seconds); can be longer	Multiple	Loud noise; pressure changes	Low-frequency conductive hearing loss; normal immittance; tinnitus; may report amplification of sound	Autophony; sensitive to loud sounds or pressure in ear; oscillopsia; drop attacks	Labyrinth
Vestibular neuritis	Rotational vertigo	30 minutes to days	Single	Sometimes preceded by illness; often idiopathic	None	Possible oscillopsia	Neural/vascular leading to labyrinthine damage
Vestibular schwannoma	Gradual imbalance or dizziness	Constant	Constant (multiple)	Not usually provoked	Unilateral hearing loss, unilateral tinnitus	Brun's nystagmus; hemifacial numbness/ weakness	Vestibular portion on CN VIII; possible labyrinth, brainstem, or cerebellum

Appendix 2–F

Genetic Disorders and Syndromes

DISORDER/ SYNDROME	INHERITANCE PATTERN	IDENTIFIERS	AUDITORY FINDINGS
Achondroplasia	Autosomal dominant	Form of short-limbed dwarfism Enlarged heart Depressed nasal bridge Short, stubby hands Lordotic lumbar spine Protruding abdomen	Ear infections CHL or SNHL
Alport syndrome	Primarily X-linked, but can be autosomal recessive or dominant	Males more affected Abnormal retina color Kidney abnormalities (glomerulonephritis)	SNHL, progressive
Apert syndrome	Autosomal dominant	Fused fingers and toes (syndactyly) Possible stenosis or atresia	Bilateral flat CHL; can be SNHL
AUNA1	Autosomal dominant	Nonsyndromic	ANSD with late teen onset Progress to profound
CHARGE	Autosomal dominant	Ocular abnormality (coloboma) Heart defects Abnormal nasal structure (atresia chonae) Delayed growth and puberty Genital abnormalities	SNHL or MHL
Congenital unilateral lower lip palsy (CULLP)	Autosomal dominant Also due to birth trauma (compression of nerves)	Unilateral facial paralysis seen when baby cries	Possible SNHL
Connexin 26 (GJB2)	Autosomal dominant; can be autosomal recessive	Nonsyndromic	Progressive bilateral SNHL

continues

APPENDIX 2–F. *continued*

DISORDER/ SYNDROME	INHERITANCE PATTERN	IDENTIFIERS	AUDITORY FINDINGS
Connexin 30 (GJB6)	Autosomal dominant; can be autosomal recessive	Nonsyndromic	Progressive high-frequency SNHL with adolescent onset
Connexin 31 (GJB3)	Autosomal dominant	Nonsyndromic Can occur with peripheral neuropathy	Bilateral SNHL
DFNA1	Autosomal dominant	Nonsyndromic	Low-frequency SNHL progressing to flat severe SNHL May have vestibular symptoms
DFNA2A	Autosomal dominant	Nonsyndromic	Tinnitus in some Progressive high-frequency SNHL
DFNA5	Autosomal dominant	Nonsyndromic	Progressive high-frequency SNHL that moves to mid- and low frequencies Onset between 11 and 50 years
DFNA6/14/38	Autosomal dominant	Nonsyndromic	Low-frequency SNHL Progressive Tinnitus in some
DFNA8/12	Autosomal dominant	Nonsyndromic	Mid-frequency SNHL HL is stable or progressive
DFNA13	Autosomal dominant	Nonsyndromic	Mid-frequency SNHL (cookie bite) Stable Possible tinnitus
DFNB4	Autosomal recessive	Nonsyndromic	Inner ear malformations Fluctuating and/or progressive SNHL Vestibular anomalies
DFNB9	Autosomal recessive	Nonsyndromic	Mid-frequency SNHL (cookie bite) or ANSD

DISORDER/ SYNDROME	INHERITANCE PATTERN	IDENTIFIERS	AUDITORY FINDINGS
DFNB21	Autosomal recessive	Nonsyndromic	Severe to profound mid-frequency SNHL
DFNX2	X-linked	Nonsyndromic	Males: Temporal bone deformity; progressive MHL Females: Possible mild HL
DFNX4	X-linked	Nonsyndromic	Males: Progressive high-frequency SNHL (onset 3–7 years) Females: Possible HL (onset childhood–40s)
Jervell & Lange-Nielsen	Autosomal recessive	Prolonged heart QT interval Repeated syncope attacks Seizures	Bilateral profound SNHL
MTRNR1 & MTTS1	Mitochondrial	Nonsyndromic	Causes enhanced susceptibility to aminoglycoside ototoxicity (progress to profound SNHL) Possible constant tinnitus
Noonan syndrome	Autosomal dominant	Short stature Widely spaced eyes (usually pale blue or green) High-arched palate Downward palpebral fissures Short nose Broad or webbed neck Hypotonia Cardiac anomalies Normal intelligence	Middle and inner ear anomalies CHL, MHL, SNHL
Pendred syndrome	Autosomal recessive	Goiter (enlarged thyroid)	Bilateral high-frequency SNHL, progressive Enlarged vestibular aqueducts Possible vestibular anomalies

continues

APPENDIX 2–F. *continued*

DISORDER/ SYNDROME	INHERITANCE PATTERN	IDENTIFIERS	AUDITORY FINDINGS
Stickler syndrome	Autosomal dominant	Flat facial profile Mandibular hypoplasia Cleft palate Musculoskeletal and joint issues Joint hypermobility Osteoarthritis Long limbs Slender bones Nearsighted Retinal detachment Cataracts Blindness	Type 1—high-frequency SNHL Type 2—severe and progressive SNHL Type 3—mild to moderate SNHL
Treacher Collins syndrome	Autosomal dominant or recessive	Craniofacial abnormalities Pinna deformities	Primarily CHL, can be MHL or SNHL
Usher syndrome Type I—age 10 Type II—early 20s Type III—puberty	Autosomal recessive	Retinitis pigmentosa (progressive eye disease)	Bilateral SNHL (progressive—Types I & III) Dizziness and/or imbalance
Waardenburg syndrome	Autosomal dominant (Types I & II) Autosomal recessive (Types III & IV)	White forelock Upper limb abnormalities (Type III) Hirschprung disease (Type IV) Dystopia canthorum (wide nasal bridge) Synophrys (unibrow) Heterochromia (Type II) Musculoskeletal (Type III)	SNHL, nonprogressive Vestibular dysfunction

Chapter 3

Acoustics, Psychoacoustics, and Instrumentation

Jenna Cramer, Katharine Fitzharris, and Jeremy J. Donai

Principles of Sound

Three attributes commonly used to characterize sound (including speech) are frequency, amplitude, and phase. Each of the three contribute to the accurate perception of speech and other auditory signals in different ways.

Frequency

- Frequency is the number of complete cycles that occur during a specified amount of time, usually 1 second, measured in hertz (Hz). Frequency of a sound is described in terms of its fundamental, or lowest frequency, and formants (natural resonances of the vocal tract in the case of speech) or harmonics (integer multiple of the fundamental), which are successively higher frequencies that help distinguish sounds (e.g., phonemes) from one another.
- The perceptual correlate of frequency is pitch, which is defined as an attribute of auditory sensation in which a sound may be ordered on a scale extending from low to high. Biological male voices are often characterized as having a low pitch (with fundamental frequencies between 100 and 175 Hz) and biological female voices as having a relatively higher pitch (with fundamental frequencies between 200 and 300 Hz).

Amplitude

Amplitude refers to the maximum displacement of the particles of a medium, measured in decibels (dB). Perceptually, it is related to the magnitude (e.g., loudness) of a signal.

- Peak Amplitude
  - Peak amplitude refers to the maximum positive or negative deviation of a sound from its zero-reference level or baseline. For an undamped pure tone, this value remains constant throughout the signal. For complex signals such as speech, peak amplitude varies throughout the signal.

- Peak-to-Peak Amplitude

  □ Amplitude measurements that are made from the point of maximum displacement in one direction to the point of maximum displacement in the other direction. This value can be informative for tonal signals that repeat consistently over time but is less helpful for measuring the amplitude of more complex signals such as music or speech.

- Root Mean Square (RMS) Amplitude

  □ Root mean square (RMS) amplitude of a signal can provide valuable information about the average signal strength across the entire signal. Calculating RMS amplitude involves (1) squaring the amplitude values over the length of the signal, (2) calculating the average of all amplitude values, and (3) finding the square root of the average.

  □ RMS amplitude values are helpful when determining the amplitude of complex signals such as music or speech. Because natural speech signals fluctuate in amplitude from moment to moment and the waveform does not consistently repeat, using a value such as peak or peak-to-peak amplitude is not recommended, as it often does not provide an amplitude value representative of the entire signal. For these types of signals, RMS amplitude values are more informative and commonly measured.

Phase

Phase represents the point in a cycle at which a vibrating object is located at a given instant in time. Phase is often described as a location or degree of radians of a circle. The topic of phase has significant implications for clinical and research activities performed by audiologists and hearing scientists.

- One example relates to the phase of a signal (i.e., condensation vs. rarefaction) and auditory system stimulation. Recall that the rarefaction phase of a signal leads to depolarization (increased firing) of the neural system due to an upward movement of the basilar membrane, movement of the hair cells toward the modiolus, shearing of the stereocilia toward the stria vascularis, opening of the mechanically gated channels, and release of the neurotransmitter glutamate.

- Conversely, the condensation phase leads to hyperpolarization (reduced firing) of the neural system due to a downward movement of the basilar membrane, movement of the hair cells toward the stria vascularis (lateral wall), shearing of the stereocilia toward the modiolus, and a compression of the mechanically gated channels (see Musiek & Baran, 2020, for additional information).

- Clinically, signal phase influences the latency of waves during the auditory brainstem response (ABR) evaluation in that the rarefaction phase will elicit waves with shorter latencies due to depolarization occurring during rarefaction phase.

Phase Cancellation

Phase cancellation, also commonly referred to as phase inversion, is a popular technique used to reduce acoustic feedback in hearing aids.

- When feedback is detected by a hearing aid, a signal of the same frequency that is 180° out of phase with the feedback signal is used to create a cancellation effect and reduce feedback.

Q & A

Question: When conducting a pure-tone threshold evaluation in the audiology clinic using audiometric earphones, does signal phase affect hearing thresholds in the ear being tested?

Answer: No, phase does not affect the perception of a signal when presented monaurally. Phase becomes increasingly important when conducting binaural testing (because phase is important when listening with both ears, as in the Masking Level Difference [MLD] test). In other words, the phase of a sine wave is irrelevant when testing one ear at a time, as is done in a traditional audiological evaluation. However, phase differences can enhance the detection of a signal when presented binaurally and out of phase. It is thought that the superior olivary complex (SOC) is primarily responsible (at least early in auditory perception) for detecting and processing these phase differences in terms of the interaural timing difference (ITD) or interaural phase difference (IPD) used for localization.

Lead and Lag

Most surfaces reflect sounds and influence the acoustic environment of a room. When an auditory signal is present, a listener hears both the initial and reflected signal. Sound coming from an initial source arrives at the ears first (lead). The echo, or reflected sound, subsequently arrives at the ears (lag).

- In Figure 3–1, the solid gray line leads the black dashed line by 90°. The starting phase of the solid line is 90°, and the starting phase of the dashed line is 0°. It should be noted that the current visual is an example of one reflected signal. In reality, additional reflections would occur in a typical acoustic environment.

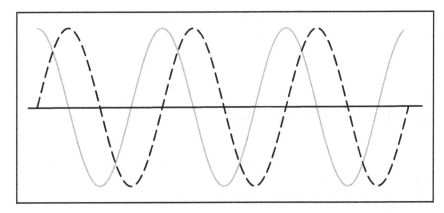

FIGURE 3–1. Example of lead and lag.

AUDIOLOGY NUGGET

Recall that in the traditional soundfield set up in the audiology clinic, the use of pure-tone signals to measure hearing sensitivity is not advisable due to the possibility of reduced signal amplitude in locations within the testing area resulting from standing waves. Standing waves result when signal reflections interact with an original signal in the same location with a 180° phase difference. A more complex signal such as a warbled or frequency modulated (FM) tone or narrowband noise to avoid this deleterious phase interaction is recommended in these situations.

Precedence Effect

In reverberant environments, sounds reach the ears through several paths. Although the direct sound is followed by multiple reflections, which would be audible in isolation, the first-arriving (lead) sound dominates many aspects of auditory perception. The precedence effect refers to a phenomenon that is thought to be involved in resolving competition for perception and localization between a direct sound and subsequent sound reflections.

- In binaural hearing, a slightly delayed signal is not entirely ignored but may influence the precise localization of the sound source. Because of the precedence effect, echoes and reverberated sounds are minimized for a short period after the original sound.

Q & A

Question: An educational audiologist is tasked with determining the reverberation time of a classroom to provide a rationale for ear-level versus soundfield FM systems for students with hearing loss. What guidelines would they use for their measurement?

Answer: ANSI S12.60: ANSI Standard for Classroom Acoustics specifies that classrooms less than 10,000 cubic feet have RT60 (time it takes from sound cessation to decay by 60 dB) values of ≤0.6 second and ambient noise levels ≤35 dBA.

Digital Signal Processing (DSP)

Digital signal processing (DSP) involves creating a digital code (0s and 1s) from an auditory signal. This requires taking amplitude measurements of a continuous signal at discrete points in time. DSP is routinely used in consumer products such as cell phones, personal tablets, televisions, and most clinical/research equipment used by speech and hearing professionals, including hearing aids (HAs) and cochlear implants (CIs).

- Two important factors in this process are accurately capturing the amplitude of the signal (amplitude quantization or amplitude resolution) and the rate at which the process occurs (sampling frequency). In simpler terms, these two processes are related to how accurately and how quickly the analog signal is sampled to reduce error and preserve the original signal to the highest degree possible.

Amplitude Resolution and Sampling Frequency

One important factor in DSP is accurately capturing the amplitude of the signal through a process called amplitude quantization. The other is the rate at which this process occurs, often referred to as sampling frequency or sample rate.

- Amplitude quantization refers to the process of using binary numbers (0s and 1s) to represent the amplitude of a signal. The term bit refers to the size of the series of 0s and 1s used to describe the amplitude of a signal. This is commonly displayed at 2^x, with the exponent (x) representing the number of bits. As such, a 4-bit system (2^4) allows for 16 potential combinations of 0s and 1s to represent amplitude values. Please refer to Figure 3–2 for an example of a 2- and 4-bit system. Sixteen-bit (65,535 potential amplitude values) is the most often used value; however, 24- and 32-bit are also available.

  □ Each bit provides for approximately 6 dB in dynamic range for a digital system. Thus, a 16-bit system (commonly used in audio applications) has a 96 dB dynamic range ($16 \times 6 = 96$).

- Sampling frequency or sample rate refers to the number of times per second amplitude quantization occurs. Thus, with a sampling frequency of 44.1 kHz (or 44,100 Hz), the amplitude of the continuous signal is quantified 44,100 times per second, creating 44,100 discrete numerical values.

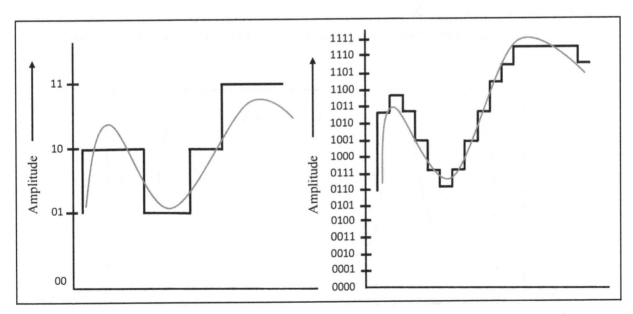

FIGURE 3–2. Visual representation of amplitude resolution. *Source:* Adapted from *Hearing Science Fundamentals, Second Edition* (pp. 1–370) by Lass, N. J., & Donai, J. J. Copyright © 2023 Plural Publishing, Inc. All rights reserved.

AUDIOLOGY NUGGET

DSP routinely involves a significant number of trade-offs. In simple terms, the more complex processing that takes place, the longer the processing time and the more significant the digital storage requirements. To increase clarity of music processing through hearing aids, most manufacturers have increased the bit resolution used in their devices (more specifically at the analog-to-digital converter or ADC). Recall that an increase in one bit increases the dynamic range of a digital system by 6 dB. Thus, by increasing the bit resolution by a value of 2 (from 16-to 18-bit, for example), these devices allow for an additional 12 dB of input with less distortion by increasing the input dynamic range from 96 to 108 dB. Given the significant fluctuations in sound level associated with many forms of music, this increase in dynamic range is intended to enhance music perception for hearing aid users.

Nyquist Theorem and Aliasing Distortion

Effective sampling of a continuous signal requires at least two samples per cycle. This equates to effective sampling occurring at one half of the sampling frequency, commonly referred to as the Nyquist frequency. Or put another way, a sampling frequency must be at least twice the highest frequency of interest in a signal. If an insufficient sampling frequency is used, distortion (i.e., aliasing distortion) will occur at or near the frequency that is one half the sampling frequency.

- Aliasing distortion (shown in Figure 3–3) is the introduction of lower-frequency components to a signal that are not present in the original signal.

- According to the Nyquist theorem, using a sampling frequency of 44.1 kHz can provide accurate frequency representation to approximately 22 kHz. Frequencies near or above 22 kHz

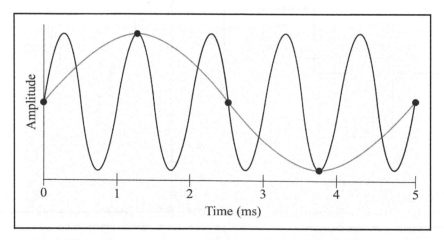

FIGURE 3–3. Example of aliasing distortion. *Source:* Adapted from *Hearing Science Fundamentals, Second Edition* (pp. 1–370) by Lass, N. J., & Donai, J. J. Copyright © 2023 Plural Publishing, Inc. All rights reserved.

are of concern due to the possibility of aliasing distortion. This is precisely the reason that most audio applications use at least a 44.1 kHz sampling frequency (22 kHz is above the frequency range of human hearing and thus any distortion should be undetectable).

■ There are two ways to reduce the effects of aliasing distortion. One is to low-pass filter the signal below the Nyquist frequency to eliminate distortion. This type of filter is often referred to as an anti-aliasing filter. The other solution is to increase the sampling frequency to increase the frequency at which aliasing distortion occurs.

DSP Stages

■ Refer to Figure 3–4 for a simplified visual representation of common DSP that occurs in HAs. Initially, a sound input is detected and processed by a microphone, converted into an electrical signal, and then amplified by a preamplifier. Then the electrical signal (i.e., continuous signal) is converted into a digital (i.e., discrete) signal, which is performed by the analog-to-digital converter (ADC).

□ During this, sampling frequency and amplitude resolution parameters are of paramount purpose and should be specified to meet the needs of the application.

■ Once the signal is in a digital format, it is processed by the DSP chip, where its frequency and amplitude characteristics are modified based on patient factors such as type and degree of hearing loss as well as patient characteristics such as previous HA use and uncomfortable listening levels (for digital hearing aid processing). Next, the digital signal is processed by the digital-to-analog converter (DAC), where the digital signal is converted back to an analog signal. In this last stage, the analog signal is amplified and transmitted to a receiver (i.e., speaker) and is then presented to the patient.

■ In CIs, the same procedure is followed, but instead of the creation of an acoustic analog signal as the final step, the signals are further broken down into frequency components, which are then assigned to different electrodes within the cochlea. At these electrode locations, electrical pulses are produced. These impulses then electrically stimulate the auditory nerve.

□ Auditory signals are coded in intensity, frequency, and time. The primary goal of CI programming is to provide audibility for low-level and conversational-level speech across the speech frequency range without exceeding the patient's comfort or creating a spread of electrical activity outside of CN VIII (Wolfe & Schafer, 2020).

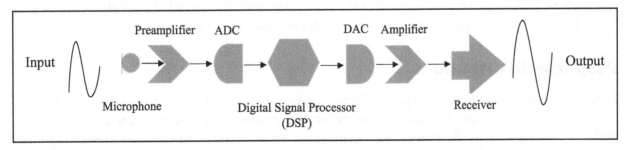

FIGURE 3–4. Digital signal processing (DSP) process. *Source:* Adapted from *Hearing Science Fundamentals, Second Edition* (pp. 1–370) by Lass, N. J., & Donai, J. J. Copyright © 2023 Plural Publishing, Inc. All rights reserved.

KNOWLEDGE CHECKPOINT

Multiple options exist for amplifying high-frequency sensorineural hearing loss. These include traditional bandwidth amplification, extended bandwidth amplification, and frequency-lowering techniques (see Chapter 9). In general, traditional bandwidth hearing aids have an upper frequency limit of approximately 6 to 7 kHz. Extended bandwidth systems, conversely, purport an upper frequency limit of approximately 9 to 10 kHz. As such, the sampling frequency (according to the Nyquist theorem) must be higher for the extended bandwidth devices to allow for accurate processing of information in the 9 to 10 kHz frequency range. To accurately process information at or near 10 kHz, a sampling frequency of *at least* 20 kHz is required.

Signal Detection Theory (SDT)

Signal detection theory is a conceptual framework used to describe decision-making in conditions of uncertainty or "noise." Noise in this instance refers to the uncertainty associated with decision-making rather than traditional acoustic sources of noise. When performing a discrimination experiment, listeners develop a response bias (sometimes referred to as a response proclivity) that creates a corresponding response pattern of hits, misses, false alarms, and correct rejections. Think of the response bias as a relationship between the level of signal and the listener's willingness to say "yes" or respond that a signal is present or different.

Response Types

There are four response types: hits (true positives), misses (false negatives), false alarms (false positives), and correct rejections (true negatives).

- Hits are defined as a correct response when the stimulus is present. This occurs when the sound is present and the individual responds.
- Misses occur when a sound of sufficient intensity (i.e., above threshold) is present but no response to the sound is provided.
- False alarms occur when the signal is absent, but the individual responds as it if were present.
- Correct rejections occur when the signal is absent, and no response is provided.

Response Distributions

Figure 3–5 provides a visual of response distributions used to model the responses associated with a discrimination task. Responses that occur in the left distribution (Noise) represent responses obtained without a signal present. Responses that occur in the right distribution (Signal + Noise) represent responses obtained with a signal present (the noise or uncertainty is always present). The x-axis represents the internal response, with responses to lower-level signals occurring to the left and responses to

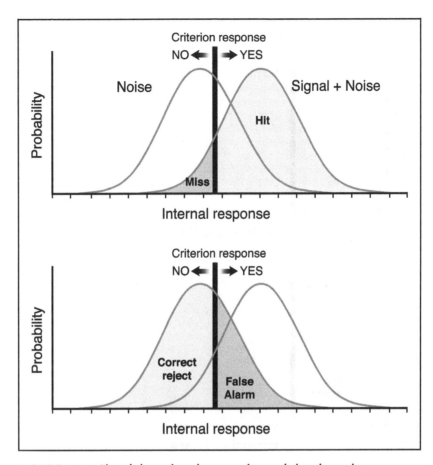

FIGURE 3–5. Signal detection theory noise and signal + noise response distributions. *Source:* Adapted from *Hearing Science Fundamentals, Second Edition* (pp. 1–370) by Lass, N. J., & Donai, J. J. Copyright © 2023 Plural Publishing, Inc. All rights reserved.

high-level signals occurring to the right of the *x*-axis (e.g., softer sounds to the left and louder sounds to the right). The criterion response (represented by the vertical black line) refers to the point at which the individual responds ("yes" responses to the right and "no" responses to the left).

Response Biases

As previously noted, when performing a detection or discrimination task (e.g., hearing test), individuals will typically develop a response bias, which is an internal judgment of how often and at what level is required for them to respond. These biases can be divided into three types: liberal, conservative, and neutral. The type of bias directly influences the distribution of hits, misses, false alarms, and correct rejections.

- Liberal response bias refers to when listeners are more likely to respond even if they are uncertain if the signal is present. This results in an increase in hits and a decrease in misses due to an increase in the number of overall positive responses. This also results in an increase in the number of false alarms and fewer correct rejections. A visual is provided in Figure 3–6.

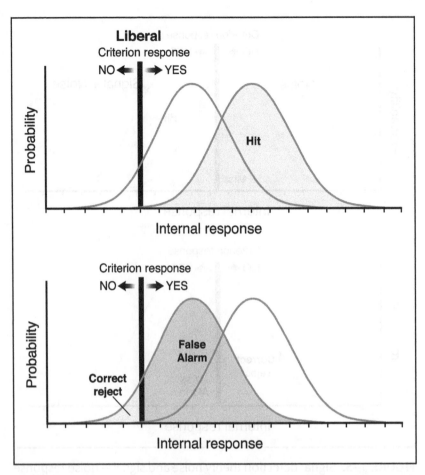

FIGURE 3–6. Liberal response bias. *Source:* Adapted from *Hearing Science Fundamentals, Second Edition* (pp. 1–370) by Lass, N. J., & Donai, J. J. Copyright © 2023 Plural Publishing, Inc. All rights reserved.

- □ A drawback to the liberal response bias is the increased number of false positives, which can create difficulty and unreliable findings during hearing testing if the false alarms are misinterpreted as hits or correct responses.

- ■ Conservative response bias refers to when a listener cautiously responds, often waiting to respond until the signal is above threshold. This results in an increased number of misses and a decrease in hits due to the conservative approach to responding. This also results in an increase in correct rejections and fewer false alarms. A visual is provided in Figure 3–7.

  - □ A drawback to a conservative response bias is that the responses deemed as "threshold" are often not representative of a true threshold (e.g., suprathreshold or minimal response levels).

- ■ Neutral response bias refers to when a listener responds in a more impartial way, not waiting until a signal is louder or surely present to respond or responding when the signal is soft and questionable. This leads to a more even distribution of hits, misses, false alarms, and correct rejections as shown in Figure 3–5.

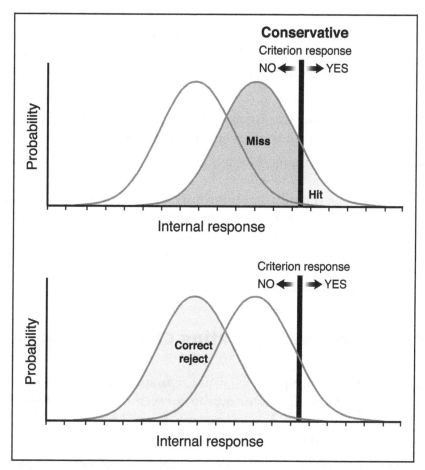

FIGURE 3–7. Conservative response bias. *Source:* Adapted from *Hearing Science Fundamentals, Second Edition* (pp. 1–370) by Lass, N. J., & Donai, J. J. Copyright © 2023 Plural Publishing, Inc. All rights reserved.

 Q & A

Imagine the situation where a clinician has an adult patient, Joe, who has a developmental disability and is eager to please. The clinician begins testing and realizes Joe's eagerness is impairing his ability to obtain valid thresholds due to a strong tendency to rapidly respond whether the sound was present or not.

Question: What response bias is Joe exhibiting, and what would you expect in terms of hits, misses, false alarms, and correct rejections?

Answer: In this case, Joe is demonstrating a liberal response bias. A liberal response bias typically leads to many hits and false alarms but few correct rejections and misses. The clinician may have a difficult time determining true threshold and may underestimate the patient's audiometric thresholds (assume thresholds are better than they actually are).

Now imagine there is a pediatric patient, Juan, who is distracted and not terribly interested in the game being used for conditioned play audiometry. Juan looks at the clinician at lower intensities but does not respond in play until about 10 dB higher intensity.

Question: What response bias is Juan exhibiting, and what would you expect in terms of hits, misses, false alarms, and correct rejections?

Answer: Juan is demonstrating a form of conservative response bias. He signals that he detects the signal by looking at the clinician but does not engage in the response behavior (play) until a higher intensity is presented (similar to someone waiting until he or she is absolutely sure the stimulus is present). These responses should not be recorded as true threshold, but rather minimal response levels. Juan's response pattern would show fewer hits, fewer false alarms, but more misses and more correct rejections.

d-prime (*d'*) and Receiver Operating Characteristic (ROC) Curves

Signal discriminability is dependent upon the relative separation between the noise (N) and signal + noise (S+N) distributions. Thus, significant overlap between the two distributions increases task difficulty and decreases discriminability. A value known as *d'*, also known as the discrimination index, quantifies the relative ease or difficulty of the discrimination task.

- *d'* values are shown in Figure 3–8 (*left*). As can be seen, lower *d'* values are associated with substantial overlap in the distributions (increased difficulty with discrimination), whereas larger *d'* values are associated with less distribution overlap (less difficulty with discrimination). These values can also be plotted on receiver operating characteristic (ROC) curves.

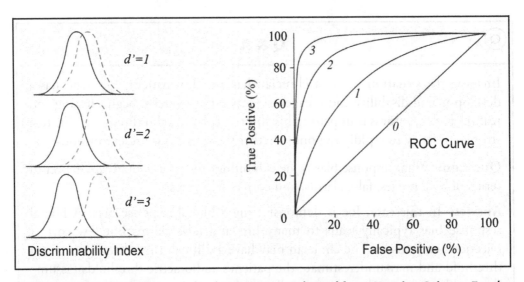

FIGURE 3–8. ROC curves and *d'* values. *Source:* Adapted from *Hearing Science Fundamentals, Second Edition* (pp. 1–370) by Lass, N. J., & Donai, J. J. Copyright © 2023 Plural Publishing, Inc. All rights reserved.

■ As can be seen in Figure 3–8 (*right*), false-positive (false alarm) values are displayed on the *x*-axis and true positives (hits) are displayed on the *y*-axis. Ideally, a test with a low false-positive rate and high true-positive rate (d' of 3 as shown in the figure) is desirable. In clinical terms, a test with a high hit rate and low false alarm rate suggests good diagnostic utility. Conversely, a test with a 50% true-positive (hit) rate and 50% false-positive (false alarm) rate (d' of 0 shown in the figure) lacks utility because the yes/no outcome is essentially left to chance. Imagine being tested for a significant medical condition and only 50% of the time the condition is correctly detected when it is indeed present (hit) and 50% of the time it is falsely detected when it is absent (false alarm).

■ ROC curves are graphical representations of the performance on a discrimination task with a binary outcome (e.g., yes/no, present/absent, condition/no condition). It can be plotted visually and as distributions with associated d' values. Notice the leftward deviation of the ROC curves as d' increases from 0 to 3 and the resulting separation of the distributions on the left (d' from 1 to 3). As d' increases, the discrimination task decreases in difficulty (signal detectability becomes easier), shown as a reduction in overlap in the two distributions (S+N and N).

Psychophysical Methods

An individual's psychological state when performing a perceptual task can drastically influence the physical response. The methods utilized for obtaining these responses are commonly referred to as psychophysical methods. Psychophysical methods are means of coupling physical properties of a stimulus to the perception of and response to that stimulus. Many factors affect perception, including motivation, alertness, and response preference or bias (refer to the Signal Detection Theory section of this chapter).

Method of Limits

The method of limits entails changing one parameter of a stimulus, intensity in the case of auditory testing, by the person performing the assessment (i.e., examiner), with the subject masked to indicate in some way when they detect the stimulus. This technique is commonly used to obtain hearing thresholds during an audiological evaluation performed in a hearing clinic (e.g., Hughson Westlake procedure).

■ Advantages: Time efficient (observations are concentrated around threshold); no need to determine a range of potential thresholds to begin testing (i.e., at what level to begin testing)

■ Disadvantages: Thresholds may be recorded without evidence that the person was listening

Method of Adjustment

The method of adjustment involves the subject adjusting some parameter of a stimulus. For example, the intensity of a stimulus may be adjusted to a point where it is barely audible, or the frequency adjusted to match the pitch of a reference tone. The changes made by the subject are recorded and analyzed by the examiner. Thresholds obtained using this method vary depending on exactly where on the recorded observations the examiner marks threshold. An example of the method of adjustment being used in behavioral testing is in Békésy audiometry.

- Advantages: Easy; appealing to the subject
- Disadvantages: May produce unreliable results

 AUDIOLOGY NUGGET

In Békésy audiometry, a listener is given a response button and instructed to depress it for as long as they hear a signal; the audiometer first ascends in intensity (typically in 2.5 dB steps) until the button is depressed, then decreases in similar step sizes until the button is released. This procedure is repeated several times and the results are plotted. Though Békésy audiometry is not commonly used in most clinics today, it is often used in military or other hearing conservation settings to monitor hearing thresholds. Historically, it has been used in detecting conductive, cochlear, and retrocochlear hearing loss, as well as in testing malingering patients.

Method of Constant Stimuli

The method of constant stimuli uses a two-alternative forced-choice (2AFC) procedure. This process requires a subject to make a choice from two options (same/different or yes/no, for example). Several stimulus levels or characteristics (e.g., intensity, brightness) above and below a predetermined criterion are selected for use in the task. The listener is asked to indicate yes/no or same/different during each period when a stimulus is presented. Results are plotted as the percentage of time each level of stimulus was detected. Plotting the response data provides the examiner with a psychometric function, which is a graphical display of how responses vary with changes in a parameter of the stimulus. A clinical example of this method is matching the pitch or loudness of tinnitus (although it includes aspects of the method of adjustment as well).

- Advantages: Easy to conduct; provides complete picture of responses (i.e., number of responses obtained above and below threshold to determine actual threshold)
- Disadvantages: Time-consuming; need a good estimation of the threshold before you start; many trials are wasted

Validity and Reliability

Validity refers to the accuracy or how well the measure assesses what it is intended to measure. Reliability refers to the consistency of a measure or the ability to obtain similar results when repeating the measure over time. Figure 3–9 provides a visual representation of reliability and validity. The leftmost visual demonstrates high reliability because all circles are located in a concentrated area but low validity because they are located away from the center of the target. The central figure conveys low reliability and low validity because the circles are widespread over the target and outside of the center of the target. The rightmost figure shows high reliability and high validity due to a concentration of circles occurring within the center of the target.

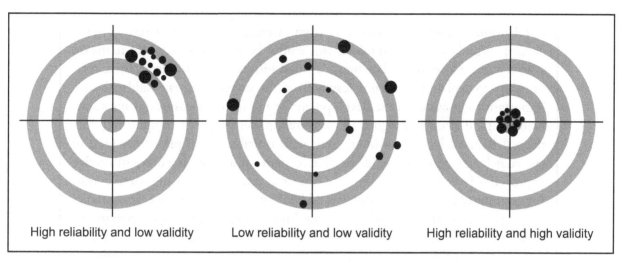

High reliability and low validity   Low reliability and low validity   High reliability and high validity

FIGURE 3–9. Visual representation of reliability and validity.

Measures of Validity

- Internal validity refers to the degree of confidence that the causal (cause-effect) relationship being tested is trustworthy and not influenced by other factors or variables.

- External validity refers to the extent to which results from a study can be applied (generalized) to other situations, groups, or events.

- Ecological validity refers to if test findings can be applied to real-world situations.

- Construct validity refers to a test's content, structure, variable associations, and responses.

- Content validity refers to if a test measures what it is intended to measure.

- Face validity refers to if a test appears to measure what it is intended to measure.

- Predictive validity refers to a test's ability to predict future behavior or performance.

- Concurrent validity of a test measures the ability to predict similar outcomes using different tests at the same time.

 KNOWLEDGE CHECKPOINT

Internal validity can be evaluated in electrophysiological measures—some measures, like the auditory brainstem response (ABR), are unchanged based on the patient's state; however, other measures, like the P300 cortical response, are greatly impacted by the patient's attentional state. External validity is exemplified by tests developed within the VA system: The normative values established in this population may not be applicable to younger patients, female patients, non-noise-exposed patients, and so on. An ecologically valid measure of speech in noise would be the QuickSIN; here, real-word stimuli (sentences) are presented to listeners. This is a more valid way of measuring patients' primary complaints of difficulty in noisy environments than a traditional word recognition test in quiet. Construct validity is what is completed when a test is being developed/updated. An example of this would be the examination of items on a survey to explore their relatedness, divided into themes, and using these relationships to explain the variable results from the survey. Content validity is also important to consider in the development or use of test measures or questionnaires (e.g., if a test is designed to measure a patient's speech recognition, does the test item analysis result in an equivalent distribution of phonemes used in everyday language?). Face validity is like content validity but is a more subjective approach—from a quick review of a test, is it testing what it purports to test? An example of predictive validity would be how well pure-tone averages predict hearing aid satisfaction in patients—hint, hint, not very well. Finally, concurrent validity would be measured between two tests, for instance, the Dichotic Digits and the Competing Sentences Test, to see how well the patient's performance aligns on measures of similar auditory processing skills.

Reliability

- Test-retest reliability measures the consistency or results when repeating the same test on the same sample at a different point in time. An example of test-retest reliability assessment is seen in the common clinical procedure of retesting 1000 Hz at the beginning of pure-tone threshold testing.

- Interrater reliability (between-rater reliability) is a measure of consistency used to evaluate the extent to which different judges agree in their assessment. A common example is determining the reliability between two "judges" in defining when a behavioral response (e.g., head turn) is present during visual reinforcement audiometry.

- Intrarater reliability (within-rater reliability) refers to the consistency of observations or judgments of one rater over several trials and is best determined when multiple trials are administered over a short period of time.

Sensitivity and Specificity

- Sensitivity refers to the relationship between a true positive (i.e., hit) and a false negative (i.e., miss) when the condition is positive. Sensitivity describes how well a condition is detected when the condition is present.

- Specificity refers to the relationship between false positives (i.e., false alarms) and true negatives (i.e., correct rejections) when the condition is negative. Specificity describes how well a condition is rejected when the condition is absent.

CASE EXAMPLE

An audiologist working in a hospital-based clinic is tasked with evaluating oto-acoustic emission (OAE) equipment for purchase. The audiologist requests data (shown below) from the manufacturer of two models (Model A and Model B) and finds the following information for each. In each box are the number of individuals who meet the response types (e.g., listeners with hearing loss who refer on the test) and listeners with normal hearing who pass the test. Based on these data, the audiologist decides to calculate the sensitivity and specificity of the two units. Both models are identical in cost at $10,000, which includes all equipment and fees associated with initial training.

Hearing Status

Model (A)	Hearing Loss	Normal
Refer	40 (a)	100 (c)
Pass	2 (b)	1000 (d)

Hearing Status

Model (B)	Hearing Loss	Normal
Refer	70 (a)	20 (c)
Pass	2 (b)	1200 (d)

To calculate sensitivity, listeners who have hearing loss and do not pass the screening (refer) are of concern. In the table for Model A, this is calculated using the formula a/(a + b) or 40/(40 + 2) = .95 or 95% sensitivity. Specificity is concerned with those that do not have a condition (normal) and do not test positive for the condition (pass). In the table for Model A, this is calculated using the formula d/(c + d) or 1000/(1000 + 100) = 0.91 or 91% specificity.

Calculating the sensitivity and specificity for Model B yields different results. Sensitivity was calculated at 97% (70/[70 + 2] = 0.97), with specificity at 98% (1200/[1200 + 20] = 0.98). Comparing these results to Model A, the sensitivity of both models is similar (95% vs. 97%), but the specificity for Model B is much higher than Model A (98% vs. 91%). This means that Model B is more effective at determining those who do not have hearing loss as not having hearing loss (pass). Given that both pieces of equipment are equivalent in cost and produce similar sensitivity results, the audiologist selects Model B based on the specificity data.

Psychoacoustics

Psychoacoustics is the study of the psychological response to acoustic signals. In addition to the profession of audiology, fields including engineering, cognitive and experimental psychology, and telecommunications are concerned with psychoacoustic principles and their applications.

Power Spectrum Model and the Critical Band

One of the most important findings influencing the study of hearing was the discovery of the auditory critical band by Fletcher (1940). In his experiments, Fletcher measured the effects of masking noises with various spectral bandwidths on the detection of a pure tone. While holding the spectrum level of the noise constant, Fletcher observed increasing thresholds with increases in masker bandwidth up to a certain point (a certain masker bandwidth), and beyond which, minimal threshold shift occurred. This is shown by the dashed line in Figure 3–10 (dashed line represents the bandwidth of the critical band) where increases in threshold occur (increases in circle height on the *y*-axis) with increasing noise bandwidth until the critical band is reached (represented by the dashed line). Please note the minimal increase in threshold following the critical band (because additional noise masking is outside of the critical band) demonstrated by thresholds of similar value on the *y*-axis.

- Fletcher referred to the bandwidth at which negligible increases in masking occurred as the critical band and suggested that only masking signals falling within the critical band would influence perception of the signal tone.

- Fletcher's findings are considered instrumental to understanding auditory masking and have subsequently shaped the understanding of effective masking and frequency selectivity in the auditory system.

  □ The power spectrum model of masking resulted from Fletcher's early work and posited that the auditory system acted as a series of bandpass filters (commonly referred to as

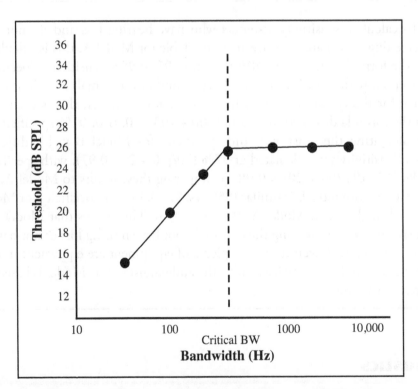

FIGURE 3–10. Effects of masker bandwidth on audibility (threshold detection). *Source:* Adapted with permission from Fletcher, H. (1940). Auditory patterns. *Reviews of Modern Physics, 12,* 47–66. Copyright 1940 by the American Physical Society.

auditory filters) that are tuned to specific frequencies. This model also stated that masking effectiveness is determined by the power of a masker falling within an individual auditory filter (or critical band) near the test signal (for steady-state maskers). See the upcoming Knowledge Checkpoint for a calculation related to masker bandwidth and critical auditory filter bandwidth—a computational example intended to strengthen the reader's understanding of masking effectiveness relative to masker bandwidth.

 KNOWLEDGE CHECKPOINT

At its core, masking procedures in clinical audiology are guided by discoveries that lead to development of the power spectrum model. Specifically, the use of narrowband maskers for masking pure-tone signals and wideband signals for masking speech signals (signals that extend to numerous critical bands) coincides with the power spectrum model and concept of the critical band. The calculation provided here is from an undergraduate hearing science text by Lass and Donai (2023), which demonstrates the relationship between effective masking of wideband signals when obtaining pure-tone thresholds. Note that toward the end of the calculation the critical band value for 1000 Hz is specified at 64 Hz. This calculation demonstrates that only a portion of the 6000 Hz bandwidth masker is effective at masking a 1000 Hz tonal signal (because only maskers falling within the 1000 Hz critical band of 64 Hz provide effective masking).

Question: What is the effective masking value of a wideband noise (e.g., bandwidth of 6000 Hz) with an overall sound pressure level of 80 dB SPL for a 1000 Hz pure tone?

Answer: First, determine the level per cycle (LPC):

$$\text{LPC} = 80 \text{ dB SPL} - 10(\log_{10} 6000)$$
$$= 80 \text{ dB SPL} - 10(3.77)$$
$$= 80 \text{ dB SPL} - 37.7 = 42.3 \text{ dB SPL}$$

Now apply the formula for effective masking (EM):

$$42.3 \text{ dB SPL} + 10(\log_{10} \text{CB})$$

The critical band for a 1000 Hz pure tone is 64 Hz:

$$\log_{10} \text{ of } 64 = 1.81$$

Therefore:

$$\text{EM} = 42.3 \text{ dB SPL} + 10(1.81) = 42.3 + 18.1 = 60.4 \text{ dB SPL}$$

This means that in the presence of 80 dB SPL wideband noise, the threshold for a 1000 Hz tone will be elevated to 60.4 dB SPL. This will vary slightly among individuals because of differing abilities to detect a signal in noise. In

> testing hearing, however, hearing level (HL) measures are used. Audiometric zero at 1000 Hz is approximately 7 dB SPL (for headphones). Therefore, the threshold for a 1000 Hz tone in the presence of this noise will be approximately 53.4 dB HL (60.4 dB SPL – 7 dB SPL).
>
> Now to demonstrate effective masking using a masker bandwidth that is identical to the bandwidth of the critical filter, perform the same calculation using a masker bandwidth of 64 Hz (instead of 6000 Hz) again with an overall sound pressure level of 80 dB SPL. What is the expected finding? If the critical band for 1000 Hz is 64 Hz and a masker of 64 Hz centered at 1000 Hz is used, all 80 dB SPL is effective at masking the pure-tone signal because all of the frequency components contributing to masking fall within the critical band.

Frequency Selectivity

Fletcher discovered that the auditory system acts as a series of band-pass filters centered at specific center frequencies. Later, it was discovered that these filters increase in width with increasing frequency. Patterson (1976) was influential in developing the notched-noise technique (which is a variation on Fletcher's early techniques) for measuring auditory filter width.

- Figure 3–11 provides the authors' interpretation of the notched-noise method. The left portion of the figure shows a tonal signal centered at a given frequency and various notch bandwidths (#1–4). On the right, corresponding thresholds for tone detection for each notch bandwidth (labeled #1–4) are provided. As shown, when the notch bandwidth is small (more noise contained within the critical band shown in #1), higher sound levels are required for threshold detection. As the notch bandwidth increases, lower sound levels are required for threshold detection (due to less noise within the critical band as shown in #4).

Frequency selectivity refers to the ability of the auditory system to process or resolve individual frequency components contained within a complex signal. This ability is influenced by the width of the auditory filter in that portions of the auditory system with narrower filter widths provide for better frequency selectivity than those with broader filtering. On a linear scale, low-frequency auditory filters are narrower and exhibit better frequency resolution than broader high-frequency auditory filters. Auditory filter width is quantified using equivalent rectangular bandwidth (ERB) values, with lower ERB values representing narrow auditory filter with and higher ERB values representing broader filter width.

- Harmonic resolvability refers to auditory system ability to resolve (or individually process in distinct auditory filters) the harmonic structure of a signal. Harmonic resolvability is often displayed using an auditory/basilar membrane excitation pattern shown in Figure 3–12.

- When viewing auditory excitation patterns, harmonics creating distinct peaks are considered resolved, with those not creating distinct peaks in the pattern being considered unresolved. As shown in Figure 3–12, lower-frequency harmonics are resolved along the basilar membrane, with higher-frequency harmonics remaining unresolved in a normal auditory system. This is why, in part, lower-frequency tonal signals evoke a stronger perception of pitch than high-frequency signals.

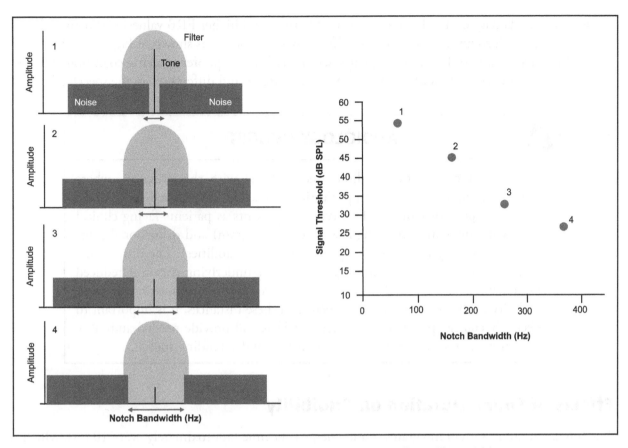

FIGURE 3–11. Illustration of notched-noise method for deriving auditory filter width.

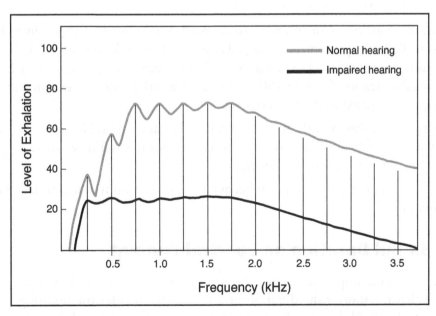

FIGURE 3–12. Excitation pattern demonstrating resolved and unresolved harmonics for normal hearing and hearing-impaired individuals. *Source:* Adapted from *Hearing Science Fundamentals, Second Edition* (pp. 1–370) by Lass, N. J., & Donai, J. J. Copyright © 2023 Plural Publishing, Inc. All rights reserved.

- Cochlear damage creates broader auditory filtering (and higher ERB values) and reduced frequency selectivity across the range of frequencies involved, as shown in Figure 3–12 (Impaired Hearing). Reduced frequency selectivity leads to poorer speech recognition abilities due to decreased processing of the fine acoustic features and differences in the speech signal.

AUDIOLOGY NUGGET

Often in clinical practice, audiologists are faced with the situations where increased audibility through amplification is needed, but speech recognition abilities are poor or reduced. This typically presents as patients facing clinical issues with attenuation (hearing loss on the audiogram) and distortional components of hearing loss (reduced speech recognition abilities). The distortional component is caused by several factors, but one underlying reason is reduced frequency selectivity, which cannot be improved with amplification (as with audibility or the attenuation component). In these instances, it is important to effectively counsel patients to the fact that HAs will provide needed audibility while providing realistic expectations regarding understanding speech.

Effects of Sound Duration on Audibility

The human auditory system integrates sound energy over time (approximately every 10 ms), which is often referred to as a sliding temporal integration window. Auditory sensitivity (threshold detection) improves as the duration of a stimulus is lengthened from the shortest duration that produces a perception of tonality up to a certain point.

- As shown in Figure 3–13, once a tonal signal reaches a duration of approximately 300 to 400 ms, negligible improvements in signal detection threshold are observed. Significant reductions in the sound level required for audibility occur for changes in very brief signals (e.g., a signal increasing from 5 to 50 ms sees a substantial improvement in audibility for the 50-ms signal compared to the 5-ms signal).

- This change in sensitivity with duration is referred to as temporal integration (summation). The temporal integration function for persons with normal auditory function appears to be constant over a wide range of frequencies.

- This concept is important in terms of behavioral and electrophysiological threshold determination.

Effects of Sound Duration on Spectral Content

Similar to the effects on amplitude, signal duration impacts the spectral content of a signal. It is well established that the shorter the duration of a signal, the broader the resulting spectral content. For example, a click stimulus is usually a very brief signal (0.1 ms) with a rapid onset and offset time, yielding a rectangular pulse and spectral pattern similar to that of white noise. This is used in electrophysiology (specifically, ABR) for its stimulation of a large area of the cochlea and its advantage in producing higher neural synchrony than other stimuli. Another stimulus used in ABR is the tone pip, which is still a brief signal (often < 10 ms), but with a tighter, frequency-specific center. Through

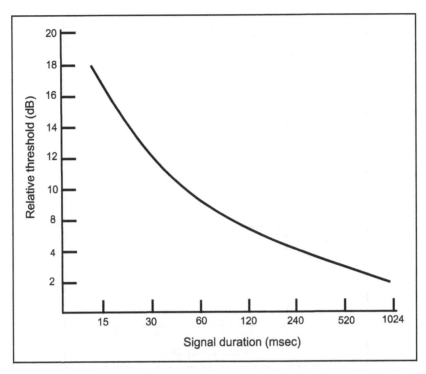

FIGURE 3–13. Effect of signal duration on audibility. *Source:* Adapted from *Hearing Science Fundamentals, Second Edition* (pp. 1–370) by Lass, N. J., & Donai, J. J. Copyright © 2023 Plural Publishing, Inc. All rights reserved.

windowing (e.g., Blackman window), spectral splatter (acoustic energy falling outside of the center frequency) can be reduced, but still, the duration of a pip yields a less "pure" tone than the tonal stimuli used in behavioral audiometry. As a side note, the variability in the duration and windowing of ABR stimuli is why they oftentimes cannot be universally calibrated to ANSI standards.

 KNOWLEDGE CHECKPOINT

In behavioral testing, stimuli are presented with a relatively long rise and fall time to ensure frequency-specific signals are presented to the listener. However, in electrophysiological measures, such as the ABR, a longer rise/fall time significantly degrades the quality of the recorded response. Thus, the trade-off is between producing a frequency-specific signal (which is more place specific along the basilar membrane) and obtaining a usable recorded ABR waveform. With rapid onsets and offsets, the frequency spectrum is broad, as shown at the top of Figure 3–14 (1-ms rise and fall time), but through ramping, or more slowly turning the signal onto full amplitude and slowly turning the signal off, the frequency spectrum becomes tighter, or more "pure," as shown in the 4-ms rise and fall time example (Figure 3–14). Windowing a signal with a Blackman window, for example, produces similar effects to increasing the rise and fall time of a signal, which is why this type of window is commonly used in ABR testing.

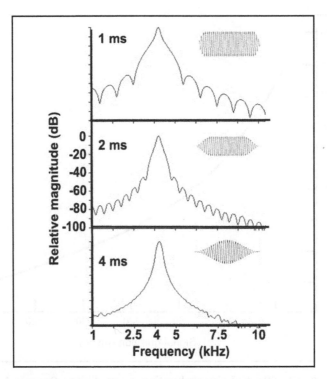

FIGURE 3–14. Effect of rise-fall time on the spectrum of a 2000 Hz tone burst. *Source:* Adapted from *Auditory Brainstem Evoked Potentials: Clinical and Research Applications* (pp. 1–379) by Krishnan, A. Copyright © 2023 Plural Publishing, Inc. All rights reserved.

Masking: Effects of Masker Location, Type, and Amplitude Modulation

Masking is defined as the process of one signal obscuring the perception of another signal. Numerous signals are used as maskers by the profession of audiology. Some examples include narrowband noise, wideband noise (e.g., white or pink noise), speech-shaped noise, International Collegium of Rehabilitative Audiology (ICRA) noise, and multitalker babble.

- Masking is generally reduced to two types: energetic and informational.
  - Energetic masking: any kind of acoustic energy that is obscuring a target auditory signal, such as white noise; occurs in the peripheral auditory system
  - Informational masking: acoustic energy (i.e., energetic masking) with meaningful content, such as speech; occurs in both the peripheral and central auditory systems
- Spatial release from masking (SRM) refers to the phenomenon where changes in masker location relative to the location of a signal of interest (often speech) "release" or enhance the perception of the signal. For example, if a speech signal and masker are co-located at 0° azimuth, it will be more difficult to recognize the signal than if the masker was moved to 90° while maintaining the position of speech at 0°. This advantage occurs due to an increase in spatial and interaural cues. For additional details, please review Litovsky (2012).

- Modulation masking release (MMR) and temporal glimpsing/dip listening occur when a masker fluctuates in amplitude over time (a modulated masker) and creates transient breaks in the noise from which information (tones or speech) can be quickly extracted. Early research by Hall et al. (1984) found improvements in detection of a pure tone in modulated background masker compared to a steady-state (unmodulated) masker.

 AUDIOLOGY NUGGET

Extracting information during temporal dips in background noise has clinical implications for the use of dynamic amplitude compression parameters in hearing aids (release time in particular). A trade-off exists between signal distortion and increasing the speed at which gain is restored following compression by decreasing the release time of a compressions system. In other words, as the release time is decreased (making the release time shorter and increasing gain to precompression levels more quickly), there is an increase in distortion of the overall shape of the signal (temporal envelope) that may negatively impact signal intelligibility. This quick increase in gain may, however, lead to an improved chance of temporal glimpsing/dip listening due to an increase in audibility (because of quickly increasing gain) during the reduced amplitude of background noise. For a thorough review of compression parameters, the trade-offs that exist related to compression speed, and their effects on the recognition of auditory signals, please review Moore (2008).

Binaural Hearing

It is well established that for most individuals, listening with two ears is preferable to one. Binaural hearing allows for improved localization of stimuli, better (lower) thresholds (also known as binaural summation), better hearing in noise, and better frequency selectivity. A summary of the benefits to binaural hearing is shown in Table 3–1. Binaural hearing can also be referred to as diotic listening (same signal delivered to both ears at the same time) or dichotic listening (different signals delivered to both ears at the same time).

Localization

Binaural signals are first processed at the level of the SOC in the auditory brainstem, as this is the first place that receives input from both peripheral auditory pathways. Vertical localization relies on spectral changes in acoustic signals, as a function of head, torso, and pinna, as signal sources change in elevation. The pinna is primarily effective at altering the frequency spectra above 3 kHz, where the head and torso are impactful below 3 kHz. Horizontal localization primarily relies on a combination of interaural intensity (level) differences (IID/ILD) and interaural timing (phase) differences (ITD/IPD) between the ears.

- High-frequency information (>1500 Hz) is responsible for IID/ILDs, mostly due to the head shadow effect. When a signal is coming from precisely in front of a listener (0° azimuth),

TABLE 3–1. Binaural Advantage Table

BINAURAL TASK	ADVANTAGE	AUTHORS
Loudness summation (noise)	Doubling	Marks (1980)
Absolute threshold (noise)	2–3 dB	Pollack (1948)
Absolute threshold (tonal stimuli)	2–3 dB	Shaw et al. (1947)
Threshold in noise	0–2 dB	Hirsh (1948)
Intensity discrimination	~60% improvement	Jesteadt and Wier (1977)
Frequency discrimination	~60% improvement	Jesteadt and Wier (1977)
Speech (speech recognition threshold)	~2.5 dB	Shaw et al. (1947)

it arrives to both ears at the same intensity; however, if the signal moves off to one side or the other (even by 1°), these higher-frequency sounds will arrive at a higher intensity to the ipsilateral ear. The contralateral ear will receive a lower-intensity signal (as much as 20 dB lower at 6 kHz and higher) due to the absorption and reflection of sound around the head and torso (i.e., shorter wavelengths deflect away from the contralateral ear while longer wavelengths will "wrap around" the head and torso). Across different frequencies and stimuli, humans are able to detect IID/ILDs as little as 0.5 to 3 dB.

■ Lower-frequency information (<1500 Hz) will be affected by ITD/IPDs for localization. These occur because of the time (maximum of 600 μs between ears) it takes for the signal to reach the contralateral ear, which also translates into a different phase of the signal arriving to the contralateral as opposed to the ipsilateral ear. A difference in the cochlear and central transmission of the auditory signal can help a listener identify the location of a sound source.

    □ Greatest ITD/IPDs are present at approximately 90° and 270° (directly to the right or left, respectively).

 AUDIOLOGY NUGGET

Most, if not all, prescriptive HA formulae (i.e., NAL-NL2, DSL, IHAFF, and manufacturer specific) prescribe increased gain in cases of monaural fittings. This is accounts for the lack of binaural input and reduced loudness perception associated with a monaural fitting. An additional amount of gain (ranging from 3 to 10 dB depending on the input level) is often prescribed in these instances. Newer HA technology has begun taking advantage of binaural cues by pairing the aids together and transferring data between them to help in gain adjustments, localization cues, and speech in noise enhancements.

MAF vs. MAP Curves

Human auditory sensitivity varies by frequency and method of presentation (headphones or speakers). When auditory sensitivity is evaluated through a speaker, the results are referred to as the minimum audible field (MAF) curve. Signals presented through headphones provide what is known as the minimum auditory pressure (MAP) curve. These curves were derived many years ago by measuring auditory sensitivity (by frequency) for thousands of otologically normal listeners. Figure 3–15 provides an example of the sensitivity by frequency of the MAF and MAP.

- Sensitivity shown on the MAF curve is approximately 6 dB better than that shown on the MAP curve. This is often referred to as the "missing 6 dB." However, in practical terms, this is most likely to be a 2 to 3 dB difference at maximum when accounting for specific recording parameters and accounting for the reflective effects of the head commonly referred to as the head-related transfer function (Yost, 2013). As such, about half of the 6 dB difference is related to the binaural advantage and the remainder created by calibration effects.

Effects of Frequency and Amplitude on Loudness Perception

The perception of loudness varies across the range of audible frequencies. These are visualized via phon curves and are often referred to as equal loudness contours (Figure 3–16). Horizontal lines along the equal loudness contours visually represent each phon level (10–120 phon). At any point along a single curve, the perceived loudness of that tone will be judged to be of equal loudness to a 1000 Hz tone on that same curve. Of note, at higher intensities, the phon curve is flatter, suggesting more equal perception of loudness across frequencies at higher intensities than at lower intensities.

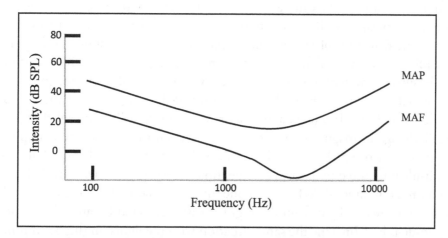

FIGURE 3–15. MAP vs. MAF curve. *Source:* Adapted from *Hearing Science Fundamentals, Second Edition* (pp. 1–370) by Lass, N. J., & Donai, J. J. Copyright © 2023 Plural Publishing, Inc. All rights reserved.

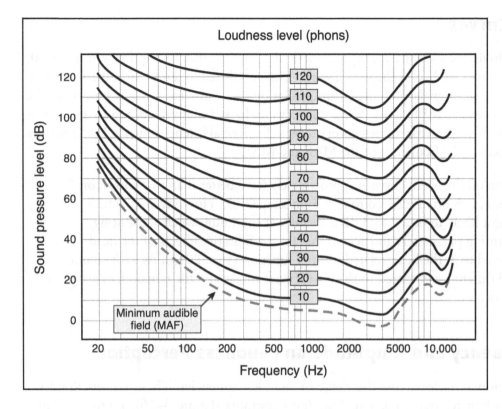

FIGURE 3–16. Equal loudness contours (phon curves). *Source:* Adapted from *Hearing Science Fundamentals, Second Edition* (pp. 1–370) by Lass, N. J., & Donai, J. J. Copyright © 2023 Plural Publishing, Inc. All rights reserved.

 AUDIOLOGY NUGGET

The ability to discern minimal differences in intensity is often measured using a just noticeable difference (JND) task that involves comparing loudness or pitch between two sounds (a standard sound and comparison sound). The outcome is often referred to as the difference limen for intensity (or difference limen for frequency if measuring JND for frequency). Weber's law is relevant to discussions of the detection of changes in perceived loudness. In short, Weber's law (or applied as the Weber fraction) states that a change in a perceived attribute (e.g., brightness, weight, loudness) is directly proportional to the magnitude of the original stimulus or object. In other words, if the magnitude of the original stimulus or object is low (e.g., a dull light, soft sound, or light [weight] object), a small change in magnitude is discernible between the two. If the magnitude is high (e.g., a bright light, loud sound, or heavy object), a larger change in magnitude is required to detect a change. Imagine a classroom with the lights off (low number of lumens). When someone turns on a flashlight in the front of the room, the increased light from flashlight is easily detected because the original magnitude is low. Imagine the same situation with the lights on (higher number of lumens), with the same flashlight lit. It is likely that the extra light due to the flashlight will go undetected because the original magnitude of the light is high. Similarly, a change from 20 to 21 dB SPL is typically discernible, whereas a change from 80 to 81 dB SPL is not.

Auditory Recruitment and Outer Hair Cell (OHC) Function

Recruitment is characterized by an abnormal growth of perceived loudness. Due to a loss of OHC function (the active mechanism/cochlear amplifier), soft sounds are inaudible and thus require increased intensity to reach threshold; loud sounds are perceived to be approximately as loud as they would be to individuals with normal hearing or at levels reported prior to hearing loss. The perceptual result of recruitment is a reduced dynamic range, which is often described as the intensity difference between a listener's threshold and his or her uncomfortable listening level. These values are often obtained using a process called loudness scaling commonly used during the fitting of HAs or CIs.

- Reductions in dynamic range cause specific problems for fitting HAs. Listeners with recruitment require more gain for low-level sounds, due to the loss of the OHC active mechanism, and less gain for moderate to loud sounds.

- One processing feature in current HAs to account for this need is called wide dynamic range compression (WDRC). WDRC attempts to account for the loss of OHC function associated with sensory hearing loss by quickly providing more gain for soft inputs and less gain for increasingly louder signals. This reduces the need for the patient to consistently increase and decrease the volume of the HA.

- WDRC adjusts the gain of the device automatically once the HA is programmed to account for differences in input levels and the patient's loudness needs.

 KNOWLEDGE CHECKPOINT

Recall that WDRC provides increased gain for lower-level inputs and less gain as input levels increase. While this is beneficial for maintaining comfort and more normal perception of loudness, this difference distorts the natural interaural-level differences present without amplification. Imagine the level of sound at the right ear being 55 dB SPL and due to the head shadow effect, the level of the same sound being 45 dB SPL at the left ear (a 10 dB difference). WDRC will provide more gain for the sound arriving at the left ear (where the sound is 45 dB, i.e., 10 dB less than the right ear). Less gain is provided for the sound at the right ear (due to a higher input level of 55 dB). Thus, the original 10 dB interaural difference will be reduced (to 5 dB, for example), thus providing an unnatural and less pronounced interaural cue for the listener. However, current technology allows communication and the sharing of information between the two HAs, thus ameliorating this potential issue to some degree.

Perception of Pitch and Timbre

Human listeners continuously make perceptual judgments regarding the pitch (perceived on a scale from low to high) and timbre (a qualitative description of complexity or quality) of sounds in their auditory environments. From recognizing the sex of a talker (which often relies on voice pitch typically associated with fundamental frequency [F0]) to recognizing musical instruments in a musical selection, these perceptual tasks are completed with minimal effort or attention. For a comprehensive review of the process of pitch perception and evidence regarding how human listeners perceive pitch, please review Yost (2009).

Theories of Pitch Perception

There are two generally accepted theories of pitch perception related to tonal stimuli: spectral (place) and temporal theory. Spectral theory posits that pitch is derived based on place of maximum basilar membrane excitation for tonal stimuli and multiple locations of basilar membrane excitation for complex signals. Temporal theory posits that pitch is extracted from the temporal patterns of neural impulses evoked by the signal. In general, it is accepted that spectral theory allows for the perception of pitch for high-frequency signals and temporal theory produces pitch sensation for low-frequency signals due to better phase locking (i.e., the synchronicity of neural firing with the frequency of the stimulus) of the auditory nerve below 1 kHz (see Figure 3–17 for a visual adapted from Palmer & Russell, 1986).

Spectral (Place) Theory

Spectral (place) theory of pitch originated in the fact that the auditory system acts as a frequency analyzer and performs a Fourier analysis (frequency analysis along the basilar membrane) of the incoming stimulus. The pitch of a signal is thought to be associated with the point at which maximum basilar membrane displacement occurs.

- A spectral (place) mechanism is thought to allow for the perception of high-frequency signals due to an inability of the auditory system to efficiently phase lock to signals above 1 kHz and a complete inability to phase lock to signals above 5 kHz (Palmer & Russell, 1986). Note the decrease in synchronization strength (synchronization index) of auditory nerve firing with increasing frequency in Figure 3–17. As such, because phase locking is poor for high-frequency signals (above approximately 1–5 kHz), the place of auditory excitation provides the perceptual information to discern signal pitch.

Temporal Theory

Temporal theory of pitch proposes that individual nerve fibers synchronize (fire) to the periodic (phase) properties of a signal at low frequencies (below approximately 1 kHz). As frequency increases, individual neurons are unable, due to refractory periods and other neural processes, to fire to each phase of a periodic signal.

- When this occurs, neighboring frequencies fire at alternating phases, commonly referred to as the volley principle (Wever & Bray, 1937). This process allows for the encoding of signal frequency due to a pooled neural response (from which pitch is derived).

Residue Pitch and Case of the Missing F0

While it is the case that F0 plays a role in the perception of pitch, it is also true that pitch can be preserved in the absence of the F0. Commonly referred to as residue pitch or the case of the missing

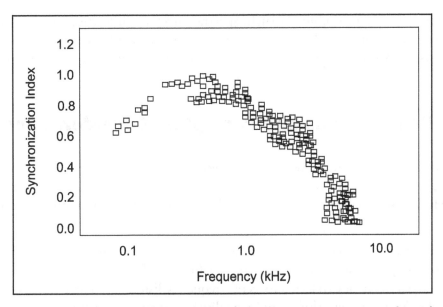

FIGURE 3–17. Phase locking strength by frequency. *Source:* Adapted with the permission of Elsevier, from Palmer, A. R., & Russell, I. J. (1986). Phase-locking in the cochlear nerve of the guinea-pig and its relation to the receptor potential of inner hair-cells. *Hearing Research, 24*(1), 1–15; permission conveyed through Copyright Clearance Center, Inc.

fundamental, this phenomenon lends support to the temporal theory of pitch perception as the removal of frequency component(s), F0 in this case, does not significantly alter the perception of pitch (although it is possible that the signal may not evoke as strong a sensation of pitch). In this phenomenon, the relative distance between adjacent harmonics in frequencies above F0 creates a periodicity (pitch period) in the signal associated with F0, and from that, pitch is preserved and extracted.

Q & A

Question: What is a real-world example of residue pitch?

Answer: Historically, the effective bandwidth of most telephones ranged from approximately 300 to 3400 Hz. As such, spectral energy at F0 for most adult male and female speakers was outside of the bandwidth of most telephones, and therefore information at this frequency was not available to listeners. Because the temporal information (period) associated with F0 is preserved in the signal, the listener on the other end could determine the sex of the talker (F0 being a salient cue for talker sex) with little difficulty.

Perception of Timbre

The perception of timbre is a qualitative judgment regarding sound quality or complexity. Timbre is derived from the spectral envelope of a signal. In other words, two identical harmonic complexes (i.e., signal with F0 with subsequent harmonics) with varying harmonic peak energy (e.g., peak energy of one signal is the second harmonic and peak energy of the other signal is at the sixth harmonic) will have similar pitch but will vary in timbre. As such, spectral envelope differences (peak harmonic energy) among these types of signals provide salient acoustic information for the perception of timbre. Timbre perception allows listeners to detect two different musical instruments simultaneously playing the same musical note.

Cochlear Dead Regions and Perceptual Considerations

When cochlear damage becomes severe and involves both the OHCs and inner hair cells (IHCs), cochlear dead regions occur. A cochlear dead region is a portion of the cochlea void of functioning OHCs and IHCs. Perceptual consequences of cochlear dead regions commonly include (but are not limited to):

- Loss of sensitivity: particularly to low-level sounds, damaged hair cell areas may still be able to detect sounds at high sound levels due to the vibration of the basilar membrane at frequencies near the signal frequency (referred to as off-frequency listening). These tonal signals are often described as having a "scratchy" or noise quality versus a tonal quality.

- Loudness recruitment: damage to the OHCs resulting in an abnormally rapid growth in loudness, due to change in slope of the response of the basilar membrane (becoming more linear)

- Reduction in frequency selectivity: the damaged cochlea results in a reduced ability to separate or resolve the different frequency components in sounds, leading to poorer frequency discrimination and speech perception abilities

- Effects on pitch perception: reduction in the precision of neural phase locking and neural representation of the temporal fine structure of sounds

---

 AUDIOLOGY NUGGET

The threshold-equalizing noise (TEN) test is a clinical behavioral test for cochlear dead regions wherein a wideband noise is spectrally shaped to give a constant masked threshold for a pure tone presented in the noise. The primary purpose of the TEN test is to determine if the obtained response is representative and being elicited by the frequency of interest or a result of excitation of a neighboring frequency (or off-frequency listening). If the frequency of the tone falls within a dead region, then the threshold will be higher ($\geq$10 dB) with the noise present (masked) than without (unmasked) and/or the threshold will be at least 10 dB higher than the presentation level of the TEN. With TEN noise present, the test tone activity will be masked and the response is actually being elicited from a neighboring area of the cochlea (which is not masked by the noise). The threshold for the tone will be higher (poorer) than if the tone was detected at the area of the cochlea tuned to the frequency since the basilar membrane is moving less at the adjacent areas than the presentation frequency. The presence of a cochlear dead region has implications for the fitting of amplification, specifically the type of processing required to account for the dead region (frequency lowering vs. traditional amplification). For additional details, please refer to Moore (2010).

- Effects on speech perception: some parts of speech are inaudible, which decreases ability to understand speech; also smears (distorts) spectrum leading to poorer resolution of formants and other important frequency cues

Instrumentation in Audiology

The provision of audiological diagnostic and rehabilitative services is highly dependent upon the use of technical equipment. Proper equipment function is determined by standards developed by organizations such as the American National Standards Institute (ANSI) and the International Organization for Standardization (ISO). Periodically, this equipment requires exhaustive calibration, which is typically completed by a calibration company with extensive experience in this process. The following sections include information regarding commonly used instrumentation in audiology service provision but are not intended to be an exhaustive review.

ANSI and ISO Specifications

Table 3–2 (ANSI) and Table 3–3 (ISO) contain standards relevant to the profession of audiology. ANSI and the ISO publish a wide range of standards that include determining audiometric zero (0 dB HL) and the calibration of audiological testing equipment to maximum allowable ambient noise levels for sound-treated test rooms, among others.

Audiometry Transducers

- Air-conduction transducers include supra-aural (e.g., TDH-39, TDH-49), circumaural (e.g., Sennheiser HDA 200 or 300, Koss HV/1A), insert earphones (e.g., Etymotic ER-3A), and soundfield speakers. Ultra-high-frequency audiometry (9–20 kHz) is traditionally administered using Sennheiser HDA 200 or 300 due to a flatter frequency response above 8 kHz compared to supra-aural and insert options, which have significant frequency response roll-off above 8 kHz.

  - One advantage of insert earphones is higher levels of interaural attenuation than that found with supra-aural earphones. Interaural attenuation represents the decibel reduction of a sound as it crosses the head from the test ear to the non–test ear. The average increase in interaural attenuation is approximately 15 to 30 dB HL (from approximately 40 dB HL for supra-aural to a conservative 50 to 70 dB HL for inserts if properly inserted). Insert earphones also protect against collapsing canals common in certain populations (e.g., young children and elderly individuals).

  - Using transducers with increased levels of interaural attenuation reduces the need for masking in cases of asymmetrical hearing loss and instances of masking dilemmas (e.g., significant bilateral conductive hearing loss), which is helpful in fast-paced clinical environments. Detailed information on interaural attenuation and masking is provided in Chapter 5.

- Bone-conduction oscillators deliver a calibrated amount of force to stimulate the bone-conduction auditory pathway. Theoretically, bone-conduction oscillators can be placed anywhere on the skull; however, a mastoid or forehead placement is most common.

  - Interaural attenuation for bone oscillators is conservatively set at 0 dB HL, when in fact it varies depending upon age and other physical factors.

TABLE 3-2. Relevant ANSI Standards for Audiology

NUMBER	NAME	DESCRIPTION
ANSI S3.1-1999 (Revised 2018)	Maximum permissible ambient noise for audiometric test rooms	For MPANLs allowed in a test room that produce negligible masking (2 dB) of test signals presented at reference level equivalent threshold levels
ANSI S3.2-1999(R2020)	Method for measuring the intelligibility of speech over communication systems	For English word lists, methods for selecting and training the talkers and listeners, for designing and reporting test conditions, for calculating the intelligibility score, for analyzing and reporting the test results
ANSI S3.6-2018	Specification for audiometers	For use in determining the threshold level in comparison with chosen standard reference threshold level, including pure tone, speech, and masking signals
ANSI S3.7-2016	Method for Measurement of Calibration of Earphones	For use with circum-aural, supra-aural, and insert-type headphones
ANSI S3.13-1987(R2020)	Mechanical Coupler for Measurement of Bone Vibrators	For calibrating bone conduction audiometers and making measurements on bone vibrations and bone conduction hearing aids
ANSI S3.20-1995(R2003)	Bioacoustical Terminology	For definitions for terms including hearing, speech, psychoacoustics, and physiological acoustics
ANSI S3.21-2004	Methods for Manual Pure-Tone Threshold Audiometry	Procedure for pure-tone testing for persons conducting in industry, schools, medical settings, and other areas
ANSI S3.25-1989(R2003)	Occluded Ear Simulator	Designed to stimulate the acoustic portion of the ear canal between the earmold and the eardrum, from 100 Hz to 10 kHz
ANSI S3.36-1985(R2006)	Specification for Manikin for Simulated In Situ Airborne Acoustic Measurements	For various uses including measurement of hearing aid gain under simulated conditions and other head-related transfer functions (HRTFs), and based on anthropomorphically average adult manikin head, ear, and torso
ANSI S3.39-1987(R2007)	Specification for Instruments to Measure Aural Acoustic Impedance and Admittance (Aural Acoustic Immittance)	For measurements of acoustic impedance, and acoustic admittance within the ear canal
ANSI S1.4-1983(R2006)	Specification for Sound Level Meters	For performance specifications for sound-measuring instruments, including transient sound signals and digital techniques and displays

TABLE 3–3. Relevant ISO Standards for Audiology

NUMBER	NAME	DESCRIPTION
ISO 8253-1, 2010	Acoustics—Audiometric Test Methods—Part 1: Basic Pure Tone Air and Bone Conduction Threshold Audiometry	Procedures and requirements for screening purposes only, including air conduction, pure-tone audiometric test, speech audiometry, electrophysiological audiometry, and procedures
ISO 389-1, 2017	Acoustics—Reference Zero for the Calibration of Audiometric Equipment—Part 1: Reference Equivalent Threshold Sound Pressure Levels for Pure Tones and Supra-Aural Earphones	A standard reference zero for the scale of hearing threshold level, for pure-tone air conduction audiometers, to promote agreement and uniformity in the expression of hearing threshold level measurements throughout the world
ISO 389-2, 1994	Acoustics—Reference Zero for the Calibration of Audiometric Equipment—Part 2: Reference Equivalent Threshold Sound Pressure Levels for Pure Tones and Insert Earphones	Levels supplementary to those specified in ISO 389:1991 (to be reissued as ISO 389-1), applicable to insert earphones of type Etymotic Research ER-3A, coupled to the human ear by ear inserts of type ER-3-1
ISO 389-3, 2016	Acoustics—Reference Zero for the Calibration of Audiometric Equipment—Part 3: Reference Equivalent Threshold Vibratory Force Levels for Pure Tones and Bone Vibrators	Calibration of bone vibrators for pure-tone bone-conduction audiometry: (a) reference equivalent threshold vibratory force levels (RETVFL), for threshold of hearing of young otologically normal persons by bone-conduction audiometry; (b) essential characteristics of the bone vibrator and the method of coupling to the test subject, and to the mechanical coupler
ISO 389-4, 1994	Acoustics—Reference Zero for the Calibration of Audiometric Equipment—Part 4: Reference Levels for Narrow-Band Masking Noise	Reference levels for narrow-band masking noise presented for air conduction in pure-tone audiometry, in terms of levels to be added to the reference equivalent threshold sound pressure levels for the corresponding pure-tone frequencies
ISO 389-5, 2006	Acoustics—Reference Zero for the Calibration of Audiometric Equipment—Part 5: Reference Equivalent Threshold Sound Pressure Levels for Pure Tones in the Frequency Range 8 kHz to 16 kHz	Reference equivalent threshold sound pressure levels (RETSPLs) of pure tones in the frequency range from 8 to 16 kHz applicable to the calibration of air-conduction audiometers for specific earphones

Calibration Considerations

The information provided in this section is an overview of issues related to the calibration of audiological equipment. For a comprehensive review of topics related to calibration, please refer to Champlin and Letowski (2014) for details on air conduction, Margolis and Popelka (2014) for details on bone conduction, and Frost and Levitt (2014) for information on calibrating the speech signal. A significant portion of the information below is found in the abovementioned articles.

Calibration Equipment

Calibration procedures are accomplished using acoustic couplers to mimic the human ear and head. These procedures are designed with specific shapes and volumes to allow for sound measurements using a calibrated microphone. A primary function is to provide a standardized and reproducible recording mechanism that mimics the impedance of the auditory system to the best degree possible. Couplers vary in their volume depending on the transducer and its location relative to the tympanic membrane.

- 6-cc couplers (e.g., IEC 318; NBS 9–A) are used with supra-aural headphones to calibrate frequencies from 125 to 8000 Hz. The 6-cc volume simulates the average volume of the adult ear canal with a supra-aural headphone place on the ear. A 500-gram weight is used to mimic the pressure induced by the supra-aural headband. To calibrate frequencies above 8000 Hz, an adapter plate is used with circumaural headphones such as the HDA 200 or HDA 300.

- 2-cc couplers (e.g., IEC 126; IEC 711; Zwislocki occluded ear simulator) are commonly used to calibrate insert earphones due to the reduced volume of air in the ear canal associated with placement of the insert earphones (versus the 6-cc associated with supra-aural headphones). HA-1 and HA-2 couplers commonly used for electroacoustic analysis of hearing aids are variants of the previously noted couplers.

- Artificial mastoid couplers (e.g., Bruel and Kjaer 4390; Larson Davis AMC493B) are used to calibrate bone-conduction oscillators (Margolis & Popelka, 2014). These devices convert mechanical energy from the oscillator to an electrical signal that is recorded by the sound-level meter. An oscillator is coupled to the artificial mastoid with 5.4 newtons (± .5 newtons) as specified in ANSI standard S3.6 (2010).

Sound-level meters (SLMs) are used to measure the output level of earphones, inserts, and loudspeakers. These devices are calibrated using a pistonphone set to a fixed frequency and fixed level of either 94 or 114 dB SPL. Pressure microphones are used for calibrating earphones while random incidence microphones are used for calibrating soundfield speakers.

- Type 1 SLMs provide the most precise measurements and are required for exhaustive electroacoustic calibration. SLMs can be set to "fast" or "slow" recording times. Fast recording times analyze the incoming signal every 0.125 ms (or eight times per second). Slow weighting is recommended for calibration purposes.

- Various weightings are available depending on the purpose of the measurements. Figure 3–18 provides example dBA, dBB, and dBC weightings. dBA weightings are used to mimic human auditory sensitivity by frequency at low intensities where low and high frequencies are attenuated (inverse of the MAF curve). This scale is commonly used in industrial settings for hearing conservation purposes.

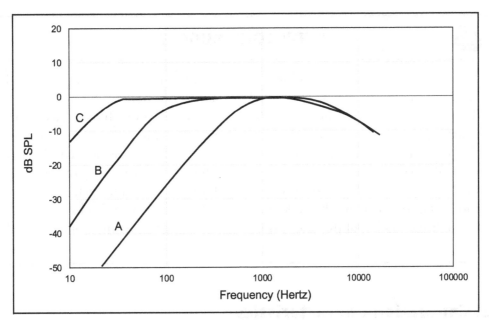

FIGURE 3–18. Sound-level meter weightings.

■ SLMs also have filter characteristics that allow for the precise analysis of frequency and reduction in ambient noise from frequencies neighboring the test frequency. These filters are typically one octave or one-third octave wide. One-third octave filters are more common in sophisticated (and more expensive) SLMs.

 KNOWLEDGE CHECKPOINT

SLMs have numerous options from which to choose when analyzing sound levels. One option relates to how the equipment weights the incoming frequencies contained within a signal. The dBA weighting is commonly used in industrial audiology when evaluating noise levels and exposure for employees because the response mimics the human auditory system and provides the best estimate of what the employee is experiencing. The dBC weighting should be used when a more equal weighting of frequencies is desired. Additional details on sound-level recording and its associated equipment are discussed in Chapter 8.

■ Multimeters are used to measure the linearity of the attenuator or the change in output level of the audiometer with changes in the HL dial. These devices measure three electrical properties, including resistance, current, and voltage, with voltage being of interest for determining output level.

■ Frequency counters are used to evaluate the integrity of the tone generator by connecting directly to the audiometer.

■ Oscilloscopes are used to visualize the waveform (output over time) of tonal signals.

AUDIOLOGY NUGGET

Extensive calibration of audiological equipment is required to be conducted annually, but it is good practice to do daily calibration checks of the audiometer. These include cycling through the different frequencies for each transducer type, listening to the changes in intensities presented, listening for intermittency in the signal, and checking for any distortion in the signal. These daily checks alert the audiologist to any potential problems with equipment prior to testing their first patient that may skew the test findings. Individuals with normal hearing are those who routinely run the biologic checks. Records of these checks may prove useful if the validity of the results obtained from a clinic are questioned in legal proceedings.

General Calibration Characteristics

Calibrating audiological equipment is a technical process requiring attention to detail. The following information provides some general topic areas involved in the calibration of hearing testing equipment.

- Output levels are measured for transducers, including earphones, inserts, bone oscillators, and soundfield speakers, using the appropriate coupler and a SLM. Calibration of these transducers is designed to match the normal pattern of human auditory sensitivity by frequency. Reference equivalent threshold sound pressure levels (RETSPLs) and reference equivalent threshold force levels (RETFLs) are used to calibrate air-conduction and bone-conduction signals, respectively, and represent the signal levels required to reach absolute thresholds of hearing among otologically normal listeners (0 dB HL or audiometric zero).

  □ Over the years, RETFLs were remeasured and converted to RETSPLs (Margolis & Popelka, 2014). For a comprehensive review of RETSPLs for air- and bone-conduction transducers, please review Table 2 in both Champlin and Letowski (2014) and Margolis and Popelka (2014). Note specific RETSPL values for mastoid vs. forehead placement in the latter.

  □ RETSPLs for signals presented via soundfield speakers require a reference point at least 1 meter away from the speaker at which all signals are measured. The signals can include FM tones (commonly referred to as warble tones) or one-third octave band noise. The angle of incidence also plays a role in RETSPL values, with specific values contained in Table 4 of Champlin and Letowski (2014). Specific angles specified are 0°, 45°, and 90°. Note the lowest RETSPL levels between 3 and 4 kHz for all angles due to the natural resonant properties and sensitivity to frequency of the human auditory system that coincides to the lowest point on the MAF curve.

- Attenuator linearity refers to the predictable (and equal) change in audiometer output with changes in dB HL (a decrease from 70 to 65 dB HL should result in a commensurate reduction in output on the multimeter). This should be checked across output levels to ensure proper function at low, mid, and high output levels. A change of 5 dB requires the output to be with ±1.5 dB of this decibel change.

- Frequency integrity should be assessed using a frequency counter to ensure proper function of the pure-tone generator. Frequency values must be within ±1% of the test frequency (e.g., if 1000 Hz is the intended frequency, the output must be within 990 and 1010 Hz).

- Harmonic distortion (often referred to as total harmonic distortion or THD) is defined as distortion occurring at integer multiples (harmonics) of a test frequency (e.g., distortion at 2, 3, and 4 kHz with a 1 kHz test frequency). This is measured using a SLM set to one-third octave filters and tested at the highest audiometer level setting. THD of greater than 2.5% is considered out of calibration.

- Signal presentation via the interrupter switch is evaluated in three ways, including the on-off ratio, crosstalk, and rise-fall time.

  □ On-off ratio refers to the output level of the signal with the tone on (interrupter button pressed) and the tone off (interrupter button not pressed). This ratio is considered out of compliance if the value is less than 70 dB.

  □ Crosstalk refers to the situation where signal information from one channel is present and can be heard in the other channel. The output is measured in one earphone (test) and compared to the output of the other earphone (nontest). Significant crosstalk is present if the difference between these two measurements is less than 70 dB.

  □ Rise-fall time refers to the time it takes for the signal to go from off to on (rise time) and from on to off (fall time). To measure this, the signal is monitored using a digital oscilloscope to monitor the rise and fall time. Rise-fall times generally cannot be less than 20 ms or greater than 200 ms for pure-tone signals.

- Masking noises commonly used in audiological testing include speech noise, narrowband noise, and sometimes pink or white noise. For narrowband noise maskers, the frequency range (band limits in Hz) and band reference levels (levels in dB) are specified and evaluated using a spectrum analyzer. For broadband maskers (white noise), the frequency distribution from 250 to 5000 Hz must be within 5 dB of the level at 1000 Hz.

- Ambient noise levels may have a dramatic effect on the validity of audiological testing. ANSI S1.1-1999 (R2003) specifies maximum permissible ambient noise levels (MPANLs) for audiometric test suites. These values are found in Table 3–4 and are specified for ears covered (earphones or inserts) and ears uncovered (soundfield speakers). As can be seen, lower ambient levels are required for ears uncovered due to a lack of passive attenuation provided when using a transducer on or in the ear. These levels have been determined to produce negligible masking of equal to or less than 2 dB when testing tonal signals at 0 dB HL (or RETSPL values) specified by ANSI S3.6 (2010).

Immittance Equipment

A tympanometer (sometimes referred to as an immittance bridge) is a piece of equipment used for the measurement of acoustic impedance within the human external ear canal and is helpful in the evaluation, identification, documentation, and diagnosis of external and middle ear disorders. Examples of clinically available tympanometers include the GSI Tympstar Pro™, the Interacoustics Titan™, and the Maico TouchTymp™. Many tympanometers analyze middle ear function using tests such as tympanometry, acoustic/middle ear muscle reflex threshold, acoustic reflex decay, and Eustachian tube

TABLE 3–4. ANSI Maximum Permissible Ambient Levels for Audiometric Test Rooms (Comparison of Ears Covered and Ears Uncovered)

OCTAVE BAND CENTER FREQUENCY (Hz)	MAX dB SPL WITH EARS COVERED	MAX dB SPL WITH EAR UNCOVERED
125	39	35
250	25	21
500	21	16
1000	26	13
2000	34	14
4000	37	11
8000	37	14

Source: American National Standards Institute. (2003). *Maximum permissible ambient noise levels for audiometric test rooms* (Rev. ed.) (ANSI S3.1-1999).

function testing. A probe tone frequency of 226 Hz is regularly used for patients older than 6 months of age (due to a stiffness-dominated middle ear system), but 678 Hz and 1000 Hz are also available stimulus frequencies (which evaluates for mass-related conditions). Wideband tympanometry is an available measurement that uses a wideband click as a stimulus. Additional details on tympanometry are provided in Chapters 5 and 6 of this text.

- A test cavity is typically included to verify the calibration of the tympanometer and is recommended to be part of a daily calibration routine. A biological calibration check is also recommended for tympanometry and reflex tests by performing a daily check on an otologically normal ear. Extensive calibration is recommended under ASNI S3.39-1987 (R2020) Standard Specifications for Instruments to Measure Aural Acoustic Impedance and Admittance (Aural Acoustic Immittance).

Hearing Aid Verification Equipment

A hearing instrument analyzer is used in the process of fitting and verifying the electroacoustic performance of hearing instruments connected to a standard acoustic coupler (test box measures) or while worn on the ear by the HA user (on-ear or probe microphone measures). Examples of this manufactured equipment are called Audioscan™ Verifit 1 and 2, Natus Aurical™ Hearing Aid Fitting System, MedRX™ Avant Arc, and Rem + Real Ear Measures and Live Speech Mapping Systems.

- On-ear measures provide information regarding HA function while the HA is being used by an individual. Examples of these measures include the real ear unaided response (REUR), real ear unaided gain (REUG), real ear aided response (REAR), real ear insertion gain (REIG), real ear saturations response (RESR), and real ear to coupler difference (RECD), all of which are commonly used.
  - □ REUR—SPL, as a function of frequency, at a specified measurement point in the ear canal for a specified auditory signal with the unoccluded ear canal

    ☐ REUG—difference, in dB as a function of frequency, between the SPL at a specified measurement point in the ear canal and the SPL at a field reference point, for a specified auditory signal with the ear unoccluded; amount of natural gain provided by the resonance properties of the external auditory system

    ☐ REAR—SPL at a specified measurement point in the ear canal for a specified sound field, with the HA in place and turned on

    ☐ REIG—difference between aided and unaided ear canal SPL; amount of gain provided by an amplification device found using the formula: REAR – REUR.

    ☐ RESR—value obtained using a narrowband signal at a high level to saturate the HA (usually 85–90 dB SPL)

    ☐ RECD—difference between the SPL in an occluded ear and the SPL in the HA-1 (2 cc coupler) produced by the same sound source with the same acoustic coupling

    ☐ Most systems come with the equipment needed to perform daily/weekly calibration checks for both on-ear and test box measures. For instance, the Verifit 2 has specific ANSI couplers (blue) to be used for test box calibration.

■ Test box measurements provide information about HA performance such as measures of gain, distortion, input/output, compression, directionality, and digital noise reduction measured in a coupler (not in situ or in the ear).

■ Speechmap fitting environment is also commonly used as it provides various stimuli, including speech and noise, for fitting HAs and testing their performance. These stimuli are available in the test box or on-ear test environment. Verification software can also calculate a Speech Intelligibility Index (SII), valued in percentages, using unaided or aided thresholds to estimate the audibility of speech. Please review Amlani et al. (2002) for a comprehensive review of the SII and its uses. Comparing unaided and aided SII results and meeting prescriptive targets at various input levels is commonly used to counsel patients on HA performance.

    ☐ Figure 3–19 provides an example of a probe-microphone (on-ear) analysis. The figure is labeled and notes important information such as UCLs, prescriptive targets, SII values (for 55, 65, and 80 dB input), and audiometric (threshold) information. To the top right are the characteristics of the fitting such as HA style, coupling (occluding in this case), real ear to coupler difference (RECD), binaural or monaural fitting, and patient age, among others. It is important to enter this information as each parameter influences prescriptive targets for the fitting.

    ☐ In interpreting Figure 3–19, one should note a few items. For most frequencies, prescriptive targets are not being met (except for approximately 2 kHz), which is the reason for lower obtained SII values (39 for 55 dB SPL input and 43 for 65 dB SPL input). This translates to 39% of the speech signal at 55 dB SPL being audible to the listener and 43% audibility at 65 dB SPL (average conversational intensity level). These values can be used to estimate speech recognition performance of various stimulus types (e.g., digits, words, sentences) by referring to page 55 of the Verifit 2 manual (which is freely available at https://docs .audioscan.com/userguides/vf2manual.pdf)

        ● Rounding to an SII of 45 (from 43), it can be estimated from the data that 100% of digits, 94% of IEEE sentences, and 63% of NU-6 words would be correctly identified at 65 dB SPL. As demonstrated in this example, SII values alone do not provide a percent correct value for recognizing the speech signal but rather a measure of audibility that is

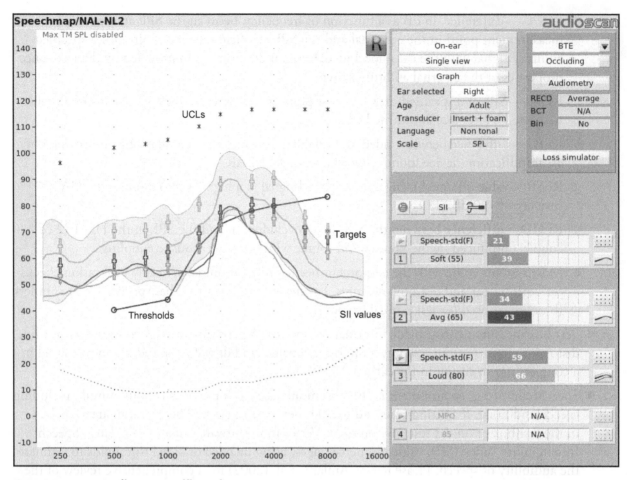

FIGURE 3–19. Audioscan Verifit2 printout.

then used to estimate speech recognition performance. It is important to note that these speech recognition values are estimates and are influenced by a host of factors, including degree of hearing loss, auditory processing capabilities, environmental acoustics (noise and reverberation), and cognitive abilities of the listener.

☐ The readers are encouraged to review the Audioscan Verifit 2 manual (as one example) for detailed information regarding testing protocols, technical details related to available signals, and interpretation of findings.

■ On-ear calibration compares the probe microphone response with the flat calibrated response of the on-ear reference microphone. It then compensates all probe-tube measurements for the difference noted. This is done by positioning the probe tube in front of the reference microphone and holding the probe dock 15 to 90 cm (depending upon the equipment) away from and directly in front of the speaker. The microphone to be calibrated faces the speaker. It is recommended to be performed daily or weekly.

■ Ambient-level check measures can also be done to measure the ambient noise level in the room where the real ear measurement is performed. Similarly, the test box also establishes a correction curve for an uncalibrated test box reference microphone. This is done by positioning the reference microphones about 1 to 2 mm from the coupler microphone. It is recommended to be performed daily or weekly. ANSI standards exist for many of the specific tests.

Signals Used in Verification

- Narrowband signals
  - □ Sinusoidal (pure tones): used in ANSI HA tests, frequency response tests, insertion gain tests (e.g., MPO stimulus contains a series of 128-ms tone bursts with 128-ms gaps at an SPL of 90 dB SPL in the test box and 85 dB in the sound field, uses 1/12 octave frequencies or 1/3 octave frequencies for MPO)
- Broadband signals
  - □ Pink noise signal: pseudo-random signal composed of 1,024 simultaneous tones summed to provide a crest factor of 12 dB; spectrum is controlled by the reference microphone with a digital feedback loop. Spectrum of pink noise decreases at approximately 3 dB per octave.
  - □ Real-speech signals: in Speechmap for on-ear and test box measurements, using four speech passages, the International Speech Test Signal (ISTS), and the single-talker International Collegium of Rehabilitative Audiology (ICRA) noise
    - Examples: ISTS consists of 500-ms segments from recording of six female talkers reading the same passage in English, Arabic, Chinese, French, German, and Spanish. Segments are spliced together to maintain appropriate pauses and filtered to be representative of the long-term average spectrum reported in Byrne et al. (1994). ICRA noise is a recording of an English-speaking talker that has been digitally modified to make the speech largely unintelligible while preserving the temporal and spectral properties of the signal.

For additional information, please review the Audioscan Verifit 2 manual (https://docs.audioscan .com/userguides/vf2manual.pdf) for one verification tool example currently utilized in clinical practice. Verification equipment from other manufacturers is available; however, the authors are most familiar with the Audioscan Verfit and its mention in this chapter is not an endorsement of the product.

Recommended Readings

Akeroyd, M. A. (2006). The psychoacoustics of binaural hearing. *International Journal of Audiology, 45,* S25–S33.

Lentz, J. L. (2020). *Psychoacoustics: Perception of normal and impaired hearing with audiology applications.* Plural Publishing.

Moore, B. C. J. (2022). Listening to music through hearing aids: Potential lessons for cochlear implants. *Trends in Hearing, 26,* 1–13.

Musiek, F. E., & Baran, J. A. (2020). Cochlear physiology I: Mostly mechanics. In *The auditory system anatomy, physiology, and clinical correlates* (2nd ed., pp. 117–132). Plural Publishing.

Oxenham, A., & Bacon, S. (2003). Cochlear compression: Perceptual measures and implications for normal and impaired hearing. *Ear & Hearing, 24*(5), 352–366.

References

Amlani, A. M., Punch, J. L., & Ching, T. Y. (2002). Methods and applications of the audibility index in hearing aid selection and fitting. *Trends in Amplification, 6*(3), 81–129.

Byrne, D., Dillon, H., Tran, K., Arlinger, S., Wilbraham, K., Cox, R., . . . Ludvigsen, C. (1994). An international comparison of long-term average spectra. *Journal of the Acoustical Society of America, 96*(4), 2108–2120.

Champlin, C. A., & Letowski, T. (2014). Audiometric calibration: Air conduction. *Seminars in Hearing, 35*(4), 312–328.

Fletcher, H. (1940). Auditory patterns. *Reviews of Modern Physics, 12,* 47–66.

Frost, G., & Levitt, H. (2014). Audiometric calibration: Speech signals. *Seminars in Hearing, 35*(4), 346–360.

Hall, J. W., Haggard, M. P., & Fernandes, M. A. (1984). Detection in noise by spectro-temporal pattern analysis. *Journal of the Acoustical Society of America, 76*(1), 50–56.

Hirsh, I. J. (1948). The influence of interaural phase on interaural summation and inhibition. *Journal of the Acoustical Society of America, 68*(2), 446–454.

Jesteadt, W., & Wier, C. C. (1977). Comparison of monaural and binaural discrimination of intensity and frequency. *Journal of the American Acoustical Society of America, 61*(6), 1599–1603.

Lass, N. J., & Donai, J. J. (2023). *Hearing science fundamentals.* (2nd ed., pp. 1–370). Plural Publishing.

Litovsky, R. (2012). Spatial release from masking. *Acoustics Today* (April), 18–25.

Margolis, R. H., & Popelka, G. R. (2014). Bone-conduction calibration. *Seminars in Hearing, 35*(4), 329–345.

Marks, L. E. (1980). Binaural summation of loudness: Noise and two-tone complexes. *Perception and Psychophysics, 27*(6), 489–498.

Moore, B. C. J. (2008). The choice of compression speed in hearing aids: Theoretical and practical consideration and the role of individual differences. *Trends in Amplification, 12*(2), 103–112.

Moore, B. C. J. (2010). Testing for cochlear dead regions: Audiometer implementation of the TEN (HL) Test. *Hearing Review, 17*(1), 10–16.

Musiek, F. E., & Baran, J. A. (2020). Cochlear physiology I: Mostly mechanics. In *The auditory system anatomy, physiology, and clinical correlates* (2nd ed., pp. 117–132). Plural Publishing.

Palmer, A. R., & Russell, I. J. (1986). Phase-locking in the cochlear nerve of the guinea-pig and its relation to the receptor potential of inner hair-cells. *Hearing Research, 24*(1), 1–15.

Patterson, R. D. (1976). Auditory filter shapes derived with noise stimuli. *Journal of the Acoustical Society of America, 59,* 640-654.

Pollack, I. (1948). Monaural and binaural threshold sensitivity for tones and for white noise. *Journal of the Acoustical Society of America, 20*(1), 52–57.

Shaw, W. A., Newman, E. B., & Hirsh, I. J. (1947). The difference between monaural and binaural thresholds. *Journal of the American Acoustical Society of America, 19*(4), 734.

Wever, E. G., & Bray, C. W. (1937). The perception of low tones and the resonance-volley theory. *Journal of Psychology: Interdisciplinary and Applied, 3,* 101–114.

Wolfe, J., & Schafer, E. (2020). Basic terminology of cochlear implant programming. In *Cochlear implants: Audiologic management and considerations for implantable hearing devices* (pp. 191–227). Plural Publishing.

Yost, W. A. (2009). Pitch perception. *Attention, Perception, & Psychophysics, 71*(8), 1701–1715.

Yost, W. A. (2013). *Fundamentals of hearing: An introduction* (5th ed.). Brill Academic Publishing.

Practice Questions

1. Otoscopy outcomes for pediatric patients are displayed in the tables using "effusion" or "no effusion" criteria to identify possible otitis media with effusion. With the population of 200, what is the calculated specificity of otoscopy for detecting "no effusion" in cases of suspected otitis media with effusion?

<table>
<tr><td></td><td></td><td colspan="2">Predicted</td></tr>
<tr><td></td><td></td><td>Effusion</td><td>No Effusion</td></tr>
<tr><td rowspan="2">Actual</td><td>Effusion</td><td>96</td><td>22</td></tr>
<tr><td>No Effusion</td><td>4</td><td>78</td></tr>
</table>

   a. 4%

   b. 22%

   c. 78%

   d. 22%

Explanation: Remember that specificity is how false alarms are related to true negatives. In most matrices, this is completed by using the calculation d/(c + d) where box d is the true negative value (here, 78) and box c is the false-positive value (here, 22). 78/(78 + 22) = 78/100 = 0.78 or 78%. Therefore, the answer is c, 78%.

2. From the visual below, what is the phase difference between the two tonal signals?

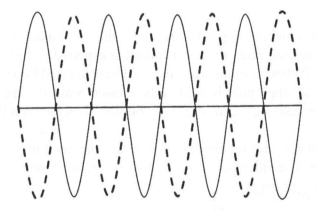

   a. 90°

   b. 180°

   c. 270°

   d. 360°

Explanation: In the figure, when one signal is at its maximum positive displacement, the other is at its maximum negative displacement. This represents a phase difference of 180°. Therefore, the correct answer is b.

3. Mr. Miller is a 34-year-old patient scheduled for a workers' compensation examination. He is a mechanic who reports hearing loss in his left ear following a tire exploding to that side when he was working on a vehicle. The right ear had normal hearing thresholds, but the left ear was consistent with a flat severe to profound hearing loss (unmasked and at levels exceeding interaural attenuation). Mr. Miller had very few false-positive responses on the left ear and a positive Stenger; speech reception threshold was not in agreement with the pure-tone average for the left ear. What form of response bias did he likely demonstrate?

   a. Conservative

   b. Hypoactive

   c. Liberal

   d. Neutral

Explanation: Mr. Miller is likely exaggerating a hearing loss in the left ear, which can be assumed given the amount of hearing loss exceeding interaural attenuation levels, SRT not agreeing with PTA, and the positive Stenger. Other tests that could confirm malingering would include objective measures such as middle ear muscle reflexes and otoacoustic emissions. Behaviorally, with the low false positives and suprathreshold responses (misses), Mr. Miller likely demonstrated a conservative response bias by waiting until the signal is above threshold to respond to the presented tones (equating to a miss), so a is the correct answer.

4. A calibration company has contacted an audiologist reporting that they only had 6-cc couplers available for use for an upcoming appointment. What devices could be sufficiently calibrated?

   a. Insert earphones

   b. Immittance probes

   c. OAE probes

   d. None of the above

Explanation: 2-cc couplers are used when the ear canal volume is expected to be reduced as opposed to 6-cc couplers, which are used when the canal volume is expected to be larger (e.g., in the case of supra-aural headphones). Probes for immittance and OAEs are inserted into the ear canal, reducing its volume, so 2-cc couplers are appropriately used in those cases. Similarly, insert earphones reduce the ear canal volume, which necessitate the use of a 2-cc coupler. Therefore, d is the correct answer.

5. A clinician runs a real ear aided response (REAR) and compares it to a real ear unaided response (REUR) for a patient. The difference between those two values is referred to as:

   a. Real ear insertion gain (REIG)

   b. Real ear saturation response (RESR)

   c. Real ear to coupler difference (RECD)

   d. Real ear occluded response (REOR)

Explanation: REIG is a measure of gain provided by amplification placed in the ear and turned on. It is calculated by subtracting REUR from the REAR. Therefore, a is the correct answer.

6. Assuming equal auditory sensitivity between the right and left ear, at which of the following degrees are interaural phase/timing differences the greatest?

   a. 45°

   b. 90°

   c. 130°

   d. 180°

Explanation: Research has shown that the strongest IPDs/ITDs occur at 90° and 270°. Thus, b is the correct answer.

7. An audiologist is conducting speech recognition in noise testing and wishes to use a masker that provides a high degree of informational masking. Which of the following would meet the audiologist's need?

   a. White noise

   b. Pink noise

   c. 2-talker babble

   d. 20-talker babble

Explanation: Recall that instances of informational masking contain meaningful content. White and pink noise provide energetic masking due to a lack of meaningful content. While 20-talker babble is composed of speech from 20 talkers and individually their productions would provide informational masking, when combined, the effects of informational masking are lost due to a loss of intelligibility of speech from any speaker. In the case of 2-talker babble, a significant amount of meaningful content is perceptible. Thus, c is the best answer.

8. During a biological check, an audiologist notices that a signal presented through one channel of the audiometer to the right headphone is heard in the left headphone, which is set to the second channel. Which of the following potential calibration issues should the audiologist report to the calibration company?

   a. Crosstalk

   b. Rise-fall time

   c. Ambient level

   d. On-off ratio

Explanation: Recall that crosstalk occurs when the presentation of a signal through one channel of the audiometer is present (and often audible) in the transducer set to the other channel. The output is measured in one earphone (test) and compared to the output of the other earphone (nontest). Significant crosstalk is present if the difference between these two measurements is less than 70 dB. Thus, a is the correct answer.

9. A new hearing aid has a sampling rate of 22 kHz. Using the Nyquist theorem, at which frequency is distortion most likely to occur?

a. 4 kHz

b. 6 kHz

c. 9 kHz

d. 11 kHz

Explanation: The Nyquist theorem/frequency is a sampling rate that is double the highest frequency of a signal that will be encoded. Thus, half the reported rate (22 kHz) would be 11 kHz. The closer you get to the maximum frequency that is encoded, the more likely the signal is going to be distorted. In this question, the frequency closest to that maximum frequency of 22 kHz is 11 kHz. Therefore, d is the correct answer.

10. An audiologist is asked to perform sound-level measurements at a local factory. The company is concerned that a new piece of equipment is exposing an employee to excessive levels of noise. The audiologist is at the site and setting the decibel scale for recordings. Which scale is the most appropriate to use?

a. dBA

b. dBB

c. dBC

d. All of the above are equivalent

Explanation: Recall that the dBA weighting provides a measurement that weights the input similarly to the response of the human auditory system. Thus, if the goal is to estimate sound levels experienced by the worker, dBA would provide the most accurate estimate. Thus, a is the correct answer.

Chapter 4

Communication Across the Lifespan: Typical vs. Disordered

Angela Van Sickle and Brittany Hall

Typical Language Development

"Communication is part of what makes us human" (Owens & Farinella, 2019, p. 2). Although humans communicate in a variety of ways (e.g., speech, gestures, facial/body expressions), language and speech are used to convey most messages. Communication and language begin to develop at birth, even though the first words may not be spoken for 10 months.

Milestones for language development (i.e., receptive and expressive) provide information related to skills that should be mastered within specified age ranges. It is important to understand language development milestones and age ranges for milestones to determine delays and disorders. Appendix 4–A outlines milestones for receptive and expressive language. Tables included in this section outline more specific components of language, such as phonology, morphology, syntax, and pragmatics.

Owens and Farinella (2019) describe three main components that are part of all human languages: content, form, and use.

- Content: information to be communicated; includes the semantics or the meaning of the message.
- Form: involves the words used to convey a message and includes phonology, morphology, and syntax.
  □ Phonology: the sound system of a specific language (i.e., 43 sounds in English) that form words.
    • Phonemes are the smallest unit of speech sounds that change meaning (e.g., changing one phoneme for "in" and "on" changes the meanings of the words).
    • Counting phonemes: for example, "kicks" contains four phonemes.
  □ Morphology: the use of grammatical structures to form and vary words. Morphemes are the smallest grammatical units that have meaning. There are free and bound morphemes.
    • Free morphemes: independent and cannot be partitioned into smaller units without losing the meaning, such as "dog."

- Bound morphemes: cannot be independent; they are attached to free morphemes and change the meaning, such as "dogs." "Dog" is a free morpheme, and "s" is a bound morpheme that changes the meaning.
- Counting morphemes: "Audiologists love studying the topics of speech." There are 10 morphemes: Audiologist, -s, love, study, -ing, the, topic, -s, of, and speech.
   □ Syntax: involves the rules for organizing and combining words to form sentences.
- Use: involves pragmatics or different ways language is utilized.

 KNOWLEDGE CHECKPOINT: Content, Form, and Use

1. A child says, "The ball wed." The adult version is "The red ball." This example shows an error with syntax (i.e., the order of the words, ball and red) and phonology (i.e., /w/ for /r/).
2. A child says, "Mommy cup." The adult version is "Mommy's cup." This example shows an error with morphology (i.e., exclusion of the bound morpheme, 's).
3. A child says, "Look at kitty." The adult version is "Look at the dog." This example shows a semantic error (i.e., "kitty" for "dog") and an error with morphology (i.e., exclusion of "the").

Phoneme Development

Each spoken language contains a unique set of sounds for creating words and for communication. Infants and children produce a variety of sounds and eventually master the sounds and combinations of sounds specific to the language spoken by individuals around them. Over time, meaning is attached to these sounds and combinations of sounds (Owens, 2020). Table 4–1 summarizes development for sounds in the English language.

 Q & A

Question: You see a 5-year-old child who has not mastered /k/ or /g/. Would you refer this child for a speech evaluation?

Answer: A 5-year-old child that has not mastered /k/ or /g/ should be referred for speech services. These phonemes should be mastered between ages 2 and 4.

Phonological Processes

McLeod and Baker (2017) synthesized the work of several researchers to provide an overview of the phonological processes or patterns that are evident in normal development of speech. They describe phonological processes or patterns as error patterns that occur during the normal development of

TABLE 4–1. Development of Phonemes

AGE RANGES	PHONEME DEVELOPMENT	EXAMPLES
Before 2 up to 3 years	/p/, /m/, /h/, /n/, /w/	pot, mom, hot, not, we
Before 2 up to 4 years	/b/	baby
2–4 years	/k/, /g/, /d/, /t/, /ŋ/	cat, go, dog, truck, sing
2.5–4 years	/f/, /j/	five, yellow
3–6 years	/r/, /l/	ring, lamp
3–8 years	/s/	stop
3.5–7 years	/tʃ/, /ʃ/	chair, shoe
3.5–8 years	/z/	zoo
4–7 years	/dʒ/	jacket
4–8 years	/v/	vet
4.5–7 years	/θ/	thumb
5–8 years	/ð/	this
6–8+ years	/ʒ/	television

Source: Data obtained from Sander (1972); Lanza and Flahive (2008).

speech. Table 4–2 includes normal phonological processes, examples, and ages they should diminish. In addition, processes or patterns that are not typical in normal development are included in the table. These do not include age ranges, since they are not part of normal development for speech.

Q & A
Your 5-year-old client says, "I throw a ba to my da" (i.e., he is describing that he throws a ball to his dog).
Question: What phonological process is this client demonstrating? Is this normal development for this child?
Answer: This client is demonstrating final consonant deletion (i.e., "ba" for "ball" and "da" for "dog"). Since the likely age of elimination for final consonant deletion is around 3 years of age, this child should not be deleting final consonants.

Vocabulary Development

Kaderavek (2011) stated that children typically begin producing words between 10 and 16 months of age. Several resources have outlined vocabulary development from first words through over 50,000

TABLE 4–2. Development of Phonological Processes or Patterns

LIKELY AGE OF ELIMINATION (YEARS)	PROCESS/PATTERN	DESCRIPTION	EXAMPLE
3	Final consonant deletion	Deletion of final consonant of a word	ba for ball
3	Consonant assimilation	A sound changes due to presence of another sound in the word	gog for dog
3	Reduplication	Repetition of the first syllable (usually) in a multisyllabic word	wawa for water
4	Weak/unstressed syllable deletion	Unstressed syllable deleted	tato for potato
4	Velar fronting	Velar sound replaced with a front sound	take for cake
/f, s/: 3 /z, v/: 4 /ʃ, tʃ, dʒ, θ/: 5	Stopping	Fricative or affricate replaced with a stop	tay for say
Without -s: 4 With -s: 5	Cluster reduction	Consonant clusters simplified to a single consonant	go for grow
6–7	Gliding	liquids replaced by glides	lello for yello
Rare or atypical processes/ patterns	• Initial consonant deletion • Backing • Gliding of fricatives • Denasalization • Affrication • Glottal insertion	• Delete initial consonant • Using a back sound for a front sound • Using glide for a fricative • Nonnasal consonant for a nasal consonant • Using an affricate for a nonaffricate • Consonant is substituted with a glottal stop	• up for cup • key for tea • woot for foot • be for me • chew for shoe • /pɛʔɪŋ/ for petting

Source: Data obtained from ASHA (n.d.-c); Lanza and Flahive (2008); McLeod and Baker (2017).

words (e.g., Kaderavek, 2011). Using several resources (Child Development Institute, n.d.; Lanza & Flahive, 2008), the following provides an overview of expressive vocabulary development for infants through 12 years of age.

- 10–16 months: first words; one-word utterances—usually describe or name (e.g., mama, dada, no, hot)

- 18 months (1.5 years): 50 to 150 words; beginning to combine words into two, three, or more utterances

- 24 months (2 years): 50 words consistently, producing 200 to 300 words
- 30 months (2.5 years): 450 words
- 36 months (3 years): 1,000 words
- 48 months (4 years): 1,600 words
- 60 months (5 years): 2,200 to 2,500 words
- 72 months (6 years): 2,600 to 7,000 words
- 12 years: 50,000 words

Data obtained from Lanza and Flahive (2008) and the Child Development Institute (https://child developmentinfo.com/child-development/language_development/).

Q & A

Question: You see a 24-month-old child for a hearing evaluation. The child's mother states the child has 10 words in her vocabulary. Is this cause for concern?

Answer: Yes; this should be noted in your report. The child should be referred for speech and language services.

Rationale: A 24-month-old child should consistently produce at least 50 words.

Morphological Development

Brown (1973) and Retherford (2000) outline morphological development. Once a child has approximately 50 words, which is around 24 to 27 months, it is possible to calculate a child's mean length of utterance (MLU) and examine the use of grammatical morphemes. MLU is calculated by counting the number of morphemes in several utterances (e.g., 100 utterances) and dividing the total by the number of utterances. This calculation is helpful in determining progress and development of language. Because this number does not provide information regarding the various morphemes used by a child, analyzing the morphemes provides additional information related to language development. SLPs begin analyzing grammatical morphemes at approximately 24 to 27 months. All grammatical morphemes should be mastered by age 4 in the following order (Brown, 1973):

1. Present progressive -ing (e.g., singing)
2. In
3. On
4. Plural -s (e.g., cats)
5. Past irregular (e.g., went, ate)
6. Possessive 's (e.g., cat's)
7. Uncontractible copula (e.g., am, is, are, was, were)
8. Articles (e.g., a, an, the)
9. Past regular -ed (e.g., walked)

10. Third person regular -s (e.g., she eats)

11. Third person irregular (e.g., she has)

12. Uncontractible auxiliary: am, is, are, has (e.g., He was playing. The subject and verb cannot be contracted, "He's playing," without changing the meaning.)

13. Contractible copula: 'm, 's, 're (e.g., I am happy. "I" and "am" can be put into the contraction.)

14. Contractible auxiliary: 'm, 's with -ing, 're, 've (e.g., "She's eating." instead of "She is eating.")

 KNOWLEDGE CHECKPOINT

If you see a 4-year-old client that is not producing present progressive -ing, possessive 's, or articles, you may consider referring the child for a language evaluation. All 14 grammatical morphemes should be acquired by age 4, and these mentioned are three of the earlier grammatical morphemes to develop.

Speech Intelligibility Development

Hustad et al. (2021) examined intelligibility for single and multiword production by children between the ages of 30 and 119 months to determine intelligibility growth for children by transcribing speech samples rather than through parent reports. Speech samples were collected from typically developing children; adult listeners transcribed the speech samples, and intelligibility was measured for single-word and multiword utterances. The following results were reported:

- Single-word intelligibility
  - 31–47 months: 50% intelligible for single words
  - 49–87 months: 75% intelligible for single words
  - 83–119 months: 90% intelligible for single words
- Multiword intelligibility
  - 34–46 months: 50% intelligible
  - 46–61 months: 75% intelligible
  - 62–87 months: 90% intelligible

 Q & A

Question: During a hearing assessment, you interact with your 5-year-old patient. You are having significant difficulty understanding the majority (over 50%) of the child's speech. Should you disregard this since the client is only 5 years old?

Answer: No, you should note this in your report and refer for SLP evaluation.

Rationale: A 5-year-old should be 75% intelligible.

Pragmatic Development

Pragmatics involves use of language in changing social situations and encompasses ways of understanding others' intentions, in addition to making the speaker's intentions understood. There are changes in the way language is used during development. As outlined in Table 4–3, language is initially used to gain attention and make requests and eventually develop complex abilities to tell stories and engage in conversations, including abstract topics.

TABLE 4–3. Pragmatic Development

Birth–6 months	• Responds and turns head to voice and sound • Attends to speaker's face • Discriminates between familiar and unfamiliar individuals • Stops crying and/or smiles when spoken to • Responses differ between individuals and between family members • Has a social smile • Babbles for attention and to make demands • Establishes eye contact
6–12 months	• Responds to "no" and name • Pats image in mirror • Points to objects to learn new words • Vocalizes for attention • Laughs • Uses actions and gestures to communicate • Smiles at image of self in mirror • Plays simple games, such as pat-a-cake • Imitates simple actions • Shouts for attention
1–2 years	• Waves • Indicates, such as when pants are wet • Repeats an action that results in laughter by another person • Parallel play • Uses gestures with words to communicate wants • Imitates adults during play • Refers to self by name • Engages in turn-taking • Engages in simple pretend play, such as cooking • Uses social words, such as "hi" and "bye" • Talks to self during play • Uses intonation; imitates adult intonation at times

continues

TABLE 4–3. *continued*

2–3 years	• Joins other children during play briefly • Watches other children play • Requests items or activities • Starting to use language for jokes or fantasy • Repairs communication attempts when misunderstood • Engages in longer conversations • Plays house • Engages in simple group activities • Defends own possessions • Engages in conversation with self and toys • Engages in simple make-believe activities • Begins to control behavior verbally • Uses fingers to indicate age
3–4 years	• Cooperates during play and takes turns • Verbalizes personal experiences • Practices conversation skills by talking to self or toys (e.g., dolls) • Acts out whole scenes during play • Becomes frustrated when misunderstood • Expresses ideas and feelings
5 years	• Mostly direct requests • Repeats statements that are misunderstood • Starting to use gender topics • Verbally invites others to play • Good control of the elements of conversation • Using "what if . . . " or "I hope . . . " imaginary conditions
6 years	• Repeats statements that are misunderstood with elaboration • Uses adverbial conjuncts, such as now, then, so • Word play, threats, promises • Asks questions for information • Communicating with more care with unfamiliar people • Announces topic shifts
7 years	• Uses/understands deictic words, such as here, you that one, next week • Narratives include beginning, end, problem, and resolution
8 years	• Adds to concrete topics • Recognizes nonliteral meaning • Begins considering intentions of others
9 years	• Adds to topics by taking several turns • Addresses perceived sources of communication breakdown when repairing • All elements of story grammar present
11 years	• Adds to abstract topics
12 years	• Uses conjunct words (e.g., anyway, however) • Uses disjunct words (e.g., probably)

Source: Information obtained from Lanza and Flahive (2008) and Owens (2020).

Language and Speech Disorders in Children

Language Disorders

Paul et al. (2018) identify the three categories of risk factors for language disorders as established, biological, or environmental. Established risk factors are those that are certain in an individual due to a condition, such as Down syndrome or profound hearing loss. Other risk factors include biological risk factors, such as having a family member with a language or learning problem, being born prematurely, or having otitis media. In addition, there are factors in an individual's environment that put them at risk for a language disorder, such as having extremely young parents, low socioeconomic status, or later birth order. Biological and environmental factors may put a child at risk but do not ensure a language disorder. The following is a list of syndromes, disorders, conditions, events, or circumstances that are associated with language disorders taken from Paul et al. (2018), Gejao et al. (2009), Galimberti et al. (2018), and the National Institute on Deafness and Other Communication Disorders (National Institutes of Health, 2023).

- Individuals with a genetic or chromosomal etiology—congenital or acquired; may be a disorder of number of chromosomes or structure.
  - Trisomy 21
  - Trisomy 9, 13 (Patau), 18 (Edwards)
  - Cri du chat
  - Turner syndrome
  - Klinefelter syndrome
  - Fragile X syndrome
- Metabolic etiologies
  - Phenylketonuria (PKU)
  - Thyroid disorder
  - Mucopolysaccharidosis
- Prenatal or perinatal environment (etiologies)
  - Exogenous factors—abnormal development due to something outside the organism
  - Teratogens—drug or agent causing abnormal development: mutagen (teratogen causing genetic mutation) or iatrogenic (abnormal development caused by medical intervention)
    - Examples of pre/perinatal etiologies: rubella, cytomegalovirus (CMV), maternal syphilis, HIV/AIDS, herpes simplex, varicella (chicken pox), toxoplasmosis, toxins, fetal alcohol syndrome, hyperbilirubinemia (jaundice), drugs (prescribed and unprescribed)
    - Examples of postnatal etiologies (acquired): respiratory disorders possibly due to low birth weight, infections/toxins (e.g., meningitis: bacterial or viral), and trauma (e.g., stroke, traumatic brain injury, poisoning, near-drowning, or other accidents); maltreatment (e.g., physical abuse, sexual abuse, emotional abuse, neglect)
- Neurodevelopmental disorder or developmental language disorder (DLD) information
  - One of the most common developmental disorders

- □ Has been referred to as specific language impairment (SLI)
- □ Not explained by other conditions (e.g., autism, lack of exposure to language)
- □ Word learning is difficult, which results in poor vocabulary, grammatical errors, struggles with conversation, difficulty following directions due to poor understanding of words.
- □ Continues into adulthood and demonstrates difficulties, such as difficulties using complex sentences, storytelling, reading, writing, grammar, and spelling.
- □ A child likely will not grow out of the disorder. Early treatment and treatment at any age can be beneficial.
- ■ Other conditions not mentioned above that may involve language disorders:
  - □ Seizure disorder
  - □ Intellectual disabilities (ID)
  - □ Autism spectrum disorder (ASD)
  - □ Attention-deficit/hyperactivity disorder (ADHD)
  - □ Anxiety and affective disorders
  - □ Conduct and oppositional disorders
  - □ Dyslexia

Symptoms of a Language Disorder

The following lists are common symptoms of a language disorders.

- ■ Difficulty with word meaning
  - □ One word may have multiple meanings or a word that may apply to several things is only used for one specific thing.
  - □ Answers questions incorrectly, such as answering "where" questions with time
  - □ Difficulty giving concrete definitions
  - □ Difficulty with figurative language
- ■ Difficulty with word structure
  - □ Morphological markers
  - □ May try to segment words at the phoneme levels rather than the syllable levels
- ■ Word-finding/word-retrieval difficulties
  - □ Unable to retrieve the words when needed
  - □ Often uses circumlocution or describing the word that cannot be retrieved
- ■ Difficulties with phrase and sentence structure
  - □ Difficulty with comprehension of phrases and clauses
  - □ Difficulty summarizing in their own words
  - □ Unable to say things differently or does not realize things can be said differently

Common Speech Disorders

Developmental speech sound disorders are diagnosed using normal milestones and standardized evaluation tools. Reviewing the normal milestones for phoneme and phonological process/pattern development will be helpful for referring clients to SLPs. Creating developmental charts, using the information presented previously (i.e., phoneme development, speech intelligibility, phonological processes), or purchasing charts from the American Speech-Language-Hearing Association (ASHA) or other vendors will be helpful for quick reference.

Common Assessment Tools for Language and Speech Development

SLPs will evaluate language in a natural environment that is age appropriate for the client (e.g., during play or story retell). They will analyze language using a language sample obtained during this interaction. Typically, standardized assessments are included as part of a comprehensive evaluation. These assessment tools may be included in a report sent to the audiologist. Common assessment tools include the following (Paul et al., 2018; Shipley & McAfee, 2016):

- Language
  - Preschool Language Scale-5 (PLS5): ages birth through 7 years, 11 months
  - Clinical Evaluation of Language Fundamentals-5 (CELF5): ages 5 to 21 years
  - Comprehensive Assessment of Spoken Language (CASL): ages 3 to 21 years
  - Oral-Written Language Scale II (OWLS-II): ages 5 to 21 years
- Speech
  - Goldman-Fristoe Test of Articulation 3 (GFTA-3): ages 2 years to 21 years, 11 months
  - Arizona Articulation Proficiency Scale-4 (Arizona™-4): ages 1 year, 6 months to 21 years, 11 months
  - Clinical Assessment of Articulation and Phonology-2 (CAAP-2): ages 2 years, 6 months through 11 years, 11 months

Language and Speech Disorders Throughout the Lifespan

Language and speech disorders are not limited to child development. At any age, an individual may acquire a language or speech disorder due to a neurologic event, disorder, or condition. The following sections provide information related to language and speech disorders that are seen most often after language and speech have already been developed or acquired.

Language

Hallowell (2017) described aphasia as the term used for the loss of language of varying degrees after an individual has learned language. Acquired language disorders have a neurologic etiology. Stroke is the most common cause for aphasia, but there are other causes, such as traumatic brain injury, infections, or space-occupying lesions. Aphasia can affect receptive or expressive language, reading, and writing. Table 4–4 provides information related to categories and types of aphasia.

TABLE 4–4. Overview of Aphasias

FLUENT APHASIAS	
Wernicke's aphasia	• Fluent speech • Poor auditory comprehension • Poor speech imitation skills • Produces unintended sounds or words • Produces new words that do not have meaning
Conduction aphasia	• Rare • Fluent speech • Good auditory comprehension • Poor speech imitation skills
Transcortical sensory aphasia	• Rarest form of fluent aphasia • Fluent speech • Poor auditory comprehension • Relatively good speech imitation skills • Severe anomia (word-finding difficulty)
NONFLUENT APHASIAS	
Broca's aphasia	• Halting • Effortful speech • Good auditory comprehension • Poor repetition skills • Anomia
Transcortical motor aphasia	• Halting • Effortful speech • Mildly impaired auditory comprehension • Good speech imitation skills
Global aphasia	• Profound language impairment • Halting • Effortful speech • Poor auditory comprehension • Poor repetition

Source: Data obtained from Hallowell (2017).

KNOWLEDGE CHECKPOINT

While collecting a case history from your patient with aphasia, you notice that he is answering questions with one-word responses most of the time. When he uses more than one word, utterances are not full sentences. Some words are left out of the sentences. He answers all questions correctly but has difficulty producing words. You ask him to repeat a few words, but this is difficult for your patient.

Your patient is demonstrating Broca's aphasia, a nonfluent aphasia. This person may have relatively good comprehension but difficulty producing language and imitating language. Depending on the testing materials, an audiologist should adapt the evaluation to exclude expressive language tasks. For example, if the person is required to produce a word they hear, the audiologist may adapt the task to pointing to picture options of the word.

Speech Disorders Throughout the Lifespan

Speech disorders may be acquired throughout the lifespan due to neurological events or conditions. Freed (2020) described two neurologic motor speech disorders, apraxia of speech and dysarthria. In addition, Watts and Awan (2019) described voice disorders that can be acquired throughout the lifespan. Voice disorders may affect speech intelligibility and hinder communication. The following information provides a summary of speech disorders that may be acquired throughout the lifespan.

- Acquired apraxia of speech
  - Neurologic etiology
  - Difficulty in planning and programming the commands needed for speech
  - Characterized by slow speech (i.e., lengthened sounds), pauses within and between words, and distorted sounds within and between words
  - Speech disorders are not caused by issues with muscles, sensory deficits, or language deficits
- Dysarthria
  - Neurologic etiology
  - Difficulty with articulation caused by disturbances in the central and peripheral nervous system
  - Characterized by slow and/or slurred speech, low volume, monotone, and/or abnormal rhythm of speech
- Voice disorders
  - Functional etiology: may be caused by vocal behaviors, such as yelling, coughing, throat clearing
  - Neurologic etiology: may be caused by neurogenic events or conditions, such as stroke or Parkinson's disease
  - Organic etiology: may be caused by organic disorders, such as gastroesophageal reflux or cancer
  - Affect communication by affecting intelligibility for speech

Q & A

Question: When your client walked into your office, he shuffled his feet rather than picking up his feet for each step. While sitting for the evaluation, you noticed his hands were trembling. In addition, he showed little to no facial expression during conversations. It was difficult to understand him because he spoke with very low volume and slurred speech. Which disorder or condition do these observations describe? Which speech and voice disorder does this man display?

Answer: This client is showing many of the signs of Parkinson's disease (PD). The speech and voice disorder associated with PD is hypokinetic dysarthria. A referral for speech-language services would be appropriate for this patient.

Auditory Hierarchy

Erber (1982) identified four skills within the auditory process that are commonly utilized within the auditory hierarchy framework. Garber and Nevins (2012) added the skill of patterning to the four skills identified by Erber to create a more accurate depiction of the auditory hierarchy regarding the progression of auditory skills. Each skill is listed below, including a description and behaviors that indicate a listener is demonstrating that specific auditory skill.

1. Detection
   - Definition: capacity to recognize the presence or absence of sound
   - What behaviors would indicate the listener is demonstrating the auditory skill of detection?
     - Wearing amplification all waking hours
     - A change in behavior when something is heard (e.g., head turning, eyes widening, stops crying)
     - Alerting or quieting to a loud environmental noise (e.g., a pan dropping to the ground, dog barking)
     - Alerting to spoken language at a typical volume (e.g., looking up from playing when others are talking in the room, smiling when hearing mother's voice)
     - Detection of Ling 6 sounds (ah, oo, ee, sh, ss, mm) by a change in behavior or a behavioral response (e.g., raising a hand)

2. Discrimination
   - Definition: perception of differences and similarities between two auditory stimuli (e.g., sounds, words, sentences). Auditory perception differences can be based on suprasegmental (i.e., duration, intensity, pitch) or segmental information (i.e., consonant and vowel sounds). Discrimination tasks require the listener to simply recognize that the stimuli are the same or different.

- What behaviors would indicate that the listener is demonstrating the auditory skill of discrimination?
  - □ Varying responses to two different environmental noises (e.g., doorbell ringing as compared to a door shutting)
  - □ Varying responses to two family members' voices (e.g., sibling's voice as compared to dad's voice)
  - □ Recognizing a difference in words or phrases

3. Patterning
   - Definition: differentiation between sounds based on suprasegmental patterns without true identification of the sounds
     - □ Patterning is a stage that can be a stepping stone to more complex auditory development for children with newly activated cochlear implants (CIs). Many children with new CIs can imitate a variety of suprasegmental patterns but do not necessarily have any higher-level understanding of what they are imitating.
   - What behaviors would indicate the listener is demonstrating the auditory skill of patterning?
     - □ Imitation of suprasegmental patterns of spoken language (e.g., imitating the appropriate duration and pitch of animal sounds) without identification

4. Identification
   - Definition: use of auditory stimuli to label things within the environment. Identification involves the recognition of auditory labels (e.g., identification of "meow" for a cat) typically through repetition of the word or picture/object pointing without further understanding of the single label (e.g., a cat is a pet that lives in the home).
   - What behaviors would indicate the listener is demonstrating the auditory skill of identification?
     - □ A young child responding to their own name
     - □ Pointing to a color when the color word is presented (e.g., a child points to a red toy when the word "red" is presented by the parent)
     - □ Choosing a correct object like a toy from a field of objects (e.g., a child picking up a dog when the word "dog" or "woof woof" is presented by a parent)
     - □ Identifying the Ling 6 sounds through a picture-pointing or repetition task

5. Comprehension
   - Definition: processing and understanding of spoken language and responding to the auditory information accurately
   - What behaviors would indicate the listener is demonstrating the auditory skill of comprehension?
     - □ Following simple and complex directions (e.g., a child picking up shoes when a parent says "it's time to go")
     - □ Repeating longer utterances or phrases (e.g., "The dog ran across the street.")
     - □ Answering questions within a context
     - □ Learning a new concept through audition only

Ling 6 Sounds

To develop skills for listening and talking, it is important that a child has auditory access to the full spectrum of speech sounds (Moeller & Tomblin, 2015). The Ling 6 sounds are often utilized by audiologists and other professionals who work with individuals with hearing loss as a straightforward screening to evaluate auditory access to six different phonemes. This procedure was adapted from Daniel Ling's original work targeting low-, middle-, and high-frequency phonemes that represent the various sounds that occur in running speech (Ling, 1989). The Ling 6 sounds include /a/–"ah," /u/–"oo," /i/–"ee," /s/–"ss," /ʃ/–"sh," and /m/–"mm."

Ling 6 Sound Test

The Ling 6 Sound Test is typically utilized as a quick diagnostic listening check (Smiley et al., 2004). The Ling 6 Sound Test assesses the auditory hierarchy skills of detection, discrimination, and identification. It is not a test of comprehension.

1. The audiologist presents the sounds using spoken language in random order.

   - Ensure there is no visual access to the speaker's mouth (e.g., with the use of a sound transparent hoop with opaque color).

   - Present each sound with the same duration and inflection as noted in conversational speech (e.g., do not exaggerate the loudness or length of /s/).

2. If detection is expected, the young child may indicate that they heard the sound by dropping a block in a bucket or raising a hand.

3. If discrimination or identification is expected, then the child will point to a picture that represents the presented sound or repeat back the sound heard.

 AUDIOLOGY NUGGET

There are many ways that the Ling 6 Sound Test has been utilized within the field of audiology (Glista et al., 2014).

- Using a live-voice picture-pointing or speech imitation task in real-time situations like a classroom setting as a quick check of current auditory access to assess function of amplification for children and adults

- Using a live-voice picture-pointing or speech imitation task via an audiometer within an audiological evaluation in sound field as a way to assess hearing aid functioning and current auditory hierarchy level with each sound (i.e., detection, discrimination, identification of sounds)

- Using a live-voice picture-pointing or speech imitation task as an aided outcome measurement that can support hearing aid validation as a quick assessment of speech sound access

- Using live voice to complete a listening check on an amplification device

---

Updates to the Ling 6 Sounds—The LMH Test

The LMH (Ling, Madell, Hewitt or Low, Medium, High) Test is a screening test that adds four additional consonants to the Ling 6 sounds to gain a better understanding of speech perception (Madell & Hewitt, 2022). With the LMH Test, four additional consonants, /n/, /h/, /z/, and /dʒ/, were added to the original Ling 6 consonants, /a/, /i/, /u/, /s/, /ʃ/, and /m/, to provide more information regarding a person's speech perception within the second and third formants. The LMH Test with 10 phonemes can be utilized in the same way that the Ling 6 Sound Test can be utilized to quickly screen for issues in speech perception.

Effects of Hearing Loss in Children

Hearing loss can have a profound effect on one's life and specifically one's communication. These effects on communication are noted in both children and adults with hearing loss. The effects of hearing loss vary vastly for each child. Regarding spoken language, a child's speech and language production is typically a reflection of what the child hears and perceives through auditory information (Sininger et al., 2010). There are some factors that influence the effects of hearing loss. The following variables were identified by Tye-Murray (2022) that influence speech and language development for a child with hearing loss:

- Severity of hearing loss
- Contribution and involvement of family
- Behavioral issues
- Consistency or lack thereof regarding the wear of amplification
- Noise levels in home, daycare, and school settings
- Disabilities in addition to hearing loss
- Type and value of intervention
- Type of amplification (e.g., hearing aids or CIs)

Without amplification, the severity or degree of hearing loss can have a direct effect on a person's ability to perceive auditory information. As the severity of the degree of hearing loss increases, so do the effects on auditory information. Estimated effects on auditory information based on the degree of unaided hearing loss are described below.

- Normal hearing: no perceived issues due to hearing loss
- Mild: difficulty hearing soft or quiet conversations and noises. Difficulty understanding speech in the presence of background noise or in noisy environments (e.g., restaurants).
- Moderate: difficulty understanding speech even in quiet settings. Louder volume levels are required for hearing the TV or listening to music on the radio. Many people with this level of hearing loss require several repetitions of speech during conversations for comprehension.
- Severe: difficulty with the detection of any speech produced by a communication partner. With this degree of hearing loss, a person would have to pair visual information (e.g., speechreading, sign language) with auditory information for any comprehension of speech.

- Profound: only loud environmental sounds and noises are available through audition. With this degree of hearing loss, most communication will require a visual component (e.g., lip reading, sign language).

There are positive prognostic indicators associated with some of the variables that can influence speech and language development for a child with hearing loss (Novaes et al., 2012). Some of those positive prognostic indicators were identified as:

- Early and appropriate identification of hearing loss and fitting of amplification
- Device and amplification use for all waking hours
- Effective intervention services including speech and language therapy from the time of identification
- Language and speech learning environments are favorable for auditory development
- No additional disabilities (other than hearing loss) are present

Effects of Hearing Loss on Speech and Articulation in Children

Speech and articulation production in children can be greatly affected by hearing loss. Typically, children with congenital, prelingual hearing loss have more speech production errors when compared to children with postlingual hearing loss (Pratt, 2005). Speech and articulation production in children can be separated into three different areas:

- Intelligibility: the degree to which speech is comprehendible or the degree to which speech can be understood
- Segmental information: the discrete sounds like consonant and vowel sounds that create spoken language
- Suprasegmental information: prosodic information like duration, intensity, and pitch that is superimposed on top of segmental information (Tye-Murray, 2022)

There is an evidence base that identifies a relationship between speech production and speech perception in children with hearing loss (Ching et al., 2018). Speech perception issues or lack of auditory access can create specific deficits in each of the three areas related to speech and articulation identified previously.

- Deficits related to intelligibility (Ashori, 2020)
  - Historically, children with a greater degree of hearing loss or prelingual hearing loss have poorer speech intelligibility
  - Great variability noted in this area for children with hearing loss
  - Advances in technology and more advanced hearing aids, CIs, and assistive technology systems have aided speech production in children with hearing loss
- Deficits related to segmental information (Sundström et al., 2018)
  - Children with hearing loss often demonstrate some developmental speech production errors and patterns that are typical of younger children acquiring speech.
    - For example, many children demonstrate the phonological speech production pattern of final consonant deletion (the final sound in a word is deleted or not produced). A child

might produce the word "hat" as "ha" without the final sound. For a child with hearing loss, the reason that the final consonant is not produced is different than a child without hearing loss. A child without hearing loss is probably developing speech in a way that is typical and will most likely begin producing sounds at the ends of words as development progress continues. However, for a child with hearing loss, the most likely reason they are not producing sounds at the ends of words is that the child is not perceiving the sound through audition and, therefore, not producing it. A child with hearing loss is not likely to "outgrow" developmental speech production errors without appropriate amplification and intervention.

- □ Common speech deficits with vowels
    - Vowels are typically substituted with another vowel sound or distorted rather than omitted from speech production
    - Vowels are often neutralized, if distorted
    - Without appropriately fit technology, there is more distortion with vowel production as the degree of hearing loss increases
- □ Common speech deficits with consonants
    - Consonants that are more visible on the mouth are typically produced more accurately than consonants that are less visible
    - Characteristics of consonants that are not visible (e.g., voiced and voiceless) are often produced in error
    - Consonants are often subject to substitutions, omissions, and distortions due to decreased auditory access. Specifically, many consonant errors for children with hearing loss are related to a lack of auditory access in the higher-frequency range.
- ■ Deficits related to suprasegmental information (Higgins et al., 2003)
    - □ Errors noted in prosodic information include errors in stress, rate, coarticulation, and breath support
    - □ Voice pitch can be high or monotone
    - □ Frequent pauses may occur, often at inappropriate semantic and syntactic boundaries

Effects of Hearing Loss on Receptive and Expressive Language in Children

Issues with receptive and expressive language are often categorized into the three main areas associated with language: form, content, and use (Turnball & Justice, 2013).

- ■ Form: syntax and morphology
- ■ Content: semantics
- ■ Use: pragmatics
    - □ It is important to note that the difficulty with the use of language is most likely related to decreased auditory access to spoken language and not a true deficit in pragmatic language ability.

As with speech production and speech perception, a lack of appropriate access to a language base can create specific deficits in each of the three areas related to receptive and expressive language. Explicit deficits are noted in relation to spoken language comprehension and production in children with hearing loss when compared to typical language development in children (Moeller & Tomblin, 2015; Yoshinaga-Itano et al., 2020).

- Common deficits in form
  - □ Reduced mean length of utterance
  - □ Decreased use of complex sentence structures and decreased use of clauses
  - □ Overuse of simple sentence structure (e.g., subject-verb-object)
  - □ Infrequent use of adverbs, auxiliary verbs, conjunctions
  - □ Incorrect word order
  - □ Incorrect use of verb tenses
- Common deficits in content
  - □ Reduced vocabulary
  - □ Decreased ability to label and sort words
  - □ Reduced comprehension of object function
  - □ Words are often categorized by things that can be seen
  - □ Decreased understanding of figurative language (e.g., idioms)
  - □ Difficulty with multiple-meaning words
- Common deficits in use
  - □ Restricted range of communicative intents in preschool kids with hearing loss
  - □ Lack of knowledge regarding conversational conventions (e.g., changing topics, closing conversations)
  - □ Limited understanding of communication repair strategies

Effects of Hearing Loss on Literacy in Children

Deficits in receptive and expressive language skills in written language (e.g., reading and writing) are often similar to the content, form, and use errors of receptive and expressive language in spoken language for a child with hearing loss. Mapping speech to print (i.e., orthographic mapping) is defined as the process of moving from a spoken phoneme to a grapheme (i.e., written letter), which progresses to spelling a spoken word in written form (Wasowicz, 2021). The deficits for children with hearing loss related to written language can arise from a limited development of an auditory basis for mapping speech to print. In different terms, a child with hearing loss does not auditorily perceive a sound correctly and therefore has no basis to learn the written form because of the errored processing of the spoken form. Limited auditory access due to hearing loss can result in deficits related to reading and writing such as:

- Deficits in phonological awareness (i.e., ability to recognize and manipulate the spoken parts of sentences and words)
- Deficits in phonemic awareness (i.e., ability to notice and work with the individual sounds in spoken words)

- Writing samples may contain:
  - Form errors such as the omission of articles and bound morphemes (boy vs. boys)
  - Overuse of subject-verb-object sentences
  - Lack of narrative structure (e.g., no use of signals in writing to indicate the beginning of a story)

Effects of Hearing Loss on Psychosocial Development in Children

With the recent advancements in technology and amplification, many children with hearing loss are provided auditory access that allows them to develop listening, speech, language, and literacy skills in spoken language that are comparable to children with normal hearing. As discussed previously in this chapter, pragmatics involves the use of language in changing social situations and develops in a predicted way for most children that demonstrate typical development patterns. Despite the progress many children with hearing loss demonstrate in spoken language production and understanding when provided with appropriately fit technology, many continue to struggle with two specific areas that fall under the umbrella term of pragmatics: theory of mind (ToM) and psychosocial (e.g., social-emotional) development (Rall, 2007).

- ToM is the ability to attribute emotional and mental states to oneself and to others, as well as understand that others have perceptions that are different from our own. Westby (2017) differentiated ToM into two separate areas: cognitive and affective.
  - Cognitive ToM involves the ability to attribute mental states to yourself and others.
  - Affective ToM involves the ability to recognize emotions in yourself and others.

There are precise deficits in two areas of psychosocial development (i.e., social development and emotional development) often noted in children with hearing loss.

Specific deficits related to social development include:

- Few or limited number of friendships that might result in social isolation
- Difficulty empathizing and issues related to ToM development
- Feeling intimidated by communication that requires increased social interaction
  - Lower levels of self-perceived social acceptance

Specific deficits related to emotional development:

- Decreased semantic repertoire related to emotional development
- Limited expression of emotional state
- Decreased accuracy in interpreting emotional states

There are many reasons that a child with hearing loss might have deficits in ToM and psychosocial development. One explicit reason a child with hearing loss may have difficulty with these skills relates to exposure. There are specific reasons why exposure to learning opportunities for ToM and psychosocial development might be limited for children with hearing loss (Khodeir et al., 2021).

- Decreased receptive and expressive language skills impact a person's ability to process more complex and abstract language situations. If a child with hearing loss has decreased language skills, language comprehension that requires metalinguistic processing in situations, like perspective-taking (i.e., the ability to understand something from another individual's point of view), can be difficult.

■ Lack of opportunity to overhear conversations that do not directly include the child with hearing loss. This specific lack of opportunity leads to fewer opportunities to hear others share their perspectives. This lack of opportunity leaves a hefty gap in learning experiences related to perspective-taking.

■ Decreased exposure to vocabulary related to social-emotional learning due to a communication partner (e.g., a parent) that attempts to use vocabulary that makes comprehension easier for the child with hearing loss. Similar to the lack of opportunity for perspective-taking, this lack of opportunity in learning experiences related to vocabulary for social-emotional learning creates a barrier for children with hearing loss (Morgan et al., 2014).

It is important to note that Deaf children of Deaf parents do not demonstrate this large difference in psychosocial development (Polat, 2003).

 ## AUDIOLOGY NUGGET

There are simple, informal ways an audiologist can gain information about a child's understanding of the two different areas of ToM, cognitive and affective, during an evaluation.

■ Cognitive ToM can be assessed through a false-belief task, which provides information regarding a child's understanding that other people can have beliefs about the world that are not true.

 □ Smarties Task (Perner et al., 1987)—create a box with a picture of "Smarties" candy on top. However, place a pencil inside the box rather than the candy. Ask the child with hearing loss to predict the contents of the box that appears as though it holds "Smarties." The child will typically reply by saying that the box holds Smarties due to the picture. Then, the audiologist would open the container to reveal that it actually contains a pencil. The audiologist could then ask what another child (who has been waiting outside the room and did not see what was in the Smarties container) would think the box contained.

■ Affective ToM can be assessed through formal or informal measures that relate to the identification of emotions.

 □ Brainstorm some common scenarios that a child with hearing loss might experience that elicit different feelings and ask the child how they would feel.

  • "Your mom picked you up after school and took you to get ice cream."

  • "Your classmate colored on your paper."

  • "Your brother yelled at you."

  • "Your sister wouldn't let you have a turn on the swings on the playground."

AUDIOLOGY NUGGET

Recently, two measures of hearing aid use have received significant attention as predictors of success with hearing aids and language outcomes among the pediatric population: unaided speech intelligibility index (SII) values (discussed in Chapter 3) and measures from daily use time (often referred to as auditory dosage; Wiseman et al., 2023). An unaided SII value of .80 or lower has been suggested as a cutoff in determining the need for amplification among children with mild hearing loss (McCreery et al., 2020). The authors found that children with unaided audibility values at or below .80 were at risk for language delays. Another measure, referred to as auditory dosage, reflects the intensity and duration of daily auditory access by weighting a child's hours of aided hearing by their aided speech audibility and hours of unaided hearing weighted by their unaided speech audibility (Wiseman et al., 2023). Both measures are evidence based and should be considered when fitting children with amplification.

Formal Ways to Assess Communication in Children With Hearing Loss

It is important to frequently assess the communication skills, including listening, speech, language, and cognition abilities of a child with hearing loss. Assessment of all communication skills can contribute to a child's therapeutic intervention plan by determining the need for intervention, developing therapeutic intervention goals, and evaluating the progress of a child's communication skills.

An interprofessional team is often created to effectively assess all skills that contribute to communication for a child with hearing loss. However, specific members of that interprofessional team are suited for an in-depth assessment of each area that contributes to communication. Therefore, many children with hearing loss are assessed in each area below by the following professionals.

- Listening skills: SLPs and/or audiologists
  - Any changes or fluctuations in listening skills should be reported to a child's audiologist.
- Speech production skills: SLPs
- Receptive and expressive language skills: SLPs
- Cognitive and intelligence skills: psychologists
- Communication skills utilized in a classroom setting: mainstream classroom teachers or teachers of the deaf

Evaluation of Speech and Language Skills for Children With Hearing Loss

Many standardized tests for the assessment of speech and language were listed previously in this chapter. These standardized tests can be utilized as a part of the assessment process when evaluating the communication skills of a child with hearing loss. However, it is important that the professional proceed with caution due to the changes in test administration that might be required, including the use of sign language. If standard scores are utilized, a cautionary statement must be included in the assessment report.

- Informal measures (i.e., nonstandardized measures that are typically flexible and personalized) are also often used for assessment purposes with children with hearing loss. Many checklists have been developed specifically for children with hearing loss that can provide helpful information as standardized tests do not always capture the full spectrum of strengths and weaknesses as it relates to all areas of speech and language.

- As the needs for children with hearing loss vary so greatly, so do the number of informal assessments available to clinicians. It would be impossible to develop an exhaustive list of informal assessments available; however, Supporting Success for Children with Hearing Loss has developed a fantastic resource of informal assessments for children with hearing loss and has been included in the Recommended Readings section of this chapter.

Effects of Hearing Loss in Adults

Just as in children, hearing loss for adults can have vastly different effects on each individual with hearing loss. For adults, significant hearing loss is typically acquired postlingual (i.e., after the development of language). This means that most adults with hearing loss have attained knowledge and experience in the world and have speech and language that has developed in a typical manner.

The International Classification of Functioning, Disability, and Health (ICF) system was developed by the World Health Organization (WHO) and is a framework for measuring health and disability (Threats, 2006). The ICF includes broad components that help determine the multifaceted interaction between functioning and disability. Although this is not a standardized assessment or system, this type of classification allows for the specific identification of hearing-related difficulties and how they affect each person in a vastly different way (Hickson & Scarinci, 2007). Three components of this system are:

- Body function and body structure
  - □ Example: type and severity of hearing loss
- Activity limitations—a specific skill deficit
  - □ Example: difficulty understanding speech in background noise
- Participation restrictions—how the activity limitation affects life participation in a broader sense
  - □ Example: choosing to not meet a friend for coffee for fear of not being able to understand the conversation

As each person with hearing loss functions in a variety of environments, there are certain aspects of a person's life that affect activity limitations and participation restrictions, which include:

- Personal factors: pertain to the patient and are highly individualized
  - □ Example: age, lifestyle, ethnicity, coping style, attitude, habits, preferences
- Environmental factors: external to the patient but still highly individualized
  - □ Example: physical environment, social environment, culture

Based on individualized factors and situations, hearing loss has varying effects on communication in adults. One of the main areas that hearing loss can negatively affect is conversational fluency, or how smoothly a conversation transpires, in a variety of contexts (Caissie & Tranquilla, 2010). Some negative effects of hearing loss on conversational fluency include:

- Disrupted turn taking
- Modified speaking and listening styles
  - □ Communication partners: speak slower, exaggerated/precise articulation
  - □ Person with hearing loss: reliance on gestures and facial expressions, unusual gaze patterns
- Less rich imagery in spoken language from the communication partner
- Inappropriate topic shifts
- Superficial content
- Frequent clarification
- Violation of implicit social rules
  - □ Disrupted grounding: interruption in information exchange when communication partners do not establish a body of information as shared common knowledge

Bluffing is a maladaptive strategy where the person with hearing loss pretends to understand what a conversational partner is saying by nodding, smiling, or agreeing. Each person with hearing loss has different reasons for bluffing and these are often multifaceted. In many situations, bluffing is impacted by a person's personality and their acceptance of the hearing loss. The use of bluffing may lead to a feeling of powerlessness to manage communication breakdowns for the person with hearing loss.

Communication Assessment for an Adult With Hearing Loss

A comprehensive communication assessment for an adult with hearing loss could include a needs assessment (e.g., assessment of the psychosocial impact on a person's quality of life) and screening measures for communication, including measures for cognition, speech/language, conversational fluency, and listening (Heffernan et al., 2016; Vas et al., 2017). Adults with hearing loss have immensely different needs, which means the goals of the communication assessment may vary for each patient. Some of the possible goals for a communication assessment might include:

- Identify activity limitations and participation restrictions in all settings (e.g., home, work)
- Assess conversational fluency and communication breakdowns
  - □ May vary as a function of communication partner and setting
  - □ May vary based on the topic of conversation
- Evaluate the psychosocial impact of hearing loss on everyday activities
- Assess how effectively they use communication strategies in a variety of settings

Activities Utilized for a Communication Assessment

There are many ways to evaluate the impact hearing loss has on adults' communication within a communication needs assessment. Three common tools utilized by audiologists to assess a person's communication, including activity limitations and participation restrictions, are interviews, question-naires, and unstructured communication interactions. Each tool is listed below, including a description, advantages, disadvantages, and examples of that tool.

1. Interview
   - Description: clinician asking specific questions of the individual with hearing loss regarding specific situations
   - Advantages: very specific information obtained regarding the individual
   - Disadvantages: can be time-consuming and difficult specifically for new clinicians with less experience
   - Examples: What brought you here today? Do you have to ask people to repeat what they said a lot? If so, tell me about a specific time you asked someone to repeat themselves. Are there times when you have more trouble hearing, such as in a car, restaurant, theater, or in large groups? If so, tell me about a specific time you had some trouble hearing.

2. Questionnaires
   - Description: individual answers questions on an assessment scale regarding a variety of factors (e.g., situations, emotions, strategies) related to hearing loss
   - Advantages: easy to administer for the clinician as the questionnaire is typically just provided to the patient for completion
   - Disadvantages: specificity can be lacking if the appropriate questionnaire isn't administered
   - Examples: the Hearing Performance Inventory (HPI; Giolas et al., 1979), the Hearing Handicap Inventory for Adults (HHIA; Newman et al., 1990), and the Hearing Handicap Inventory for the Elderly (HHIE; Newman & Weinstein, 1988)

3. Unstructured communication interactions
   - Description: observation of spontaneous communication interactions between the person with hearing loss and a variety of communication partners
   - Advantages: provides real-world information on how the individual with hearing loss is communicating with frequent communication partners
   - Disadvantages: may not be possible to observe during the course of a typical audiological evaluation
   - Example: observing a husband and wife or a parent and an adult child have a conversation during an audiological evaluation

Conclusions

Communication provides a connection to people and experiences. Deficits in communication hinder one's ability to build relationships and participate in life activities. It is important for audiologists to understand communication development, communication disorders, and strategies utilized to assess communication across the lifespan. With this understanding, audiologists can apply that knowledge to communication development and assessment for persons with hearing loss. This knowledge allows the audiologist to be an effective interprofessional team member and a skillful clinician.

Recommended Readings

American Speech-Language-Hearing Association. (n.d.). *How does your child talk? Birth to one year.* https://www.asha.org/public/speech/development/chart/

Kaderavek, J. (2011). *Language disorders in children: Fundamental concepts of assessment and intervention.* Pearson.

McLeod, S., & Baker, E. (2017). *Children's speech: An evidence-based approach to assessment and intervention.* Pearson.

Olusanya, B. O., Davis, A. C., & Hoffman, H. J. (2019). Hearing loss grades and the International Classification of Functioning, Disability and Health. *Bulletin of the World Health Organization, 97*(10), 725.

Owens, R., & Farinella, K. (2019). *Introduction to communication disorders* (6th ed.). Pearson.

Owens, R. E. (2020). *Language development: An introduction* (10th ed.). Pearson.

Paul, R., Norbury, C., & Gosse, C. (2018). *Language disorders from infancy through adolescence* (5th ed.). Elsevier.

Retherford, K. (2000). *Guide to analysis of language transcripts.* Thinking Publications.

Tests—Informal Assessments for Parents, Students, Teachers. (n.d.). https://successforkidswithhearingloss.com/tests-informal-assessments-for-parents-students-teachers/

van der Straaten, T. F., Rieffe, C., Soede, W., Netten, A. P., Dirks, E., Oudesluys-Murphy, A. M., . . . Frijns, J. H. (2020). Quality of life of children with hearing loss in special and mainstream education: A longitudinal study. *International Journal of Pediatric Otorhinolaryngology, 128,* 1–9. https://doi.org/10.1016/j.ijporl.2019.109701

References

American Speech-Language-Hearing Association. (n.d.-a). *How does your child talk? Birth to one year.* https://www.asha.org/public/speech/development/chart/

American Speech-Language-Hearing Association. (n.d.-b). *Language in brief.* https://www.asha.org/practice-portal/clinical-topics/spoken-language-disorders/language-in-brief/#:~:text=Language%20is%20a%20rule%2Dgoverned,e.g.%2C%20American%20Sign%20Language

American Speech-Language-Hearing Association. (n.d.-c). *Phonological Processes.* https://www.asha.org/practice-portal/clinical-topics/childhood-apraxia-of-speech/phonological-processes/

Ashori, M. (2020). Speech intelligibility and auditory perception of pre-school children with hearing aid, cochlear implant and typical hearing. *Journal of Otology, 15*(2), 62–66.

Brown, R. (1973). *A first language. The early stages.* George Allen & Unwin.

Caissie, R., & Tranquilla, M. (2010). Enhancing conversational fluency: training conversation partners in the use of clear speech and other strategies. *Seminars in Hearing, 31,* 95–103.

Child Development Institute. (n.d.). *Language development in children.* https://childdevelopmentinfo.com/child-development/language_development/

Ching, T. Y., Dillon, H., Leigh, G., & Cupples, L. (2018). Learning from the longitudinal outcomes of children with hearing Impairment (LOCHI) study: Summary of 5-year findings and implications. *International Journal of Audiology, 57*(Suppl. 2), S105–S111.

DeDe, G., & Flax, J. (2016). Language comprehension in aging. In H. H. Wright (Ed.), *Cognition, Language, and Aging.* John Benjamins Publishing.

Erber, N. P. (1982). *Auditory training.* Alexander Graham Bell Association for Deaf.

Freed, D. (2020). *Motor speech disorders: Diagnosis and treatment* (3rd ed.). Plural Publishing.

Galimberti, C., Madeo, A., Di Rocco, M., & Fiumara, A. (2018). Mucopolysaccharidoses: Early diagnostic signs in infants and children. *Italian Journal of Pediatrics, 44*(Suppl. 2), 133–142. https://doi.org/10.1186/s13052-018-0550-5

Garber, A., & Nevins, M. E. (2012, October 5). *Getting started with auditory skills.* Audiology Online. https://www.audiologyonline.com/articles/getting-started-with-auditory-skills-7034

Gejao, M., Ferreira, A., Silva, G, Anastacio-Pessan, F., & Lamonica, D. (2009). Communicative and psycholinguistic abilities in children with phenylketonuria and congenital hypothyroidism. *Journal of Applied Oral Science, 17,* 69–75. https://doi.org/10.1590/S1678-77572009000700012

Giolas, T. G., Owens, E., Lamb, S. H., & Schubert, E. D. (1979). Hearing performance inventory. *Journal of Speech and Hearing Disorders, 44*(2), 169–195. https://doi.org/10.1044/jshd.4402.169

Glista, D., Scollie, S., Moodie, S., & Easwar, V. (2014). The Ling 6 (HL) test: Typical pediatric performance data and clinical use evaluation. *Journal of the American Academy of Audiology, 25*(10), 1008–1021.

Hallowell, B. (2017). *Aphasia and other acquired neurogenic language disorders: A guide for clinical excellence.* Plural Publishing.

Heffernan, E., Coulson, N. S., Henshaw, H., Barry, J. G., & Ferguson, M. A. (2016). Understanding the psychosocial experiences of adults with mild-moderate hearing loss: An application of Leventhal's self-regulatory model. *International Journal of Audiology, 55*(Suppl. 3), S3–S12.

Hickson, L., & Scarinci, N. (2007). Older adults with acquired hearing impairment: Applying the ICF in rehabilitation. *Seminars in Speech and Language, 28*(4), 283–290.

Higgins, M. B., McCleary, E. A., Carney, A. E., & Schulte, L. (2003). Longitudinal changes in children's speech and voice physiology after cochlear implantation. *Ear and Hearing, 24*(1), 48–70.

Hustad, K., Mahr, T., Natzke, P., & Rathouz, P. (2021). Speech development between 30 and 119 months in typical children I: Intelligibility growth curves for single-word and multiword productions. *Journal of Speech, Language, and Hearing Research, 64,* 3707–3719. https://pubs.asha.org/doi/epdf/10.1044/2021_JSLHR-21-00142#url6

Kaderavek, J. (2011). *Language disorders in children: Fundamental concepts of assessment and intervention.* Pearson.

Khodeir, M. S., Moussa, D. F. E. S., & Shoeib, R. M. (2021). The effect of age at time of cochlear implantation on the pragmatic development of the prelingual hearing impaired children. *The Egyptian Journal of Otolaryngology, 37*(1), 1–9.

Lanza, J., & Flahive, L. (2008). *Communication milestones* (2012 ed.). LinguaSystems.

Ling, D. (1989) *Foundations of spoken language for hearing impaired children.* Alexander Graham Bell Association for the Deaf.

Madell, J. R., & Hewitt, J. G. (2022). *From listening to language: Comprehensive intervention to maximize learning for children and adults with hearing loss.* Thieme.

McCreery, R. W., Walker, E. A., Stiles, D. J., Spratford, M., Oleson, J. J., & Lewis, D. (2020). Audibility-based hearing aid fitting criteria for children with mild bilateral hearing loss. *Language, Speech, and Hearing Services in Schools, 51,* 55–67.

McLeod, S., & Baker, E. (2017). *Children's speech: An evidence-based approach to assessment and intervention.* Pearson.

Moeller, M. P., & Tomblin, J. B. (2015). An introduction to the outcomes of children with hearing loss study. *Ear and Hearing, 36,* 4S–13S.

Morgan, G., Meristo, M., Mann, W., Hjelmquist, E., Surian, L., & Siegal, M. (2014). Mental state language and quality of conversational experience in deaf and hearing children. *Cognitive Development, 29,* 41–49.

National Institutes of Health (NIH). (2023, May 8). *Developmental language disorder.* National Institute on Deafness and Other Communication Disorders. https://www.nidcd.nih.gov/health/developmental-language-disorder#What-are

Newman, C. W., & Weinstein, B. E. (1988). The Hearing Handicap Inventory for the Elderly as a measure of hearing aid benefit. *Ear and Hearing, 9*(2), 81–85.

Newman, C. W., Weinstein, B. E., Jacobson, G. P., & Hug, G. A. (1990). The Hearing Handicap Inventory for Adults: Psychometric adequacy and audiometric correlates. *Ear and Hearing, 11*(6), 430–433.

Novaes, B. C., Versolatto-Cavanaugh, M. C., Figueiredo, R. D. S. L., & Mendes, B. D. C. A. (2012). Determinants of communication skills development in children with hearing impairment. *Journal da Sociedade Brasileira de Fonoaudiologia, 24,* 335–341.

Owens, R., & Farinella, K. (2019). *Introduction to communication disorders* (6th ed.). Pearson.

Owens, R. E. (2020). *Language development: An introduction* (10th ed.). Pearson.

Paul, R., Norbury, C., & Gosse, C. (2018). *Language disorders from infancy through adolescence* (5th ed.). Elsevier.

Perner, J., Leekam, S. R., & Wimmer, H. (1987). Three-year-olds' difficulty with false belief: The case for a conceptual deficit. *British Journal of Developmental Psychology, 5*(2), 125–137. https://doi.org/10.1111/j.2044-835x.1987.tb01048.x

Polat, F. (2003). Factors affecting psychosocial adjustment of deaf students. *Journal of Deaf Studies and Deaf Education, 8*(3), 325–339.

Pratt, S. R. (2005). Aural habilitation update: The role of speech production skills of infants and children with hearing loss. *The ASHA Leader, 10*(4), 8–33.

Rall, E. (2007). Psychosocial development of children with hearing loss. *The ASHA Leader, 12*(13), 5–43.

Retherford, K. (2000). *Guide to analysis of language transcripts.* Thinking Publications.

Sander, E.K., (1972). When are Speech Sounds Learned? *Journal of Speech and Hearing Disorders, 37*, 55–63.

Shipley, K., & McAfee, J. (2016). *Assessment in speech-language pathology: A resource manual* (5th ed.). Cengage Learning.

Sininger, Y. S., Grimes, A., & Christensen, E. (2010). Auditory development in early amplified children: Factors influencing auditory-based communication outcomes in children with hearing loss. *Ear and Hearing, 31*(2), 166.

Smiley, D. F., Martin, P. F., & Lance, D. M. (2004, May 3). *Using the Ling 6-sound test every day.* Audiology Online. https://www.audiologyonline.com/articles/using-ling-6-sound-test-1087

Sundström, S., Löfkvist, U., Lyxell, B., & Samuelsson, C. (2018). Prosodic and segmental aspects of nonword repetition in 4-to 6-year-old children who are deaf and hard of hearing compared to controls with normal hearing. *Clinical Linguistics & Phonetics, 32*(10), 950–971.

Threats, T. T. (2006). Towards an international framework for communication disorders: Use of the ICF. *Journal of Communication Disorders, 39*(4), 251–265.

Turnball, K. L. P., & Justice, L. M. (2013). *Language development from theory to practice.* Pearson Education.

Tye-Murray, N. (2022). *Foundations of Aural Rehabilitation: Children, adults, and their family members* (6th ed.). Plural Publishing.

Vas, V., Akeroyd, M. A., & Hall, D. A. (2017). A data-driven synthesis of research evidence for domains of hearing loss, as reported by adults with hearing loss and their communication partners. *Trends in Hearing, 21*, 2331216517734088.

Wasowicz, J. (2021). A speech-to-print approach to teaching reading. *LDA Bulletin, 53*(2), 10–18.

Watts, C., & Awan, S. (2019). *Laryngeal function and voice disorders.* Thieme.

Westby, C. (2017). Keep this theory in mind. *The ASHA Leader, 22*(4), 18–20. https://doi.org/10.1044/leader.AEA.22042017.18

Wingfield, A., & Grossman, M. (2006). Language and the aging brain: Patterns of neural compensation revealed by functional brain imaging. *Journal of Neurophysiology, 96*, 2830–2839. https://doi.org/10.1152/jn.00628.2006

Wiseman, K. B., McCreery, R. W., & Walker, E. A. (2023). Hearing thresholds, speech recognition, and audibility as indicators for modifying intervention in children with hearing aids. *Ear and Hearing.* Advance online publication. https://doi.org/10.1097/AUD.0000000000001328

Yoshinaga-Itano, C., Sedey, A. L., Mason, C. A., Wiggin, M., & Chung, W. (2020). Early intervention, parent talk, and pragmatic language in children with hearing loss. *Pediatrics, 146*(Suppl. 3), S270–S277.

Practice Questions

Use the following case to answer Questions 1–3.

> Your patient is a 3-year-old female. Her parents report that the child speaks but does not say as many words as her friends in kindergarten. They also report that her vocabulary is likely around 100 words. During your evaluation, she produces the following statement about her dog: "That Mommy da."

1. Which type of error is the omission of 's?
   a. Pragmatics
   b. Phonology
   c. Morphology
   d. Semantic

Explanation: The omission of 's is an error in morphology. The 's is a bound morpheme that adds meaning to the word. Therefore, c is the correct answer.

2. The likely age of elimination for the phonological process of final consonant deletion (i.e., "da" for "dog?") is _____.
   a. 2 years
   b. 3 years
   c. 5 years
   d. 8 years

Explanation: Omitting /g/ in "dog" is final consonant deletion. The phonological process of final consonant deletion is likely eliminated by 3 years of age. Therefore, b is the correct answer.

3. How many words should a 3-year-old have in their vocabulary?
   a. 50 words
   b. 500 words
   c. 1,000 words
   d. Over 2,000 words

Explanation: At 36 months or 3 years, a child should have approximately 1,000 words in their vocabulary. This child is delayed in vocabulary development if her vocabulary consists of a total of 100 words. Therefore, c is the correct answer.

Use the following case to answer Questions 4 and 5.

> Your patient is a 70-year-old adult male. Recently, your patient suffered a stroke. After introducing yourself, you start the appointment by asking a few simple questions. You quickly notice that your patient is speaking with ease, but using utterances that are not words. His answers do not answer the questions you are asking.
>
> You: How are you today?
> Patient: We have stived here for a bet and talked to them over here.
> You: Can you tell me why you are here?
> Patient: We went over there to the hands. I talk of thets and more.

4. What type of aphasia does your patient demonstrate?
   a. Broca's aphasia
   b. Conduction aphasia
   c. Wernicke's aphasia
   d. Global aphasia

Explanation: This patient has Wernicke's aphasia, which is characterized by fluent speech, jargon or new words that do not have meaning, and poor auditory comprehension. Therefore, c is the correct answer.

5. Aphasia is an acquired language disorder. This patient is having difficulty understanding language and producing language that matches his intended message. This patient continues to be just as intelligent as before his stroke. Knowing this, how might you adjust your evaluation?
   a. Use pictures, gestures, or video without language to facilitate comprehension
   b. Repeat instructions several times, until he understands
   c. Cancel the evaluation. Language comprehension is required for many tasks.
   d. Write all instructions for him to read.

Explanation: Use of pictures, gestures, or videos would not require language for comprehension. Any adjustment that did not include language may facilitate understanding for completion of your evaluation. Repeating instructions may not be helpful, since he is having difficulty comprehending language. Although writing may be helpful, writing involves language. Individuals with Wernicke's aphasia may have difficulty reading written language. Therefore, a is the correct answer.

6. Which of the following is true when considering standardized language and speech assessment measures for children with hearing loss?
   a. Standardized tests should never be used with children with hearing loss.
   b. Standardized tests should rarely be used with children with hearing loss.
   c. Standardized tests may be used with no restrictions for children with hearing loss.
   d. Standardized tests may be used but results must be reviewed with caution for children with hearing loss.

Explanation: Standardized assessment measures for language and speech may be utilized for children with hearing loss. However, the clinician must review the measure and apply any assessment results with caution. Therefore, d is the answer.

7. Joyce no longer attends a weekly board game night with her friends because she is having difficulty following along with the conversation due to her hearing loss. What is Joyce not attending the game night an example of?

    a. Participation restriction

    b. Activity limitation

    c. Bluffing

    d. Anticipatory strategy

Explanation: A participation restriction is how hearing loss affects life participation in a broader sense. Choosing not to attend a weekly game night because of deficits related to hearing loss would be a participation restriction. Therefore, a is the correct answer.

8. James demonstrated difficulty with friends in part because of his difficulty with skills related to theory of mind (ToM). Which of the following might have contributed to his difficulty with ToM skills?

    a. Difficulty using functor words when communicating

    b. Difficulty using appropriate word order when creating sentences

    c. Lack of an age-appropriate language base to mediate ToM skills

    d. Lack of phonological awareness skills

Explanation: One reason ToM skills can be difficult for children with hearing loss is due to deficits in expressive and receptive language. Without an adequate language foundation, it can be difficult for children with hearing loss to utilize metalinguistic and metacognitive skills to process a concept like ToM. Therefore, c is the correct answer.

9. An audiology patient nods in agreement during an audiological evaluation but does not understand what was said. What is this an example of?

    a. Acknowledgment gesture

    b. Bluffing

    c. Anticipatory strategy

    d. Message tailoring strategy

Explanation: Bluffing is a maladaptive strategy where the person with hearing loss does not understand what was said by a conversational partner but nods or smiles in agreement. This contrasts with and hinders the use of supportive strategies that a person with hearing loss might utilize during a conversation. Therefore, b is the correct answer.

10. A preschool child demonstrated a conditioned play response to a pure tone presented in the sound booth. What level of auditory skill development was demonstrated?

    a. Identification

    b. Comprehension

    c. Discrimination

    d. Detection

Explanation: Conditioned play audiometry involves game or play-like activities (e.g., dropping a block into a bucket or placing a ring on a ring stacker) to elicit a response from a child to determine if they detect a sound. A conditioned play response would only indicate the detection of a sound without higher-level auditory skills required. Therefore, d is the correct answer.

Appendix 4–A

Overview of Language Development Across a Lifespan

AGE RANGE	RECEPTIVE LANGUAGE	EXPRESSIVE LANGUAGE
Birth to 3 months	• Infants startle to loud noises • Listens and/or turns to voices • Beginning to distinguish speech sounds • Eye contact (Kaderavek, 2011)	• Cooing sounds • Specific cries based on different needs • Smiles
4–6 months	• Infants look toward the direction of sounds • Respond to noises from toys • Attends and respond to sounds, speech, music, and other noises	• Cooing and babbling when alone or with others • Speech-like babbling sounds, such as /ma/ or /pa/ • Laughs • Produces sounds when happy or upset
7 months–1 year	• Turns and looks in the direction of sounds • Looks when someone points • Responds to name • Understands words for common items and names (e.g., mama, cup, dog) • Starts to respond to simple words and phrases (e.g., "no," "want more?") • Interacts during games • Listens to music or stories for short periods of time • Joint visual attention between 10 and 12 months (Kaderavek, 2011) • Understands common words and names	• Linking sounds together, such as /mamama/ or /dadada/ • Uses sounds to gain and maintain attention of others • Points or uses gestures to communicate, such as nodding for yes or pointing to objects • Imitates speech sounds • Begins producing a few words, but may not be intelligible
1–2 years	• Responds to some simple verbal commands (one-step commands) • Responds to simple questions, such as "Where is the ball?" • Points to pictures in books or a few body parts when named	• Uses new words • Increasing number of words that can be produced • Starts to name pictures • Asks simple questions, such as "Where's doggy?" • Begins to put two words together, such as "no eat" or "more cookie"

AGE RANGE	RECEPTIVE LANGUAGE	EXPRESSIVE LANGUAGE
2–3 years	• Understands opposites, such as stop and go • Follows two-step commands, such as "Get the doll and put her in the bed." • Comprehension exceeds expression • Listens to stories for longer periods of time • Comprehends simple humor	• Provides labels for most objects • Refers to things not in immediate area or out of sight • Uses prepositions (e.g., "in," "on," "over") • Puts two to three words together • Uses statements and questions
3–4 years	• Understands words for some colors • Understands words for some shapes • Understands words for family members	• Responds to simple questions: who, what, where • Produces rhyming words • Uses pronouns • Begins using some plurals • Asks simple "when" and "how" questions • Puts more words together for utterances (i.e., four words) • Talks about events in the day • Able to use four sentences at a time
4–5 years	• Understands words for order, such as first, last, and next • Understands words for time, such as today and tomorrow • Responds to longer commands, such as simple three-part commands • Able to follow directions in the classroom • Understands the majority of information at home and in school	• Able to name letters and numbers • Able to use sentences with more than one action, such as "I play with her, and we jump." • Able to tell a story • Participates in conversation • Changes the way of talking for different situations or with different people (e.g., talking quieter inside and louder outside)
School-age	• Reading skills improve • Understands 60,000 words by sixth grade and 80,000 words by the end of high school • Comprehension becomes adult-like	• Vocabulary of 25,000–30,000 • Understands and uses slang • Written language is more complex than spoken language • Content is broad and expanding
Early and middle adulthood	• Comprehension continues to increase	• Content includes a full range of topics • Vocabulary may be reflective of education and occupation • Written language continues to improve

continues

APPENDIX 4–A. *continued*

AGE RANGE	RECEPTIVE LANGUAGE	EXPRESSIVE LANGUAGE
Advanced age	• Comprehension may decrease with hearing loss • Typically remains preserved • Possible changes in comprehension possibly associated with changes in cognitive processing and hearing	• Naming and word-finding decrease

Sources: Information obtained and adapted from ASHA (n.d.-a), DeDe and Flax (2016), Kaderavek (2011), Owens and Farinella (2019), Wingfield and Grossman (2006).

Section III

Assessment and Differential Diagnosis

Chapter 5

Adult Assessment and Differential Diagnosis

Karah Gottschalk and Trey Cline

Introduction

Aging adults are commonplace in audiology practices. The Administration for Community Living (2019) reported that there were 54.1 million adults over the age of 65 years. Adults over the age of 65 years represented 16% of the population, and this is expected to grow to 21.6% by 2040 (Administration for Community Living, 2019).

Audiology Case History

In audiology, each appointment should begin with a thorough case history of the patient. A thorough case history will serve many purposes, including test battery selection for diagnostic assessment, informing the process of differential diagnosis, and assessing a patient's progress during a rehabilitative process. Taking an initial case history and asking the necessary follow-up questions informs the audiologist for selection of the best test battery moving forward in order to efficiently and accurately arrive at a diagnosis. At subsequent follow-up appointments, a proper case history allows the audiologist to assess the patient's progress from any provided treatments, the disease progression, and the need for any additional/new tests. Additionally, in a situation where an audiologist may be audited by an insurance company or other payor, having a proper and detailed case history allows the audiologist to provide adequate medical justification for the test battery they have completed. The overarching theme with a thorough case history is that it allows the audiologist to make educated, informed decisions regarding the care they are about to provide with a medical justification.

Otoscopy

Prior to any testing procedures, a proper otoscopic inspection should be conducted. The primary purpose of this evaluation is to evaluate the external auditory canal's (EAC) suitability for audiological testing (i.e., is the ear free from cerumen or other foreign objects and a clear and open path to the tympanic membrane visible?). A secondary purpose of otoscopy is to evaluate the status of the pinna, EAC, and tympanic membrane (TM). Anomalies that can be viewed via otoscopy are described in Chapter 2.

- While diagnostic or video otoscopes are most commonly used by audiologists, there are also surgical microscopes or pneumatic otoscopes that can be used to more closely evaluate the external ear and, in the case of pneumatic otoscopes, test for TM motility.

- For adults, pulling up and back on the pinna helps to straighten the ear canal and make viewing the tympanic membrane easier. Remember to use other fingers on the hand holding the otoscope to brace against the head—this way, if the patient suddenly moves, the otoscope will move with them and prevent harm. Some issues that may affect testing are excessive or impacted cerumen, foreign objects, and collapsing canals.

- If excessive cerumen is found, depending on the licensure laws of the state in which the audiologist practices, cerumen removal may be conducted. Special concern should be taken for patients with diabetes or those prescribed blood thinners; these individuals are more prone to injury or infection and can still be treated but will often sign a waiver acknowledging these risks.

  □ A brief mention of cerumen management techniques is provided in Chapter 2.

- Otoscopic results also shape recommendations for further treatment. While audiologists cannot diagnose medical disorders, they can refer to otolaryngologists who may diagnose and treat disorders such as otitis externa, otitis media, and other external and middle ear conditions.

- For additional details see Falkson, S. R., and Tadi, P. (2022, October 31). *Otoscopy.* https://www.ncbi.nlm.nih.gov/books/NBK556090/

Adult Behavioral Techniques

Pure-Tone Audiometry

The hallmark procedure in most audiology practices is pure-tone audiometry (as part of a comprehensive audiologic evaluation). Pure-tone audiometry is utilized to quantify hearing thresholds via air and bone conduction (AC and BC, respectively) at various frequencies in each ear individually. AC thresholds can be established via circumaural, supra-aural, and/or insert earphones, while BC thresholds are established via the bone oscillator. AC thresholds could also be established via frequency-modulated, also known as warbled, tones, or filtered noise in the soundfield, but this method does not allow for ear-specific threshold determination. The first question that may arise is why audiologists are concerned with pure-tone thresholds versus speech stimuli given that speech is generally the signal of interest as people move about their day-to-day lives.

- Pure-tone testing allows for determination of type of hearing loss by comparing AC and BC.
  □ Site of lesion (outer, middle, inner ear) can be inferred.
  □ Appropriate treatment plan for audiologists and otolaryngologists can be made.
- Pure-tone testing allows for quantification of the frequency-specific degree of hearing loss.

- □ Informs treatment plan for the type of rehabilitation (e.g., amplification, cochlear implants)

- □ Appropriate programming for hearing aids (HAs) and implants

- □ Baseline measures for a hearing conservation program

- □ Hearing sensitivity monitoring for disease progression or recovery (e.g., Ménière's, autoimmune inner ear disease, acoustic neuroma/vestibular schwannoma)

The process of establishing pure-tone thresholds is completed via pure-tone audiometry. Historically, there was not a standardized method of pure-tone audiometry. Carhart and Jerger (1959) suggested a standardization for establishing pure-tone thresholds in order to relieve potential confusion and complication. They suggested the adoption of the Hughson-Westlake procedure for establishing pure-tone thresholds. In today's clinical practice, the modified Hughson-Westlake procedure is used for obtaining audiometric thresholds. This procedure is based on the principle that minimum audibility is measured only by progressively increasing the stimulus intensity, meaning the threshold must be established in an ascending approach moving from an inaudible stimulus to the first intensity level that the stimulus is perceived (Carhart & Jerger, 1959). The ascending approach may also be labeled as a down-up procedure.

- ■ Modified Hughson-Westlake procedure

  - □ Begins with the audiometer set to 30 dB HL, usually at 1000 Hz, AC

  - □ The patient is instructed to respond (e.g., pressing a response button, hand raise, verbal confirmation) any time they think they perceive a sound, no matter how faint. The notion of responding when they think they hear a sound is important because otherwise, patients may wait until the sound stimulus is obvious, and thus, the obtained "thresholds" may be elevated.

  - □ If the patient responds to the initial tone, indicating that they heard the sound, the intensity level of the pure tone is decreased by 10 dB steps to the point that the patient stops responding.

- ■ If the patient fails to respond at the initial 30 dB HL level, the stimulus should be increased in 20 dB steps until an initial response is obtained and then the decrease in 10 dB steps is initiated.

  - □ Once the patient stops responding in 10 dB decrements, the stimulus is increased in 5 dB steps until a response is reestablished.

- ■ Known as the "down 10, up 5" rule

- ■ This should be repeated multiple times until a response is obtained on at least two ascending runs.

  - □ Once a response is obtained on two ascending runs, this value can be taken as the audiometric threshold for this specific frequency.

  - □ The examiner would then move on to the next frequency with repetition of the same procedure.

  - □ The frequencies that are typically examined during a conventional audiometric evaluation would be octave frequencies from 250 through 8000 Hz.

- ■ If there is an interoctave difference between frequencies of more than 20 dB HL, it is recommended that the interoctave frequency be examined.

- For example, if a threshold is obtained at 15 dB HL at 2000 Hz and 35 dB HL at 4000 Hz, it is recommended that the threshold also be established at the interoctave frequency of 3000 Hz.
  □ The procedure is followed for both AC and BC.

Bone-Conduction Audiometry

To obtain BC pure-tone thresholds, there are additional considerations. Traditional testing procedures begin with placing the bone oscillator on the mastoid of the better-hearing ear, if known, or the forehead, if necessary, and evaluating frequencies 250 through 4000 Hz. However, ASHA (2005b) recommends testing the frequencies in the following order: 1000, 2000, 3000, 4000 Hz, and then doing a retest of 1000 Hz to establish reliability, before testing 500 and 250 Hz. A consideration when testing below 500 Hz via BC is the level of ambient noise present as this can elevate very low-frequency thresholds during BC testing (ASHA, 2005b). Additionally, if the patient is set up for masking, there is potential for increased occlusion effect at lower frequencies. When establishing thresholds for BC, the same modified Hughson-Westlake procedure can be used with the "down 10/up 5" rule still in effect.

Masking Considerations

- When establishing pure-tone thresholds, the examiner must consider any asymmetries that are present on the audiogram to determine if masking (the presentation of one-third octave noise centered around the test frequency, which encompasses the critical band, to the nontest ear [NTE]) is necessary. Determining whether masking is necessary depends on several factors, including the transducer used, the frequency tested, and the degree of asymmetry between the ears. There are additional considerations regarding BC masking that will be discussed later in the section titled BC Masking Procedures. Masking procedures are utilized to prevent cross-hearing in which the NTE is contributing to a response in the test ear.
  □ Plateau method: one of the most commonly used methods of clinical masking in audiology, the plateau method entails putting an initial amount of masking in the NTE (AC threshold plus 10 dB) and then retesting the AC or BC threshold in the test ear. If a response is obtained, the masking is increased by 10 dB and the test ear threshold is rechecked. Once the masking can be increased in the NTE twice (20 dB above the initial masking level), the pure-tone threshold in the test ear can be accepted. Some audiologists will increase masking in three steps of 5 dB above initial masking levels.
  □ Alternatively, for the sake of time, some audiologists will place all of the effective masking in the NTE initially versus rechecking pure-tone thresholds after each successive 10-dB increase in masking (sometimes referred to as the "dump" method). For example, if the initial masking level is 10 dB above the NTE AC threshold and then two subsequent steps of 10 dB would be added after each recheck of the pure-tone threshold in the test ear (30 dB total of effective masking), some audiologists would put 30 to 40 dB of effective masking in the NTE from the start and then recheck the test ear threshold. This method eliminates the need for the two steps of increased masking by placing all masking in at the beginning. As a note of caution, the audiologist would need to consider the possibility of overmasking. If overmasking is suspected, a more traditional plateau method of masking should be used.

- Cross-hearing occurs when sound is sufficiently loud enough and is transmitted transcranially (BC), stimulating the cochlea in the NTE (opposite/contralateral) ear. This occurs when a sound is loud enough that the earphone vibrates with enough force to stimulate the opposite cochlea.

- Additionally, cross-hearing can also occur via AC in which the sound travels from the test ear around the head to the opposite ear. Generally speaking, because the opposite ear also has a transducer covering or in the ear canal, cross-hearing via AC is usually minimal.

- The chosen transducer is a vital element when examining auditory thresholds as to whether or not masking is necessary. This is due to the fact that each transducer has a different interaural attenuation (IA) value. IA is the amount of sound energy that is lost as it is traveling from the test ear to the NTE.

  □ When using supra-aural headphones, the generally accepted IA is 40 dB (Yacullo, 2015). If the difference between AC in the test ear and the AC value in the NTE exceeds 40 dB, then masking is necessary.

  □ IA value for inserts varies by frequency, and research has shown that IA values can range from 50 to 110 dB if properly inserted (Gumus et al., 2016). However, the generally accepted, conservative value in clinical practice is 55 dB (Perkins & Mitchell, 2022). Table 5–1 demonstrates IA values based on transducer, including the value for speech testing to be discussed later. Table 5–2 summarizes masking rules for clinical practice.

Q & A

Question: If the AC threshold in the test ear is at 70 dB HL with an insert earphone and the AC threshold in the NTE is at 10 dB HL, is masking of the NTE required?

Answer: The answer is yes because there is a difference in thresholds of 60 dB, which meets or exceeds the IA value of 55 dB, and thus masking is necessary. IA = 70 dB – 10 dB = 60 dB.

TABLE 5–1. Interaural Attenuation Values

	INTERAURAL ATTENUATION VALUES (dB)
Supra- or Circumaural Headphones	40
Insert Earphones	55–70 (can range from 50 to 110 dB)
Bone Oscillator	0–10
Speech Testing	45

TABLE 5–2. Masking Rules

Rule 1	$AC_{TE} - AC_{NTE} \geq IA$
Rule 2	$AC_{TE} - BC_{TE} \geq IA$
Rule 3	$AC_{TE} - BC_{NTE} \geq IA$

- In addition to comparing the AC thresholds between ears, one additional rule must also be considered. The AC threshold of the test ear must be compared to the BC threshold of the NTE to verify if this difference exceeds the IA value of the transducer. Keep in mind that cross-hearing is primarily occurring through BC and is stimulating the cochlea in the opposite ear (Yacullo, 2015).

- Remember that the focus of masking is keeping the NTE from contributing to the response of the test ear so that clinicians can verify that the response obtained is accurate for the ear being evaluated.

BC Masking Procedures

While the procedure for establishing audiometric thresholds via BC is similar to the procedure for AC, there are some key points and observations that the examiner must make. Primarily, when obtaining BC thresholds, the clinician must determine if there is more than a 10 dB difference between the AC and BC thresholds in the same ear, also known as an air-bone gap. If an air-bone gap is present, masked BC much be completed to verify whether the air-bone gap is real.

- This allows the clinician to determine a site of lesion with a conductive or mixed hearing loss (CHL; MHL) or a sensorineural hearing loss (SNHL).

- In theory, the IA for BC is 0 dB since the bone oscillator is vibrating the skull, but it is generally accepted that if the AC and BC thresholds are within 10 dB of each other (i.e., within test-retest reliability), masking is not necessary.

- As a reminder, there are couple of points to keep in mind when setting up and completing BC audiometry.

  - When placing the bone oscillator on the mastoid process, special care needs to be taken to make sure that the oscillator is not touching the pinna and that there is minimal, if any, hair between the skin and the surface of the bone oscillator.

  - A bone oscillator has a much lower output limit (by as much as 50 dB) compared to AC earphones. In cases of severe hearing losses, it may become difficult to determine if an air-bone gap is present due to the limits of the bone oscillator.

  - Because the bone oscillator is vibrating against the skull, the patient can perceive vibrotactile responses. Vibrotactile responses are responses from the patient due to a sensation of feeling the vibrations of the bone oscillator versus actually hearing the stimulus. It is important to verify with the patient when a response is obtained as to whether or not they felt the vibration or heard the tone. If the patient indicates that they felt the vibration of the bone oscillator as opposed to hearing the tone, this must be notated on the audiogram. If it is simply marked as an auditory threshold, there are two possible negative outcomes that can occur as a result: First, this may be interpreted as an incorrect air-bone gap and thus the patient may be misdiagnosed, leading to the wrong treatment plan and/or delaying appropriate treatment; second, this may also suggest auditory function in patients with profound SNHL and the patient is actually anacusic.

    □ In cases of maximum CHL, the air-bone gap is expected to be in the 50 to 60 dB range.

Masking for pure-tone thresholds via BC is very similar to masking for AC thresholds. However, there is a slight addition to the procedure. When masking for BC, the test ear is unoccluded by the headphone, whereas the NTE will be occluded in order to introduce the masking noise. This covering of the NTE creates what is known as an occlusion effect (OE), or an enhancement in bone conduction sounds, in the NTE. Therefore, this OE must be accounted for when completing masking procedures for frequencies below 2000 Hz.

- The occlusion effect can range from as much as 30 to 10 dB from 250 to 1000 Hz with supra-aural headphones.

- Utilizing deeply inserted insert earphones, the clinician can greatly reduce the OE. With properly inserted earphones, the OE can be reduced to 20 dB at 250 Hz, 10 dB at 500 Hz, and 0 dB for 1000 Hz.

- The OE is accounted for when calculating the initial masking levels. Therefore, for BC, the initial masking level is the AC threshold in the NTE plus 10 dB plus the OE.

    □ For example, if testing at 1000 Hz:

        • The NTE threshold was found at 10 dB using insert earphones. Add 10 plus the OE, which is 5 dB.

        • 10 dB + 10 dB + 5 dB = 25 dB for the initial masking level.

- After the initial masking level is employed, the plateau method can be utilized in the same manner as is used for masking AC thresholds.

Speech Audiometry

Speech audiometry can be broken down further into specific tests, including speech recognition threshold (SRT), speech detection/awareness threshold (SDT or SAT), and word recognition scores (WRS). Information on speech-in-noise testing will be provided later in the section Speech Testing in Noise.

- Speech testing is ideally completed with recorded and calibrated stimuli due to the variability inherent to monitored live voice (MLV; speech stimuli presented verbally while monitoring the energy of the tester's voice using a VU meter). Variation can stem from the gender of the talker, dialects, personal characteristics to their speech patterns, and how well they are able to monitor and control their voices.

- Procedure: patients are asked to verbally repeat the word that they hear, or if they cannot verbalize their response, they can write their answers (significantly increases test time and depends on the patient's spelling and writing abilities) or point to pictures (often used in pediatrics or individuals with intellectual disabilities).

Speech Recognition Threshold (SRT)

The SRT can be defined as the lowest level (most commonly in dB HL) at which a patient can correctly identify spondaic words, otherwise known as spondees, 50% of the time. Spondee words are two-syllable words (in English; other languages vary in the number of syllables included) that apply equal emphasis to each syllable (e.g., baseball, cowboy, sidewalk, toothbrush). The SRT can serve several functions within the comprehensive audiological evaluation:

- Cross-check principle to validate pure-tone thresholds. In this capacity, the SRT can serve as a metric of response reliability in patients who appear to be malingering.

- Reference measure for completion of future suprathreshold speech measures (WRS).

- Provide an extremely gross measure of degree of hearing loss in the absence of pure-tone thresholds.

SRT Procedures

- Explain to the patient the stimuli that will be used and that they are to verbally repeat the words heard.
  - □ It is important to inform the patient that the words will become softer as the test continues and that they should guess at the word even if not heard completely.
- The patient should be familiarized with the spondee word list that will be used at an intensity level that is easily audible to the patient and all of the words are correctly repeated.
  - □ Familiarization of the words is vitally important as previous research has shown that patients performed almost 5 dB HL worse on SRT without familiarization (Tillman & Jerger, 1959).
- Present an initial spondee word approximately 30 to 40 dB above the expected SRT (sensation level; SL).
  - □ If the patient responds correctly, the audiologist should begin descending in 10 dB steps, with one spondee word at each step, until the patient responds incorrectly.
- Present a second spondee word at the same level.
  - □ If the second word is repeated correctly, then continue descending in 10 dB steps until two consecutive words are missed.
- Once two consecutive words are missed, the audiologist should increase the level by 5 dB.
- The "down 10/up 5" rule is typically used with two to four words at each level with the SRT corresponding to the lowest level at which the patient can correctly repeat 50% of the words. This is sometimes referred to as the bracketing method and is similar to the previously described Hughson-Westlake procedure that is utilized for obtaining pure-tone AC thresholds.
- Alternatively, ASHA (1988) recommends presenting two words at each 2 dB descending increment with the calculation of the SRT being based on the Spearman-Kärber equation. However, this technique is less commonly used.

Speech Detection Threshold (SDT)

In place of an SRT, the examiner may only be able to obtain a speech detection threshold (SDT), also referred to as a speech awareness threshold (SAT), due to the patient's inability to complete SRT testing.

- The SDT is defined as the lowest intensity level at which a patient can just notice, detect, or be aware of the speech signal in 50% of the speech presentations.

- The significant difference between an SRT and the SDT is that in an SRT, the patient is able to repeat the words 50% of the time, whereas with the SDT, the patient is only aware of the sound 50% of the time and repetition is not expected.

- SDT is often completed in patients who are unable to complete SRT testing such as infants, young children, or older children or adults who are unable to do SRT because of some other reason (e.g., developmental delay, cognitive delay, spondee words are unintelligible due to severity of hearing loss).

- The stimuli for SDT will likely be words that are familiar to the patient (e.g., their name, "uh oh," "bye bye"), connected speech or spondee words, or nonsense syllables (baba . . .), and the stimuli are most often presented via MLV.

- In most cases, the SDT typically will agree with the patient's best pure-tone thresholds, whereas often with SRT, this measure is expected to align with the patient's pure-tone average (PTA). For example, if a patient has normal peripheral hearing from 250 to 1000 Hz that precipitously slopes to a moderately severe to severe SNHL, the audiologist should expect that the SDT will likely be in the normal hearing range corresponding to the thresholds in the 250 to 1000 Hz range. The SDT is typically about 10 dB better (lower) than the SRT; this would be highly dependent on the configuration of the hearing loss.

SDT Procedures

The procedure for obtaining an SDT is very similar to the Hughson-Westlake procedure for obtaining pure-tone thresholds.

- The initial level of presentation should be 30 to 40 dB above the estimated threshold so that audibility is ensured to the patient.
  - □ If no response is obtained at this level, increase the intensity by 20 dB until the patient provides a response.
- The first level that the patient provides a response is the starting level.
- From here, the threshold search follows the previously discussed "down 10/up 5" rule. A speech stimulus is presented, and for each response, that intensity level is decreased by 10 dB until the patient fails to respond. The stimuli are then increased in 5-dB steps until a response is obtained.
- The "down 10/up 5" portion should be repeated several times with the SDT being taken as the level at which the patient responds approximately 50% of the time.

Speech Recognition

Speech recognition testing in quiet is used to assess how well a person can repeat speech when the stimulus is loud enough that the patient can obtain a maximum score (also referred to as PB$_{max}$).

- Speech recognition testing in quiet is often referred to as a word recognition score (WRS); to avoid confusion, WRS will be used.

- WRS testing is presented suprathreshold to ensure audibility to the patient since the clinician is concerned about the patient achieving maximum speech scores.

- Once a suprathreshold presentation level is selected, the audiologist will generally present a list of at least 25 monosyllabic words (in English; the number of syllables varies by language) to the patient and have the patient verbally repeat the words (or point to pictures in the case that verbal repetition is not an option). Note that some tests, like the NU-6, have options to present the 10 most difficult words instead of a full list of 25 or 50.

☐ The test is scored as a percentage of words correct. There are many variables that must be determined with completing word recognition testing:

- Stimulus delivery: recorded stimuli are preferred for reasons previously discussed.
- Type of stimuli: monosyllabic words; sentences; nonsense syllables/phonemes
- Response method: verbal (most circumstances); alternate forms (written or picture pointing)
- Presentation levels and number of presentation levels: consider the purpose of the test—if PB_{max} is being sought or if the patient's performance at typical conversational levels is being examined.
- Presence of competing noise: again, consider the purpose of the test.
- Masking: generally accepted speech testing IA is 45 dB HL for supra-aural headphones and approximately 60 dB HL for insert earphones.

Speech Testing Considerations

The advantages and disadvantages of using MLV versus recorded speech material were previously discussed, so this section will discuss the stimuli used in WRS.

Speech Stimuli

The most common stimulus used as part of the comprehensive audiologic evaluation is the monosyllabic word. Common word lists utilized are the:

- Phonetically Balanced 50 (PB-50) (Egan, 1948)
  - ☐ Created in the Psychoacoustic Laboratory at Harvard
  - ☐ A 1,000-word bank was divided into 20 different lists of 50 words each that were built so that the phonetics aspects of the English language were proportionally represented in each list.
- CID Auditory Test W-22 (W-22) (Hirsh et al., 1952)
  - ☐ Evolved from initial PB-50 word lists
  - ☐ Based on familiarity ratings of the 1,000 words that initially were used by in Harvard Psychoacoustic Laboratory
  - ☐ Took 120 original words plus 80 new words to develop four 50-word lists known as the CID W-22 lists
- Northwestern University Auditory Test Number 6 (NU-6) (Lehiste & Peterson, 1959)
  - ☐ Developed with focus on a phonemically balanced word list as opposed to phonetically balanced lists used with the PB-50 and W-22
  - ☐ Phonemic balancing could be accomplished using the consonant-vowel-consonant structure by using the frequency of each initial consonant, the vowel, and final consonant across word lists. The NU-6 comprises four 50-word lists.

While monosyllabic words are likely the most commonly utilized stimulus for word recognition testing, sentences and nonsense syllables can also be used.

- Sentence testing was initiated during World War II as a method to evaluate military communication equipment.

- Introduced into clinical practice with the CID Everyday Sentences with 10 lists of 10 sentences (Silverman & Hirsh, 1955)

- Each list of the CID Everyday Sentences Test has 50 key words with the responses being scored as a percentage of key words correctly identified. The thought process was that monosyllabic words provided useful information in regard to the patient's hearing status, but not representative of daily speech.

- The Nonsense Syllable Test (NST) was introduced with the goal to examine the usefulness of nonsense stimuli as a component of speech audiometry (Lawson & Peterson, 2011).

  □ There are two forms of NST with six randomizations of 25 high-frequency consonant-vowel-consonant-vowel stimuli in each form. The patient is instructed to repeat the nonsense syllable heard. The test is scored based on each phoneme identified as a function of intensity.

  □ The NST test could provide some differentiation of listeners with normal hearing and those that were hearing impaired. This test was thought to be beneficial in examining auditory, speech reading, and audiovisual abilities (Lawson & Peterson, 2011).

Presentation Level

In choosing a presentation level, most audiologists choose a sensation level in reference to the SRT as their presentation level to achieve maximum word recognition. However, other approaches include using a fixed sound pressure level (SPL) or on the basis of loudness measures such as most comfortable loudness level (MCL).

- Most researchers recommend utilizing different word lists at multiple presentation levels to determine PB_{max} (Beattie & Raffin, 1985).

- Approximately 74% of practicing audiologists only present at one presentation level (40 dB SL re: SRT) (Guthrie & Mackersie, 2009).

  □ This presentation level is thought to correspond to a level that normal-hearing individuals could achieve maximum speech understanding, but research has shown that the presentation level necessary for PB_{max} is variable across individuals (Beattie & Raffin, 1985).

  □ A 40 dB SL presentation level can also encroach on a patient's uncomfortable loudness level/loudness discomfort level (UCL/LDL).

- In a study of individuals with different degrees of hearing loss, PB_{max} was achieved at 5 dB below UCL and an SL re: 2000 Hz threshold. The SL re: 2000 Hz thresholds varied 10 to 25 dB SL depending on the 2000 Hz pure-tone threshold (Guthrie & Mackersie, 2009).

When necessary, during SRT or WRS, the masking rules still apply and therefore must be implemented when necessary to prevent cross-hearing. Remember that the commonly accepted IA for speech testing is 45 dB for supra-aural headphones or 60 dB for insert earphones.

AUDIOLOGY NUGGET

One additional phenomenon that can be captured with multiple presentation levels during WRS is rollover. The rollover effect can be seen in individuals with retrocochlear pathology in which the WRS will decrease with increased intensity on speech presentation levels. With retrocochlear pathology, patients can show improved WRS with increasing intensity of the presentation level. However, at a certain point, the patient may begin to show decreasing WRS with subsequent increases in presentation level. This is the rollover effect.

For example: If the clinician is completing multiple word lists, creating PI-PB function in which word recognition score is measured as a function of presentation level, to determine PB_{max} let us look at an example. If a patient obtain a WRS of 76% at 65 dB HL, but then scores 40% at 85 dB HL, this would indicate rollover and may be suggestive of retrocochlear pathology. Significant rollover for identifying retrocochlear pathology has been suggested to be greater than 0.35 to 0.45 when using the formula: $(PB_{max} - PB_{min}) / PB_{max}$ (Meyer & Mishler, 1985). In this example, $(76 - 40) / 76$ equals 0.47, which would be significant for suspected retrocochlear involvement.

Speech Testing in Noise

The main concern for most patients with hearing impairment is not being able to understand speech in the presence of background noise. Available information through speech-in-noise testing can provide valuable insight in managing a patient from a rehabilitation standpoint, which can include selection of appropriate technology with HAs, cochlear implants, and assistive listening devices. Additionally, this can also help guide appropriate counseling techniques to help the patient understand realistic expectations and appropriate use of communication strategies.

- The most common speech-in-noise tests that are clinically available are the Quick Speech-in-Noise Test (QuickSIN), the Words-in-Noise Test (WIN), the Bamford-Kowal-Bench Speech-in-Noise Test (BKB-SIN), and the Hearing-in-Noise Test (HINT); the QuickSIN and the WIN have been shown to be the most sensitive of the four tests to speech recognition performance in background noise (Wilson et al., 2007).

- QuickSIN (Killion et al., 2004):
  - Twelve six-sentence lists that can be utilized with individuals with normal hearing or hearing impairment and is time efficient for clinical use as each list takes approximately 1 to 2 minutes to complete.
  - Each word list presents sentences at varying SNRs ranging from 25 dB to 0 dB that decrease in 5 dB steps with five target words in each sentence.
  - At the end of the list, the audiologist scores the number of target words that were correctly repeated, and a SNR loss can be calculated with scores ranging from normal to severe SNR loss.
  - The SNR loss is defined as the increase (improvement) in the SNR that is required for a listener to obtain 50% correct words or sentences versus a normal performance.

□ The lower the score, the better the patient performs in noise.

□ One of the goals of the QuickSIN was to provide a more valid representation of daily speech discourse than what could be accomplished with isolated monosyllabic words in quiet. This evaluation can be used as part of the diagnostic audiometry evaluation or in conjunction with the rehabilitative process in an aided or unaided configuration (Killion et al., 2004).

■ WIN (Wilson & Burks, 2005)

□ Words-in-noise test with 35 NU-6 words in a background of multitalker babble at varying SNRs ranging from 24 dB to 0 dB; the SNR changes in 4 dB increments.

□ The test is scored in terms of the SNR that the patient is able to achieve 50% correct. As with the QuickSIN, this test can also be used with individuals with normal hearing and hearing loss (Wilson & Burks, 2005).

Ultra/Extended High-Frequency Audiometry

The frequencies that correspond to a conventional audiologic evaluation are 250 to 8000 Hz, but humans are capable of hearing ultra- or extended high frequencies (UHF or EHF; UHF will be used) up to 20,000 Hz.

■ It is well documented that hearing loss in adults that occurs with age, known as presbycusis, begins in the highest frequencies and, over time, progress downward (rather, upward along the basilar membrane) to lower frequencies.

■ While UHF may not add much diagnostic value with some patients, in cases of monitoring hearing due to continued noise exposure or ongoing treatment with ototoxic medications (cisplatin/chemotherapy or aminoglycosides), UHF may provide crucial information regarding early detection of changes in the auditory system.

■ This would allow for early preventative measures to be instituted, especially in the case of noise exposure, which is a preventable contributor to hearing loss.

■ In conjunction with physicians, early detection of hearing loss secondary to ototoxic medication exposure can lead to changes in treatment plans to prevent further deterioration of hearing and detrimental effects on daily listening abilities.

■ Research has demonstrated that individuals who reported difficulty with speech understanding in background noise, as well as performed poorly on sentence-in-noise testing, demonstrated significantly poorer UHF thresholds compared to controls (Badri et al., 2011).

□ The two groups demonstrated clinically normal hearing thresholds with no significant differences between them on standard audiometric frequencies.

□ Additionally, Braza et al. (2022) found benefits associated with audibility of UHF for speech-in-speech recognition and noted the potential benefits of clinical evaluation of thresholds above 8 kHz.

■ One difficulty with UHF is the lack of normative data with which to compare thresholds obtained clinically. Traditionally, because of the variability of the UHF thresholds with the age of the listeners, UHF thresholds are often plotted in dB SPL versus dB HL. Plotting thresholds in dB SPL also does not allow for labeling of the thresholds (normal, mild, moderate, severe, etc.) in the same way as thresholds plotted in dB HL. However, some clinically used audiometers will plot UHF thresholds in dB HL.

■ One additional area of use for UHF audiometry is in patients presenting for management of tinnitus, which is discussed later in this chapter.

CASE EXAMPLE: OTOTOXICITY

Patient is a 65-year-old male who presented with bilateral hearing loss, tinnitus, and occasional dizziness. The patient reported that he is currently undergoing chemotherapy with cisplatin for the past 8 months. He noted that these issues started approximately 4 months ago. He denied noise exposure, aural fullness, and otalgia.

■ Otoscopy revealed clear canals and normal tympanic membranes bilaterally.

■ Audiometric testing revealed a normal sloping to severe SNHL bilaterally. SRT and PTA were not in agreement bilaterally due to the sloping nature of hearing loss. WRS was fair (72%) bilaterally. The audiometric findings can be seen in Figure 5–1.

■ DPOAEs were not completed due to patient's age.

  □ Note: This is an area of debate—whether to perform OAEs on older adults for monitoring purposes. In this case, given that the patient has documented high-frequency SNHL and OAEs are not as reliable in frequencies <2 kHz, it is unlikely that DPOAEs would add value to the differential diagnosis.

■ The overall clinical impression is bilateral SNHL related to ototoxicity.

■ The patient's oncologist should receive a copy of the results.

■ With medical clearance, amplification should be pursued.

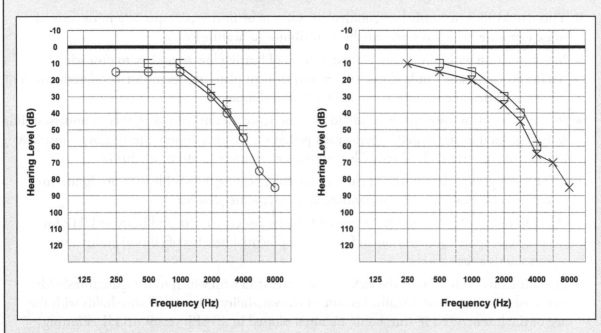

FIGURE 5–1. Ototoxicity case audiogram.

> ■ There should be a plan for routine follow-up audiograms while the patient is taking cisplatin and every 3 months for a year after he ceases treatment, then once or twice per year to monitor.

Specialty Tests

In addition to a standard comprehensive audiologic evaluation that includes pure-tone air and bone conduction, as well as speech recognition threshold and word recognition testing, there are a number of specialty tests that may be of use to the audiologist.

Stenger

The first of the specialty tests is the Stenger test. The Stenger test can only be used in cases of unilateral hearing loss or significant asymmetry. To complete the Stenger test, the asymmetry between ears needs to be at least 20 dB between AC thresholds. This test is based in the Stenger effect and binaural fusion. The Stenger effect states that if the same tone is presented simultaneously to the two ears, one tone is perceived at the midline (binaural fusion); a fused tone is only localized to the ear that would be better able to perceive it. This is the premise for the Stenger test. Based on the Stenger effect, the ear that is better able to detect the tone is where the pure tone should be heard (Durmaz et al., 2009.

- ■ Stenger test administration
  - □ The tone in the "good" ear is presented approximately 10 dB above the pure-tone threshold and the tone in the "poorer" ear is presented approximately 10 dB below the pure-tone threshold.
  - □ The patient is instructed to respond if they hear the tone.
  - □ The clinician presents two tones simultaneously to the ears.
  - □ Negative Stenger: if the hearing loss in the poorer ear is real, then the patient will only hear the tone in their good ear and should respond appropriately.
  - □ Positive Stenger: if the hearing loss in the poorer ear is not real, then the patient will perceive the presented tone in their poorer ear only, as it is the louder of the two tones and would be completely unaware of the tone in their good ear. In this case, the patient would not respond as the tone would be perceived in the poorer ear (the ear in which the patient is falsifying threshold(s)).
  - □ See example of Stenger administration in Figure 5–2 and Table 5–3.

Threshold Equalizing Noise (TEN) Test

- ■ Utilized to detect cochlear dead regions (areas of the cochlea with loss of inner hair cell connection)
- ■ Patients are instructed to detect a pure tone with the presence of a masking background noise.
- ■ The noise is a spectrally shaped, broadband noise designed so that pure-tone thresholds 250 to 10,000 Hz are essentially equal.
- ■ When cochlear function is normal, the pure-tone threshold should be within a few dB of the noise intensity.

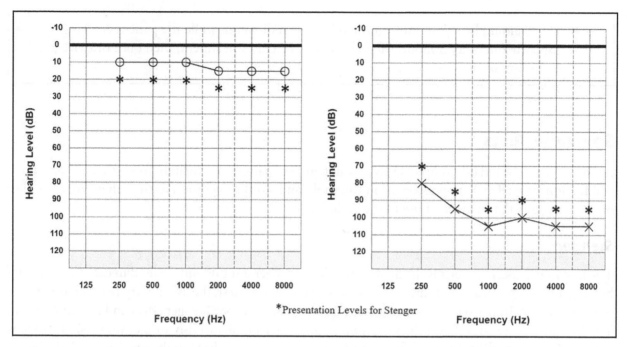

FIGURE 5–2. Stenger audiogram.

TABLE 5–3. Stenger Case Presentation Levels

		FREQUENCY (Hz)			
		500	**1000**	**2000**	**4000**
PRESENTATION LEVEL (dB HL)	Better Ear (Right Ear)	20	20	25	25
	Poorer Ear (Left Ear)	95	95	95	95

- However, if the pure-tone threshold is >10 dB above the noise intensity, this is diagnosed as a cochlear dead region and the signal is only being detected by nearby areas of the cochlea due to increased vibrations of the basilar membrane with surviving inner hair cells and neurons (Moore et al., 2000).

Binaural Loudness Balance Test

- Created to measure the presence of loudness recruitment or the abnormally rapid growth of loudness as intensity is increased above the threshold.
- It is used in cases of unilateral SNHL and can help to differentiate between cochlear and retrocochlear pathology.
- The test entails balancing the loudness of a tone in one ear against the fixed loudness of a reference tone in the opposite ear to obtain a sensation of equal loudness.

- The good ear uses a reference tone that is fixed while the listener is asked to indicate when the tone being adjusted in the poorer ear is perceived to be of equal loudness to the reference tone.
- After completing this at multiple intensities, if the dynamic range in the poorer ear is the same as the good ear (reference tones), then no recruitment is present. However, if the dynamic range is reduced in the poorer ear, this would indicate a degree of recruitment (Sung & Sung, 1976).

Tuning Forks

Tuning fork testing is a fundamental clinical screening tool that is still regularly used since its inception during the 19th century. Prior to the introduction of audiology as a field after World War II, tuning forks were the primary form of hearing testing. These measures are often used bedside by otolaryngologists to screen for the presence of hearing loss, confirmation of already completed diagnostic audiometric testing, estimation of hearing loss severity, and as part of the surgical candidacy workup.

- Tuning fork testing is completed by striking the fork approximately two thirds of the way along the fork tines against a hard but elastic object (e.g., rubber pad), which in turn produces a pure-tone stimulus that will decay over time.
- Each tuning fork corresponds to a specific pure-tone frequency with the most commonly used forks representing 256 and 512 Hz.
  - Low-frequency forks may produce vibrotactile sensations and can provide misleading information.
- Inferences regarding hearing status are made by comparing hearing with the tuning fork via AC (holding the fork near the external auditory canal [EAC]) versus BC (placing the fork on the mastoid or forehead) or with the emphasis on lateralization of the sound via BC.

Two of the most commonly used tuning fork tests currently are the Rinne and the Weber.

Rinne Test. The Rinne tuning fork test, first described by Heinrich Adolf Rinne in 1855, focuses on the loudness of the stimulus comparing AC to BC. The tuning fork is first held near the opening of the EAC and then immediately placed on the mastoid process. The patient is asked to indicate if the pure-tone stimulus is louder by AC or BC. Results would indicate a positive Rinne (normal or SNHL) if the patient reports that the tone is louder by AC than by BC. In a positive Rinne, AC is perceived as being louder because of a normal ear canal and middle ear functioning (thus no impedance of the AC sound) with air being a less dense medium (and thus easier transmission) compared to the higher density of bone. The test is considered negative (conductive component) if the pure-tone stimulus is softer via AC when compared to BC. There are two reasons why BC is heard louder than AC:

- Outer and/or middle ear involvement will likely attenuate a stimulus traveling by AC.
- Outer and/or middle ear disorder can essentially trap pure tones presented via BC, which would serve to intensify a bone-conducted signal. This is also known as the occlusion effect.

Weber Test. The Weber tuning fork test was first introduced by C. T. Tourtual and Charles Wheatstone in 1827; it is most clinically relevant in cases of unilateral hearing loss with the goal of identifying the better-hearing cochlea. The test begins by striking and placing the tuning fork on a midline bony structure, such as the forehead or incisors. The patient is asked to indicate if the pure tone is heard

TABLE 5–4. Tuning Fork Test Table

TUNING FORK TEST	FINDINGS	
Rinne	Positive test: AC is louder than BC. Most commonly associated with normal peripheral hearing or sensorineural hearing loss.	Negative test: BC is louder than AC Most commonly associated with a conductive component to the hearing (loss).
Weber	Sensorineural hearing loss: tone will lateralize to the better-hearing ear. In cases of normal-hearing sensitivity: tone will remain centralized and be heard at the midline.	Conductive hearing loss: tone will lateralize to the poorer hearing ear.

equally in both ears or if it is louder in one ear versus the other. If the peripheral hearing sensitivity is normal, the pure tone is heard centrally in the head. In the presence of a CHL, the pure tone should lateralize to the poorer hearing ear due to the occlusion effect. However, in cases of SNHL, the tone should lateralize to the better-hearing ear. A summary of the Rinne and Weber tests along with corresponding results can be found in Table 5–4.

Obvious limitations of tuning fork testing would be the limited number of frequencies examined and difficulty determining the audiometric threshold. Additionally, about 5% of patients with normal hearing or SNHL are misdiagnosed as having a CHL using the Rinne test, and this test has been shown to miss patients with significant CHL by as much as 50% of cases (Schlauch & Nelson, 2015). Therefore, it is important to remember that tuning fork tests are one clinical tool, primarily used by otolaryngologists, but are not a replacement for conventional pure-tone audiometry.

Potential Age Effects

In any population, challenges may arise that an audiologist or clinician must recognize and adapt in order to ensure accurate test results. The adult population is no exception. Testing procedures can be altered based on anatomical changes and cognitive changes/abilities. Later in this chapter, the latter will be discussed more in detail.

- Remember that the outer one third of the external auditory canal is made of cartilage and the inner two thirds is made of temporal bone.

- With time, that cartilaginous tissue can change: There are degenerative changes in the elastic tissues associated with the pinna and cartilaginous portion of the external ear canal. With these changes, the pressure of the earphone against the pinna can cause a closing or collapsing of the ear canal, thus creating a false air-bone gap, typically in the high-frequency region, and a patient incorrectly diagnosed with C/MHL.

- Comparing pure-tone testing using a supra-aural headphone, causing ear canal collapse, and an insert earphone showed an improvement of 15 to 30 dB in thresholds from 250 Hz through 2000 Hz when using insert earphones (Mahoney & Luxon, 1996). Collapsing ear canals should always be considered with findings that include unexpected air-bone gaps, especially in the presence of normal acoustic immittance.

Other considerations that should be made during audiometric testing can include response mode.

- Many clinicians will have adults push a response button during pure-tone audiometry.
- There should also be consideration for patient dexterity and other response modes may be necessary such as hand raising or verbal confirmation.
- Verbal responses to speech stimuli may not always be possible, and therefore, written responses or a picture-pointing task, such as the Word Intelligibility by Picture Identification (WIPI) Test, may be necessary.

Physiological Techniques

Physiological or objective measures are a useful tool to utilize on patients of all ages. Physiological techniques such as immittance, otoacoustic emissions (OAEs), and evoked potentials are a vital cross-check principle to use on patients throughout the lifespan. A cross-check principle means that findings from a single test are checked and confirmed against another test to ensure that results are accurate. This principle is particularly important when working with children or individuals with developmental delays and is also discussed in Chapter 6.

Immittance

The transmission of sound requires movement through the outer and middle ear space before ending in the inner ear and auditory cortex. To perceive sound, sound energy is required to be transmitted from an air medium (with low impedance) to a fluid medium (high impedance).

- The middle ear acts as an impedance matching transformer to account for this difference in impedance.
- To assess the outer and middle ear space, the objective measurement of tympanometry was created. Tympanometry refers to the measurement of how the middle ear system responses to both sound energy and atmospheric pressure.
- Tympanometry is obtained by utilizing a probe tip that contains both a stimulus (226 Hz pure-tone or wideband clicks for adults) and a microphone.
- In addition to sound being presented, air pressure is varied from ambient pressure to positive pressure to negative pressure. The fluctuation in pressure causes the ossicular chain and tympanic membrane (TM) to stiffen, which impacts the admittance, or flow of energy through the system. This pressure change causes the TM to move, increasing and decreasing the volume of the external auditory meatus. The resultant intensity changes in the pure tone are then transformed into plotted data.
- The changes are typically plotted on a graph called a tympanogram, where admittance is plotted on the y-axis and middle ear pressure is on the x-axis.
- There are five tympanometry classifications based on the Linden-Jerger classification scheme, which can be found in Figure 5–3 (Jerger, 1970; Liden et al., 1969).

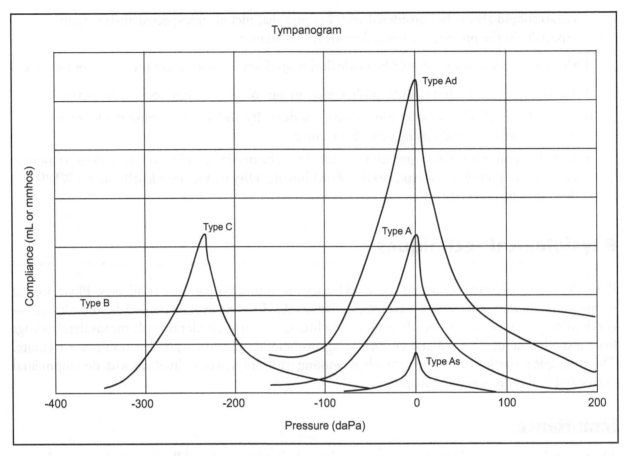

FIGURE 5–3. Tympanometry classification types.

Audiologists must judge not only the tympanogram but also the four values provided: equivalent ear canal volume (ECV), static-compensated acoustic admittance (Ytm), tympanometric peak pressure (TPP), and tympanometric width (TW) or gradient. A variety of researchers have found different

CASE EXAMPLE: CERUMEN IMPACTION

Patient is a 38-year-old female who presented with left otalgia, plugged feeling, and drainage. She stated that symptoms started approximately 1 week ago. She denied hearing loss, ear infections, and any recent health concerns but did report that she has had to have her ears cleaned out due to cerumen.

- Otoscopy revealed clear right canal and normal tympanic membrane. Left otoscopy revealed occluding cerumen.

- Tympanometry revealed a flat Type B tympanogram with an ECV of 0.17 cm³.

- The overall clinical impression is left cerumen impaction. Patient wished to have cerumen removed at the clinic and was not diabetic or taking blood thinners. Cerumen was successfully removed using irrigation and patient reported immediate relief of symptoms.

normative ranges based on age (Hunter & Sanford, 2014). Table 5–5 displays the normative ranges while Table 5–6 shows the classification types of tympanograms regarding their values.

The ECV measurement is vital when assessing Type B tympanograms since different pathologies can impact ECV. A breakdown of the variations of Type B tympanograms can be seen in Table 5–7.

TABLE 5–5. 90% Measurement Ranges for Tympanometric Values for Males and Females

ARTICLE	ECV (cm³)	ADMITTANCE (mmho)	TPP (daPa)	TW (daPa)
Wiley et al., 1996	0.9–2.0	0.2–1.5	—	35–135
Roup et al., 1998	0.9–1.80	0.30–1.19	−103.5–4.2	32.8–95.0

TABLE 5–6. Measurement, Classification, Description, Pathology, and Type of HL Expected

MEASUREMENT	TYPE A	TYPE As	TYPE Ad	TYPE B	TYPE C
ECV	WNL	WNL	WNL	Depends	WNL
Admittance	WNL	Shallow (under normative range)	Deep (over normative range)	NP	WNL
TPP	WNL	WNL	WNL	NP	Negative pressure present
Description	Normal middle ear function	Stiff middle ear system	Hypercompliant middle ear	Flat/nonmobile TM	Negative middle ear pressure
Pathology	Normal	Otosclerosis, ossicular fixation, or low-lying otitis media	Ossicular disarticulation or TM pathology	Fluid, OME, PE, TM perforation, occluding cerumen	Eustachian tube dysfunction
Type of HL	SNHL	SNHL, mixed, CHL	SNHL, mixed, CHL	Mixed or CHL	SNHL, mixed, CHL

Note. WNL: within normal limits; NP: not present; SNHL: sensorineural hearing loss; CHL: conductive hearing loss; OME: otitis media with effusion; PE: pressure equalizing tube; TM: tympanic membrane.

TABLE 5–7. ECV variations in Type B Tympanograms

ECV	PATHOLOGY
Normal ECV	Fluid/otitis media
Small ECV	Occluding cerumen
Large ECV	TM perforation or PE tube

Wideband Tympanometry

An expansion in technology occurred that created wideband tympanometry (WBT) as well as multifrequency tympanometry (MFT). Both of these techniques will be discussed in Chapter 6. WBT provides additional information not available in traditional tympanometry by utilizing a transient stimulus at a variety of frequencies, which makes WBT useful in diagnosing middle ear pathologies.

- The range of frequencies tested include 226 to 8000 Hz delivered via click stimuli.
- Measurement data obtained from this includes admittance (Ya), conductance (Ga), susceptance (Ba), and phase angle (ϕa), which allow for a clearer picture of admittance properties of the middle ear.

CASE EXAMPLE: OTOSCLEROSIS

Patient is a 43-year-old female reporting a left hearing loss, intermittent tinnitus, and difficulty hearing when chewing. She stated that these issues have been present for the last 2 years and appear to be getting worse. She denied aural fullness, otalgia, and dizziness. The patient reported that she is in the beginning stages of perimenopause.

- Otoscopy revealed clear and normal canal in the right ear and a reddish (Schwartz/e sign) tympanic membrane in the left ear.
- Tympanometry revealed a Type A tympanogram in the right ear and a Type As tympanogram in the left ear. The tympanometry can be seen in Figure 5–4.

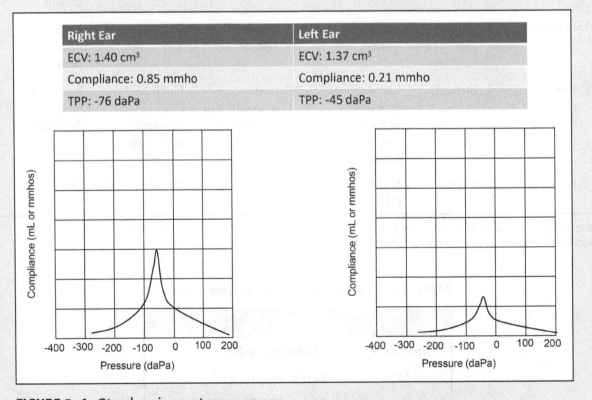

Right Ear	Left Ear
ECV: 1.40 cm³	ECV: 1.37 cm³
Compliance: 0.85 mmho	Compliance: 0.21 mmho
TPP: -76 daPa	TPP: -45 daPa

FIGURE 5–4. Otosclerosis case tympanogram.

- Audiometric findings demonstrate normal hearing in the right ear with a moderate rising to normal CHL in the left ear. Additionally, a Carhart's notch is present. SRT and PTA are in agreement. WRS is excellent bilaterally. The audiometric findings can be seen in Figure 5–5.

- The overall clinical impression is consistent with left otosclerosis due to the presence of a Schwartz/e sign, Carhart's notch, and low-frequency CHL.

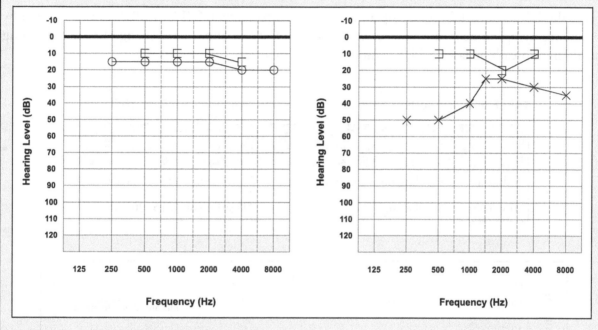

FIGURE 5–5. Otosclerosis case audiogram.

- Instead of the typical tympanogram, normal WBT tympanograms are "M" shaped.
- The most useful portion of WBT is the ability to calculate resonant frequency (RF). RF varies from high to low based on different pathologies.
  □ Pathologies with high RF: otosclerosis
  □ Pathologies with low RF: ossicular discontinuity and external otitis media

Eustachian Tube Testing

Immittance testing also includes Eustachian tube function (ETF) tests.

- The Eustachian tube (ET) is important in both mucus drainage and pressure equalization between the air and middle ear space.

- Typically, the ET is closed in order to protect the middle ear, but it does open when swallowing, yawning, and chewing.

- Sickness, such as ear infections, barotrauma, upper respiratory infections, and allergies, can cause ET dysfunction (ETD) where the tube is unable to open.

- There are two tests that can be completed to assess ETF. These tests require a traditional tympanogram to be completed where the patient is sitting still, then having the patient either blow air while holding their nose (Valsalva maneuver) and then having them swallow (Toynbee maneuver).

■ Once all three are completed, TPP is assessed to see if there are any changes.

■ If a shift in pressure is not seen in the different test conditions, than it is thought that there is ETD. Table 5–8 highlights what is seen during testing, and Figure 5–6 reveals normal and abnormal ETD findings and test conditions (normal breathing, forced breathing through both nostrils, and forced breathing through one nostril).

If the ET remains abnormally open, it is termed a patulous ET (PET). PET can be assessed by completing tympanometry during different breathing tasks. If admittance changes are noted during the different breathing tasks, a PET is thought to be occurring.

TABLE 5–8. ETF Testing, Patient Condition, and Tympanogram Peak Shift

ETF TEST	PATIENT CONDITION (MOUTH CLOSED)	TPP FROM RESTING TYMPANOGRAM
Valsalva	Holding nose and blowing air	Positive shift >15–20 daPa
Toynbee	Swallowing	Negative shift >15–20 daPa

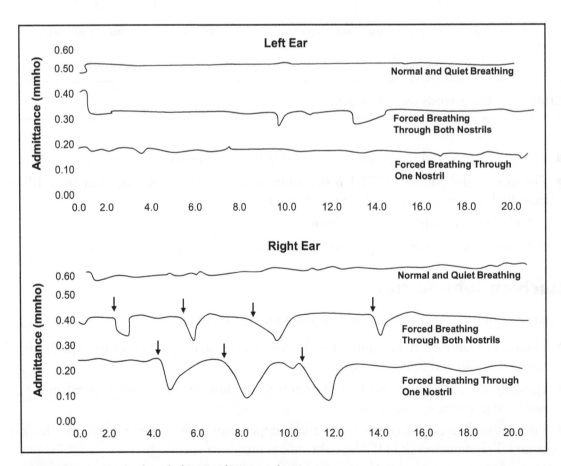

FIGURE 5–6. Normal and abnormal PET tracings.

Middle Ear Muscle Reflex (MEMR) or Acoustic Reflex (AR)

Another useful objective tool audiologists can utilize is the MEMR (sometimes referred to as the acoustic reflex or AR). This can assist in the differential diagnosis of a retrocochlear versus cochlear site of lesion. Further, MEMR is used as a part of the cross-check principle, as well as in cochlear implant testing. While there are two middle ear muscles located in the human ear (tensor tympani and stapedius muscle), there is only one that is the main contributor to the MEMR or acoustic stapedial reflex.

- The stapedius is the smallest skeletal muscle in humans and contracts when exposed to loud sounds, creating a stiffer TM and ossicular chain, decreasing the amount of energy reaching the stapes footplate and oval window.

- This change can be measured via a tympanometer and reflex activator stimulus.
  - □ The activator frequencies include 500, 1000, 2000, and 4000 Hz. There is also the option for broadband noise (BBN).

- MEMRs can be obtained ipsilaterally and contralaterally. Due to this bilateral response, there are four pathways in what is known as the reflex arc, which is shown in Figure 5–7.

- During the measurement, a probe tone (226 Hz) is responsible for the admittance, while the activator is responsible for creating the change in admittance. This means that the MEMR is a measurement of the decrease in admittance when an activator frequency is presented. One can see this change via the growth chart in Figure 5–8.

When testing, one can begin the intensity around 70 to 80 dB HL to start assessing for a response.

- If no response is noted, then increase the intensity by 5 dB HL until a response growth is noted.

- A reflex threshold is obtained at the level between a no response run and an enlarged deflection.

- The absolute mmho value is not necessarily the most important determinant of the reflex presence; instead, it is the evidence of a growth in the response. Some audiologists in practice utilize a value of 0.02 to 0.03 mmho to show evidence of growth.

- Normal MEMR thresholds can range between 70 and 100 dB SPL. See Table 5–9 for normal MEMR thresholds.

- Responses above 100 dB SPL are considered elevated, and absent responses occur when there is no response even at equipment limits (110 or 115 dB SPL).

As shown in the table, ipsilateral responses occur at lower intensities than contralateral thresholds. This is due to the different pathways that these must take.

- Research has suggested that MEMR thresholds are approximately 70 to 90 dB HL above behavioral thresholds obtained, hence why it can be used for as a cross-check.

- While obtaining MEMRs is quite easy, the terminology surrounding the reporting of results still causes confusion to this day.

- It is important to remember that one must use ANSI S3.39 standards terminology (Feeney & Schairer, 2014), which states that recording and naming is based on the stimulus ear, not the probe ear. Table 5–10 highlights the ANSI standard for reporting MEMRs with normative values.

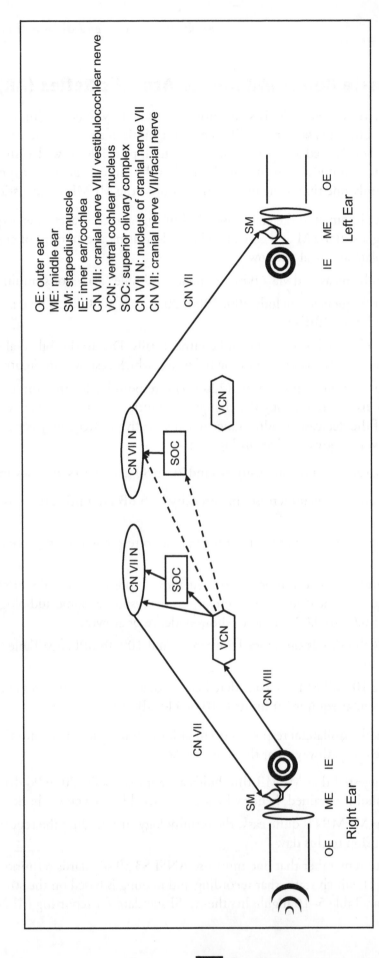

OE: outer ear
ME: middle ear
SM: stapedius muscle
IE: inner ear/cochlea
CN VIII: cranial nerve VIII/ vestibulocochlear nerve
VCN: ventral cochlear nucleus
SOC: superior olivary complex
CN VII N: nucleus of cranial nerve VII
CN VII: cranial nerve VII/facial nerve

FIGURE 5–7. Reflex arc diagram. Solid lines represent ipsilateral pathways and dashed lines represent contralateral pathways.

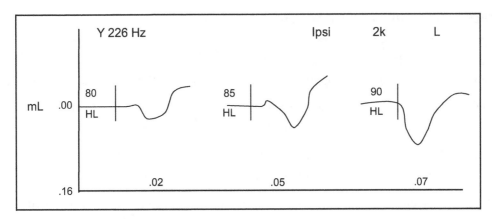

FIGURE 5–8. AR growth chart.

TABLE 5–9. Mean Normal MEMR Thresholds

ACTIVATOR	IPSILATERAL (dB HL)	CONTRALATERAL (dB HL)
500 Hz	79.9	84.6
1000 Hz	82.0	85.9
2000 Hz	86.2	84.4
4000 Hz	87.5	89.3
BBN	64.6	66.3

TABLE 5–10. ANSI Standards for Probe and Stimulus Placement for Ipsilateral vs. Contralateral MEMR and Sample MEMR Threshold

MEMR	PROBE	STIMULUS	500 Hz	1000 Hz	2000 Hz	4000 Hz
Right Ipsilateral	Right Ear	Right Ear	85	85	85	85
Right Contralateral	Left Ear	Right Ear	95	95	90	95
Left Ipsilateral	Left Ear	Left Ear	85	85	85	85
Left Contralateral	Right Ear	Left Ear	100	95	100	95

Different pathologies reveal different responses for MEMRs. Table 5–11 demonstrates pathologies and expected reflex patterns for MEMRs.

Decay

Another objective test that could be completed to assess for retrocochlear pathologies is decay testing. Decay is assessing if the MEMR is sustained for a specific duration or if it decreases by half of its magnitude.

TABLE 5–11. MEMR Reflex Patterns and Pathologies

PATHOLOGY	IPSILATERAL	CONTRALATERAL
None	Right: Normal Left: Normal	Right: Normal Left: Normal
Right Cochlear	Right: Elevated/Absent Left: Normal	Right: Elevated/Absent Left: Normal
Left Vestibulocochlear	Right: Normal Left: Elevated/Absent	Right: Normal Left: Elevated/Absent
Right Middle Ear (Mild)	Right: Elevated/Absent Left: Normal	Right: Normal/Elevated Left: Elevated
Left Middle Ear (Severe)	Right: Normal Left: Absent	Right: Absent Left: Absent
Left Facial Nerve	Right: Normal Left: Absent	Right: Absent Left: Normal
Right Brainstem	Right: Normal Left: Normal	Right: Absent Left: Absent

- In this test, a 226 Hz probe tone is used with either a 500 or 1000 Hz activator that is presented for 10 seconds.
- Completed contralaterally
- The intensity of the activator is decided by the MEMR threshold obtained, usually 10 dB above the threshold obtained at that frequency.
- If admittance (the MEMR) is sustained for 10 seconds, that is labeled as a negative or normal decay. If admittance is not sustained, that is a positive or abnormal decay.
  - □ Abnormal decay is consistent with retrocochlear disorders.
- This is noted by assessing the reflex magnitude seen in Figure 5–9.

Both MEMR and decay testing can be impacted by abnormal tympanometric findings such as Type B tympanograms (e.g., fluid or perforation). As such, it is important to complete tympanometry, then MEMR, then decay.

Otoacoustic Emissions (OAEs)

OAEs were discovered by Dr. David Kemp, a British physicist, in the late 1970s (Dhar & Hall, 2018). OAEs are an objective, acoustical measure generated in the cochlea as a by-product of the cochlear amplifier and outer hair cell motility.

- The two common forms of OAEs are distortion product (DPOAEs) and transient evoked (TEOAEs).
- There are three main anatomical portions of the ear that are involved in the generation of OAE responses: the external ear, middle ear, and the cochlea.
  - □ The pinna has very little, if any, effect on OAE responses, and the external auditory canal can modify OAE responses.

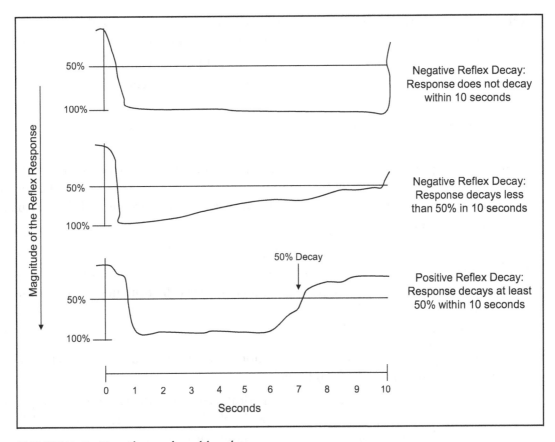

FIGURE 5–9. Negative and positive decay.

- □ The OAE probe is placed in the ear canal and the stimulus is delivered toward the TM. The variations in ear canal geometry can significantly influence the quality of OAE results. This is also true of cerumen or debris present in the canal that can impede OAE stimuli or recordings (Dhar & Hall, 2018).

- ■ The middle ear plays two critical roles in OAE generation and recording: propagation of the signal toward the cochlea and the outward movement of the OAE into the ear canal for recording.

  - □ The stimulus, as with all sounds, utilizes the area ratio between the TM and the oval window and the lever advantage from the ossicular chain to create an advantage as the stimulus moves inward.

  - □ As the emission moves outward, the middle ear will impede the emission, which contributes to the low levels with which OAEs are typically recorded (Dhar & Hall, 2018).

  - □ OAEs are heavily influenced by middle ear status; therefore, if the patient has middle ear pathology (otitis media, middle ear effusion), the OAE responses are likely to be reduced or absent.

- ■ The OHCs in the cochlea serve as the third major anatomic site involved in OAE responses and the generation source for OAEs.

- ◻ OHCs have an active mechanical component to their function as the cells have been shown to change length and shape in response to depolarizing and hyperpolarizing currents.
- ◻ As a sound wave travels (traveling wave) through cochlear fluid creating displacement of the basilar membrane, there is an increase in viscous drag, and subsequent loss of energy, due to the motion of the wave.
- ◻ The cochlear amplifier, created by OHC motility, is a necessary to amplify the wave as it loses energy.
- ◻ OAEs are a by-product of the cochlear amplification process as there is displacement of the basilar membrane that creates energy movement back toward the basal end of the cochlea generating vibration on the oval and round windows and thus vibration of the ossicular chain and tympanic membrane.
- ◻ If there is dysfunction with the cochlear amplifier, OAEs cannot be generated.
- ■ DPOAEs are generated by a mechanical process within the cochlea with intermodulation between two tones (f_1, f_2), relatively close in frequency, that will create new frequency-specific components.
  - ◻ Measured based on frequency and dB SPL
  - ◻ These new frequency components are distortion products of the interaction between the two initial tones on the basilar membrane.
  - ◻ The new frequency components are mathematically related to the two initial tones. The mathematical relationship that generally provides the largest DPOAE response is $2f_1 - f_2$ and is the most common formula used in generation of DPOAEs.
  - ◻ Normative values: no universal standard exists for DPOAEs but a general recommendation is an SNR of ≥6 dB and additional considerations for emission level (i.e., the emission must be of a certain level in dB). Normative data are typically specified by the manufacturer of OAE testing equipment.
  - ◻ Figure 5–10 demonstrates clinical DPOAE measurements.
- ■ TEOAEs
  - ◻ TEOAEs are generated using a broadband click stimulus.
  - ◻ After the presentation of a brief click stimulus, time-synchronous averaging allows for appropriate measurement of the response. This averaging method allows for removal of noise within the recording but maintains the emission response.
  - ◻ The TEOAE response is analyzed using a fast Fourier transform (FFT) technique, which converts a time-domain response into a frequency-domain response. This is important because utilizing a broadband stimulus will elicit different portions of the TEOAE response at different latencies due to the tonotopicity of the cochlea.
  - ◻ The TEOAE recording will feature two waveforms that are averaged over time. During analysis, those two waveforms are compared to each other with the difference between them being attributed to noise levels. Therefore, displayed TEOAE results will feature the TEOAE-level waveform with a second (and hopefully smaller) waveform superimposed representing the noise level of the response.

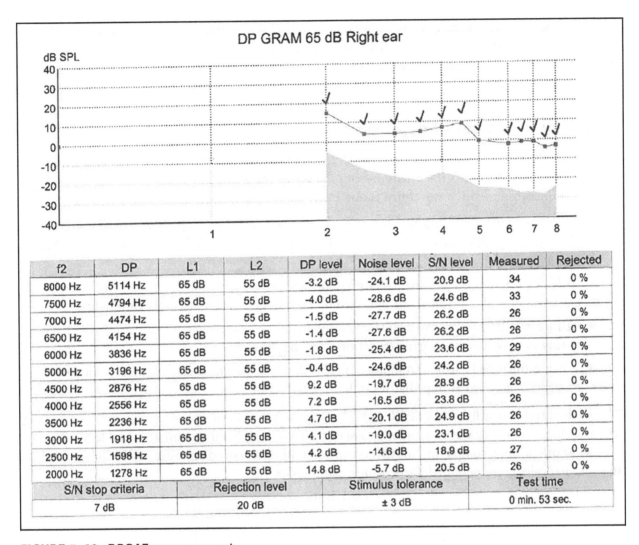

FIGURE 5–10. DPOAE measurement.

While DP and TEOAE responses represent cochlear function and are widely used clinically, there are differences between the two methods that offer some clinical utility.

- DPOAEs can utilize a wide-frequency spectrum for observation and can be seen up to 10 kHz.

- Due to the continuous tone presentation associated with DPOAEs, they tend to be impacted less by subtle ear conditions compared to TEOAEs. Therefore, DPOAEs can be recorded in individuals with up to moderate hearing losses, whereas TEOAEs are typically absent in individuals with more than a mild hearing loss (20–30 dB HL).

- Clinically, both tests offer similar reflection of the cochlea's frequency resolution and are good indicators of hearing loss.

- Common utilization of OAEs include newborn hearing screening and part of the test battery for differential diagnosis of hearing loss (cochlear vs. retrocochlear).

- It must be remembered the OAEs are not a test of hearing but a test of cochlear physiology.

□ The intensity of the OAE response relates to cochlear function but can be influenced by other nonauditory factors such as the probe fit in the ear canal. Therefore, the focus of the response should be on the presence of the emission and not necessarily the strength of the response.

Auditory Brainstem Response (ABR)

Auditory brainstem response (ABR) is an objective tool that has been utilized for decades to evaluate auditory function. ABR tests the function from the peripheral auditory system to the lower brainstem. When completing an ABR, a waveform is obtained (Figure 5–11).

■ Each waveform will have a number of peaks (Jewett waves), typically five, that are marked I to V. Each of the different waves represents different generator sites along the auditory pathway (Appendix 5–A).

■ ABRs are often utilized in the pediatric population to estimate hearing sensitivity when behavioral thresholds cannot be obtained or are thought to be inaccurate thresholds.

■ ABRs can still be utilized to estimate hearing in adults who are unable to complete behavioral testing or may have nonorganic/functional hearing loss.

■ When estimating hearing thresholds via ABR in adults, similar electrode placement and procedures are used as in pediatrics (refer to Chapter 6).

Each waveform will be assessed for the latency, amplitude, morphology (shape), and latency-intensity function of the waves in order to assign a type of peripheral hearing loss (Table 5–12).

Most often, when completing an ABR on an adult, often a neurodiagnostic ABR will be completed in order to evaluate for potential retrocochlear pathologies.

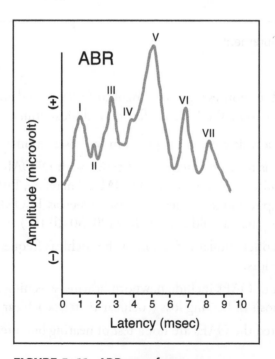

FIGURE 5–11. ABR waveform.

TABLE 5–12. Waveform Patterns and Correlating Hearing Loss

	MORPHOLOGY	WAVE LATENCIES	WAVE AMPLITUDE	LATENCY-INTENSITY FUNCTION
Normal Hearing	Good	All within normal limits	Normal	Falling within normal range
CHL	Good	Interwave within normal limits Waves I–V delayed	Normal	Outside of normative range
Sensory HL	Poor	Interwave within normal limits Waves I–V slightly delayed	Waves I–III: small to absent	High-intensity responses would be within normal range but all others would be outside.
Neural HL	Poor	Interwave delayed Waves III and V delayed	Normal	High-intensity responses would be within normal range but all others would be outside.

■ Electrode placement is similar to pediatric ABR, but procedures are different since thresholds are not being obtained.

□ Electrodes are placed with the noninverting electrode at the forehead midline (Fz) or vertex (Cz) with the inverting electrode at the ipsilateral earlobe or mastoid (A1/A2).

■ In a neurodiagnostic ABR, the amplitude and latencies of the waves are being assessed using a high-intensity click stimulus (80–85 dB nHL) with different stimulus polarities and rates. The polarity will be altered from rarefaction and condensation and click rate will be adjusted from slow (e.g., 21.1 clicks/s) to fast (e.g., 71.1 clicks/s).

□ Varying the polarity allows one to assess for auditory neuropathy spectrum disorder (ANSD), which is uncommon to have an adult onset but has been related to genetic causes (AUNA1). If a cochlear microphonic is the only aspect visible when completing an ABR, the resultant waveforms will "flip" when polarity is changed. Adding the rarefaction and condensation tracings will yield an absent or highly abnormal ABR, indicative of ANSD. OHC are depolarized to rarefacting stimuli and hyperpolarized to condensing stimuli; this creates a slight latency difference between the polarities. The morphology should not change drastically between rare and con, but most normative data were collected using rarefacting clicks.

□ Increasing the click rate allows for the tester to "stress" the auditory system by increasing the number of presentations within 1 second. The neural refractory period will often not allow the neural components to respond as quickly as the presentations are arriving, which can lead to a poorer waveform morphology as well as an increased latency in wave V. Abnormally prolonged wave Vs or abnormally poor morphologies can be associated with demyelinating diseases or neoplasms along the central auditory pathway. Slow presentation rates allow for the greatest amount of neural synchrony, which is why they can be used to measure the "best-case" scenario in the ABR.

- Suggested filter settings: a high-pass filter of 30 Hz to a low-pass filter of 1500 Hz; note, if "peakier" waves are desired, the low-pass filter can be increased to 3000 Hz and if muscular movement interference needs to be minimized, the high-pass filter can be raised to 100 Hz.

  □ Negative consequences of changing the filter settings include altering the waveform morphology (making it more difficult to peak pick and altering waveform latencies), ablating the waveform altogether, allowing high-frequency noise into the recording (e.g., WiFi), or including frequencies that lead to artifact-contaminated runs.

- Once these are obtained, the absolute latencies are assessed (Table 5–13).

- Interaural absolute wave V latency and wave I to V interpeak latencies should be ≤0.4 ms. With the change in click rate from slow to fast, it is expected to see an increase in wave V latency of approximately ≤0.5 ms (or 0.1 ms per 10 clicks/s increase in rate).

- Latency intensity function (LIF) can also be assessed, which is a graphical representation of wave V latency (*y*-axis) over different intensities (*x*-axis). It is well documented that the latency of wave V increases as stimulus intensity decreases due to reductions in neural synchrony and neural firing. Here, remember that "low is long." There is a normal, though nonlinear, range for this latency shift to occur with relation to the decrease in intensity with an approximate average of a 0.4-ms increase in latency for every 10-dB decrease in intensity.

  □ In individuals with normal hearing, one would note that as intensity decreases, latency increases, with all responses falling inside a normative range.

  □ For individuals with CHL, all latency values for every intensity are outside of normal (i.e., pushed to the right of the normal range).

  □ In the presence of SHNL, wave V at high intensities will fall in the normal range, but as threshold is approached, the latencies prolong abnormally (moving to the right of the normal range). The slope in SNHL is often steeper than for normal hearing or CHL.

  □ In retrocochlear hearing loss, there is no predictable pattern of the LIF.

TABLE 5–13. Normal Latencies for ABR

WAVE AND INTERPEAK WAVES	MEAN LATENCIES (MS)
I	1.54
III	3.70
V	5.60
I–III	2.20
III–V	1.84
I–V	4.04
Interaural Absolute V	≤0.4
Interaural Interpeak I–V	≤0.4

Source: Hall and Mueller (1998).

  ☐ Note that the LIF is not used as often any more since there are frequency-specific tests and bone-conduction measures that are utilized. However, some hardware such as the Interacoustics Eclipse will still plot the LIF.

 Comparison between latencies and morphologies will assist in determining the site of lesion. In retrocochlear pathologies, one might see a complete absence of waves, poor morphology, interaural differences, abnormal prolongation in latency of wave V at a faster rate, prolongation of waves III and V, and prolongation of interpeak waves I to V.

 ## CASE EXAMPLE: RETROCOCHLEAR PATHOLOGY

Patient is a 53-year-old female who reported progressive right-sided hearing loss and tinnitus. Patient stated that hearing has declined over the last 7 years. She stated that she has difficulty with speech understanding. Patient does note mild imbalance but denied aural fullness, otalgia, and noise exposure.

 Otoscopy revealed normal ear canals and tympanic membranes bilaterally. Audiometric findings demonstrate normal to mild hearing sensitivity in the left ear and a mild sloping to severe SNHL in the right ear. WRS were excellent (100%) in the left ear and poor (52%) in the right ear. The patient audiogram can be seen in Figure 5–12.

 Acoustic reflexes were present in the left conditions and absent in the right conditions and can be seen in Table 5–14.

- Based on the findings of an asymmetrical SNHL, asymmetrical word recognition scores, and acoustic reflex pattern, an ENT referral was made.

- ENT requested a neurodiagnostic ABR testing to assess for further pathologies.

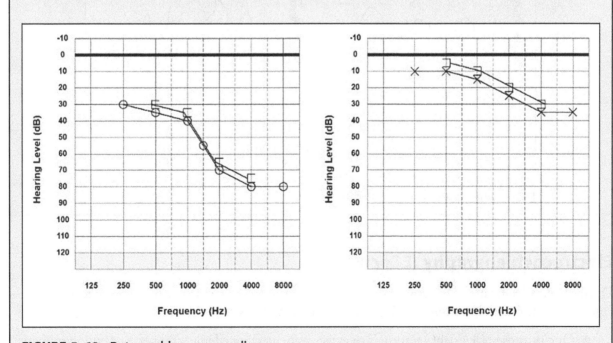

FIGURE 5–12. Retrocochlear case audiogram.

- ABR testing revealed normal absolute and interpeak latencies for a high-intensity click in the left ear. Testing in the right ear revealed normal absolute wave I latency with a prolonged absolute wave V latency. Additionally, wave I to V interpeak latency was prolonged in the right ear. There were significant interaural latency differences. Poor morphology was noted in the right ear. The patient ABR tracings can be seen in Figure 5–13.

- The overall clinical impression is consistent with a right acoustic neuroma.

TABLE 5–14. Retrocochlear Case MEMRs

ACTIVATOR	RIGHT IPSILATERAL (dB HL)	RIGHT CONTRALATERAL (dB HL)	LEFT IPSILATERAL (dB HL)	LEFT CONTRALATERAL (dB HL)
500 Hz	Absent	Absent	Present	Present
1000 Hz	Absent	Absent	Present	Present
2000 Hz	Absent	Absent	Present	Present
4000 Hz	Absent	Absent	Present	Present

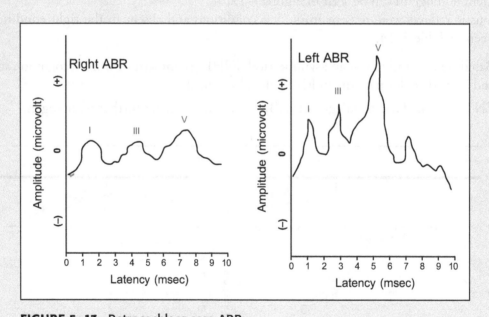

FIGURE 5–13. Retrocochlear case ABR.

Electrocochleography (ECochG)

During neurodiagnostic ABR testing, if wave I is not present, it may be useful to complete electrocochleography (ECochG) testing, which is a variation of ABR testing.

- One purpose of ECochG testing is to assist in identifying Ménière's disease or endolymphatic hydrops.

- ECochG testing can assist in increasing the amplitude of wave I due to different click rates, intensity levels, and transducers utilized.
- The 100-μs click rate is typically at 7.1 clicks/s, intensity is at 90/95 dB nHL, and transducer is a tiptrode, tymptrode, or transtympanic needle.
  □ The active electrode is usually placed on the tympanic membrane (tymptrode) or the skin of the outer ear canal (tiptrode). The active electrode can be placed at the niche of the round window or the promontory of the cochlea (transtympanic needle electrode), but this requires anesthesia and physician assistance and is a much more invasive procedure. It can be done during intraoperative monitoring.
  □ The close placement of the transducer aids in the ability to see wave I. Placement of the electrodes includes the test ear (nape/mastoid), vertex (forehead), and ground (cheek below the eye).
- Filters settings can range from a high-pass filter of 0 to a low-pass filter of 3000 Hz.
- An ECochG is displayed on a graph with amplitude and latency (Figure 5–14).
- Assessment occurs by labeling the base, summating potential (SP), and action potential (AP).
  □ Base: placed prior to or at the onset of the stimulus; serves as a reference amplitude for other measures
  □ SP: cochlear response (IHCs, OHCs, spiral ganglion); occurs approximately 0.8 ms after stimulus onset
  □ AP: synchronous firing of CN VIII; same as wave I of the ABR; occurs approximately 1.5 ms after stimulus onset
- The main result of interest is the amplitude ratio between SP and AP.

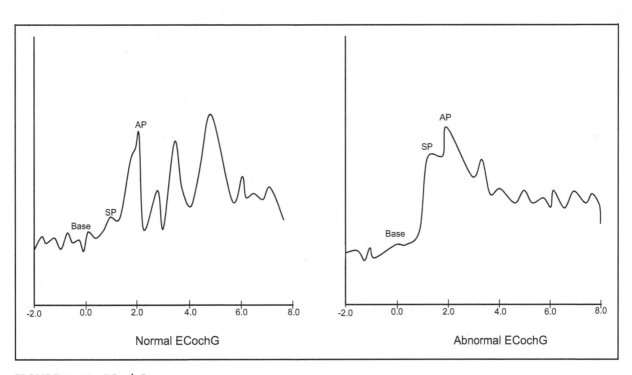

FIGURE 5–14. ECochG.

- Research suggests that normal ratio should be approximately ≤40% (0.4) for tymptrode and ≤50% (0.5) for tiptrodes (Chung et al., 2004).

- In Ménière's disease, the ratio is going to be above normative ranges. The difficulty with this testing and Ménière's is that if the patient is not actively experiencing symptoms, results are likely to be within normative ranges.

- ECochGs are becoming less prevalent in clinical settings due to a lack of reliable norms and standards and a lack of sensitivity for detecting pathologies.

- The CM can also be elicited with an ECochG of a constant (either rarefacting or condensing runs) polarity. The CM represents OHC function, which produces a response that mimics stimulus polarity. This, plus the remainder of the ECochG, can be important in identifying the site of lesion for ANSD.

KNOWLEDGE CHECKPOINT

When completing this testing, it is important to note that hearing loss from 2000 to 4000 Hz can lead to an absent ECochG. As such, audiograms to confirm hearing sensitivity should be completed prior to any testing. ECochG can also be used for threshold testing, but this is not common.

Middle Latency Response (MLR)

Following the ABR, the middle latency response (MLR) is an auditory evoked potential reflective of thalamocortical function that is composed of two negative and two positive peaks occurring between approximately 15 and 75 ms. It comprises four peaks: Na (first negative peak, 15–20 ms), Pa (first positive peak, 25–35 ms), Nb (second negative peak, 40–50 ms), and Pb (second positive peak, 50–60 ms).

- The Na/Pa complex amplitude is the most commonly used waveform for analysis of the MLR, specifically comparing between ears.

- The MLR can be elicited using a click- or frequency-specific stimulus (500 Hz gives very robust waveforms).

- Filter settings generally can be set at 5 to 30 Hz for the high-pass and 1500 Hz for the low-pass filters.

- The MLR will utilize a much slower stimulus rate (< 10 per second) when compared to the ABR.

- Electrode placement for the MLR will yield the greatest response at Cz (vertex) with the reference electrode at the mastoid or earlobe of the stimulated ear. Multichannel recordings can also be made using site C3, T3, or C5 in the left hemisphere or C4, T4, or C6 over the right.

Clinically, the MLR can serve multiple purposes:

- Most commonly is for site-of-lesion testing within the central auditory nervous system and for threshold estimation.

- In threshold estimation, the MLR is better utilized for estimating lower-frequency thresholds due to less dependence upon neural synchronization compared to the ABR. Therefore, in cases of insult to the central auditory system that may impact neural synchrony, the MLR may be a viable option for threshold estimation and can generally be obtained within approximately 10 dB of behavioral thresholds.

- In cases with cerebral lesions, the MLR can provide information regarding the physiological integrity of the underlying neural generators site and inform the clinician regarding possible insult at anatomical sites. The MLR may provide information in cases of injury, stroke, neurodegenerative diseases, seizure disorders, and tumors.

- When analyzing the MLR response, latency and amplitude are both monitored. However, amplitude, specifically interaural or interelectrode montage, is considered the best indicator of functional changes in the MLR as the latency of the response has very large variations even among individuals with normal central auditory systems.

Key concepts of the MLR that clinicians must consider:

- Response maturation. Like other auditory evoked potentials, the MLR does not fully mature in terms of latency, amplitude, and morphology until approximately 8 to 10 years of age, which is much later than the ABR.

- The Pb component (which is also referred to as the P50 or P1 response) of the MLR may not reach adult-like maturation until approximately 15 years of age.

- In younger populations, responses will occur at longer latencies and generally have smaller amplitudes.

- In cases of hearing loss, there may be delayed maturation of the MLR.

- The MLR, unlike the ABR, is susceptible to the patient's state of arousal and can be influenced (responses absent/reduced) by sleep, sedation, and various forms of anesthesia. This requires patient cooperation for testing to be completed and is of particular importance if utilizing the MLR for threshold estimation, especially in a pediatric population.

Auditory Long/Late Latency Responses (LLR)

One of the most common auditory long latency responses (LLR) is the P1-N1-P2 waveform complex and typically begins around 50 ms in mature adults.

- The P1 waveform is suspected to be generated by the primary auditory cortex with possible contributions from the hippocampus, planum temporale, and lateral temporal cortex. It occurs around 50 ms and is the same wave as Pb in the MLR.

- The N1 component is likely generated in the auditory cortex in the superior temporal lobe (Heschl's gyrus). The N1 response occurs at approximately 100 ms.

- The P2 waveform is suspected to have multiple generator sites, including the primary and secondary auditory cortices in Heschl's gyrus. The P2 waveform occurs at approximately 150 to 200 ms.

- Similar to the ABR, the P1-N1-P2 response has exogenous characteristics, meaning that the response will vary based on stimulus characteristics such as tonal or speech stimuli.

The LLR can be used to estimate hearing thresholds, similar to the ABR and MLR, but there are aspects of the response to consider.

- The response does not fully mature until individuals reach their late teenage years.
- One advantage of the LLR has over the ABR is that the response amplitude is much greater and therefore can be obtained in fewer sweeps.
- The LLR reflects physiology at the level of the primary auditory cortex, providing the clinician a broader picture of the central auditory nervous system versus the ABR, which only reflects the central auditory system through the level of the brainstem.
- The disadvantage of this response is the previously discussed maturation of the response (late teens), as well as sleep state, which can diminish the response.
- Finally, there are currently no norms published for the LLR.

Utilization of the LLR can be as follows:

- Quantify the effects of HAs or cochlear implants through recording aided responses by presenting stimuli through the soundfield.
- The use of aided evoked responses is a way to potentially verify HA and implant programming.
- Aided LLR responses contribute to monitoring neuroplastic changes in the central nervous system.
- Finally, the LLR has been used to monitor neural change in response to auditory training/rehabilitation.

P300

The P300 is unique in relation to other electrophysiologic auditory measures in that it requires the patient or participant to be actively engaged with the task.

- The auditory P300 is an electrophysiological test that reflects physiological function of the primary auditory cortex (superior temporal gyrus), hippocampus, and the frontal cortex and is observed around 300 ms after stimulus onset.
- The response is elicited through an oddball paradigm in which the patient hears two stimuli: a target/rare/oddball stimulus (approximately 20% of the time) and a nontarget/standard/common stimulus (approximately 80% of the time).
- The patient is often instructed to count the target stimuli.
- The P300 can be elicited in other modalities, such as vision, but acoustically, it is traditionally elicited with either tonal or speech stimuli at 60 to 80 dB peSPL.
- As the P300 task complexity increases, the response latency will also increase with similar effects seen on response amplitude (reductions). As the discrimination task becomes easier, the latency should decrease while the amplitude should increase. Contrastingly, when the discrimination tasks become more difficult, latency will increase (up to approximately 600 ms) while amplitude decreases.
- Latency is associated with processing speed while the amplitude is associated with the attentional resource allocation used in the processing.

The utilization of the auditory P300 clinically in audiology is often debated as generation of the response requires active participation in the discrimination task by the patient. The debate focuses on the principle that if the patient is reliably able to do the task necessary to obtain a P300 response, then what is the diagnostic value added to the case as the patient should be able to provide reliable behavioral responses. Additionally, the P300 can be affected by state of arousal and fatigue, age, attention, task complexity, handedness, depression, and dyslexia. While the auditory P300 is a clinically available assessment, its use and diagnostic value is often questioned. For comparison, Figure 5–15 demonstrates the ABR, MLR, and auditory P300 responses.

Mismatch Negativity

Mismatch negativity (MMN) is another electrophysiologic auditory measure that assesses higher-level auditory function.

- The MMN is an electrophysiological test that reflects physiological function of the primary auditory cortex, frontal cortex, hippocampus, and the thalamus at approximately 100 to 300 ms.
- The response is elicited through an oddball paradigm in which a deviant stimuli is presented alongside a standard stimulus (tone burst, speech vowels, or consonant-vowel combinations). The MMN response is seen by subtracting responses seen from the standard stimuli to the deviant stimuli.
- Unlike P300, MMN is independent of attention.
- Can be elicited with either tonal or speech stimuli at 60 to 80 dB peSPL
- Recommended to tell the patient to ignore the stimuli during testing
- Electrode placement is the same as P300.
- Measurements are labeled as N1, P2, and MMN.

Similar to P300, MMN is not widely used clinically due to poor repeatability and applicability.

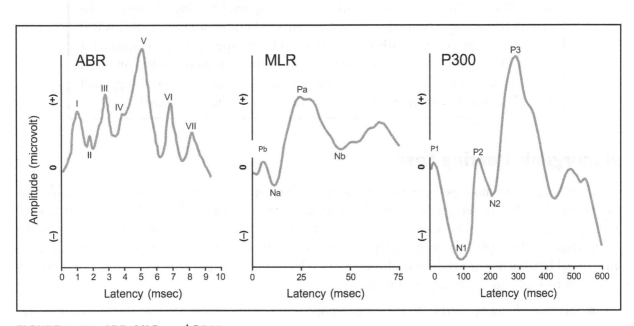

FIGURE 5–15. ABR, MLR, and P300.

Testing for Specific Pathologies

Adult (Central) Auditory Processing Disorder

Beyond the standard comprehensive audiologic evaluation is central auditory processing disorders ([C]APD), which will be discussed in more detail in Chapter 6, as it is more common in the pediatric population. Central auditory processing ([C]AP) is defined as the processing of auditory information in the central auditory nervous system and the underlying activity that gives rise to electrophysiologic potentials (ASHA, 2005a). (C)AP can be subdivided into specific skills, as shown in Table 5–15.

Individuals with (C)APD will often have normal hearing sensitivity on a standard audiologic evaluation but will report many symptoms consistent with those individuals with hearing loss. For a complete list of symptoms, see Chapter 6 and AAA (2010). Management of (C)APD is variable and very much dependent on the specific deficit as described in Chapter 6 but may include:

- Direct therapy
- Indirect therapy
- Environmental modifications

While it is beyond the scope of this chapter to have an in-depth discussion of (C)APD, the goal is to provide a brief overview of the condition and consideration of evaluation for individuals for which their difficulties cannot be explained using the standard audiologic evaluation. These concerns can arise in adults and especially older adults.

AUDIOLOGY NUGGET

Many patients will present to an audiology clinic reporting difficulties with hearing and believing they have hearing loss. However, their audiologic evaluation will generally be consistent with normal peripheral hearing sensitivity. The standard audiologic evaluation (pure-tone air and bone conduction, SRT, WRS) does not assess central auditory function and it is appropriate to consider a (C)APD evaluation or make an appropriate referral to someone who can assess auditory processing function. Screening tests and batteries have been suggested (e.g., Dichotic Digits and Gaps in Noise; first page of the SCAN-3A).

Nonorganic Hearing Loss

While not very common, perhaps one of the most challenging situations in terms of audiological assessment is with patients who have pseudohypoacusis, have nonorganic hearing loss (NOHL), or are malingering. NOHL is the presence of a behavioral hearing deficit that is more significant or greater than what can be attributed to pathology within the auditory system; it can also be referred to as functional hearing loss or psychogenic hearing loss. The common thread with NOHL is that it exceeds what can be explained by an organic/medical cause.

- The prevalence of NOHL in the general population is 2% to 9%, with females twice as likely than males to exhibit NOHL (Mathai et al., 2021).

TABLE 5–15. (Central) Auditory Processing Skills Information

	PERFORMANCE WITH DEGRADED SIGNALS (AUDITORY CLOSURE)	PERFORMANCE WITH COMPETING SIGNALS (DICHOTIC LISTENING)	TEMPORAL PROCESSING	LOCALIZATION AND LATERALIZATION	DISCRIMINATION
Definition	Ability to complete distorted or missing parts of the acoustic signal and recognize the message	Different auditory stimuli presented simultaneously to both ears	Perception of alteration of sound within a given sound domain	Representation of auditory space due to interaural timing and intensity cues in order to separate auditory signals from competing noise	Ability to tell the difference between sounds
Further divisions		Binaural integration: report back both ears (no order) (CW-FR, DD) Binaural separation: report back one ear, then the other or one ear instead of the other (CW-DE, CST)	Temporal integration: summation of neuronal activity with duration of sound energy (not often tested clinically) Temporal masking: masking of one sound with an addition sound presented immediately prior to or following the target sound (not often tested clinically) Temporal ordering: processing two or more auditory stimuli in order of occurrence temporal resolution: shortest duration of time that is discriminable between two auditory signals		

continues

TABLE 5–15. *continued*

	PERFORMANCE WITH DEGRADED SIGNALS (AUDITORY CLOSURE)	PERFORMANCE WITH COMPETING SIGNALS (DICHOTIC LISTENING)	TEMPORAL PROCESSING	LOCALIZATION AND LATERALIZATION	DISCRIMINATION
Tests	Low-pass filtered speech, time-compressed speech, speech-in-noise tests, synthetic sentence identification with ipsilateral competing message	Integration: Competing Words–Free Recall; Dichotic Digits; Dichotic Rhyme; Dichotic Consonant-Vowels; Dichotic Sentence Identification Separation: Competing Words–Directed Ear Competing Sentences: Staggered Spondaic Words; Synthetic Sentence Identification with Contralateral Competing Message	Ordering: Duration Patterns: Frequency Patterns, Duration Patterns Resolution: Gaps in Noise; Random Gap Detection	Listening in Spatialized Noise	Component of all (C)AP tests

- Adults are often seeking compensation or financial gain, but also could be due to psychosocial factors or situational avoidance.

- Individuals scoring lower on measures of socioeconomic status have also been shown to more likely be associated with NOHL (Mathai et al., 2021).

AUDIOLOGY NUGGET

Many individuals, both children and adults, who present with NOHL or intentionally malinger during an audiologic evaluation will often have an ulterior motivation for the evaluation. Those motivations for adults may include some type of financial compensation or incentive. For example, individuals who are presenting for evaluation as part of a workers' compensation claim, military service, motor vehicle accident, disability payment, or any other (legal) claim in which they stand to receive financial compensation may provide motivation for that individual to elevate or exaggerate hearing loss (if hearing loss is present at all).

When completing a conventional audiological assessment, there are many signs or "red flags" of NOHL and, subsequently, ways to approach further assessment:

- Poor agreement between the SRT and the PTA: generally, a clinician should expect the SRT and PTA to be within approximately 8 to 10 dB of each other with a few exceptions (precipitous or reverse slope configurations). In cases of NOHL, the SRT will often be obtained at a much lower (better) threshold compared to the PTA.

- Additionally, air- and bone-conduction thresholds may not occur as expected based on objective testing (tympanometry or MEMRs).

- Patient behaviors: patients may exhibit excessive listening effort or appear to be trying extremely hard to hear the stimulus.

- Financial incentive: any assessment that is being completed for which the patient has a financial interest (e.g., workers' compensation claim, motor vehicle accidents, military service) may also introduce a conflict of interest for the patient and should be approached with caution.

- Aberrant unilateral test results: in cases of unilateral hearing loss, patients with NOHL may never exhibit a shadow curve, meaning an unmasked stimulus is loud enough for cross-hearing (exceeds interaural attenuation). No response is obtained from the patient with NOHL. Figure 5–16 demonstrates a typical shadow curve when appropriate masking is not applied to the NTE.

- Testing considerations: patients may exhibit fewer false-positive responses as well as have a low test-retest reliability.

- Abnormal speech testing results: word recognition abilities may be much better than expected at reduced SLs.

- Objective test results disagreeing with behavioral results: normal MEMR thresholds at values lower than would be expected with presenting behavioral thresholds or the presence of OAEs in light of the severity of behavioral thresholds can indicate NOHL.

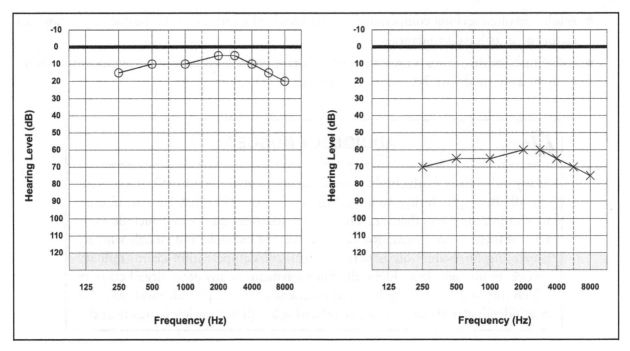

FIGURE 5–16. Audiogram shadow curve.

- General theme: poor reliability throughout testing and poor consistency/agreement within and between behavioral and objective findings.

Testing for NOHL includes reinstruction, altering test parameters (e.g., ascending compared to descending thresholds—should be within 10 dB, but more exaggerated in NOHL), and the utilization of the Stenger test, which can only be used in cases of unilateral hearing loss or significant asymmetry. To complete the Stenger test, the asymmetry between ears needs to be at least 20 dB where it is expected that the hearing loss is intentionally elevated and inaccurate. Please refer to the Specialty Tests section for a description of Stenger test administration.

In addition to alterations and reinstructions that can be made as part of the behavioral audiologic evaluation, there is a battery of objective tests that clinicians have at their disposal to provide additional information regarding the physiology of the auditory system. The available objective tests include:

- Acoustic immittance: MEMR thresholds that are approximate to the behavioral audiometric thresholds (within 10–15 dB) are indicative of NOHL.

- OAEs: present OAEs in the presence of more than a mild hearing loss (40 dB HL) are indicative of NOHL.

- Electrophysiological measures: thresholds measured via ABR or ASSR (as discussed in Chapter 6) are a close representation of true auditory thresholds when using correction factors; if these objective thresholds are lower than the behavioral findings, it is safe to suspect NOHL.

CASE EXAMPLE: NOHL

Patient is a 24-year-old male who was referred to the clinic by the Department of Workers' Compensation. He reported a left unilateral hearing loss and tinnitus, which began after a workplace accident 4 months ago. Patient is a carpenter and experienced noise exposure due to use of a nearby nail gun at a work site. He stated that he is currently on administrative leave to assess the damages that occurred. He stated that his hearing loss and tinnitus is debilitating and has severely impacted his quality of life.

- Audiometric findings using insert earphones demonstrated normal hearing in the right ear and a profound hearing loss in the left ear. Unmasked bone-conduction thresholds are worse than air-conduction thresholds in the right ear. There should be bone-conduction responses near the right air-conduction thresholds. SRT and PTA were in agreement for the right ear only with no response to SRT in the left ear. Word recognition scores were good (88%) in the right ear and poor (0%) in the left ear. His initial audiometric thresholds are presented in Figure 5–17.

- Based on the case history and workers' compensation claim in conjunction with inconsistent behavioral audiologic results, it is reasonable to suspect a NOHL or malingering.

- In this particular case with a patient presenting with a unilateral hearing loss, the Stenger test is appropriate and would provide the audiologist a relatively quick insight into the validity of the thresholds.

- Figure 5–18 and Table 5–16 demonstrate the appropriate presentation levels for the Stenger test in this particular case.

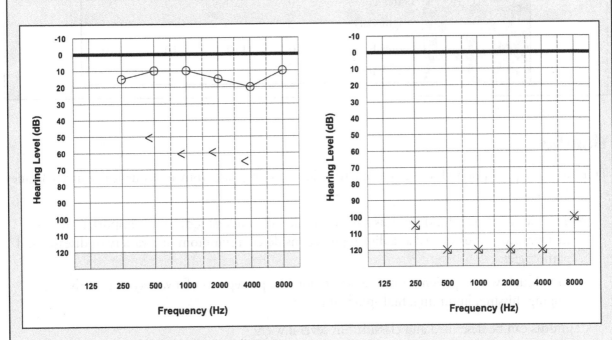

FIGURE 5–17. Stenger case initial audiogram.

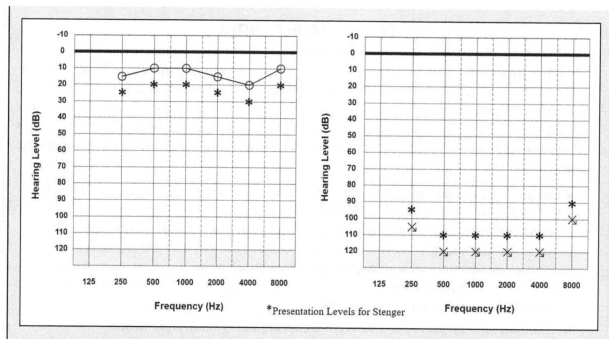

FIGURE 5–18. Stenger case presentation-level audiogram.

TABLE 5–16. Stenger Case Presentation Levels

		FREQUENCY (Hz)			
		500	**1000**	**2000**	**4000**
PRESENTATION LEVEL (dB HL)	Better Ear (Right Ear)	20	20	25	30
	Poorer Ear (Left Ear)	110	110	110	110

Tinnitus

Tinnitus is the perception of sound or noise that does not originate from an acoustical source (Baguley et al., 2013).

■ The mechanisms behind tinnitus have yet to be fully understood, so it is important to note that tinnitus is not viewed as a disease; it is considered a symptom of a variety of diseases and pathologies.

■ Individuals who experience tinnitus will report the perception of a variety of sounds (e.g., ringing, hissing, humming, high-pitched tone).

Tinnitus can be described and classified in several ways:

1. Subjective or objective: subjective tinnitus is heard only by the patient, while objective tinnitus is heard by the patient and others.

2. Primary or secondary: primary tinnitus is either associated with an unknown cause or SNHL, whereas secondary tinnitus has identifiable causes.

   ■ Noise-induced hearing loss (NIHL) and hearing loss have been highly correlated with primary tinnitus. It is suggested that 90% of individuals with chronic tinnitus have hearing loss (Hoffman & Reed, 2004; Wang et al., 2020).

   ■ Secondary tinnitus is typically caused by medical conditions (i.e., middle ear myoclonus). This can also be described as somatosensory, where the perception of tinnitus is due to issues in the somatosensory afference from the temporomandibular area or cervical spine (Michiels et al., 2018).

 AUDIOLOGY NUGGET

Somatosensory tinnitus can present as pulsatile, meaning that the tinnitus matches an individual's pulse. This patient should be immediately referred to otolaryngology. Further, secondary tinnitus can have auditory-related causes, such as cerumen impaction, cochlear abnormalities, and auditory nerve pathologies, to nonauditory causes, such as middle ear myoclonus, vascular abnormalities, and temporal mandibular joint disorder.

To describe the tinnitus, it is important to understand what the patient is experiencing. Table 5–17 displays the different ways that tinnitus can be described.

There are numerous factors and causes that are associated with the development of tinnitus. Associated factors can include:

■ Mental health: depression, attentional issues, anxiety, stress

■ Auditory concerns: presbycusis, noise exposure

TABLE 5–17. Description of Tinnitus on Different Parameters

Unilateral or Bilateral	Right
	Left
	Bilateral
Temporal Characteristics	Spontaneous
	Temporary
	Occasional
	Intermittent
	Constant
Duration	Recent/acute (<6 months)
	Persistent/chronic
Impact	Nonbothersome
	Bothersome

- Other medical phenomena: hormonal changes, thyroid issues, diseases of the heart/blood, medication interaction, ear and sinus infections, Ménière's disease, tumors, obesity

Research has suggested that there are definitive and possible risk factors for tinnitus (Hoffman & Reed, 2004). These are discussed in Table 5–18.

Prior to the start of any assessment, case history is important to obtain.

- Useful in understanding any definite or possible risk factors that may be present
- Allows for the patient to share the chief complaint (CC), which can impact procedures and diagnosis

TABLE 5–18. Risk Factors for Tinnitus

RISK	FACTORS
Definite Risk Factors	• Cardiovascular/cerebrovascular disease • Drugs such as salicylate analgesics, anti-inflammatory drugs, antibiotics, loop diuretics & chemotherapy agents) • Ear infections • Head/neck trauma or injury • Hyper and hypothyroidism • Noise exposure • Meniere's disease • Otosclerosis • Presbycusis • Sudden SNHL • Vestibular schwannoma
Possible Risk Factors	• Alcohol • Anxiety • Depression • Familial inheritance • Geographic region • Health status of fair-poor • Obesity • Limited education • Low height • Low socioeconomic status • Low weight • Lyme disease • Rural residence • Smoking

Source: Adapted from Hoffman, H. J., & Reed, G. W. (2004). Epidemiology of tinnitus. *Tinnitus: Theory and Management, 16,* 41.

CASE EXAMPLE

Patient is a 36-year-old male who presents with hearing loss and tinnitus concerns. Patient stated that his main concern is understanding the noises that he hears. During case history, you learn that he has high blood pressure and is now in high-stress scenarios at work, which has increased his anxiety and depressive symptoms. Additionally, you learn that he does not sleep well at night.

The information gained during your case history can help you present your findings and recommendations to the patient.

In addition to case history, questionnaires and inventories are a vital part of any tinnitus assessment. Since tinnitus perception is variable in patients, questionnaires can assist the audiologist to understand to full impact of tinnitus on each individual. Questionnaires and inventories can assist individuals in describing the nature of their tinnitus, medical and psychological impacts, medication use, history of hearing loss and/or noise exposure, and overall impact on the individual. There are a variety of validated questionnaires that pose questions, scored into a numerical value to quantify the impact of tinnitus. The outcomes of the inventories can be used to assist in treatment planning. Inventories include:

- Tinnitus Reaction Questionnaire (TRQ; Wilson et al., 1991)
- Tinnitus Severity Index (TSI; Meikle et al., 2008)
- Tinnitus Handicap Inventory (THI; Newman et al., 1996)
- Tinnitus Functional Index (TFI; Meikle et al., 2012)

Although there is no diagnostic criterion when working with tinnitus, there are clinical assessments that can be utilized to address patient concerns (Deshpande & Hall, 2022).

- Otoscopy: assess for any external/middle ear disorders or diseases
- Immittance: evaluate potential middle ear issues that could indicate a potential diagnosis and/or referral
- DPOAEs: determine cochlear (OHC) integrity and function
- Pure-tone audiometry (250–20,000 Hz with interoctaves): identify presence of hearing loss since the pitch of tinnitus often aligns with elevated thresholds on pure-tone testing
- Speech audiometry: testing may not be as important as the other methods suggested in terms of measuring tinnitus
- ABR: assess peripheral and central auditory function. This testing is not a typical component of a tinnitus assessment.

The psychoacoustic assessment of tinnitus includes loudness discomfort levels (LDLs), pitch matching, loudness matching, minimal masking levels (MML), and residual inhibition. The psychoacoustic assessment can only be completed if the individual is currently experiencing tinnitus at the time of the visit. Table 5–19 highlights what is completed during the test and why each is used (Deshpande & Hall, 2022).

TABLE 5–19. Aspects of Psychoacoustic Assessment

ASSESSMENT	STIMULI AND IMPORTANCE	ASSESSMENT PROCEDURE
Loudness Discomfort Levels (LDLs)	• Stimuli: tonal and speech signals • Assesses: recruitment and sound sensitivity	• Completed in right and left ear conditions • Patient listens to stimuli and tells the audiologist to stop when the stimuli become uncomfortably loud

Pitch Matching	• Stimuli: pure tones, FRESH noise, or narrowband noise (NBN)
	• Assesses: frequency range of an individual's tinnitus
		• Completed: in right, left, and binaural conditions depending on individual complaints
		• Assessment:
		  1. Completed in the opposite ear than the tinnitus ear (if unilateral) at a comfortable level. If bilateral, start in one ear, complete the other ear, and complete in binaural conditions
		  2. Present signal at 1000 and 2000 Hz. Matching should occur using a two-alternative approach, which forces the individual to decide which stimuli presented is closer in frequency.
		  3. Depending on patient response, either present a lower or higher frequency until it is reported that the stimuli sound like the tinnitus.
		  4. Complete in other ear and in binaural condition if necessary.

Loudness Matching	• Stimuli: pure tones, FRESH noise, or NBN
	• Assesses: loudness of the perceived tinnitus
		• Completed: right, left, and/or binaural conditions depending on individual complaints
		• Assessment:
		  1. At the frequency where the individual pitch matched their tinnitus, start around their pure-tone threshold.
		  2. In 2-dB steps, increase loudness until the individual tells you to stop.
		  3. Repeat at least two times and obtain the average.
		  4. Repeat in opposite ear and binaural conditions if necessary.

Minimal Masking Levels (MML)	• Stimuli: NBN or white noise (WN)
	• Assesses: if masking noise is beneficial to the individual experiencing tinnitus; to determine the amount and type of noise needed for masking individual's tinnitus
		• Completed in right, left, and binaural conditions.
		• Assessment:
		  1. Some audiological practices have you complete MML at all frequencies, where some only have you complete at the frequency that was matched for the individual's tinnitus.
		  2. Increase masking noise in 2 dB steps and have the individual tell you to stop when the masking noise just covers up their tinnitus.
		  3. Repeat in opposite ear and binaural conditions if necessary.

TABLE 5–19. *continued*

ASSESSMENT	STIMULI AND IMPORTANCE	ASSESSMENT PROCEDURE
Residual Inhibition	• Stimuli: BBN or NBN • Assesses: amount of noise needed to suppress perception of tinnitus	• Completed in binaural condition • Assessment: 1. At the pitch and MML level of the individual's tinnitus, present noise for 60 seconds. 2. After that time, the patient is asked to describe if their tinnitus changed/was not noticeable.

Sound Sensitivity

Noise, defined as acoustic energy that interferes with hearing, is subjective and individuals will describe different things as "noise." Some individuals, however, are more sensitive to or intolerant to sounds, which are often described as having hyperacusis. As is evident, there is not agreement on the presence and degree of distress that is present for the diagnosis of hyperacusis.

Hyperacusis can be defined in a variety of ways, such as a poor tolerance to everyday sounds, an intolerance to environmental sounds, and/or inappropriate responses to these sounds (Aazh et al., 2018; Klein et al., 1990; Vernon, 1987).

- Research suggests that there are four categories of hyperacusis: loudness, fear, pain, and annoyance (Tyler et al., 2014).
  □ These categories are based on the reaction that patients have to sounds.
- Like tinnitus, hyperacusis is considered a symptom of a medical condition.
- Audiometrically, these patients will typically have normal pure-tone thresholds, speech thresholds, and word recognition scores but will have abnormally low UCLs. An individual without hyperacusis with normal hearing will typically have UCLs around 100 dB HL (Tyler et al., 2014).
- Questionnaires regarding hyperacusis include the Hyperacusis Questionnaire (HQ; Khalfa et al., 2002) and the Multiple Activity Scale for Hyperacusis (MASH; Dauman & Bouscau-Faure, 2005).
- Table 5–20 displays a breakdown of the type of hyperacusis, the reaction, and findings.

In addition to hyperacusis, individuals can also experience misophonia.

- Misophonia is described as the hatred of sound in which individuals have a strong emotional reaction such as anger, disgust, hate, and rage toward the individual emitting the sounds, most commonly people eating and breathing.
- The perceived loudness of these sounds does not typically matter to an individual's reaction.
- Similar to hyperacusis, misophonia is a hearing disorder that may be associated with a mental health condition/disorder such as attention-deficit/hyperactivity disorder (ADHD), obsessive compulsive disorder (OCD), and mood and/or panic disorders (Ferreira et al., 2013).
- Questionnaires for misophonia include the Amsterdam Misophonia Scale (A-MISO-S; Schröder et al., 2013), Misophonia Questionnaire (MQ; Wu et al., 2014), and the Selective Sound Sensitivity Scale (S-Five; Vitoratou et al., 2020).

TABLE 5–20. Types of Hyperacusis and Patient Reactions

TYPE OF HYPERACUSIS	REACTION
Loudness	Sounds are deemed to be uncomfortably/painfully loud even when it is not
Fear	Dread of certain sounds which causes abnormal behaviors such as avoidance
Pain	Perception of pain in response to sounds that are not typically perceived as loud.
Annoyance	Regardless of loudness level, negative emotional response to sounds

AUDIOLOGY NUGGET

Misophonia and hyperacusis are often confused for one another. An easy way to remember the difference is that misophonia has more of an extreme emotional response to sounds than hyperacusis. A typical trigger for misophonia is chewing and breathing sounds.

Assessment for tinnitus and other sound sensitivity can be completed quite quickly, typically in under 90 minutes. Time should be built into any appointment for counseling. While the psychoacoustic assessment provides useful information, clinicians must leave ample time to address the individual's complaints and concerns.

- A medical referral should be provided immediately if the patient is complaining of secondary tinnitus, suicidal thoughts, rapid onset of tinnitus, and other medical issues.

Tinnitus Treatment

- Typically, tinnitus cannot be cured unless there is a treated medical condition present. There are a variety of options that can be utilized to assist a patient managing and learning about their tinnitus.
- First, counsel the patient about their tinnitus. Counseling should address the individual's CC, review audiogram and findings, and information about tinnitus/sound sensitivity,
- Counsel on current trends in therapies and/or mindfulness techniques (cognitive behavioral therapy [CBT], mindfulness therapy, tinnitus retraining therapy [TRT], progressive tinnitus management [PTM]).
  - Audiologists should refer to appropriate mental health providers who specifically work with tinnitus for these therapies.

- Additionally, one can consider utilizing devices and applications (HAs, ear level maskers, phone applications/noise generators), and referrals to other health professions for medical and/or psychological management.

- Alternative treatments include hypnotherapy, neuromodulation, biofeedback, transcranial magnetic stimulation (TMS), and vagus nerve stimulation (VNS).

- It is important to remember that not one therapy or device may work for each patient, so it is critical to discuss a variety of options with the patient.

Sound Sensitivity Treatment

- Treatments for sound sensitivity disorders are similar to those used in tinnitus.

- Informational counseling, CBT, and sound therapy (such as music, broadband noise, and exposure therapy to bothersome sounds) are all possible treatment options.

- Individuals with either hyperacusis or misophonia may find hearing protection alleviates their symptoms, however this is not a viable long-term treatment plan.

- Referrals to other healthcare providers (e.g., psychologists, psychiatrists, primary care physicians, occupational therapists) to create an interprofessional team for the treatment of sound sensitivity disorders is important as well.

Special Populations

Developmental/Neurodevelopmental Issues

A population that is commonly seen in audiology settings due to its comorbidity with hearing loss are individuals with intellectual and developmental disabilities (IDDs). To begin, a thorough case history is necessary. The case history should include questions surrounding previous medical history, including surgeries and interventions, communication strategies, and caregiver/individual concerns.

- Sometimes a thorough case history is not available if the individual is brought by a case worker who is not familiar with the individual's medical history.

- Through the case history, the examiner is able to start to assess what tests and procedures may need to be completed by the patient's responses or lack thereof.

- Case history can also provide the audiologist with information on how the patient may respond to testing and what modifications may need to be made.

Testing individuals with IDDs may require modified testing techniques in order to make certain that behavioral thresholds are accurate. Although individuals with IDDs are adults, their mental and physical capacity may not match their chronological age. As such, it is important to assess everyone's mental and physical function. Individuals with IDD have the possibility of CHL, MHL, and SNHL (Willems et al., 2022).

- A retrospective study of Special Olympics athletes over a 10-year period determined that cerumen impaction was found in 40.7%, middle ear issues in 29.5%, and confirmed hearing loss in 26.9% of athletes (Willems et al., 2022).

  □ Otoscopy is an imperative part of testing this population. During otoscopy, it is important to assess for microtia/atresia, stenosis, cerumen impaction, otitis media with effusion (OME), and tympanic membrane landmarks.

  □ When performing otoscopy, it is important to be cognizant of touch sensitivities that an individual with IDD may have. As such, clinicians may have to deviate from typical testing technique to leave otoscopy and immittance testing for the end so as to not upset the patient prior behavioral testing.

  □ Due to the high prevalence of middle ear issues, immittance testing should be completed. It can provide insight into the probable type of hearing loss even if masking cannot be accomplished.

  □ Depending on the individual patient, it may be difficult to obtain reliable behavioral testing, so OAEs should also be utilized.

- Some individuals with IDD can complete the typical comprehensive audiological testing with no issues, whereas others may need modifications to testing, conditioned play audiometry (CPA), or visual reinforced audiometry (VRA) for pure-tone assessment.

- Once the testing technique is decided on, it is suggested to complete control trials that require the audiologist to not provide any stimuli to see if there may be false positives due to the patient's wishing to please others (i.e., liberal response bias).

  □ For speech testing, individuals may not have sufficient language abilities to complete adult speech tasks such as the NU-6, so alternate lists may be used: Phonetically Balanced Kindergarten (PBK), Northwestern University of Children's Perception of Speech (NU-CHIPS), Word Intelligibility by Picture Identification (WIPI), or spondee board picture pointing.

- It is important to consistently monitor the hearing status of an individual with IDDs, since minor changes in middle or inner ear status may not be accurately expressed by the individual.

 AUDIOLOGY NUGGET

The American Association on Intellectual and Developmental Disabilities (AAIDD, 2023) describes IDDs as differences that impact one's physical, intellectual, and/or emotional development that are typically present at birth. IDDs can impact the nervous system, sensory system, and metabolism. Some IDDs can also be degenerative disorders, where individuals meet developmental milestones and then lose certain abilities, whereas others can be fully present at birth. IDDs can include individuals with autism spectrum disorders (ASDs), brain injuries, cerebral palsy, Down syndrome, and fragile X syndrome (AAIDD, 2023).

Diminished Cognitive Function

Cognition includes the different processes that allow humans to function on many different levels on a daily basis. This allows for individuals to do such things like learn, solve problems, and memorize materials. As one ages, there are both normative and nonnormative changes to cognitive functioning (Harada et al., 2013).

- Normal age-related brain changes can have an impact on an individual's quality of life and day-to-day functioning; it is becoming far more important to understand these changes. Numerous studies show a correlation between age and cognitive decline, but the age at which a cognitive decline becomes evident is a subject of considerable debate (e.g., Salthouse, 2009).

- Typically, these cognitive changes are noted to be a decline in cognitive functioning, but it is crucial to note that not all cognitive changes result in a decline, since some cognitive functions (e.g., language) improve with age or are resilient in the aging brain.

- Memory (most common cognitive complaint among aging adults): declines typically beginning around the age of 60 (Hedden & Gabrieli, 2004).

- Complex attention: declines around the age of 30 beginning with processing speed (Salthouse & Meinz, 1995).

- Executive function and perceptual motor function: peak in the third decade of life and then steadily decline (Salthouse, 2012).

- Vocabulary and general knowledge: remain stable or even improve until the sixth to seventh decade of a person's life (Lezak et al., 2012; Salthouse, 2012).

- These normative cognitive changes can potentially have a minor impact a person's daily activity of living.

There are a variety of factors that produce additional nonnormative changes in the brain, which can increase the degree of cognitive decline (Murman, 2015).

- Nonnormative changes include cerebral ischemia, mild cognitive impairments, dementias (e.g., Alzheimer's disease), and head traumas.

- A variety of different impacts can be seen on cognitive function, including increased memory issues, poor attention, and executive function, as well as a decline in language abilities, perceptual motor function, and social cognition.

- Depending on the severity of cognitive decline, the individual may experience major impacts on their activities of daily living and may require long-term care.

 KNOWLEDGE CHECKPOINT

The fifth edition of the *Diagnostic and Statistical Manual of Mental Disorders* (*DSM-V*) determined that cognitive functioning can be separated into six key domains: executive functioning, complex attention, learning and memory, language, perceptual motor function, and social cognition (Silverman et al., 2015). Each domain has various subthemes associated with it. Such separation allows clinicians and researchers to establish the etiology and severity of each neurocognitive disorder.

Research trends over the past 20 years have suggested that there is a relationship between hearing loss and cognitive decline (e.g., Lin et al., 2013; Surprenant & DiDonato, 2014).

- Research suggests that those with hearing loss are at a greater risk for cognitive decline and dementia even when sex, age, race, diabetes, smoking history, education, and cardiovascular issues are controlled (Lin et al., 2013).

- When compared to normal-hearing individuals, individuals with a mild, moderate, and severe hearing impairment, respectively, had a two-, three-, and fivefold increased risk of incident all-cause dementia over >10 years of follow-up (Lin et al., 2011).

The exact relationship is not fully understood, but research does suggest that one exists. Due to the current trends, it is important to understand that cognitive functioning can have an impact on your patients with hearing loss. Cognition is needed to process all sensory information. When there is diminished cognitive functioning, it can impact how sensory information, such as auditory information, is processed.

- The Framework for Understanding Effortful Listening (FUEL) was adapted from the capacity theory (Kahneman, 1973; Pichora-Fuller et al., 2016).

- FUEL incorporates the aspect of cognitive demand and the supply of cognitive capacity available to listening situations.

- Persons with hearing loss must allocate more resources to comprehend, remember, and respond to events and auditory information, which could negatively impact working memory and attention, similar to what those with normal hearing experience in difficult listening environments (Pichora-Fuller et al., 2016).

- It may be beneficial for audiologists to complete cognitive screenings on their patients, which may help understand why certain patients experience more difficulties than others.

- There are a variety of screening measures that are sensitive enough to mild cognitive changes, such as the Mini-Mental State Exam (MMSE), Montreal Cognitive Assessment (MoCA), Mini-Cog, or clock drawing.

Differential Diagnoses

Common auditory and vestibular pathologies are discussed in Chapter 2. For a list of the clinical utility of audiological tests and their corresponding anatomical area of evaluation, see Appendix 5–A. Appendix 5–B provides a series of common pathologies with common or expected patterns of adult diagnostic results.

Conclusions

While many focus on a comprehensive audiologic evaluation as the main form of an adult diagnostic assessment, it is important to remember that clinicians have access to an extensive battery of tests, including many objective assessments. Each test has its own unique contribution to the adult diagnostic assessment, and each will provide a certain amount of value dependent upon the individual case.

Recommended Readings

American Speech-Language-Hearing Association. (2005). *Guidelines for manual pure-tone threshold audiometry* [Guidelines]. http://www.asha.org/policy

Baguley, D., McFerran, D., & Hall, D. (2013). Tinnitus. *The Lancet, 382*(9904), 1600–1607.

Braza, M. D., Corbinm, N. E., Buss, E., & Monson, B. B. (2022). Effect of masker head orientation, listener age, and extended high-frequency sensitivity on speech recognition in spatially separated speech. *Ear & Hearing, 43*(1), 90–100.

Deshpande, A. K., & Hall, J. W. (2022). *Tinnitus: Advances in prevention, assessment, and management.* Plural Publishing.

Katz, J., Chasin, M., English, K. M., Hood, L. J., & Tillery, K. L. (Eds.). (2015). *Handbook of clinical audiology* (Vol. 7). Wolters Kluwer Health.

Lightfoot G. (2016). Summary of the N1–P2 cortical auditory evoked potential to estimate the auditory threshold in adults. *Seminars in Hearing, 37*(1), 1–8.

References

Aazh, H., Knipper, M., Danesh, A. A., Cavanna, A. E., Andersson, L., Paulin, J., . . . Moore, B. C. J. (2018). Insights from the third international conference on hyperacusis: causes, evaluation, diagnosis, and treatment. Noise & health, 20(95), 162–170. https://doi.org/10.4103/nah.NAH_2_18

Administration for Community Living. (2019). *Profile of older Americans.* https://acl.gov/aging-and-disability-in-america/data-and-research/profile-older-americans

American Academy of Audiology. (2010). *Diagnosis, treatment and management of children and adults with central auditory processing disorder* [Clinical practice guidelines]. https://www.audiology.org/practice-resources/practice-guidelines-and-standards/

American Association on Intellectual and Developmental Disabilities. (2023). *Defining criteria for intellectual disability.* AAIDD. https://www.aaidd.org/intellectual-disability/definition

American Speech-Language-Hearing Association. (1988). *Determining threshold level for speech* [Guidelines]. http://www.asha.org/policy

American Speech-Language-Hearing Association. (2005a). *(Central) auditory processing disorders—the role of the audiologist* [Position statement]. http://www.asha.org/policy/

American Speech-Language-Hearing Association. (2005b). *Guidelines for manual pure-tone threshold audiometry* [Guidelines]. http://www.asha.org/policy.

Badri, R., Siegel, J. H., & Wright, B. A. (2011). Auditory filter shapes and high-frequency hearing in adults who have impaired speech in noise performance despite clinically normal audiograms. *The Journal of the Acoustical Society of America, 129*(2), 852–863. https://doi.org/10.1121/1.3523476

Baguley, D., McFerran, D., & Hall, D. (2013). Tinnitus. *The Lancet, 382*(9904), 1600–1607.

Beattie, R. C., & Raffin, M. J. M. (1985). Reliability of threshold, slope, and pb max for monosyllabic words. *Journal of Speech and Hearing Disorders, 50*(2), 166–178.

Braza, M. D., Corbin, N. E., Buss, E., & Monson, B. B. (2022). Effect of masker head orientation, listener age, and extended high-frequency sensitivity on speech recognition in spatially separated speech. *Ear and Hearing, 43*(1), 90–100. https://doi.org/10.1097/AUD.0000000000001081

Carhart, R., & Jerger, J. (1959). Preferred method for clinical determination of pure-tone thresholds. *Journal of Speech and Hearing Disorders, 24*(4), 330–345.

Chung, W. H., Cho, D. Y., Choi, J. Y., & Hong, S. H. (2004). Clinical usefulness of extratympanic electrocochleography in the diagnosis of Ménière's disease. *Otology & Neurotology, 25*(2), 144–149.

Dauman, R., & Bouscau-Faure, F. (2005). Assessment and amelioration of hyperacusis in tinnitus patients. *Acta Oto-Laryngologica, 125*(5), 503–509.

Deshpande, A. K., & Hall, J. W. (2022). *Tinnitus: Advances in prevention, assessment, and management.* Plural Publishing.

Dhar, S., & Hall, J. W., III. (2018). *Otoacoustic emissions: Principles, procedures, and protocols* (2nd ed.). Plural Publishing.

Durmaz, A., Karahatay, S., Satar, B., Birkent, H., & Hidir, Y. (2009). Efficiency of Stenger test in confirming profound, unilateral pseudohypacusis. *The Journal of Laryngology & Otology, 123,* 840–844.

Egan, J. P. (1948). Articulation testing methods. *Laryngoscope, 58*(9), 955–991.

Feeney, M., & Schairer, K. (2014). Acoustic stapedius reflex measurement. In J. Katz, M. Chasin, K. English, L. Hood, & K. Tillery (Eds.), *Handbook of clinical audiology* (7th ed., pp. 165–186). Lippincott Williams and Wilkins.

Ferreira, G. M., Harrison, B. J., & Fontenelle, L. F. (2013). Hatred of sounds: Misophonic disorder or just an underreported psychiatric symptom? *Annals of Clinical Psychiatry, 25*(4), 271–274.

Gumus, N. M., Gumus, M., Unsal, S., Yuksel, M., & Gunduz, M. (2016). Examination of insert ear interaural attenuation (IA) values in audiological evaluations. *Clinical and Investigative Medicine, 39*(6), 27507.

Guthrie, L. A., & Mackersie, C. L. (2009). A comparison of presentation levels to maximize word recognition scores. *Journal of the American Academy of Audiology, 20*(6), 381–390.

Hall, J. III, & Mueller, G. (1998). *Audiologists' Desk Reference* (Vol. 2). Singular Publishing Group.

Harada, C. N., Love, M. C. N., & Triebel, K. L. (2013). Normal cognitive aging. *Clinics in Geriatric Medicine, 29*(4), 737–752.

Hedden, T., & Gabrieli, J. D. (2004). Insights into the ageing mind: A view from cognitive neuroscience. *Nature Reviews Neuroscience, 5*(2), 87–96.

Hirsh, I. J., Davis, H., Silverman, S. R., Reynolds, E. G., Eldert, E., & Benson, R. W. (1952). Development of materials for speech audiometry. *Journal of Speech and Hearing Disorders, 17,* 321–337.

Hoffman, H. J., & Reed, G. W. (2004). Epidemiology of tinnitus. *Tinnitus: Theory and Management, 16,* 41.

Hunter, L., & Sanford, C. (2014). Tympanometry and wideband acoustic immittance. In J. Katz, M. Chasin, K. English, L. Hood, & K. Tillery (Eds.), *Handbook of clinical audiology* (7th ed., pp. 137–163). Lippincott Williams and Wilkins.

Jerger J. (1970). Clinical experience with impedance audiometry. *Archives of Otolaryngology, 92*(4), 311–324. https://doi.org/10.1001/archotol.1970.04310040005002

Kahneman, D. (1973). *Attention and effort.* Prentice-Hall.

Khalfa, S., Dubal, S., Veuillet, E., Perez–Diaz, F., Jouvent, R., & Collet, L. (2002). Psychometric normalization of a hyperacusis questionnaire. *Journal for Oto-Rhino-Laryngology and Its Related Specialties, 64*(6), 435–442.

Killion, M. C., Niquette, P. A., Gudmundsen, G. I., Revit, L. J., & Banerjee, S. (2004). Development of a quick speech-in-noise test for measuring signal-to-noise ratio loss in normal-hearing and hearing-impaired listeners. *Journal of the Acoustical Society of America, 116,* 2395–2405.

Klein, A. J., Armstrong, B. L., Greer, M. K., & Brown, F. R., 3rd (1990). Hyperacusis and otitis media in individuals with Williams syndrome. *Journal of Speech and Hearing Disorders, 55*(2), 339–344. https://doi.org/10.1044/jshd.5502.339

Lawson, G. D., & Peterson, M. E. (2011). *Speech audiometry.* Plural Publishing.

Lehiste, I., & Peterson, G. (1959). Linguistic considerations in the study of speech intelligibility. *Journal of the Acoustical Society of America, 31,* 280–286.

Lezak, M. D., Howieson, D. B., Bigler, E. D., & Tranel, D. (2012). *Neuropsychological assessment* (5th ed.). Oxford University Press.

Lidén, G., Peterson, J. L., & Björkman, G. (1969). Tympanometry. A method for analysis of middle-ear function. *Acta Oto-Laryngologica. Supplementum, 263,* 218–224.

Lin, F. R., Yaffe, K., Xia, J., Xue, Q. L., Harris, T. B., Purchase–Helzner, E., . . . Health ABC Study Group, F. T. (2013). Hearing loss and cognitive decline in older adults. *JAMA Internal Medicine, 173*(4), 293–299.

Mahoney, C. F. O., & Luxon, L. M. (1996). Misdiagnosis of hearing loss due to ear canal collapse: A report of two cases. *Journal of Laryngology and Otology, 110,* 561–566.

Mathai, J. P., Aravinda, H. R., Appu, S., & Urs, H. R. (2021). Prevalence and audiological findings of functional hearing loss: A retrospective study. *Journal of Indian Speech Language & Hearing Association, 35*(2), 33–38.

Meikle, M. B., Stewart, B. J., Griest, S. E., & Henry, J. A. (2008). Tinnitus outcomes assessment. *Trends in Amplification, 12*(3), 223–235. https://doi.org/10.1177/1084713808319943

Meyer, D. H., & Mishler, E. T. (1985). Rollover measurements with Auditec NU-6 word lists. *Journal of Speech and Hearing Disorders, 50,* 356–360.

Meikle, M. B., Henry, J. A., Griest, S. E., Stewart, B. J., Abrams, H. B., McArdle, R., . . . Vernon, J. A. (2012). The tinnitus functional index: Development of a new clinical measure for chronic, intrusive tinnitus. *Ear and Hearing, 33*(2), 153–176.

Michiels, S., Ganz Sanchez, T., Oron, Y., Gilles, A., Haider, H. F., Erlandsson, S., . . . Hall, D. A. (2018). Diagnostic criteria for somatosensory tinnitus: A Delphi process and face-to-face meeting to establish consensus. *Trends in Hearing, 22*, 2331216518796403.

Moore, B. C., Huss, M., Vickers, D. A., Glasberg, B. R., & Alcántara, J. I. (2000). A test for the diagnosis of dead regions in the cochlea. *British Journal of Audiology, 34*(4), 205–224.

Murman, D. L. (2015, August). The impact of age on cognition. *Seminars in Hearing, 36*(3), 111–121.

Newman, C. W., Jacobson, G. P., & Spitzer, J. B. (1996). Development of the Tinnitus Handicap Inventory. *Archives of Otolaryngology-Head & Neck Surgery, 122*(2), 143–148.

Perkins, C. J., & Mitchell, S. (2022). *Audiology clinical masking*. StatPearls Publishing.

Pichora-Fuller, M. K., Kramer, S. E., Eckert, M. A., Edwards, B., Hornsby, B. W., Humes, L. E., . . . Wingfield, A. (2016). Hearing impairment and cognitive energy: The framework for understanding effortful listening (FUEL). *Ear and Hearing, 37*, 5S–27S.

Salthouse, T. (2012). Consequences of age-related cognitive declines. *Annual Review of Psychology, 63*, 201.

Salthouse, T. A. (2009). When does age-related cognitive decline begin? *Neurobiology of Aging, 30*(4), 507–514.

Salthouse, T. A., & Meinz, E. J. (1995). Aging, inhibition, working memory, and speed. *The Journals of Gerontology Series B: Psychological Sciences and Social Sciences, 50*(6), P297–P306.

Schlauch, R. S., & Nelson, P. (2015). Puretone evaluation. In J. Katz, M. Chasin, K. English, L. J. Hood, & K. L. Tillery (Eds.), *Handbook of clinical audiology* (7th ed., pp. 29–47). Wolters Kluwer.

Schröder, A., Vulink, N., & Denys, D. (2013). Misophonia: Diagnostic criteria for a new psychiatric disorder. *PLoS ONE, 8*(1), e54706.

Silverman, S. R., & Hirsh, I. J. (1955). Problems related to the use of speech in clinical audiometry. *Annals of Otology, Rhinology, and Laryngology, 64*(4), 1234–1244. https://doi.org/10.1177/000348945 506400424

Silverman, J. J., Galanter, M., Jackson-Triche, M., Jacobs, D. G., Lomax, J. W., Riba, M. B., . . . Yager, J. (2015). The American Psychiatric Association practice guidelines for the psychiatric evaluation of adults. *American Journal of Psychiatry, 172*(8), 798–802.

Sung, R. J., & Sung, G. S. (1976). Study of the classical and modified alternate binaural loudness balance tests in normal and pathological ears. *Journal of the American Audiology Society, 2*(2), 49–53.

Surprenant, A. M., & DiDonato, R. (2014). Community-dwelling older adults with hearing loss experience greater decline in cognitive function over time than those with normal hearing. *Evidence-Based Nursing, 17*(2), 60–61. https://doi.org/10.1136/ eb-2013-101375

Tillman, T. W., & Jerger, J. F. (1959). Some factors affecting the spondee thresholds in normal-hearing subjects. *Journal of Speech and Hearing Research, 2*(2), 141s146. https://doi.org/10.1044/jshr.0202.141

Tyler, R. S., Pienkowski, M., Roncancio, E. R., Jun, H. J., Brozoski, T., Dauman, N., . . . Moore, B. C. (2014). A review of hyperacusis and future directions: Part I. Definitions and manifestations. *American Journal of Audiology, 23*(4), 402–419.

Vernon, J. A. (1987). Pathophysiology of tinnitus: A special case—hyperacusis and a proposed treatment. *The American Journal of Otology, 8*(3), 201–202.

Vitoratou, S., Hayes, C., Uglik–Marucha, E., & Gregory, J. (2020). Selective sound sensitivity syndrome scale (s–five): A psychometric tool for assessing misophonia. Summary on three waves of sampling and analysis. *Prominent Papers in Psych, 1*–29.

Wang, T. C., Chang, T. Y., Tyler, R., Lin, Y. J., Liang, W. M., Shau, Y. W., . . . Tsai, M. H. (2020). Noise induced hearing loss and tinnitus—new research developments and remaining gaps in disease assessment, treatment, and prevention. *Brain Sciences, 10*(10), 732.

Willems, M., Acke, F., Lannon, B., Leyssens, L., Maes, L., & Marks, L. (2022). Global data on ear and hearing screening in an intellectual disability population. *American Journal on Intellectual and Developmental Disabilities, 127*(2), 125–134. https:// doi.org/10.1352/1944–7558–127.2.125

Wilson, P. H., Henry, J., Bowen, M., & Haralambous, G. (1991). Tinnitus Reaction Questionnaire: Psychometric properties of a measure of distress associated with tinnitus. *Journal of Speech, Language, and Hearing Research*, *34*(1), 197–201.

Wilson, R. H., & Burks, C. A. (2005). The use of 35 words to evaluate hearing loss in terms of signal-to-babble ratio: A clinical protocol. *Journal of Rehabilitation Research and Development*, *42*, 839–852.

Wilson, R. H., McArdle, R. A., & Smith, S. L. (2007). An evaluation of the BKB-SIN, HINT, Quick-SIN, and WIN materials on listeners with normal hearing and listeners with hearing loss. *Journal of*

Speech, Language, and Hearing Research, *50*, 844–856.

Wu, M. S., Lewin, A. B., Murphy, T. K., & Storch, E. A. (2014). Misophonia: Incidence, phenomenology, and clinical correlates in an undergraduate student sample. *Journal of Clinical Psychology*, *70*(10), 994–1007.

Yacullo, W. S. (2015). Clinical masking. In J. Katz, M. Chasin, K. English, L. J. Hood, & K. L. Tillery (Eds.), *Handbook of clinical audiology* (7th ed., pp. 77–111). Wolters Kluwer.

✎ Practice Questions

1. A 37-year-old female is on your schedule for a comprehensive audiological evaluation. Which assessments should be completed as part of this evaluation?

   a. Pure-tone air and bone conduction, SRT, and word recognition

   b. Pure-tone air conduction, SRT, and word recognition

   c. Pure-tone air and bone conduction, SRT, and acoustic immittance

   d. Pure-tone air conduction, SRT, word recognition, and acoustic immittance

Explanation: To be considered a full comprehensive audiologic evaluation, all four assessments of pure-tone air- and bone-conduction audiometry along with SRT and word recognition must be completed. When all four are completed in one session, this is defined as a comprehensive audiologic evaluation and billed using the CPT code 92557. Acoustic immittance is billed under separate codes and is not necessary for a comprehensive evaluation. Therefore, answer a is the correct answer.

2. The speech recognition threshold (SRT) can be best defined as:

   a. The lowest level an individual can understand at least one NU-6 word

   b. The lowest level that an individual can understand at least 50% of spondee words

   c. The lowest level that an individual can understand at least 75% of spondee words

   d. The lowest level that an individual can understand at least 50% of NU-6 words

Explanation: The SRT is defined as the level that a patient can understand a closed set of words 50% of the time. Familiarization and verification of the words to the patient is an important step in SRT testing as it has been shown to influence the threshold by as much as 5 dB. This is important because one of the most common clinical uses of SRT is cross-check validation of pure-tone thresholds. Therefore, answer b is the correct answer.

3. Your next patient of the afternoon is a 58-year-old male who was referred to you with the complaint of right constant acute tinnitus. Based on your knowledge of tinnitus, the time frame for acute tinnitus would mean that the patient has been suffering from tinnitus for:

   a. Three months or less

   b. Six months or less

   c. Six months or more

   d. A year or less

Explanation: When describing the duration of tinnitus, the terms chronic and acute are used. When an individual is experiencing acute tinnitus, that means they have experienced these symptoms for 6 months or less. With that in mind, answer b is the correct answer.

4. Mr. Friedman, a right-handed 24-year-old male with complaints of difficulty listening in background noise and on the phone, is seen for an audiological evaluation. Otoscopy was clear bilaterally, and the next test was immittance. Type A tympanograms were recorded bilaterally. On reflex testing, there are present responses in the left ipsilateral and contralateral conditions, but absent responses in the right ipsilateral and contralateral conditions. Without further testing, where would the suspected lesion be?

   a. CN VIII right

   b. CN VIII left

   c. CN VII right

   d. CN VII left

Explanation: First, we must remember that ANSI standards for MEMRs are based on the stimulus ear. Present left ipsilateral responses suggest that the middle ear, cochlea, cranial nerve (CN) VIII, ventral cochlear nucleus (VCN), superior olivary complex (SOC), facial nerve nuclei (FNN), and the facial nerve (CN VII) are functioning properly on that side. Absent right ipsilateral responses suggest that there is an issue in one of those structures on the right side. Present left contralateral responses suggest that the left cochlea, left CN VIII, left VCN, right and left SOC, right FNN, and right CN VII are functioning. Absent right contralateral responses suggests that the issues are either in the right CN VIII or VCN, so a is the correct answer.

5. A 42-year-old male presents to your office with complaints of right hearing loss and tinnitus. He stated that he is a factory worker and noted the issues suddenly after work one day when an explosion occurred. Tympanometry revealed Type A tympanograms bilaterally. DPOAEs were present and robust. MEMRs were present bilaterally. Audiometry revealed a unilateral moderate to moderately severe sensorineural hearing loss in the right ear. You completed the Stenger test, during which the patient did not respond. What would be your diagnosis?

   a. Conductive hearing loss

   b. Presbycusis

   c. Retrocochlear hearing loss

   d. Nonorganic hearing loss

Explanation: Although the patient presented with hearing loss and tinnitus in the right ear, the objective tests (tympanometry, DPOAEs, and MEMRs) do not align with our subjective findings (audiometry). Additionally, the patient did not respond during the Stenger test (positive Stenger). As such, the patient would be diagnosed with nonorganic hearing loss and would be referred for further testing such as an ABR, ENT, and/or psychology. Therefore, d is the answer.

6. Which of the following is true of otoacoustic emissions?

   a. They are impacted by disorders of the auditory nerve.

   b. They are by-products of OHC function and the cochlear amplifier.

   c. They are not impacted by middle ear dysfunction.

   d. The strength of the emission is the most important quality of the response.

Explanation: The cochlear amplifier is created by OHC motility. As the traveling wave moves through cochlear fluid creating displacement of the basilar membrane, there is a significant energy loss due to viscous drag. Because of this energy loss, the cochlear amplifier is a necessary component of cochlear function. The cochlear amplifier enhances the traveling wave as it loses energy. As a result of the cochlear amplifier, there is displacement of the basilar membrane that creates energy movement back toward the basal end of the cochlea generating vibration on the oval and round windows and thus vibration of the ossicular chain and tympanic membrane. Therefore, answer b is the correct answer.

7. What is one of the main advantages of DPOAEs over TEOAEs?
   a. DPOAEs offer better cochlear frequency resolution.
   b. Middle ear status does not impact DPOAE responses.
   c. DPOAEs can be observed with higher degrees of hearing loss.
   d. DPOAEs are a better predictor of behavioral hearing thresholds.

Explanation: Due to the continuous tone presentation used with DPOAEs, they tend to be impacted less by subtle ear conditions compared to TEOAEs. Therefore, DPOAEs can be recorded in individuals with up to moderate hearing losses, whereas TEOAEs are typically absent in individuals with more than a mild hearing loss (20–30 dB HL). Therefore, answer c is the correct answer.

8. You completed a neurodiagnostic ABR on a 49-year-old male patient. You noted that wave __ was absent. As such, you completed an ECochG to attempt to see this wave, which is generated where?
   a. I; distal end of the VIIIth nerve
   b. I; proximal end of the VIIIth nerve
   c. III; distal end of the VIIIth nerve
   d. III; caudal brainstem; near superior olivary complex (SOC) and trapezoid body

Explanation: An ECochG is a variation of an ABR, which increases the amplitude of wave I due to different click rates, intensity levels, and transducers. When wave I is not present, an ECochG can be utilized. Wave I (also referred to as AP) is generated at the distal end of the VIIIth nerve, which would make a the correct answer.

9. A 36-year-old male presents with an onset right hearing loss and tinnitus in the last 2 days. He denied any hearing loss, tinnitus, and other audiologic symptoms prior to this occurrence. He denied recent noise exposure, otalgia, aural fullness, and dizziness. Audiological testing revealed normal hearing in the left ear and a moderate flat SNHL in the left ear. Tympanometry was normal. Ipsilateral MEMRs were present in the left ear and absent in the right. Clinically, this is most consistent with which pathology?
   a. Otosclerosis
   b. Sudden SNHL (SSNHL)
   c. Otitis media with effusion
   d. Ménière's disease

Explanation: Based on patient complaints, timeline (of 2 days), and audiological findings, the most consistent pathology is SSNHL. Therefore, b is the correct answer. It is imperative for audiologists to refer these patients to ENT for treatment as soon as possible. Treatment should be initiated as soon as possible after the onset of the hearing loss and generally consists of systemic (oral pill) or intratympanic injection of corticosteroids in order to reduce inflammation or swelling. Treatment is difficult because only about 10% of patients with SSNHL have an identifiable etiology. When treatment is delayed by 2 weeks or more, it becomes less likely that permanent hearing loss will improve.

10. A 48-year-old female presented in the clinic with the following findings: normal hearing sensitivity in the right ear and a mild sloping to moderate SNHL in the left ear. Word recognition scores were 92% in the right ear and 24% in the left ear. High-intensity ABR testing revealed normal findings in the right ear and prolonged wave V latency in the left ear with a prolonged wave I to V interpeak latency. These findings would be most consistent with which pathology?

    a. Ménière's disease

    b. Otosclerosis

    c. Otitis media

    d. Acoustic neuroma

Explanation: The patient is presenting with left SNHL, poorer than expected word recognition scores, and prolonged absolute and interpeak latencies on an ABR. Additionally, findings are asymmetrical for all testing completed. Therefore, these findings point to a suspected acoustic neuroma, which is answer d.

Appendix 5–A

Objective Assessment, Clinical Utility, and Anatomical Sites of Testing

OBJECTIVE ASSESSMENT	CLINICAL UTILITY	ANATOMICAL SITE
Tympanometry	Tympanic membrane mobility Ossicular/middle ear pathologies	Tympanic membrane Middle ear
Wideband Tympanometry	Tympanic membrane mobility Middle ear pathologies	Tympanic membrane Middle ear
Middle Ear Muscle Reflex	Diagnosis of a retrocochlear versus cochlear site of lesion Used as a cross-check principle for cochlear implant testing	Stapedial muscle Low auditory brainstem pathway
Acoustic Reflex Decay	Diagnosis of a retrocochlear versus cochlear site of lesion	Stapedial muscle Low auditory brainstem pathway
Otoacoustic Emissions	Reflect the frequency resolution of the cochlea Can be a predictor of hearing loss Newborn hearing screenings Aid in differential diagnosis between cochlear and retrocochlear pathology	Outer hair cells and cochlear amplifier Highly influenced by outer and middle ear systems
Auditory Brainstem Response (Waves I–V)	Threshold estimation Site-of-lesion testing and physiological integrity of auditory pathways	Wave I: Distal end of CN VIII Wave II: Proximal end of CN VIII Wave III: Caudal brainstem; near cochlear nucleus Wave IV: Superior olivary complex (SOC) Wave V: Lateral lemniscus (LL) with contributions of the inferior colliculus (IC) Trough after V: IC
Middle Latency Response (Na-Pa-Nb-Pb)	Threshold estimation site-of-lesion testing and physiological integrity of auditory pathways	Thalamocortical pathways (thalamus through primary auditory cortex)

continues

APPENDIX 5–A. *continued*

OBJECTIVE ASSESSMENT	CLINICAL UTILITY	ANATOMICAL SITE
Late Latency Response (P1-N1-P2)	Threshold estimation Physiological integrity at the level of the primary auditory cortex Monitoring neural plasticity and maturation of auditory pathways, especially after cochlear implantation Amplification verification through aided responses	P1: Primary auditory cortex (hippocampus, planum temporale, lateral temporal cortex) N1: Primary auditory cortex and superior temporal gyrus (Heschl's gyrus) P2: Primary and secondary auditory cortices
MMN	Reflects the cerebral response of auditory memory, discrimination, and processing abilities	Auditory cortex, frontal cortex, hippocampus, thalamus
P300	Reflects processing speed and neural effort on various auditory processing tasks	Primary auditory cortex, frontal cortex, hippocampus

Appendix 5–B

Differential Diagnosis

PATHOLOGY	COMPLAINTS/ HISTORY	OTOSCOPY	IMMITTANCE	OAES	PURE-TONE AUDIOMETRY	SPEECH AUDIOMETRY	ELECTRO-PHYSIOLOGY	INTERVENTION
Cerumen Impaction	Decreased hearing; aural fullness; otalgia	Occluding Cerumen	Tymp: Type B tympanogram with small ECV MEMR: WNT Decay: WNT	Reduced to absent	CHL or mixed HL	SRT-PTA match Good to excellent WRS	TABR & NABR: absolute latencies prolonged; normal interpeak latencies; reduced amplitude ECOG: reduced SP/AP	Cerumen removal ENT referral
Exostoses	No major complaints	Bony growths in EC	All normal	Present	Normal	SRT-PTA match Good to excellent WRS	All normal	ENT referral
Otitis Externa (OE)	Drainage; aural fullness; otalgia; foul smell; decreased hearing	Red EC; debris in EC	Tymp: Type As or B tympanogram with normal ECV MEMR: WNT Decay: WNT	Reduced to absent	CHL or mixed; max conductive component of 60 dB HL	SRT-PTA match Good to excellent WRS	TABR & NABR: absolute latencies prolonged; normal interpeak latencies; reduced amplitudes ECOG: WNT; reduced to absent SP/AP	ENT referral Retest after medical management

continues

241

PATHOLOGY	COMPLAINTS/ HISTORY	OTOSCOPY	IMMITTANCE	OAES	PURE-TONE AUDIOMETRY	SPEECH AUDIOMETRY	ELECTRO-PHYSIOLOGY	INTERVENTION
Otitis Media with Effusion (OME)	Aural fullness; otalgia; drainage, decreased hearing; foul smell; tinnitus	Red EC and TM; no landmarks visualized; air bubbles; debris in EC	Tymp: Type As or B tympanogram with normal ECV MEMR: WNT Decay: WNT	Reduced to absent	CHL or mixed; max conductive component of 60 dB HL	SRT-PTA match Good to excellent WRS	TABR & NABR: absolute latencies prolonged; normal interpeak latencies; reduced amplitudes ECOG: WNT; reduced to absent SP/AP	ENT referral Retest after medical management
Tympanic Membrane Perforation	Aural fullness; otalgia; drainage, decreased hearing; tinnitus	Red EC; visualize perforation; debris in EC (may be related to OME or OE)	Tymp: Type B tympanogram with large ECV MEMR: WNT Decay: WNT	Reduced to absent	CHL or mixed; max conductive component of 60 dB HL	SRT-PTA match Good to excellent WRS	TABR & NABR: absolute latencies prolonged; normal interpeak latencies; reduced amplitudes ECOG: WNT; reduced to absent SP/AP	ENT referral Retest after medical management
Ossicular Chain Disarticulation	Decreased hearing; possible previous trauma	Generally normal	Tympanogram: Type A or Ad MEMR: WNT Decay: WNT	Reduced to absent	CHL; max conductive component of 60 dB HL	SRT-PTA match Good to excellent WRS	TABR & NABR: absolute latencies prolonged; normal interpeak latencies; reduced amplitudes ECOG: WNT; reduced to absent SP/AP	ENT referral Retest after medical management

PATHOLOGY	COMPLAINTS/ HISTORY	OTOSCOPY	IMMITTANCE	OAES	PURE-TONE AUDIOMETRY	SPEECH AUDIOMETRY	ELECTRO-PHYSIOLOGY	INTERVENTION
Otosclerosis	Decreased hearing; aural fullness	Generally normal	Tympanogram: Type A or As MEMR: WNT Decay: WNT	Reduced to absent	CHL; max conductive component of 60 dB HL Carhart's notch noted in BC at 2 kHz	SRT-PTA match Good to excellent WRS	TABR & NABR: absolute latencies prolonged; normal interpeak latencies; reduced amplitudes ECOG: WNT; reduced to absent SP/AP	ENT referral Retest after medical management
Tinnitus	Perception of noise; decreased hearing	Generally normal	Generally normal MEMR: normal to absent Decay: normal to abnormal	Normal to absent	Normal to SNHL	SRT-PTA match Poor to excellent WRS (dependent on degree of HL)	TABR & NABR: dependent on degree/configuration of HL ECOG: WNT; normal to absent SP/AP	ENT/mental health professional referral Tinnitus therapies
Conductive Hearing Loss	Decreased hearing; aural fullness	Normal to abnormal depending on pathology	Tymp: any type depending on pathology MEMR: normal to absent Decay: normal to abnormal	Reduced to absent	Hearing loss with ABG; max conductive component of 60 dB HL	SRT-PTA match Good to excellent WRS	NABR: absolute latencies prolonged; normal interpeak latencies; reduced amplitude ECOG: reduced to absent SP/AP	ENT referral Retest after medical management Amplification/cochlear implant/OID

continues

PATHOLOGY	COMPLAINTS/ HISTORY	OTOSCOPY	IMMITTANCE	OAES	PURE-TONE AUDIOMETRY	SPEECH AUDIOMETRY	ELECTRO- PHYSIOLOGY	INTERVENTION
Mixed Hearing Loss	Decreased hearing; aural fullness	Normal to abnormal depending on pathology	Tymp: any type (depending on pathology) MEMR: normal to absent Decay: normal to abnormal	Reduced to absent	SNHL with ABG	SRT-PTA match Poor to excellent (dependent on degree of SNHL)	NABR: absolute latencies prolonged; small—no wave I; prolonged interpeak latencies; reduced amplitude ECOG: reduced to absent SP/AP	ENT referral Retest after medical management
Sensorineural Hearing Loss	Decreased hearing; tinnitus; poor word understanding; difficulty communicating	Normal	Tymp: Type A MEMR: normal to absent (depending on degree of HL) Decay: normal to abnormal	Reduced to Absent	HL with no ABG	SRT-PTA match Poor to excellent (dependent on degree of HL)	NABR: absolute latencies normal to prolonged; small—no wave I; normal interpeak latencies; reduced amplitude; poor morphology ECOG: reduced to absent SP/AP	ENT referral for unilateral/ asymmetrical findings Amplification/ cochlear implant
Noise- Induced Hearing Loss (NIHL)	Decreased hearing; tinnitus; poor word understanding; difficulty communicating; noise exposure	Normal	Tymp: Type A MEMR: normal to absent (depending on degree of HL) Decay: normal to abnormal	Reduced to absent	SNHL with notch at 3–4 kHz	SRT-PTA match Poor to excellent (dependent on degree of HL)	NABR: absolute latencies normal to prolonged; small—no wave I; normal interpeak latencies; reduced amplitude; poor morphology ECOG: reduced to absent SP/AP	ENT referral for unilateral/ asymmetrical findings Amplification/ cochlear implant

PATHOLOGY	COMPLAINTS/ HISTORY	OTOSCOPY	IMMITTANCE	OAES	PURE-TONE AUDIOMETRY	SPEECH AUDIOMETRY	ELECTRO-PHYSIOLOGY	INTERVENTION
Sudden Sensorineural Hearing Loss (SSHL)	Sudden HL; tinnitus	Normal	Tymp: Type A MEMR: normal to absent (depending on degree of HL) Decay: normal to abnormal	Reduced to absent	HL with no ABG	SRT-PTA match Poor to good (dependent on degree of HL)	NABR: absolute latencies normal to prolonged; small—no wave I; normal interpeak latencies; reduced amplitude; poor morphology ECOG: reduced to absent SP/AP	Immediate ENT referral Should be seen within 48 hours of onset of complaints
Retrocochlear Pathology	Decreased hearing; tinnitus; poor word understanding; difficulty communicating	Normal	Tymp: Type A MEMR: elevated to absent Decay: Abnormal	Normal	Normal to SNHL	SRT-PTA match Poor to fair (dependent on pathology) WRS is often poorer than expected with degree of HL	NABR: prolonged Wave III, V, and/ or interpeak Waves I–V • absence of waves • poor morphology • significant interaural differences	ENT referral

Note. WNT: would not test; PTA: pure-tone average; WRS: word recognition score; TABR: threshold ABR; NABR: neurodiagnostic ABR.

Chapter 6

Pediatric Assessment and Differential Diagnosis

Tori J. S. Gustafson and Candace Bourland Hicks

Case History Considerations

The case history is an important part of a pediatric audiological evaluation, one that provides information that the audiologist must consider related to risk factors for hearing loss and developmental factors. The case history assists the audiologist in planning or modifying plans for testing, along with assisting with recommendations and referrals following the testing.

Parent/Caregiver Concerns

The audiologist can gauge the parent/caregiver concerns by starting with a general question (e.g., what do you think of your child's hearing?). This provides a way to determine concerns without leading them to answer a certain way (e.g., only answering the specific questions given by the clinician, which may not relate to the true concern) or to answer only yes/no.

Pregnancy/Birth

Case history questions should address pregnancy, including maternal sicknesses and exposure to drugs or alcohol. Questions related to pregnancy can provide the audiologist with considerations for embryological development of infant in the womb.

- For a review of embryological development, see Chapter 2 of this text or Hill (2017).
  - □ Insults during the first trimester lead to greater risk for development of the inner ear.
  - □ Depending on timing of fetal insult, may lead to a lack of development of portions of the ear. Examples of inner ear aplasia (which would lead to sensorineural hearing loss) include:
    - Michel Aplasia/Complete Labyrinthine Aplasia: inner ear does not develop; insult in third week of pregnancy
    - Common cavity: aplasia with a single auditory/vestibular cavity; insult in fourth week
    - Mondini's Aplasia/Incomplete Partition: small cochlea, 1 to 1.5 cochlear turns (classical Mondini's); insult in seventh week (Jackler et al., 1987)

- □ Maturation continues into the second and third trimesters.
- ■ Ask questions related to the birth, including information such as:
  - □ Premature birth
  - □ Gestational age at birth
  - □ Birth weight
  - □ Neonatal intensive care unit (NICU) stay
    - If yes, how long was the stay and what type of treatments did the child receive?

These questions can provide insight into other possible developmental delays and comorbidities the child may have.

Risk Factors for Hearing Loss

Questions should also address risk factors for hearing loss (Joint Committee on Infant Hearing, 2019), such as anoxia, NICU stay of > 5 days, hyperbilirubinemia treated with exchange transfusion, syndromes associated with hearing loss, craniofacial anomalies, and ototoxic medications.

- ■ Consider risk factors of delayed onset or progressive hearing loss, such as family history of progressive or delayed-onset childhood hearing loss, extracorporeal membrane oxygenation (ECMO), and (s)TORCH infections.
- ■ Always consider caregiver concern for hearing or speech-language development.
- ■ Another risk factor is a family history of permanent childhood hearing loss; see Chapter 2 for a review of genetic disorders and patterns.
- ■ Questions for the family should include if loss is potentially progressive.

Medical History

In planning testing and prioritizing the ordering of testing, the medical history is an important part of the pediatric audiologic assessment. The medical history includes both otologic-related history and general medical history.

- ■ Otitis media (ear infections)
  - □ Gather information on how many infections the child has had in various age ranges, how these infections were treated, and when the most recent infection was.
  - □ Treatment questions can include whether the child received pressure equalization (PE) tubes. If so, questions would relate to when the PE tubes were received, how many sets the child has had, and if they know if the PE tubes are still in place.
  - □ Information regarding otitis media can assist with the testing plan by allowing the audiologist to consider if the child may have sensitivity to having their ears touched, to consider if drainage may be present that could impact the transducer chosen, and to consider if the order of testing needs to be modified to prioritize collecting of low-frequency thresholds.
- ■ Hospitalizations and reasons
  - □ Questions can address areas such as if head trauma was present and if treatment included use of ototoxic medications.

- Other diagnoses
  - □ Some diagnoses could show a connection to hearing loss.
    - Craniofacial disorders—often associated with conductive hearing loss
    - Certain syndromes associated with sensorineural hearing loss (e.g., Waardenburg)
    - See Etiology of Pediatric Hearing Loss section later in this chapter for additional information.
  - □ Some diagnoses could impact the plan of testing.
    - Syndromes associated with atresia can impact plan of testing (e.g., which transducer to use).
    - Visual impairment can change the plan for visual reinforcement audiometry (VRA) and conditioned play audiometry (CPA) testing.
    - Children with anxiety and sensory sensitivities may need adjustments to testing approaches.

Other Developmental Areas

- Speech-language development, which is often a primary concern for toddlers who are seen for audiological testing
  - □ Inquire about information about expressive and receptive abilities, including questions such as what percentage of the child's speech is understandable to a familiar adult (e.g., a parent) and for an unfamiliar adult. Questions can also include if the child can understand one- or two-step directions.
  - □ Ask if certain sounds or concepts are missing.
  - □ Speech-language ability could also impact the plan of testing. For example, is the child's language appropriate for the word recognition list chosen based on developmental age rather than chronological age? Is the child's speech intelligible, which could impact if you choose a word repetition versus a picture-pointing task?

 AUDIOLOGY NUGGET

As a general rule, by 24 months of age, a child should be able to produce 70% of consonants correctly and will have two- to three-word phrases. The child's speech should be 26% to 50% intelligible at this age. By 36 months of age, speech should be 75% intelligible, and by 48 months of age, speech should be 100% intelligible (Bleile, 2015).

- Motor and cognitive development
  - □ Development of motor or cognitive function may provide clues as to the overall developmental age of the child. This information helps determine what behavioral testing is appropriate and what should be included in the test battery.
    - Consider motor problems if picture pointing or body part identification will be part of speech testing.

- Problems in motor coordination can impact response times for VRA and CPA. If motor issues are present, care must be taken in the choice of appropriate CPA toys.
  - Cognitive delays can impact the choice of test (i.e., base the test on developmental age) and may lead to modification of instructions.
- Other areas of development can impact testing, such as social development. For example, a child with autism spectrum disorder (ASD) could benefit from a task such as tangible reinforcement operant conditioning audiometry (TROCA) that provides tangible reinforcement rather than CPA.

 AUDIOLOGY NUGGET

The developmental age of a child, as opposed to chronological age (i.e., birth date to current date), should be considered in planning for audiological testing. The parent may be able to report developmental age (for example, from a physician or from assessments completed by an early intervention program). However, in many cases, the clinician must estimate developmental age from development in other areas. Motor and cognitive milestones can provide information, which can help the audiologist plan testing. Some important milestones from the Centers for Disease Control and Prevention (CDC, n.d.) include:

- 4 months: when held, the child can hold their head without support.
- 6 months: the child can roll from front to back; the child reaches for objects.
- 9 months: the child can sit up independently without support and will look when their name is called.
- 12 months: the child will wave and pull to a standing position; the child can walk with support.
- 15 months: the child can take steps independently and will try to use objects in a correct manner.
- 18 months: the child walks independently and can climb (e.g., on furniture); the child can copy activities and will point at objects to direct a person's attention to the object.
- 2 years: the child can run, kick a ball; the child can identify at least two body parts.

Support Services

- Early intervention services
  - Can include speech-language therapy, physical therapy, or occupational therapy
  - Information can help the audiologist in planning testing

- Example: if the child cannot sit without support and does not have head/neck control, testing with VRA may be impacted.

    □ Referrals to early intervention services may be recommended if the child is not receiving services.

- ■ Educational services

    □ Can include Individualized Education Program (IEP) or a 504 plan

    □ Ask questions about the educational setting.

    - Daycare; self-contained classroom

    □ Ask questions about the child's progress in the different academic subjects.

    □ Answers to these questions can lead to additional testing.

    - Is testing in background noise needed to make recommendations for services or for hearing assistive technology (HAT)?

    □ Answers to these questions can allow the audiologist to consider specific educational recommendations based on test results.

Functional Questionnaires

Functional testing is important in determining impact of hearing loss and in determining if treatment (hearing aid, cochlear implant, etc.) is providing functional benefit. Examples of functional questionnaires include:

- ■ Little Ears

    □ Parent questionnaire designed for children birth to 24 months of age

    □ Includes yes/no responses to questions such as children responding to distant sounds or looking for sound sources

- ■ Infant-Toddler Meaning Auditory Integration Scale (IT-MAIS)

    □ Parent questionnaire that addresses how/if the child responds spontaneously to sounds

- ■ PEACH/TEACH

    □ Parents' Evaluation of Aural/Oral Performance of Children (PEACH)

    - Parents rate the child on communication behaviors in quiet (e.g., responding to their name in quiet or talking on the telephone) and in noise (e.g., responding to their name in noise or recognizing environmental sounds in noise).

    □ Teachers' Evaluation of Aural/Oral Performance of Children (TEACH)

    - Teacher rates the child on communication behaviors in quiet (e.g., responding to their name in quiet or talking on the telephone) and in noise (e.g., responding to their name in noise or recognizing environmental sounds in noise).

For additional information, see Bagatto et al. (2011) and Deconde Johnson and Seaton (2021). Functional assessments specific to the academic environment are addressed in the Educational Audiology section later in this chapter.

Testing Considerations

As with adults, the purpose of pediatric audiological testing is to obtain a comprehensive picture of hearing abilities. However, pediatric testing often requires modifications to allow for the child's ability to respond according to their developmental age level. Testing may require more than one appointment to obtain the comprehensive results.

Otoscopic Considerations

Otoscopy, theoretically, should be completed prior to insertion of probes and insert earphones; however, this is not always a practical approach. Despite the benefits of performing otoscopy first, audiologists routinely elect to perform it later in the test session. Common reasons for this decision include sensitivities to touch or individuals being in their personal space that result in aversion to otoscopy.

- Examination includes the preauricular area, postauricular area, and auricle to examine for dermatologic issues such as sores, rashes, pits, and tags.
- Look for auricular malformations, size (micro or macro), and location (offset, low-, or high-set ears).
  - □ These malformations may be an indication of a syndrome or genetic contribution that may be associated with specific hearing loss.
- Next, examine the external ear canal and tympanic membrane (TM) for landmarks and anomalies, especially looking for signs of otitis media and presence of PE tubes.
- Otoscopic inspection
  - □ Choose appropriate specula size for canal.
  - □ Bridge/brace against the side of the head to allow contact to absorb force if bumped or patient moves suddenly.
  - □ Infants and toddlers should be braced by the caregiver (e.g., in a "side hug" position), which reduces child movement.
  - □ Visual distractions (e.g., showing a spinning toy in front of the child) can be beneficial.
  - □ Pull auricle to the back (sometimes will be back and downward as opposed to upward in adults).
  - □ Insert speculum tip and adjust tip to view the TM.
- Note that abnormalities in the outer ear and ear canal may be one factor associated with a conductive component on the audiogram and influence immittance findings. Possible otoscopic findings include:
  - □ Blockage by cerumen or foreign body
  - □ Otitis externa as a fungal growth in the ear canal
  - □ Necrotizing otitis externa can occur in immunocompromised individuals and necrotization can progress to the point of affecting cranial nerves.
  - □ Abnormal middle ear pressure (positive = bulging TM; negative = retracted TM)
  - □ Tympanosclerosis appears as white patches on the TM, caused by plaque buildup.

□ Scarring looks like white scratches on the TM; can be the result of infections, perforations, or PE tube placement.

□ Perforations can be in any area of the TM and range in sizes; the size and location impact hearing loss differently.

□ Monomeric membranes may appear as a perforation, where the outer layers of the TM have healed but not the fibrous layer(s), so there is a clear view into middle ear space.

□ Tympanoplasty may show atypical landmarks due to repair of the TM.

□ Otitis media signs include the TM may not be translucent (possibly red and retracted) and may appear discolored with infection with possibly bubbles or a meniscus.

□ PE tubes may be visualized for children with chronic or acute otitis media and may include short-acting grommets or longer-term T tubes.

Behavioral Techniques and Procedures

Behavioral Observation (BO) [previously known as Behavioral Observation Audiometry]

The audiologist presents stimuli and is then looking for responses (e.g., eyes widening, increase or decrease in sucking) from a patient who is not actively involved in the task. BO is used in infants up to 6 months of age but may be used in older children with developmental delays or other disorders such as cerebral palsy. No reinforcement is used, as studies show infants' responses are not impacted by such reinforcement (e.g., Hicks et al., 2000; Moore et al., 1977). There can be problems with habituation, with variability of responses, with repeatability of responses, and with bias of examiner.

Also note that BO responses are considered minimal response levels (MRLs: softest intensity that the clinician sees a response), not true thresholds. The MRLs are used as a measure of responsivity and should not be used for diagnosis of hearing loss or for treatment purposes (e.g., when fitting amplification). Instead, physiologic testing and functional testing should be utilized for diagnosis and treatment purposes. The responses obtained during BO can be used as confirmation of caregiver reports and can be used to show behavioral responses in conjunction with the physiologic testing (Diefendorf & Tharpe, 2017).

■ Testing considerations:
   □ Most often conducted in the soundfield (responses not ear specific); can be conducted via headphones or insert earphones if tolerated by the child, providing ear-specific information.

   □ Stimuli should be varied (narrowband noise [NBN], FRESH noise, warble tones, filtered songs) to prevent habituation.

   □ Ascending (i.e., increasing in stimulus intensity as opposed to decreasing intensity) presentations could help prevent habituation.

   □ The Pediatric Observation, Testing, and Tallying System (POTTS) form can be beneficial to document responses.

   □ The overall goal is to obtain responses within the speech-frequency range for at least a low-frequency (500 Hz) and a high-frequency sound (2000 Hz).

☐ Speech awareness testing (note that this is not threshold, but an MRL) is beneficial with BO, as this test can be beneficial in counseling parents when used along with other counseling tools.

AUDIOLOGY NUGGET

MRLs must be compared to age-appropriate behaviors rather than defining responses as a specific degree of hearing loss. For example, expected MRLs for warble tones are 70 to 75 dB HL for infants up to 4 months of age and 45 to 50 dB HL from infants 4 to 9 months of age (Northern & Downs, 2002). If an infant who is 5 months of age exhibits MRLs of 50 dB HL to warble tones, these results would be consistent with expected responses for a 5-month-old. However, if MRLs are obtained at 70 dB HL, these responses would be poorer than expected for a 5-month-old. Again, MRLs are not used to define hearing loss, although responses can be used as part of the cross-check principle (cross-checking electrophysiologic results) or as part of counseling with the family.

Visual Reinforcement Audiometry (VRA)

Visual reinforcement audiometry (VRA) is used with slightly older infants/toddlers (i.e., those who have controllable head movements and core strength to sit with minimal support, such as in a high-chair). The typical age range for VRA is 4 to 6 months of age up to 24 months of age based on developmental age (or until they can perform a conditioned play task). The audiologist is looking for active responses to sound (e.g., head turning) either in the soundfield (younger infants/toddlers, testing the better ear only) or with earphones (ear specific) or bone oscillator (can use if the infant/toddler tolerates them), with the responses being reinforced with visual stimuli (e.g., video, mechanical toy). Note that localization is not required for VRA, though the child will turn their head. Reinforcement occurs when an infant looks for the sound, regardless of whether the response is in the correct direction of the sound. Localization is required, however, for conditioned orientation reflex (COR), which includes conditioning to the task. If the child is well conditioned to the task, responses are considered thresholds as opposed to MRLs.

- Testing considerations:
  ☐ Conditioning can occur but is not required for VRA testing.
  ☐ Stimuli can be frequency specific (e.g., warble tones, NBN) or nonfrequency specific (speech, e.g., calling the child's name, repeated syllables).
  ☐ The overall goal is to obtain frequency-specific information within the speech frequency range.
    - Typical to test octave frequencies between 500 and 4000 Hz
    - Frequency order can be modified to ensure that at least one high-frequency response and one low-frequency response are obtained if the child habituates to the task.
    - If the child is still attending, consider testing under earphones (if initially testing in soundfield) or via bone conduction.

□ Considerations for testing include use of larger step sizes (e.g., 20 down/10 up until close to threshold) or using of an ascending technique to prevent habituation.

□ Make sure to use control trials to ensure that the child is not responding to a presentation pattern rather than hearing the sound.

□ For a more in-depth discussion of testing considerations, see Diefendorf and Tharpe (2017).

 KNOWLEDGE CHECKPOINT

VRA is often conducted in soundfield. When testing in soundfield, warble/frequency-modulated (FM) tones should be used instead of pure tones. This will prevent standing waves and will allow for a consistent signal even with movement of the child (ASHA, n.d.). Narrowband noise (NBN) may also be used. The child's head must be in the calibrated position within the booth, which is often marked.

When testing in soundfield, use of an assistant can be beneficial. The assistant can help center the child to look forward, allowing for easier visualization of head turns toward sounds. When using an assistant, it is important to ensure they do not provide any cues to the child. For example, the assistant may wear headphones and listen to noise through an external device (e.g., CD player). If this is not possible, the audiologist should provide direct instructions to the assistant to not provide any cues (e.g., calling attention to the sounds, stopping movement of distractor toys) when sounds are presented. If parents are in the booth with the child during testing, they should also be instructed to not provide cues to the child.

Conditioned Play Audiometry (CPA)

With CPA, the audiologist uses a play task to obtain hearing test results. The child is taught/conditioned to respond using play task (e.g., building blocks, throwing toys into a basket) in response to sounds. This test can be used as a testing technique starting at approximately 24 months of age up to 3 years of age or as developmentally appropriate (Diefendorf & Tharpe, 2017).

■ Testing considerations:

□ Condition the child to the task.

□ Stimuli typically include frequency-specific pure tones (steady or pulsed), but other frequency-specific stimuli can be used.

□ The overall goal is to obtain ear-specific and frequency-specific information within the speech frequency range (500–4000 Hz).

• Frequency order can be modified to ensure that at least one high-frequency response and one low-frequency response are obtained if the child stops responding to the task.

• Testing can also include responses in both ears at each frequency (e.g., testing 1000 Hz in the right ear and then the left ear before moving to 4000 Hz) to ensure that some results from both ears are obtained if the child tires of the task.

□ Can use larger step sizes (e.g., 20 down/10 up until close to threshold) to prevent habituation or to allow for additional threshold estimations (e.g., both air and bone conduction).

□ Typically, ear-specific (headphones/insert earphones) or bone conduction; can use soundfield if child will not tolerate headphones.

□ Make sure to use control trials to ensure that the child is not responding to a pattern rather than hearing the sound.

□ For a more in-depth discussion of testing considerations, see Diefendorf and Tharpe (2017).

 AUDIOLOGY NUGGET

When thresholds are obtained for pediatric patients, the normative data for degree of hearing loss vary as compared to adult normative data. The primary difference is the inclusion of a "slight" or "minimal" hearing loss category. This is due to research showing the impact of slight to mild hearing losses in children (e.g., Winiger et al., 2016). The pediatric normative data are:

≤15 dB HL	Hearing within normal limits
16–25 dB HL	Slight/minimal hearing loss
26–40 dB HL	Mild hearing loss
41–55 dB HL	Moderate hearing loss
56–70 dB HL	Moderately severe hearing loss
71–90 dB HL	Severe hearing loss
≥91 dB HL	Profound hearing loss

Tangible Reinforcement Operant Conditioning Audiometry (TROCA)

For TROCA, the audiologist conditions the child to a task in which the child responds (such as pressing a button or giving a high five) when sounds are heard. The child is reinforced with a tangible object (stickers, edible reinforcements such as candy pieces) for correctly responding to sounds. This testing is typically used in children from approximately 2 years of age who cannot condition to CPA.

■ See CPA section for testing considerations.

Traditional Audiometry Considerations With Children

Traditional techniques (e.g., raising a hand) can be used as early as 3 years of age. By the time the child is school-aged, traditional techniques are commonly utilized.

■ Testing considerations:

□ With false positives, the first step is to reinstruct; ascending technique could be beneficial.

□ Stimuli typically include pure tones; the frequency and ear order are often similar to the considerations noted above for CPA.

CASE EXAMPLE

Juan is a 3-year-old child scheduled for an audiological evaluation. The audiologist has planned to test him using CPA. When seen for the appointment, Juan's parents report that he just started walking last month and that he is just beginning to say his first words. He is scheduled for a comprehensive development evaluation by a developmental pediatrician next week. Would this information change the plan of testing?

The testing plan should be reviewed to consider that motor and speech development are delayed. The reported milestones are consistent with a child who is 12 months of age, as opposed to the chronological age of 3 years. Case history questions could address cognitive development in addition to motor and speech development. Behavioral testing should be chosen based on the estimated developmental age. The audiologist's plan of testing would be modified to be VRA, which is appropriate for a child who is developmentally 12 months of age.

□ Goal is to obtain ear-specific information.
  • The child can be tested in soundfield if they will not tolerate use of headphones/insert earphones.
□ With younger children, larger step sizes (20/10 dB) can be beneficial to more quickly estimate threshold, with traditional step sizes (10/5 dB) used when closer to possible threshold.
□ With children who do not appear to be giving consistent and accurate responses, the audiologist can try the "yes/no" technique. With this technique, the audiologist instructs the child to say "yes" when a sound is heard and "no" when they do not hear the sound. Chapter 5 includes applications related to patients who do not appear to be giving true threshold information. For more in-depth information on this topic, see Peck (2017).

Screening of Pure Tones in Children

Screening of pure tones may be conducted in large-scale screening settings (e.g., in preschools). The pure-tone screenings typically use play or conventional techniques for children ≥ 3 years of age.

■ ASHA guidelines (1997) for hearing screening include screening at an intensity of 20 dB HL at 1000, 2000, and 4000 Hz. It is recommended to get two repeatable responses at the screening level in both ears at all frequencies tested in order to pass the screening.
■ Newer recommendations add 6000 Hz into the screening battery in order to detect high-frequency hearing losses due to noise exposure.

Threshold Speech Testing

Testing of pediatric patients may include speech stimuli instead of tonal stimuli. The audiological evaluation of pediatric patients may also include speech as a stimulus. Threshold speech testing is used to allow for an estimation of reliability of the threshold tonal responses (e.g., is the

SAT/SRT in good agreement, or within 7 dB, of the PTA or of the best thresholds in the speech frequency range).

- Speech awareness threshold (SAT)
  - Softest level the child responds to sound, typically lowest intensity that the child responds 50% of the time
  - Obtain MRL to speech up to 24 months of age.
  - SAT may be used up until the child can identify simple objects, which could be as early as 18 months (Northern & Downs, 2002).
  - Often running speech (repetitive syllables, "where am I?" "uh oh") or child's name delivered via live voice
- Speech reception threshold (SRT)
  - Softest level the child correctly identifies objects or repeats words
  - Spondee words are used (i.e., two-syllable words with equal emphasis on both syllables).
    - Examples of child-specific SRT words: baseball, cowboy, hotdog, airplane
  - To complete the SRT task, familiarize the child with the words, then perform the test procedure.
  - SRT is often a word repetition task but can be obtained via picture pointing.
    - Number of pictures can vary by language ability.
    - Can use spondee words with picture representations
    - Familiarize child to the pictures/words, then perform procedure with the child pointing to the picture.
    - Can use body part identification when necessary.
      - Ask parent/caregiver if child knows body parts (and which ones).
      - Familiarize at higher intensity to confirm child will respond to the body parts, then use items the child is familiar with during the identification task.

Word and Sentence Recognition Testing

Word recognition testing (WRS) and sentence recognition testing (SRS) vary by developmental/language age, articulation abilities, and auditory development. ASHA guidelines have recommendations for WRS in the 25- to 60-month age range, dependent upon the abilities of the particular child (ASHA, 2004). Word and sentence lists vary in structure (for example, phonetically or phonemically balanced) as well as language level. Developmentally appropriate lists should be used when testing a child, with considerations for receptive language ability, expressive language ability, primary language of the child, and the abilities of the audiologist to accurately and reliably judge responses. Testing may be performed in quiet, as well as in noise. Table 6–1 lists age-appropriate word lists and Table 6–2 lists age-appropriate sentence lists. The reader is also referred to Uhler et al. (2017) for information on the Pediatric Minimum Speech Test Battery.

- For closed-set word lists, one must consider chance level. For example, the NU-CHIPS has a chance level of 25% (child chooses from a set of four pictures), and the WIPI has a chance level of 16% (child chooses from a set of six pictures).

TABLE 6–1. Word Lists for Testing Children of Various Ages

CODE	TEST	AUTHOR	RECOMMENDED AGE	STIMULI	PRESENTATION FORMAT	RESPONSE	USAGE
WIPI	Word Intelligibility by Picture Identification	Ross and Leman (1970; rev. 2004)	4–6 years	Four equivalent lists of 25 monosyllabic words each	Recorded or live	Point to one of six color pictures	WRS for children who have speech difficulties
NU-CHIPS	Northwestern University Children's Perception of Speech	Elliott and Katz (1980)	3–5 years	50 monosyllabic words	Recorded or live	Point to one of four grayscale pictures	WRS for children who have speech difficulties
PSI	Pediatric Speech Intelligibility Test	Jerger and Jerger (1982)	3–6 years	20 monosyllabic words and two sentence formants in two lists of 10 sentences each	Recorded	Point to one of five pictures	WRS or SRS or APD; can be tested as performance-intensity (PI) function or message-to-competition ratio (MCR)
TAC	Test of Auditory Comprehension	Trammel (1981)	4–17 years	Environmental sounds, words, stereotypic messages arranged in 10 subtests	Recorded	Point to one of three pictures	HA or AR
PBK	Phonetically balanced kindergarten word lists	Haskins (1949)	6–12 years	50 monosyllabic words	Recorded or live Tape or CD	Repeat the words	WRS
PAL PB 50	Psychoacoustics Laboratory phonetically balanced 50-word lists	Eagan (1948)	12 years and up	Monosyllabic words	Recorded or live	Repeat the words	WRS
CID W-22	Central Institute for the Deaf W-22	Hirsh et al. (1952)	12 years and up	Monosyllabic words	Recorded or live	Repeat the words	WRS
NU-6	Northwestern University 6	Tillman and Carhart (1966)	12 years and up	Monosyllabic words	Recorded or live	Repeat the words	WRS

Source: Adapted from Thibodeau, L. M. (2007). Speech audiometry. In *Audiology Diagnosis, 2nd ed.* Eds. Ross Roeser, Michael Valente, & Holly Hosford-Dunn. New York: Thieme. Pages 300–301.

TABLE 6–2. Sentence Lists for Testing Children of Various Ages

CODE	TEST	AUTHOR	RECOMMENDED AGE	STIMULI	PRESENTATION FORMAT	RESPONSE	USAGE
BKB SIN	Bamford-Kowal-Bench Speech in Noise	Etymotic Research (2005)	5–14 years	Sentences	Recorded	Repeat the sentence	HA or APD
HINT-C	Hearing in Noise Test for Children	Nilsson et al. (1996)	6–12 years	Sentences	Recorded	Repeat the sentence	HA or APD
HINT	Hearing in Noise Test	Nilsson et al. (1994)	13 years and up	Sentences	Recorded	Repeat the sentence	HA or APD
Quick SIN	Quick Speech in Noise	Etymotic Research (2001)	12 years and up	Sentences	Recorded	Repeat the sentence	HA or APD
SPIN	Revised Speech Perception in Noise	Bilger et al. (1984)	12 years and up	High and low predictability sentences	Recorded	Repeat the final word of the sentence	HA or APD
SSI	Synthetic Sentence Identification	Speaks and Jerger (1965)	12 years and up	Sentences that do not convey meaning	Recorded	Identify the sentence from a list of ten	HA or APD

Source: Adapted from Thibodeau, L. M. (2007). Speech audiometry. In *Audiology Diagnosis, 2nd ed.* Eds. Ross Roeser, Michael Valente, & Holly Hosford-Dunn. New York: Thieme. Pages 300–301.

- Word lists that are repetition tasks (e.g., PBK) can be impacted by articulation abilities of the child's speech. If the audiologist has difficulties understanding the child and does not believe they can accurately record the responses, a closed-set task should be chosen.

- Adult lists: Sanderson-Leepa and Rintelmann (1976) showed the Northwestern Auditory Test No. 6 (NU-6) was more difficult than the PBK in children who were 7.5, 9.5, and 11.5 years of age. The authors indicated use of these tests may depend on the purpose of the assessment.

- Sentence materials are often used to examine performance in situations closer to conversational speech and are frequently used in educational environments (e.g., functional listening evaluations). More information is in the later Educational Audiology section of this chapter.

 KNOWLEDGE CHECKPOINT

According to Sanderson-Leepa and Rintelmann (1976), use of pediatric versus adult word lists can vary depending on the purpose of the testing. For diagnostic purposes, utilizing a pediatric list is appropriate to ensure that results relate to audibility of words rather than the child's language and vocabulary. However, if the purpose is more functional testing, such as comparing aided to unaided abilities in a child with a mild hearing loss, then an adult word list may be preferable. For example, a 7-year-old child with a mild hearing loss may have a very high (e.g., 96% correct) word understanding score in quiet utilizing the PBK words. This would not allow for any improvement of scores in an aided condition and may not represent actual listening conditions for the child. As such, testing in soundfield without and with hearing aids could use a more difficult adult word list, such as the NU-6 lists. The child may have more difficulty in the unaided condition, allowing the audiologist to see if there is improvement with use of amplification. This testing would be used in conjunction with additional functional assessments (including speech in noise tasks and parent/teacher rating scales).

Testing in Background Noise

Testing speech in the presence of background noise gives more ecologically valid ("real life") considerations of functional abilities, especially for school-aged children (Deconde Johnson & Seaton, 2021).

- Can use tests such as the Selective Auditory Attention Test (SAAT), the BKB-SIN, or the auditory figure-ground tests from the SCAN-3.
  - If there is a hearing loss present, the testing would be for the purpose of functional abilities only rather than diagnosis of processing difficulties. The audiologist would have to consider the intensity level chosen for the testing, as many of these tests were normed at a normal conversational level (e.g., 50–55 dB HL). For a child with hearing loss, this may be a lower sensation level (SL); as such, the testing intensity may need to be raised to take the degree of hearing loss into account.

□ When testing in noise is being used for documentation (e.g., for an IEP), then tests with age-appropriate normative data are needed. More flexibility is allowed in choice of test if the purpose is to compare performance across different listening conditions (e.g., comparison of different hearing aid settings or comparison of testing with and without a HAT system).

■ Appropriate WR list (e.g., PBK) can be used for testing in background noise. However, normative data may not be available. For example, Chermak et al. (1984) found that reliability of the NU-CHIPS was impacted when tested in background noise.

□ The background noise may be speech-shaped noise, multitalker babble, or environmental noise (e.g., cafeteria noise). Multitalker babble may be a better representation of noise in the classroom with multiple people talking (Deconde Johnson & Seaton, 2021).

Physiological Evaluation

Physiological tests allow the audiologist to objectively evaluate specific portions of the auditory system. An important concept in pediatric audiology is the cross-check principle. This principle relates to the importance of completing both behavioral testing and physiological testing to form a complete picture of the child's auditory abilities. The physiological tests do not require an active response from the child.

Immittance

See Chapter 5 for a review of immittance principles. Testing considerations for the pediatric population are included below. Recall that sound transfer depends upon:

■ Impedance (Z): the resistance of energy flow and is made up of mass and compliance reactance and resistance, which prevent movement of the system.

■ Mass reactance (X_m): the resistance of movement caused by the mass of a system

■ Compliance reactance (X_c): the resistance to movement caused by the stiffness of a system

■ Resistance (R): the opposition of movement caused by the friction within a system

■ Admittance (Y): how much movement a system will allow to pass through (made up of mass and stiffness susceptance and conductance); it is the exact opposite of impedance and is what current immittance bridges utilize for testing

■ Mass susceptance (B_m): how much movement that the mass of a system allows to pass through

■ Compliance susceptance (B_c): how much movement that the stiffness of a system allows to pass through

■ Conductance (G): how much movement that the friction of a system allows to pass through

Tympanometry

The most common tympanometric measurement uses a low-frequency probe tone (220–226 Hz) in children greater than approximately 6 to 9 months. High-frequency probe tones (e.g., 667 or 1000 Hz) can also be used. See the High-Frequency Stimuli section in this chapter for consideration of these probe tones. There are child-specific norms for peak static acoustic compliance, tympanometric width, tympanometric peak pressure, and ear canal volume. The normative values vary dependent upon the desired sensitivity/specificity.

- Current recommendations, such as the ASHA (1997) guidelines for middle ear screening, recommend utilizing normative values for static acoustic compliance or tympanometric width rather than type of tympanograms (Hunter & Blankenship, 2017; Roush & Corbin, 2017).

- ASHA (1997) guidelines include recommendations for referral for a middle ear rescreening for children older than 6 to 12 months to include static acoustic compliance of <0.3 mmho or tympanometric width >200 daPa. For infants, the recommendation is static acoustic compliance of <0.2 mmho or tympanometric width >235 daPa.

  □ The use of tympanometric peak pressure is not recommended as part of the middle ear screening protocol.

- The American Academy of Otolaryngology-Head and Neck Surgery clinical practice guidelines for PE tubes (Rosenfeld et al., 2022) includes information on Type B (flat tympanograms) that are associated with middle ear effusion in 85% to 100% of cases. The American Academy of Audiology endorses these guidelines.

- Results may be interpreted using patterns, such as described by Jerger (1970) and Feldman (1976). Tympanometric patterns are discussed in Chapter 5.

- Normative data can vary. Example normative data for a 226 Hz probe tone for children are included in Table 6–3. Compliance values below the normative range are consistent with abnormal movement of the TM (such as effusion in the middle ear), while compliance values above the normative range are consistent with increased movement of the TM (e.g., a flaccid TM or disarticulation of the ossicular chain). Widths larger than the normative range are consistent with abnormal movement of the TM.

High-Frequency Stimuli

The current recommendation is to utilize a 1000 Hz probe for children up to 9 months of age (Joint Committee on Infant Hearing, 2019).

TABLE 6–3. Pediatric Immittance Norms

	STATIC ACOUSTIC COMPLIANCE (mmho), 5TH–95TH PERCENTILES	TYMPANOMETRIC WIDTH (daPa)
6–12 months	0.20–0.50	102–234
12–18 months	0.20–0.60	102–204
18–24 months	0.30–0.70	102–204
24–30 months	0.30–0.80	96–192

Source: Information from Roush et al., 1992, as cited in Hunter & Blankenship, 2017.

	STATIC ACOUSTIC COMPLIANCE (mmho)	TYMPANOMETRIC WIDTH (daPa)
3–10 years	0.25–1.05	80–159

Source: Information from Margolis and Hunter (2000), as cited in Martin and Clark (2006).

- Low-frequency probe tones are not effective in young infants (see upcoming Audiology Nugget).
- High-frequency probe tone should have a peaked formation to be considered normal (e.g., Hoffman et al., 2013). See Figure 6–1, which shows a 226 Hz probe tone tympanogram (left panel) compared to a 1000 Hz probe tone tympanogram (right panel).

AUDIOLOGY NUGGET

Due to incomplete maturation of the external auditory canal (EAC) and middle ear, a standard 226 Hz probe tone may not provide accurate immittance results for children less than 6 to 9 months of age.

Some factors that may influence immittance results in young children are:

- Excessively compliant EAC
- Horizontal orientation of the TM
- Underossified ossicular chain
   □ Sound transfer depends on mass and stiffness properties (see Multifrequency Tympanometry section).

Wideband Acoustic Immittance

Wideband acoustic immittance (WAI) uses a wideband chirp signal that measures up to 10 kHz (range that encompasses frequencies for speech perception), which measures reflectance, absorbance, and impedance (admittance). It is a recent addition to the immittance battery and has utility in uncovering more detailed information about middle ear disorders in newborns, infants, children, and those with developmental disabilities, such as the presence of low absorbance from 1000 to 3000 Hz in individuals with otitis media with effusion (Hunter & Blankenship, 2017).

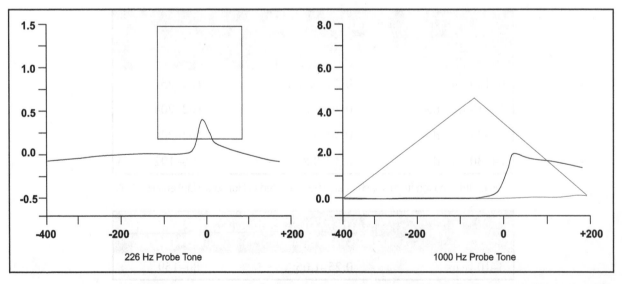

FIGURE 6–1. Example tympanograms with low-frequency (226 Hz) and high-frequency (1000 Hz) probe tone.

- Power absorbance is a WAI measure that provides information regarding the amount of acoustic power absorbed into the middle ear at the TM relative to the total power of a stimulus (typically a broadband click or chirp stimulus) in the ear canal.

- Values range from 0 to 1 or 0% to 100%, with 0 (0%) suggesting no sound energy absorbed and 1 (100%) meaning all sound energy absorbed. Results are plotted as a function of frequency and referred to as wideband absorbance (WBA).

- Recent evidence suggests WBA to be more sensitive to certain middle ear pathologies than traditional tympanometry (Shahnaz, Aithal, & Bargen, 2023).

- Please review Shahnaz et al. (2023) for detailed information regarding WAI in children.

CASE EXAMPLE

A 2-week-old infant is referred due to not passing the newborn hearing screening using otoacoustic emissions (OAEs). The infant is being seen for a rescreening appointment, and the child has absent OAEs in both ears. Tympanometric testing is completed with a 226 Hz probe tone, indicating Type A tympanograms with normal static acoustic compliance, tympanometric width, and peak pressure values. Would this indicate that the absent OAEs were consistent with abnormal outer hair cell function?

Conductive problems or abnormal movement of the TM can lead to absent OAEs. The audiologist should note that a low-frequency probe Hz is not effective in determining mobility of the TMs in young infants. As such, tympanometric testing should include a high-frequency (e.g., 1000 Hz) probe tone. If the high-frequency tympanograms are abnormal, the absent OAEs could relate to the abnormal movement of the TM rather than cochlear function. If results indicate normal movement, then a battery of tests (e.g., air-conduction and bone-conduction ABR) would be needed to determine the nature of the hearing loss.

Multifrequency Tympanometry (MFT)

MFT utilizes the properties of the middle ear (i.e., susceptance and conductance) to identify middle ear pathologies by varying the frequency of the probe tone and evaluating for the normal progression of results. MFT is used in both children and adults to more accurately determine whether middle ear abnormalities are due to mass (e.g., mucoid effusion) or stiffness (e.g., otosclerosis) related pathologies. MFT utilizes the physical components of the middle ear system.

- MFT is indicated when the following audiometric results are seen during testing:
  - Type A tympanogram with a wide width/gradient, an As or an Ad tympanogram
  - When 226 Hz (Y) admittance tympanogram has a consistent (there on repeated tympanogram) notch (i.e., 3Y). This would indicate that the resonant frequency is abnormally low (due to either mass-loading or abnormal flaccidity).
  - Type A tympanogram with a conductive hearing loss component

- □ Abnormally large acoustic reflexes at very low sensation levels
- ■ Typical patterns of results are expected related to the progress of results across frequencies and the morphology of the results.
  - □ MFT will result in multiple peaks (B and G) appearing on the tympanogram (as opposed to the single peak that is typically seen in a normal Y tympanogram).
    - B peaks represent susceptance of the mass and stiffness of the middle ear system.
    - G peaks represent conductance of the middle ear system.
  - □ At the resonant frequency, a 3B1G configuration should be noted. Resonant frequency (f_0) is defined as the point at which the middle ear mass susceptance equals that of stiffness susceptance, which leaves conductance as the only force that will act against the transfer of sound through the middle ear space. In other words, this is the frequency that will allow for the most efficient transfer of sound through the middle ear.
  - □ At a specific frequency, the configuration is labeled based on the number of peaks and valleys (or extrema) observed in the B/G tympanograms:
    - Normal results will appear in certain patterns depending on the frequency at which testing occurs.
    - Vanhuyse model predicts that in a normally functioning middle ear system, B and G peaks will appear in four distinct patterns relative to the frequency of the probe tone used.
    - The pattern progress is 1B1G, 3B1G, 3B3G, and 5B3G.
    - Figure 6–2 depicts progression through the Vanhuyse model.
  - □ For children, normal resonant frequencies occur between 800 Hz and 1800 Hz.
  - □ For adults, normal resonant frequencies may reach as high as 2000 Hz.
  - □ Configurations should progress in order from 1B1G to 5B3G as the probe tone moves from a lower frequency to a higher frequency.
  - □ Morphology
    1. There should **never** be more than 5B or 3G extrema, or
    2. There should **never** be a greater number of G than B extrema, or
    3. Outermost G extrema which do not fall within the width/gradient of the outermost B extrema.
       - ○ Three extrema configuration: the width/gradient between the outermost extrema should be <75 daPa.
       - ○ Five extrema configuration: the width/gradient between the outermost extrema should be <100 daPa.
  - □ It is important to note that while B tympanograms may appear normal, G tympanograms may still be abnormal because the conductance (friction) of the system is affected.
- ■ Clinical evaluation using MFT
  - □ To examine resonant frequency, a frequency sweep typically 500 Hz to 2000 Hz is performed.
    - Testing at lower frequencies is useful for finding stiffness-related problems such as otosclerosis.

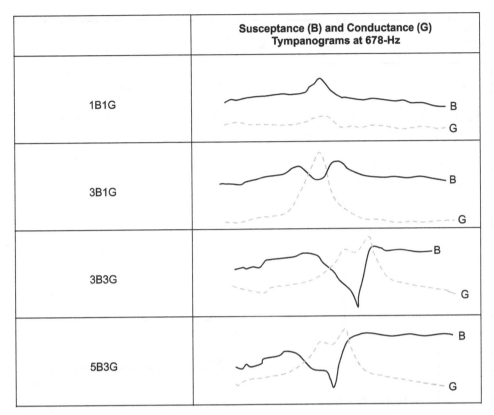

FIGURE 6–2. Pattern progression of B/G tympanograms found in Vanhuyse model.

- Testing at higher frequencies is useful for finding mass-related problems such as mucoid effusion.
  □ An abnormally low resonant frequency (<800 Hz) indicates that the middle ear space is either mass-loaded or abnormally flaccid:
    - Type Ad tympanogram with a low resonant frequency = abnormally flaccid (e.g., disarticulation of the ossicles, monomeric TM)
    - Type A tympanogram with a low resonant frequency = mass-loading (e.g., mucoid effusion adhering to the ossicles)
  □ An abnormally high resonant frequency (>1800 Hz) indicates that the middle ear space is abnormally stiff:
    - As tympanogram with a high resonant frequency = abnormally stiff (e.g., otosclerosis [ossification and immobilization of the stapes])

Middle Ear Muscle or Acoustic Reflexes (MEMR; AR)

MEMRs are discussed in Chapter 5. The information below is specific to the pediatric population.

- For infants younger than 6 to 9 months of age, use of high-frequency probe tone is recommended.
- Clinicians should be cognizant of the SPL in the ear canal (due to reduced ear canal size) of high-intensity MEMR-activating stimuli. For infants and children, the intensity should not be higher than 95 dB SPL (McCreery & Walker, 2017).

Q & A

Figure 6–3 is an example of a measure of resonant frequency.

Question: If the resonant frequency is 1000 Hz, what information does that provide regarding the middle ear system?

Answer: The mass and stiffness of the system are typical because the resonant frequency (i.e., where system shifts from mass dominated to stiffness dominated) was within the range of 800 to 1800 Hz.

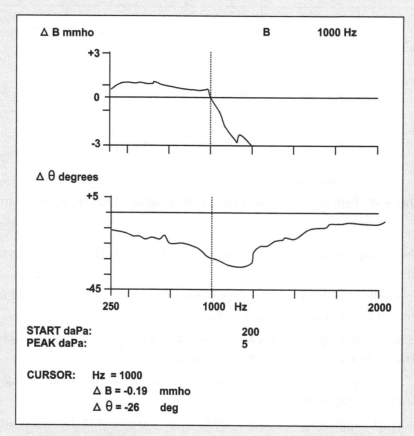

FIGURE 6–3. Case example of resonant frequency for multifrequency tympanometry.

- Sensitivity prediction with the acoustic reflex (SPAR) can be used to estimate hearing sensitivity by comparison of pure-tone MEMR thresholds (500, 1000, and 2000 Hz) and broadband threshold. This method is less effective with those with moderate hearing losses (Jerger et al., 1978, as cited in Northern & Downs, 2002). The SPAR is utilized less often with the use of more common physiologic tests (e.g., OAEs and ABR).

- MEMR, used in conjunction with tympanometric measures, can be useful in determining the presence of middle ear effusion. In addition, MEMR can be useful as part of a battery for diagnosis of auditory neuropathy spectrum disorder (ANSD), as absent or abnormal MEMR is expected in this population (Berlin et al., 2005).

Otoacoustic Emissions (OAEs) in Pediatric Assessments

OAEs measure cochlear (outer hair cell) responses to sound and can be an integral part of the pediatric screening and assessment of hearing. The child must be quiet/still, as noise levels can negatively impact the ability to see the emission response. See Chapter 5 for additional and more general information on OAEs. Absent OAEs can indicate the possibility of sensorineural hearing loss (i.e., a problem in the outer hair cells of the cochlea). However, conductive components or abnormal movement of the TM/ function of the middle ear can also lead to absent OAEs. As such, immittance testing in conjunction with testing of OAEs is an important cross-check in interpretation of absent OAEs. Children with mild hearing losses or ANSD may have present OAEs. This confirms the need for cross-checking of OAEs results with behavioral results or with ABR. In addition, OAEs are useful in monitoring of cochlear function in cases with risk factors such as ototoxic drugs, as the negative impact on the cochlea may be seen earlier with OAEs than with behavioral assessment of hearing (Dhar & Hall, 2018).

Distortion Product OAEs

- Distortion product OAEs (DPOAE)—a distortion (a third tone, typically *2f1–f2*) created by two presented tones; plotted on a DP-gram (Abdala et al., 2017)
- Must have appropriate signal-to-noise ratio (SNR) to be present, often 3 to 6 dB (Abdala et al., 2017), in addition to amplitude of the DPOAE of >0 dB SPL (Dhar & Hall, 2018).
  - Diagnostic DPOAEs are classified as present, reduced, or absent, depending on the SNR and overall amplitude of the response. Of note, for billing purposes, a diagnostic (comprehensive) DPOAE consists of at least 12 frequencies tested.
  - Screening protocols often include "pass" criteria that must be met at a minimum number of frequencies (e.g., present OAEs at three or four tested frequencies). Screeners use a more limited number of frequencies and as such do not provide the fine-grained information gathered from diagnostic DPOAEs.
- Example pediatric parameters can be found in Table 6–4 (Abdala et al., 2017).
- DPOAEs are measured over a large frequency range, with better responses than transient-evoked OAEs (TEOAEs) at higher frequencies (> 2000 Hz). DPOAEs will be absent with hearing losses from 25 dB HL up to 50 to 60 dB HL (Farinetti et al., 2018).

TABLE 6–4. Example of Pediatric Parameters for DPOAEs

STIMULUS	L1= 60–65 dB SPL; L2 SEPARATED BY 10–15 dB
Frequency Ratio	F2:F1= 1.22
Frequency Range	1500–8000 Hz

Transient-Evoked/Click-Evoked OAEs

- TEOAEs are reflection emissions produced by irregularities along the cochlea; evoked with a broadband click presented between 80 and 84 dB SPL, which is averaged for approximately 20 ms

- Present if response reproducibility is > 50% and a response is present above the noise floor (SNR)

- TEOAEs are absent if sensorineural hearing loss is more than 40 dB HL (Farinetti et al., 2018).

Electrophysiological Evaluation

Auditory Steady-State Response (ASSR)

The ASSR is an auditory evoked potential that measures neural responses to modulated auditory stimuli and can be used to predict hearing thresholds when behavioral thresholds cannot be obtained. Interpretation is mathematically based on the relationship between bioelectric events and stimulus repetition rate (Beck et al., 2007). ASSR analysis is objective and relies on determination of presence of a response based on statistical analyses (Korczak et al., 2012). For a comprehensive review, please refer to Korczak et al. (2012).

- Responses can be detected at intensity levels close to behavioral (true) threshold.
- Can include binaural presentation of stimuli
- Advantages of ASSR as compared to ABR include:
  - Testing time can be significantly shorter than ABR, as ASSR can include presentation of multiple stimuli simultaneously (up to eight frequencies; four in each ear) (Krishnan, 2023).
  - ASSR can differentiate between severe to profound hearing losses better than threshold ABR (Eder et al., 2020).
- Previously referred to as steady-state evoked potential (SSEP)
  - Other responses that follow modulations are called amplitude-modulation-following response (AMFR), envelope-following response (EFR), steady-state response (SSR), and the auditory steady-state response (ASSR).
- The ASSR has a carrier frequency (CF; the frequencies being tested) and a modulation frequency (MF).

Neural Generators of ASSR (Korczak et al., 2012)

- ASSRs elicited by stimuli presented at modulation rates < 20 Hz have responses mainly generated by activity in the primary auditory cortex.
- ASSRs elicited by stimuli presented at modulation rates 20 to 60 Hz have responses mainly in the primary auditory cortex, auditory midbrain, and thalamus.
- ASSRs elicited by stimuli at rates > 60 Hz generated primarily by contributions from the superior olivary complex, inferior colliculus, and cochlear nucleus (brainstem).

□ These are unaffected by subject state (similar to the ABR), whereas those derived from slower modulation rates (< 60 Hz) that result from activity at higher levels of the auditory system are influenced by subject state.

□ Typically, higher stimulation rates are used in children when searching for threshold.

Protocols for ASSR

■ If used as a screening tool, recommendations are to use a "pass" intensity of 40 dB HL at 2000 and 4000 Hz, 45 dB HL at 1000 Hz, and 50 dB HL at 500 Hz (Van Maanen & Stapells, 2009, 2010, as cited in Korczak et al., 2012).

■ Recommended protocols include obtaining a chirp ABR threshold in both ears; use 10 to 20 dB above this threshold to start the frequency-specific thresholds for ASSR. Obtain responses down to 10 to 20 dB nHL for stimuli frequencies of 500, 1000, 2000, and 4000 Hz (Sininger et al., 2020).

Threshold Auditory Brainstem Response (ABR)

ABRs are auditory evoked potentials that can be used to assess the neurologic status of the auditory system (i.e., neurodiagnostic) or used to estimate hearing sensitivity (threshold ABR). The primary use for the pediatric population is to determine auditory sensitivity through threshold ABR testing. For a description of abnormal auditory electrophysiological findings, see Appendix 6–A.

Stimuli for Threshold ABR

■ Clicks

□ Broadband signals that contain a wide range of frequencies and therefore not frequency specific

□ Leads to responses to a large portion of the cochlea and represents the part of the cochlea with the best hearing within 500 to 8000 Hz (Krishnan, 2023)

■ Chirps

□ Brief tonal stimuli with frequencies adjusted in timing of presentation (i.e., low frequencies presented first so that the more apical low-frequency regions of the basilar membrane are activated at the same time as the high-frequency regions near the base)

□ Improve the neural synchrony (Krishnan, 2023), providing a larger wave V amplitude compared to clicks due to how chirps simultaneously stimulate each frequency place along the basilar membrane

□ Latency of chirp responses has been shown to be longer than responses to click stimuli (Cobb & Stuart, 2016).

■ Frequency-specific stimuli

□ Tone bursts or pips (500, 1000, 2000, and 4000 Hz)

□ Narrowband chirps are filtered around center frequencies (500, 1000, 2000, and 4000 Hz) to allow more frequency-specific results (Eder et al., 2020).

• Produce larger wave V amplitude as compared to clicks and tone pips (Cobb & Stuart, 2016)

- May show decreased amplitudes and frequency sensitivity at high intensity levels (Small & Stapells, 2017)

Protocols for ABR Threshold Testing

- Single or alternating polarity is acceptable, although alternating should be used for bone-conduction testing.
- Test air conduction for each ear (2000, 500, 4000, then 1000 Hz).
- Can perform a click or chirp threshold first, then start frequency-specific testing 10 to 20 dB above this threshold. Obtain responses down to 10 to 20 dB nHL for stimuli frequencies of 500, 1000, 2000, and 4000 Hz (Sininger et al., 2020).
- To determine conductive component, especially when testing infants, can compare air- to bone-conduction ABR thresholds to determine if air-bone gaps are present
  - □ Must consider masking when testing via bone conduction to obtain ear-specific results
- Use high-intensity clicks to assess for ANSD or other neurological problems (see protocols for ANSD below).

 AUDIOLOGY NUGGET

ABR thresholds are measured in dB nHL, which has a reference to behavioral thresholds that would correspond to the intensity that elicits an ABR response (Krishnan, 2023). However, when used in determining degree of hearing loss or in fitting amplification based on ABR results, correction factors are utilized to allow for estimation of an equivalent HL value (i.e., dB eHL). For example, the British Columbia Early Hearing Program uses a correction factor of −15 at 500 Hz, −10 at 1000 Hz, and −5 at 2000 Hz (as cited in Small & Stapells, 2017). Using these correction factors, a child with an ABR threshold of 55 dB nHL at 1000 Hz would be estimated to have a 45 dB HL behavioral threshold at 1000 Hz (45 dB eHL). It is always recommended that each clinic develop their own normative values for correction factors, but most manufacturers will include presets to give an estimated audiogram depending on thresholds determined via ABR (or ASSR).

Protocols for ABR Screening

- ASHA (1997) guidelines suggest the following stimulus conditions for screening ABR: click at 35 dB nHL at rate 37/s, minimum 1,000 repetitions for operator-controlled ABR.
- For automated ABR systems, a chirp stimulus at 35 dB nHL may be used at rates up to 92 clicks/s (Krishnan, 2023).
- Similar to screening OAEs, these results are reported as a "pass" or "refer" (or "fail").
- Thresholds are not established with screeners and follow-up diagnostic testing is required to do so.

Protocols for Auditory Neuropathy Spectrum Disorder (ANSD). As ANSD has specific hallmark ABR responses, a separate protocol is necessary for testing (Norrix & Velenovsky, 2014). Other results that can indicate ANSD include present OAEs (may disappear with age), abnormal MEMRs, speech recognition that is poorer than expected, and variable pure-tone thresholds.

- Patients with ANSD have abnormal or absent ABR with present cochlear microphonic (CM).
  - CM arises from the outer hair cells and mimics the stimulus waveform/polarity (sinusoid following the repetition rate of the stimulus).
  - Measured via a high-intensity (e.g., 90 dB nHL, 2,000 sweeps, rate of 21.1 clicks/s) click with condensation and with rarefaction polarities (Krishnan, 2023).
  - Inversion of the responses with changes in stimulus polarity will be seen in normal responses (Figure 6–4, panel A); alternating polarity cancels the CM (Figure 6–4, panel B).
  - Recommendations include a control run: closing off the insert earphone to prevent the stimulus from going into the ear. This ensures the CM is no longer measured and that the appearance of a waveform is not stimulus artifact.

Frequency Following Response (FFR)

The frequency following response (FFR) reflects sustained neural activity that is phase-locked to the stimulus waveform, with the complex ABR (cABR) being a form of FFR. Although it has yet to be widely adopted clinically, the FFR has had a resurgence in research in the past 20 years. A detailed explanation of the FFR and its applications can be found in Krishnan (2023). The following information is a cursory review.

- There are two forms of the FFR: envelope FFR (eFFR) and the FFR. Each is elicited in the brainstem by harmonically related complex sounds, such as a consonant vowel (CV) stimulus (e.g., ba or da).

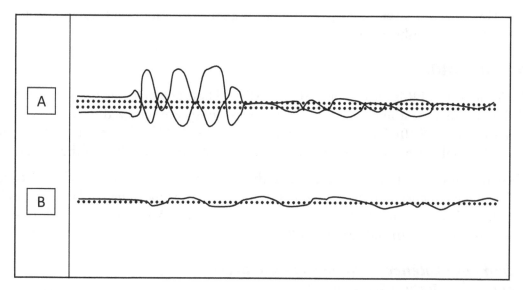

FIGURE 6–4. ABR results seen with auditory neuropathy spectrum disorder.

- □ eFFR reflects phase-locking to envelope periodicity (slow varying amplitude oscillations) of the stimulus waveform.
  - The eFFR response typically occurs after wave V of the ABR (>5.5 ms).
  - To separate the eFFR from the FFR, an alternating polarity signal can be used wherein rarefacting and condensing runs are summed.
  - The eFFR is also referred to as the auditory steady-state response (ASSR) to tonal stimuli.
- □ The ASSR, as described in this chapter, is used in threshold estimation for individuals unable to complete behavioral audiometry.
- □ FFR reflects phase-locking to the temporal fine structure (rapid amplitude oscillations) of complex sounds.
  - Response occurs simultaneously with the eFFR (i.e., onset after the cochlear microphonic and wave V of the ABR). The traditional paradigm for recording the FFR includes the use of 500 Hz tones, but tonal stimuli up to 2000 Hz or complex stimuli can be used.
  - Neural generators of the FFR have been the subject of many investigations, such that there is thought to be unique generators for different frequencies of the FFR: Low-frequency responses arise from the auditory cortex and surrounding areas while high-frequency responses are from brainstem structures and CN VIII.
  - The FFR is analyzed relative to its spectral information, like the eFFR.
  - Like the eFFR, the FFR has limited clinical utility at present but has the potential to allow for exploration of neural encoding in individuals with hearing loss, aging individuals, and those undergoing auditory training.
- □ The recording setup for these responses can be the same as the traditional ABR, but the stimuli vary based on the auditory area of interest.
- □ The recording window depends on stimuli duration: ~15-ms window for shorter tonal stimuli; ~250-ms window for longer stimuli such as speech.
  - Frequency analysis: FFT, spectral correlation, spectrogram
  - Time analysis: response latency, stimulus-response correlation; autocorrelogram, phase coherence (Krishnan, 2023)

Complex ABR (cABR)

A popular form of the FFR is the complex ABRs (cABR). These potentials are unique from the traditional ABR in that they use stimuli such as music, syllables, nonspeech vocalizations, and environmental sounds (Skoe & Kraus, 2010). Stimuli are presented at suprathreshold levels with the goal of examining the amount of neural synchrony to the onset, sustained component, and offset of the stimulus.

- ■ These responses arise from the brainstem to the cortex and have many research applications as well as clinical applications in the realm of (C)APD, training measures, and other neurological disorders (Skoe & Kraus, 2010). For more literature on the cABR, the reader is directed to Skoe and Kraus (2010) and Krishnan (2023).

Middle and Late Latency Responses in Children
(See Chapter 5 for Testing Procedures)

Middle and cortical evoked responses applications when working with children vary and are still being developed.

- Middle latency response/auditory evoked (MLR/MLAEP) (Cacace & McFarland, 2015)
  - Threshold estimation: NOT used among children because they are highly variable and, in some instances, not present when a child is asleep.
  - Central auditory processing disorders: abnormal MLRs have been seen in children with learning disabilities.
  - Cochlear implants: MLRs evoked through electrical pulses (like a cochlear implant) are similar to an acoustically evoked response.
  - Though potential is seen in these areas, there is the need for more research to verify feasibility in clinical use.
- Cortical potentials (CAEP) (Tremblay & Clinard, 2015)
  - P1-N1-P2 potential can be used as a measure of threshold for patients who are passively cooperative.
    - Thresholds have been found to be within 10 dB of behavioral thresholds.
  - CAEPs can reliably be measured in the soundfield, which allows for testing using amplification or cochlear implants; this is beginning to be used clinically as a verification measure.
    - Differences of developmental patterns of P1-N1-P2 have been seen after cochlear implantation.
  - The P1-N1-P2 has also been used to monitor performance following auditory training exercises and in (C)APD.
  - Other potentials include the P300 and MMN and are more commonly used for research. See Chapter 5 for additional information.

Etiology of Pediatric Hearing Loss

Etiology of hearing loss in the pediatric population can be related to many factors, including genetics, ototoxicity, noise-induced hearing loss, infections, and other medical conditions (e.g., otitis media with effusion or cholesteatoma). Hearing loss may also be syndromic (i.e., associated with other symptoms/disorders) or nonsyndromic. In addition, hearing loss may be prenatal (e.g., due to maternal infections), perinatal (e.g., oxygen deprivation during birth), or postnatal (e.g., bacterial meningitis). Etiologic factors may be noted in the case history, or the audiologist may detect signs/symptoms that may necessitate referral to other professions (e.g., physicians, genetic testing). It is important to consider the risk of progressive hearing loss in determining how to monitor hearing for children. Examples of syndromes and of other infections/disorders seen in the pediatric population are noted below. Readers can refer to Northern (2014) for a more comprehensive list of pediatric hearing disorders.

Syndromic Hearing Loss

Hearing loss can be associated with various syndromes. These syndromes may lead to conductive, sensorineural, or mixed hearing losses. See Table 6–5 for common pediatric syndromes that are associated with hearing loss.

TABLE 6–5. Examples of Pediatric Syndromes

SYNDROME/ DISORDER	TYPE OF HL	GENETIC INHERITANCE	CHARACTERISTICS
Alport Syndrome	Progressive SNHL	X-linked (commonly); can be autosomal dominant or recessive	Kidney failure; abnormalities of the eye (which may not impact vision)
Branchio-Oto-Renal (BOR) Syndrome	Mixed, but can be CHL or SNHL	Autosomal dominant	Preauricular pits, abnormal pinna, stenosis, atresia, fused ossicles, inner ear malformations; kidneys may be absent or underdeveloped
CHARGE (Coloboma, Heart defect, Atresia choane, Delayed growth and development, Genital abnormality, Ear abnormality)	Mild to profound HL (depending on CNS function); balance problems	Sporadic gene mutation	Hole in eye structure (coloboma); blocked or narrowed nasal passages; abnormal CNS function; auricular deformities (often asymmetrical); middle or inner ear malformations possible; vestibular system may be impacted; delayed cognitive development
Cleft Palate	CHL	Autosomal dominant	Malformed palate and/or lip; risk of Eustachian tube dysfunction and otitis media
Crouzon Syndrome	CHL	Autosomal dominant	Craniosynostosis (fused skull and facial bones); possible stenosis, atresia, middle ear deformities; high risk of otitis media
Down Syndrome	Primarily CHL; at increased risk for SNHL or mixed HL as compared to general population	Chromosomal disorder, majority are trisomy 21	Craniofacial characteristics (e.g., broad nasal bridge, almond-shaped eyes, large tongue); heart problems, ear infections; intellectual functioning is impacted
Goldenhar Syndrome	CHL, SNHL, or mixed HL	Possibly hereditary, sporadic cases	Unilateral problems with eye and facial malformations; unilateral microtia, atresia, pits/tags, middle ear problems; can impact heart, kidneys, and CNS
Jervell and Lange Nielson Syndrome (JLNS)	Profound bilateral SNHL	Autosomal recessive	Cardiac arrhythmia

TABLE 6–5. *continued*

SYNDROME/ DISORDER	TYPE OF HL	GENETIC INHERITANCE	CHARACTERISTICS
Landau-Kleffner Syndrome	Auditory agnosia; normal ABR but abnormal behavioral	Autosomal dominant	Sudden- or gradual-onset aphasia and seizures; linguistic regression
Neurofibromatosis II	Progressive SNHL	Autosomal dominant	Bilateral vestibular schwannoma; balance problems, tinnitus, facial weakness
Pierre Robin Sequence	CHL	Genetic, but usually not hereditary	Micrognathia, retroglossia; otitis media with effusion
Stickler Syndrome	Sloping HF SNHL; possible cleft palate (mixed)	Autosomal dominant	Impacts connective tissue and collagen; inner ear structures; vision may be impacted; chronic otitis media
Treacher Collins Syndrome	CHL	Autosomal dominant	Craniofacial impact; malformed ears– microtia, anotia, atresia; hypoplastic, ankylosed, or absent ossicles; may impact vision
Usher Syndrome	SNHL; degree depends on Type I, II, or III	Autosomal recessive	Retinitis pigmentosa; onset of visual impairment is in the first 10 years for Type I, with later onset for Type II. Vestibular problems are seen in Type I.
Waardenburg Syndrome	SNHL	Autosomal dominant	Pigmentation abnormalities; can impact vision
Wolfram Syndrome	Bilateral, progressive, sloping HF SNHL	Autosomal recessive	Diabetes; can impact intellectual function

Note. CHL: conductive hearing loss; SNHL: sensorineural hearing loss; HF: high frequency; CNS: central nervous system; HL: hearing loss.

CASE EXAMPLE

Edie, a 9-month-old child with Down syndrome, is scheduled for an assessment. The case history indicates that she was born full term with no pregnancy or birth complications. She is being followed for problems related to her heart. Edie has a significant history of ear infections. By parent report, the otolaryngologist reported that Edie's ear canals are too small for placement of pressure-equalization (PE) tubes. Test results show no movement of the TM (Type B tympanograms) for both 226 and 1000 Hz probe tones with ear canal volumes of 0.2, bilaterally. DPOAEs are absent in both ears. Edie would not condition to the VRA task.

What is your interpretation of the test results, and what is the next step in Edie's plan of testing?

The ear canal volumes obtained during immittance testing are at the low end of normal but could be consistent with small ear canals that can be seen in children with Down syndrome. Moreover, the tympanograms would be consistent with abnormal movement of the eardrum, consistent with middle ear infections. The absent DPOAEs could then be consistent with the abnormal movement of the eardrum. Because of developmental requirements of VRA testing, infants with Down syndrome can be delayed in their ability to successfully perform the task (Nightengale et al., 2020). Given these results, the recommendation would be to schedule ABR testing to estimate the type and degree of hearing loss. The ABR should include both air- and bone-conduction testing. In addition to the baseline ABR testing, the hearing should be monitored, given the risk for recurrent middle ear disorder and the risk for speech-language delays in this population.

Infections and Disorders

Other infections and disorders may be associated with pediatric hearing loss. Examples can be found in Table 6–6. It is important to note that certain infections (e.g., (s)TORCH infections) can be associated with progressive hearing loss. The possibility of a progressive nature of hearing loss has implications for consistently monitoring auditory status in these patients. The reader can refer to the 2019 Joint Committee on Infant Hearing revised risk indicators for recommendations regarding monitoring frequency (Joint Committee on Infant Hearing, 2019).

TABLE 6–6. Examples of Pediatric Infections and Disorders

INFECTION/DISORDER	ASSOCIATED HEARING LOSS	INFECTION/DISORDER DESCRIPTION AND IMPACT
Childhood infections		
Bacterial Meningitis	Severe to profound Bilateral/symmetrical SNHL Fluctuating or progressive	Bacterial infection that can enter and damage the inner ear; can lead to ossification of the cochlea; sequelae also include problems with vision and cognition
Mumps (Mizushima & Murakami, 1986)	Profound Unilateral SNHL Sudden onset	Viral infection that causes swollen salivary glands and can damage the inner ear
In utero infections		
Syphilis	Severe to profound Bilateral SNHL Early onset/rapid progression or late onset/sudden	STD transmitted from mother to fetus; in addition to hearing loss, can impact central nervous system (CNS) and vestibular system
Toxoplasmosis	Sensorineural HL	Parasitic infection from cat feces or litter; in addition to hearing loss, can impact vision and cognitive function; can lead to hydrocephaly, microcephaly, and cerebral palsy
Rubella	Mild to profound Bilateral SNHL Cookie bite configuration common	Risk depends on gestation of transmission; in addition to hearing loss, can impact heart function, vision, and intellectual function
CMV	Severe to profound Bilateral (symptomatic) or unilateral (asymptomatic—majority of babies) SNHL Can fluctuate or progress; delayed onset	Type of herpes that increases risk if transmitted during pregnancy or if immunocompromised; in addition to hearing loss, can impact vision
Herpes	SNHL Delayed onset, progressive	Prenatal or perinatal (more severe) transmission; in addition to hearing loss can lead to other neurologic problems

CASE EXAMPLE

Jamal is a 3-month-old infant being seen for an audiological assessment. In the hospital, Jamal was in the well-baby nursery and did not have any symptoms of infection. He passed the initial hearing screening via OAEs in the well-baby nursery. However, testing in the hospital determined that Jamal had congenital cytomegalovirus (cCMV). By parent report, he has been taking medication for the cCMV, and his viral load has decreased significantly. Jamal is being followed by early childhood intervention (ECI) due to his risk of developmental delays. Recommendations following a passed hearing screening were for Jamal's hearing to be monitored regularly. On the current test date, tympanometry using a 1000-Hz probe tone indicated normal TM mobility bilaterally. Based on this case history information, the audiologist performed threshold auditory brainstem response (ABR) testing using click and tone burst (500, 2000, and 4000 Hz in both ears). Bone conduction ABR was also completed. The ABR testing with masking revealed a moderate sensorineural hearing loss in the right ear, with responses at normal intensity levels in the left ear. Why could a hearing loss caused by cCMV be missed in a newborn hearing screening? What are the recommendations for this child?

The hearing loss with cCMV can be progressive. As such, it is possible that the right ear either had normal hearing or had a slight loss that would be missed by screening OAEs. The hearing loss could have progressed to a moderate hearing loss by the appointment when Jamal was 3 months old. Given the progressive nature of cCMV, it is important to counsel parents regarding options for a unilateral hearing loss.

In this case, Jamal was fit with a hearing aid in his right ear. His hearing continued to be monitored. At 12 months of age, Jamal's hearing had progressed to a severe-to-profound loss in the right ear and a mild loss in his left ear. At that time, he was referred to a cochlear implant team for his right ear. Due to the continued possibility of progression of hearing loss, Jamal received a cochlear implant at 14 months of age in the right ear. His hearing progressed to a moderate hearing loss in the left ear, for which he received a hearing aid. The recommendation also would include assessment and treatment by a speech-language pathologist, in addition to continuation of monitoring by the physicians on his team.

(Central) Auditory Processing Disorder ((C)APD)

(Central) auditory processing disorder presents in children with normal peripheral auditory sensitivity, yet they experience difficulty with various (and more complex) auditory tasks. Its etiology is thought to be abnormal function of the central auditory nervous system (CANS), whether due to an insult, lesion of the system, or functional difficulties related to immaturity of the CANS. Characteristics of

(C)APD are associated with difficulties not only in auditory skills but are seen in speech/language and academic difficulties.

- Common issues include difficulty in background noise, difficulty following oral directions, poor listening skills, academic difficulties, poor auditory association skills, easily distracted or inattentive to auditory signals, and hyperacusis. It is important to recognize that (C)APD is a continually evolving field of research and there are different views on causes, symptoms, and management. It is best managed by an interdisciplinary team that can examine the impact/relation to not only auditory skills but to communication and education.

Definition and Purpose of (C)APD Testing

ASHA convened a group of professionals to develop a working definition of auditory processing difficulty in 2005. In 2010, AAA released their statement, which supported this definition.

- "Difficulties in the processing of auditory information in the central nervous system (CNS) as demonstrated by poor performance in one or more of the following skills" (ASHA, 2005)
  - □ Sound localization and lateralization
  - □ Auditory discrimination
  - □ Auditory pattern recognition
  - □ Temporal aspects of audition (including temporal integration, temporal discrimination, temporal ordering, temporal masking)
  - □ Auditory performance in competing acoustic signals (including dichotic listening)
  - □ Auditory performance with degraded acoustic signals
- Purpose of (C)APD testing is to diagnose (C)APDs and identify areas of difficulty; the second purpose then is to devise management and treatment intervention programs for individuals with (C)APD.
- Categories of (C)APD include
  - □ Developmental (C)APD: present in children with normal audiometric hearing, with no known etiology or defined lesion
  - □ Acquired (C)APD: occurs in patients with no previous of history of auditory processing difficulties, who later present with auditory processing difficulties
- Diagnostic criteria
  - □ Two tests at least 2 standard deviations below the mean for at least one ear (ASHA, 2005; AAA, 2010); note that there is disagreement regarding this criterion in that some suggest the use of as little as 1 standard deviation below the mean to make a diagnosis of (C)APD.
  - □ Poor performance on one test may be considered abnormal if results are 3 standard deviations below the mean and/or consistent with severe functional difficulties (ASHA, 2005).
- Educational implications
  - □ U.S. Court of Appeals for the Ninth Circuit ruled that (C)APD can be classified as Other Health Impaired (OHI) for qualification for special education services through the Individuals with Disabilities Act (IDEA) in *E.M. v. Pajaro Valley Unified School* (2019).

- ☐ To be considered OHI for IDEA, a disorder must
  - Be a chronic or an acute health problem
  - Due to the identified problem, the student has limited strength, vitality, or limited alertness (including a heightened alertness to environmental stimuli that results in limited alertness with respect to the educational environment)

Central Anatomy and Physiology Review

For a comprehensive discussion of CANS anatomy and physiology, please refer to Chapter 2. The information provided in Table 6–7 is a brief review of important CANS structures relevant to (C)APD in children.

Approaches in Audiology

Different approaches are used to categorize (C)APDs. The approach an audiologist chooses should be founded in evidence-based practices that consider a clinical protocol based on age-based normative data with a clear indication of what the inclusion criteria are and who should be excluded based on other diagnoses. Currently, there are primarily two approaches to address (C)APDs. One is a model approach that uses scores on specific diagnostics tests to categorize the type of disorder, while the other uses deficit-specific areas to guide diagnosis and management.

Models of (Central) Auditory Processing

A model approach to examining auditory (central) processing includes testing that would place a child's performance into various categories of processing difficulties. These models are based on neurologic areas of damage and infer functional components based on scores on specific diagnostic tests or test batteries. Two common models include the Buffalo Model by Jack Katz and the Bellis/Ferre Model (Jutras et al., 2007).

The Buffalo Model

The Buffalo Model considers areas of CANS performance as measured test scores on the staggered spondaic word test (SSW; a dichotic test), phonemic synthesis test (test that blends speech sounds to form a word), and speech-in-noise test. Scores from these tests are used to divide children into four categories. Based on the category, functional skills are inferred, and therapy is conducted related to these areas.

- ■ Decoding: breakdown at the phonemic level
  - ☐ Test results include excessive errors in the SSW right competing and left noncompeting conditions, and poor phonemic synthesis.
  - ☐ Projected area of dysfunction is the left posterior temporal lobe.
  - ☐ Possible functional difficulties include weakness is expected in oral reading, word accuracy, and spelling skills due to difficulty at the phonemic level.
- ■ Tolerance fading memory: breakdown at the memory level
  - ☐ Test results include quick responses, "smushed" responses (using component of both spondees to make a single word), repeating the carrier phrase, and omissions of words on the SSW. Omissions are also seen on the phonemic synthesis test and these individuals have difficulty on the speech-in-noise test.

TABLE 6–7. Anatomical Structures Related to Auditory Processing and Sample Test Measures

ANATOMICAL STRUCTURE	ROLE IN AUDITORY PROCESSING	EXAMPLES OF (C)APD TESTS
Cochlear Nucleus	Precise timing patterns	Ipsilateral deficits on dichotic listening
Superior Olivary Complex (SOC)	Interaural timing	MLDs
	Figure-ground: reduction of low-frequency, moderately loud noise[a]	Acoustic reflexes
	Figure-ground—reduction of mid-high frequency, quiet noise[a]	Suppression of OAEs
Inferior Colliculus	Sound duration and gap detection	Contralateral deficits on dichotic listening and/or degraded signals (e.g., filtered speech, time-compressed speech)
Medial Geniculate Body	Localization interaural time and intensity differences and beginning processing of the natural speech signal	Contralateral dichotic listening deficits
Auditory Cortex right hemisphere	Temporal skills, spatial representation of stimuli, overall meaning of the message	Dichotic tests—left ear scores. Temporal patterns of pitch and duration, gap detection
Auditory Cortex left hemisphere	Language dominance and organization, details within the overall pattern of speech, perceive subtle speech cues	Dichotic tests—right ear scores
Corpus Callosum	Connection of the two hemispheres of the brain to integrate auditory information from both cerebral hemispheres	Verbal labeling pitch or duration patterns, significant deficits on left ear during dichotic listening

[a]Information from Liberman and Guinan (1998).
Source: Data primarily from Musiek and Baran (2020) and Rawool (2016).

- ☐ Projected areas of dysfunction are the frontal lobes and anterior temporal region.
- ☐ Possible functional difficulties include poor auditory memory and difficulty listening in noise, expressive language difficulties, and impulsive responses.
- ■ Integration: integration of information from both sides of the brain
  - ☐ Test results include Type A SSW pattern, as well as long response time on SSW
  - ☐ Projected areas of dysfunction are the posterior corpus callosum and/or angular gyrus of the parietal-occipital region. There is a secondary profile of integration that is more associated with the anterior region of the corpus callosum.

□ Possible functional difficulties are poor reading skills, difficulty spelling, and difficulty with visual\auditory association (e.g., dyslexia).

■ Organization: organizing what is heard

□ Test results include reversals on primarily the SSW but can be seen on the phonemic synthesis test as well.

□ Projected area of dysfunction is the anterior temporal/temporoparietal regions

□ Possible functional difficulties poor organization, planning, and sequencing

Bellis/Ferre Model

The Bellis/Ferre Model examines areas of CANS performance as measured on test scores for dichotic measures (e.g., dichotic digits, SSW, competing words), temporal tasks (e.g., pitch or duration patterns), low-redundancy speech (e.g., filtered words), and speech-in-noise tests. Scores from these tests are used to divide children into three primary categories. Based on the category, functional skills are inferred and therapy related to these areas.

■ Auditory decoding deficit: poor phonemic skills

□ Test results include poorer right ear scores on low-redundancy tests and speech-in-noise tests.

□ This is also associated with poor right ear scores (or both) on dichotic tests and/or competing sentences.

□ Projected area of dysfunction is thought to be the primary auditory cortex in the left hemisphere.

□ Possible functional difficulties include difficulty with phonemic skills, discrimination, and sound blending.

■ Prosodic deficit: difficulty recognizing the prosodic components of speech (e.g., rate, rhythm, inflection)

□ Test results include abnormal tonal patterns (e.g., pitch and duration), poor left ear skills on dichotic testing, but good speech-in-noise.

□ Projected area of difficulty is the right hemisphere.

□ Possible functional problem areas: singing, social skills, flat tone of voice, and poor visual-spatial skills

■ Integration: inter- or intrahemispheric skills

□ Test results include poor left ear on dichotic tasks and labeling of pitch or duration patterns.

□ Projected areas of difficulty would be the corpus callosum (interhemispheric transfer of auditory information).

□ Possible functional problems would include drawing, understanding someone speaking (when the child needs to take notes), and multimodality learning tasks.

Deficit-Specific Categorization

Assessing deficit-specific abilities is another viewpoint for classifying (C)APD. Some researchers suggest that specific scores on specific tests do not always correlate with specific functional areas of deficit (Gustafson & Keith, 2005). Considering tests that examine specific functional abilities is designed to address concerns related to specific areas of observed deficit. Note, however, that these areas do not all align with the specific auditory skills outlined by ASHA and AAA as underpinning auditory processing. This method allows the provider to address specific difficulties experienced by the child and apply them to the educational setting. A deficit-based "hierarchy" of auditory processing skills (adapted from English, 2001) and examples of domain-specific tests include:

- Awareness/localization: knowing that a sound has occurred and knowing where a sound source is located
    - Testing includes pure-tone testing, Listening in Spatialized Noise–Sentences (LiSN-S)— can be used to diagnose spatial processing disorder. Localization can also be assessed using an informal method of having them point to a sound source when their eyes are closed.
- Discrimination: ability to know if two sounds are the same or different
    - Tests include the Test of Auditory Processing Skills–4 (TAPS-4; subtest of discrimination) and Lindamood Assessment.
- Recognition: recognizing a word and being able to repeat it back correctly
    - Testing would include speech recognition testing at various levels such as syllables, words, and sentences.
- Auditory attention: skill of being able to attend to a particular auditory signal
    - Tests include the Auditory Continuous Performance Test (ACPT)
- Figure-ground: ability to ignore background noise (both speech or nonspeech) and repeat the desired signal; different types of noise and targets should be utilized.
    - Tests include word recognition in noise, but also the Selective Auditory Attention Task, Synthetic Sentence Index Test (SSI), and the SCAN-3 (Child or Adolescents; figure-ground section).
- Synthesis: putting sounds together and taking them apart
    - Tests include Phonemic Synthesis, Phonemic Awareness Test, or TAPS-4 (Phonological Deletion and Phonological Blending).
    - Note: when working in an interdisciplinary team, the speech-language pathologists often assess this area.
- Degraded signals: ability to fill in missing acoustic information in degraded auditory signals
    - Tests include filtered speech, SCAN-3 (Child or Adolescents; filtered speech and time compressed sentences subtests), and time-compressed speech.
- Dichotic listening tasks: examining the ability to separate and integrate information from both sides of the brain and are a measure of language dominance
    - Tests include the SSW; SCAN-3 (Child or Adolescents, competing words and sentences subtests); dichotic digits, words, or sentences; and binaural fusion.
    - Dichotic tests are often examined not just as overall scores, but by comparing the ears' performance to each other. If one ear outperforms the other, this is referred to as an ear advantage. Right ear advantages are typical to a degree.
- Memory and sequencing: remembering acoustic information and keeping it sequenced in order
    - Tests include the TAPS-4, or pitch and duration pattern sequence.

■ Temporal resolution: processing the auditory information to identify rate, pitch, and duration, at an appropriate speed

  □ Tests include gap detection (Gaps in Noise, Random Gap Detection), pitch pattern sequence, and duration pattern sequence.

Q & A

Question: A 9-year-old girl with difficulty retelling a story she has heard was tested for (C)APD using dichotic measures. She shows a right ear advantage (REA) typical of a much younger child. What does a REA tell you about her auditory development?

Answer: She still appears to be on a typical developmental path but is delayed in acquiring dichotic listening skills. Depending on the other findings, she may be diagnosed with integration-type (C)APD with training efforts focused on dichotic listening.

Testing Factors

The selection of tests used depends on the approach (model or deficit specific) used and what information is desired. An audiologist should consider the implications for the child and what information tests will supply the other members of the multidisciplinary team.

■ Factors that impact whether a child should be tested and/or influence test results

  □ Age: scores are variable below age 7 with large confidence intervals so testing is not recommended.

  □ Language: children for whom English is a second language should be tested in the child's primary language. Also, the language level of the task when testing needs to be considered for a child. Children with lower language skills may require nonverbal tasks.

  □ Global function: it is recommended that the child's global functioning (IQ) be 85 or greater. If that is not possible as a total score, a nonverbal IQ of 85 or greater could be used as the criterion. Any known executive function difficulties (e.g., working memory) should also be considered related to concerns for whether a child should be tested and/or which tests may be inappropriate to use because the skills required for testing would be highly impacted by poor executive function.

  □ ADHD: children with ADHD should be tested on medication to try to control attention impact. Later testing can be done off of medications (working with the child's doctor) to see if ADHD makes the symptoms worse or if (C)APD was the primary concern.

  □ Multidisciplinary team: a team is needed to address all areas of functional concern and coordinate management.

  □ Hearing: in pursuing a diagnosis of (C)APD, hearing needs to be within normal limits; by and large, testing norms are based off of individuals with normal hearing.

☐ Speech/language disorders: a child's speech/language abilities need to be considered so that test results will not be impacted by errors due to articulation or by language skills impacting the child's understanding of the task.

☐ Neurological disorders: since (C)APD is examining the CANS, children with known lesions of the CANS should have difficulty on the test measures, so a diagnosis of (C)APD cannot be definitively made.

The information above is related to diagnosis of (C)APD as the primary disorder. (C)APD tests of function may be given to individuals with comorbid disorders to examine the individual's functional abilities but should not change their primary diagnosis.

■ Case history risk factors (C)APD

☐ History of otitis media

☐ History of hyperbilirubinemia

☐ Family history

☐ Medical issues during pregnancy such as anoxia, bacterial/viral illness, maternal drug or alcohol abuse

☐ Severe childhood illness

☐ Neurologic issues

☐ Maternal smoking during pregnancy

☐ Smoking in the home (contribution to otitis media)

☐ Anesthesia use recently

■ Checklists can be used to get an idea of the difficulties experienced by a child with (C)APD.

☐ The Screening Instrument for Targeting Educational Risk (SIFTER) and Children's Auditory Performance Scale (CHAPS) are two that can be used. These are discussed later in the chapter in the Educational Audiology section.

☐ Fisher's Auditory Problems Checklist is a checklist of auditory characteristics where the teacher or parent checks off applicable behaviors.

☐ Children's Home Inventory for Listening Difficulties (CHILD) by Anderson and Smaldino (2011) is a checklist that parents and the child answer regarding how difficult 15 different listening situations are for the child.

☐ Other tests can be found in resources listed in the Educational Audiology section.

■ Factors to consider when testing for (C)APD

☐ Test difficulty

☐ If a lower-level problem is seen in the auditory skills hierarchy, testing at the higher levels may not be performed as they build on each other as a foundation.

☐ Functional implications in educational settings

☐ Test scores

• Some tests do not have standard scores and/or the scores have large confidence intervals, which makes diagnosis difficult. This is reflective of the fact that auditory development of complex skills varies widely as children development, with marked variability at younger ages.

- □ Validity of testing
  - Test protocol is required and testing should be performed in a controlled environment.
- □ Language load
- □ Tests contain varying language loads (language difficulty) and these need to be considered prior to testing to be sure the instructions and stimuli are appropriate for a child's language skills and cognitive level.

- ■ Peripheral audiological testing should be completed prior to (C)APD testing to not only rule out peripheral hearing loss but also examine results that impact the auditory processing. A peripheral test battery should include:
  - □ Pure-tone audiometry, including interoctave frequencies
  - □ Speech recognition in quiet and noise
  - □ Immittance measures
  - □ OAEs
  - □ Use of electrophysiology
    - There are no agreed-upon criteria as to when electrophysiology should be included in the clinical evaluation of (C)APD. However, electrophysiology assessment should be considered when results of neurologic concern are obtained, such as hearing asymmetries, abnormal MEMRs, large asymmetry between ears for word recognition scores, switching ear advantages on right ear first versus left ear first reporting of dichotic tasks, large left ear advantages, and so on.
    - Limited evidence exists to support the inclusion of these tests in cases of normal peripheral findings, with the exception of the ABR. When used with OAEs, the ABR is necessary in identifying ANSD.
    - MLR and later potentials (like the P300) can provide insight into thalamocortical and cortical functioning, respectively.

- ■ Not all testing requires an audiometer; there have been an increasing number of computer or app-based (C)APD measures recently.
  - □ Feather Squadron (Acoustic Pioneer) is an app-based system to assess auditory processing skills. Based on results, therapy programs to address areas of functional difficulties exist.
  - □ CAPDOTS (capdots.com) is an online system that includes an assessment for auditory processing disorders designed to work with children with binaural integration and separation difficulties.

- ■ Speech and language testing may cover some of the same areas, such as phonemic skills, and can be used in conjunction with (C)APD testing to look at more functional areas. Following or concurrent with (C)APD testing, advanced language assessment may help in developing strategies and determining if bottom-up or top-down training may be best. Advanced language assessment may include phonemic skills, executive function, problem-solving, theory of mind, reading skills.

Management Overview

Management of (C)APD can be grouped into modification of the environment, compensatory strategies, and direct rehabilitative services, which include perceptual/auditory training as well as cognitive training. Components of management include:

- Modifications of the environment
  - Improvement of the signal-to-ratio (SNR) by:
    - Increasing the signal loudness by increasing the teacher's loudness or decreasing the child's distance from the speaker
    - Decreasing the background noise through improving classroom acoustics (including reverberation) and controlling noise in the classroom
  - Train student to listen better by using whole-body listening, increasing the child's motivation to listen and teaching the child to advocate when struggling.
  - Hearing assistive technology systems (HATS), where the teacher is wearing a microphone that transmits to some form of receiver the child is wearing, can be used to improve environmental listening by improving SNR. (A more in-depth discussion is in the Educational Audiology section later in this chapter.)

- Compensatory strategies for children with (C)APD include improving acoustics/environment, accommodations, modifying presentation methods, providing support, maximizing other sensory cues, and providing encouragement.

- Direct services can be provided by audiologists and/or speech-language pathologist and include both perceptual and cognitive training.
  - Perceptual/auditory training is a bottom-up style therapy based on perceptual auditory skills using training to strengthen skills. It utilizes several principles in training (Musiek et al., 2014). It relies on the fact that the central auditory system is plastic and can learn auditory skills through exposure to auditory stimuli either through increased natural exposure or planned therapy. It includes the principle that active exposure for the child is more efficient when the child is active and motivated. Evidence-based research supports different perceptual trainings (Musiek et al., 2014).
    - Dichotic Interaural Intensity Training (DIID) (Moncrieff & Wertz, 2008)
    - Speech-in-noise training
    - Discrimination training
    - Temporal processing training
    - Commercial computer-based training programs
      - CAPDOTS (capdots.com)
      - Insane Airplane, Zoo Caper, Elephant Memory (Acoustic Pioneer)
  - Cognitive training is a top-down style using cognition concepts to facilitate processing. Often this is performed in collaboration with the speech-language pathologist on the team. It uses cognitive strategies, metacognitive strategies, and metalinguistic strategies to train the child to perform top-down tasks. For more information about different strategies, the reader is directed to Chermak (2014).

- Cognitive strategies include training in auditory attention and vigilance, auditory memory, mnemonics strategies, and mind-mapping.

- Metacognitive strategies areas include attribution retraining, self-instruction, cognitive problem-solving, self-regulation, cognitive strategies, cognitive style and reasoning, reciprocal teaching, and assertiveness training.

- Metalinguistic strategies include discourse cohesion devices, schema, auditory verbal closure, vocabulary building, phonologic awareness, and prosody training.

☐ There is a complementary nature of bottom-up and top-down processing. Bottom-up focuses on strategies to deal with novel or degraded incoming signals, whereas top-down uses prior knowledge for structure to process the incoming message.

Educational Audiology

Children with hearing loss are included as individuals who may need to receive services under the Individuals with Disabilities Act (IDEA) and Section 504 of the Rehabilitation Act. To qualify, a "specialist" in hearing/deafness needs to provide evidence the child has a significant difficulty in an educational system due to their hearing status. Though there are several professionals who could be a "specialist" (e.g., otolaryngologist, teachers of the deaf, speech-language pathologists), audiologists are trained to recognize the specific impact of hearing difficulties. To meet the growing needs of students with varying levels and types of hearing loss, audiologists are being more frequently employed by, or contracted with, local school districts or educational service centers to provide audiological services to children in the school systems. The audiologist will determine the nature and degree of hearing loss as well as how the child processes speech information. They will also examine amplification the child is using, as well as make recommendations for HATS. This information will help determine the level of concern for the child's educational need.

- Educational implications of hearing loss: children who are deaf or hard of hearing are at risk for educational difficulty. Educational implications vary according to degree of hearing loss; however, degree of loss does not address all listening situations. Factors not reflected on the audiogram will affect each child differently. Educational recommendations should be created based on assessment and individual needs.

- Some factors associated with children who are Deaf/Hard of Hearing (DHH):
  ☐ Poor speech production (articulation)
  ☐ Problems with expressive and receptive language skills (especially high-level skills)
  ☐ Difficulties with language often lead to delays in reading and writing.
  ☐ Poor understanding of speech in noise
  ☐ Difficulty focusing and paying close attention so as to fill in missing information
  ☐ Experience fatigue by the end of the day as hearing loss may impact listening effort, or how much effort is exerted to be able to understand speech, or listening fatigue (Hicks & Tharpe, 2002)
  ☐ Negative effects to Theory of Mind (ToM) skills
  ☐ Notable changes for mental health have been noted, as well as the impact of bullying due to being considered different by other children

      ☐ One item that is NOT a result of hearing loss is cognitive ability. Hearing loss does not lower a child's cognitive ability. As seen above, the deficit relates more to effectively communicating thoughts and developing cognitive skills due to language deprivation.

Relevant Legislation

Much of the current legislation is based on laws regarding children with disabilities in the 1970s. Example legislation, from the 1970s to current, includes:

- Section 504 of the Rehabilitation Act of 1973, which prohibits discrimination and protects individuals, including children in the schools
- PL 94-142, The Education for all Handicapped Children Act (1975)
  - ☐ Ensured "free appropriate publication in the least restrictive environment"
  - ☐ First to delineate Individualized Education Programs (IEPs) in the schools
- PL 99-457 Education of the Handicapped Act Amendments (1986)
  - ☐ Extended 94-142 to include children from 3 to 5 years of age
  - ☐ Included option for early intervention services for birth to 2 years and Individualized Family Service Plans (IFSPs) for the early intervention services
- Americans with Disabilities Act (ADA)
  - ☐ Protects against discrimination
- Individuals with Disabilities Education Act (IDEA)
  - ☐ Combined 94-142 and 99-457
  - ☐ Services for birth to 5 and preschool/school age children are included as well.
  - ☐ IDEA has different sections for school-aged children and early childhood intervention with different eligibility requirements.

Eligibility and Services

Eligibility should be determined using a multidisciplinary team to obtain information about if the child meets criteria for the description of significant hearing loss. This hearing loss needs to show an impact on educational performance, leading to a need for special education. Once a child has been identified as having hearing difficulties by a "specialist" in hearing/deafness, information will be examined by a team to determine if the child qualifies for services and, if so, what services. Using this information, the educational system (and/or early childhood program) will determine if the child qualifies under IDEA. In the educational setting, a team would comprise an administrator, a general education teacher, a special education teacher, and the child's parent(s)/legal guardian(s) but can include others such as the audiologist, teacher of the deaf, speech-language pathologist, and so on. The team members vary by state requirements.

- 504 Services
  - ☐ Considerations for 504 accommodations and modifications would be included in the IDEA determination. However, a child found to not qualify for IDEA still qualifies for 504 services.

☐ 504 services address lack of access to information in an educational setting. Reasonable accommodation would be provided to have appropriate access to general education. This may include seating assignment, HATS, and so on. However, it would not include modifications to instruction such as a special education teacher who modifies assignments or instruction or speech-language therapy.

KNOWLEDGE CHECKPOINT

Section 504 of the Rehabilitative Act of 1973 protects a child against discrimination for a disability that impacts a major life activity, which includes hearing-related disabilities. In these cases, the child would have a 504 plan but would be provided accommodations through general education. Children with slight losses or unilateral losses may not qualify for services under IDEA. In states that have not expanded the definition of DHH for IDEA to include slight or unilateral hearing loss, a 504 plan may be used to provide accommodations.

■ Services for birth to 5 and preschool/school age children
  ☐ Legislation has described how provisions should be outlined and documented.
    • IFSP—Individualized Family Service Plan for the child and family of children that are less than 3 years old
    • Provides services to train parents/caregivers and family members how to facilitate communication and development for a child with hearing loss as well as:
      ○ Teaches the family how to be an advocate for their child
      ○ Provides connections to other DHH families, mentors, and role models
      ○ Includes transition planning to move to preschool services
      ○ Different states implement these services through different programs, either through early childhood intervention (ECI) or through the area educational services.
■ Services for school-aged children
  ☐ Eligibility is covered through IDEA utilizing the criteria for hearing loss.
    • IEP—Individualized Educational Program for school-aged children up to the age of 21
      ○ Provides for educational placement
      ○ Includes FAPE (free and public education) and LRE (least restrictive environment), including opportunity to communicate with peers and staff in the child's preferred language/communication system
      ○ Directs accommodations and services the child will receive to promote educational access
      ○ A child served through IDEA (i.e., with an IEP or an IFSP) is provided accommodations and modifications through special education services. As such, they must qualify for these services through formal and informal testing indicating a significant educational impact of the hearing loss.

○ Eligibility criteria are set by each state. However, the hearing loss may still negatively impact auditory performance (e.g., difficulty understanding in background noise), even if other eligibility criteria are not met.

○ Includes audiologic services to be provided through the schools, such as programming/ verification of amplification, hearing assistive technology systems, assessment of performance with equipment, and training for families and educators. These services may be provided by an audiologist working directly for the school, contracted with the school, or the child's personal audiologist.

○ Eligibility is based on interdisciplinary coordination of assessment by different professionals

Assessment

IDEA clauses related to evaluation (300.101, 304, and 303.324) "use a variety of assessment tools and strategies to gather relevant functional, developmental, and academic information about the child, including information provided by the parent, that may assist in determining whether the child is a child with a disability" (300.304(b)(1)). Functional skills are not solely related to academic performance and cannot be measured using one assessment or criterion. Testing should include both formal as well as informal methods. The goal is to measure performance and determine functional performance. Testing should include assessment performed both in an audiometric booth and in the classroom. Multiple measures should be administered to determine how to provide free and appropriate education (FAPE) by determining services and supports that will be needed to meet the identified academic and functional needs.

- Assessment should be performed regularly to assist in development of the Individualized Education Program (IEP).
  □ Reevaluations every 3 years are required by the IEP; however, testing may be recommended more frequently. Best practice for audiologic monitoring is annually or as recommended according to the audiologist.
  □ Testing should also be considered if the child is experiencing difficulties, changing schools, changing classrooms, changing teachers, changing academic level (e.g., elementary to middle school), or if the child has a change in listening skills or amplification.
  □ Testing should also be performed if the team and parents express concerns.
  □ Addendums or modifications can be made at any time by the IEP or 504 team based on assessment data.
- An audiologist is responsible for several areas in educational assessment.
  □ The initial purpose is an assessment to determine eligibility.
  □ Further assessment provides information about the impact of the child's hearing loss and the functional difficulties associated with the loss.
  □ Other areas of assessment beyond diagnostic testing for eligibility include speech perception and auditory skills development, assessing the learning environment, determining equipment benefit, and determining functional performance.
- Basic assessment procedures start with an age-appropriate typical pediatric audiologic evaluation as discussed earlier in the chapter, with a few additions of measurement of speech

using more conversational speech measures (such as sentences) to examine more functional components. Speech perception in noise should also be performed to evaluate functional components.

☐ Additional measures should include:

- Speech recognition for sentences and phrases, with and without visual support to assess auditory-only versus auditory-visual condition

- Listening in noise at various signal-to-noise ratios with a baseline of testing in quiet for a comparison of performance

■ Measuring auditory skill development can include parent measures (especially for very young children) and measures requiring response from the child. This can be performed by the speech-language pathologist or obtained via data from other members of the team.

☐ Examples of parent/teacher measures that can be used to describe what the caregiver sees as the child's perception of sound include the IT-MAIS and PEACH/TEACH described earlier in this chapter.

☐ Examples of child perceptual measures

- Ling 6: gross determination of if a child can perceive speech sounds across the frequency spectrum, as well as being used to check equipment function

- Early Speech Perception Test (ESP; Geers & Moog, 2012): identify skills for children as young as 3 years old

- Cottage Acquisition of Speech and Language Learning (CASLLs; Wilkes, 2001): checklists that can be used to report if a child has age-appropriate auditory perceptual skills

- Developmental Approach to Successful Listening II (DASL II; Stout & Windle, 1986): checklist that corresponds to a stimuli booklet to help examine perceptual skills

■ An audiologist is also needed to examine the child's learning environment to determine the impact of reverberation and noise in a classroom. The audiologist will perform assessment to determine the signal-to-noise ratio (SNR) by examining the qualities of the class environment that may impact hearing and provide recommendations to improve the acoustic environment. Performance in the classroom for listening comprehension (recognition) in the classroom (e.g., speech recognition, functional listening evaluation [FLE]) should also be assessed. Assessment includes:

☐ Classroom acoustic measures including noise levels, reverberation, critical distance, SNR, and the distribution of speaker's voice in the classroom. These should be examined in light of the ASHA/ANSI recommendations of:

- Unoccupied classroom level should be ≤35 dBA

- SNR of at least +15 dB at the child's ears

- Reverberation time for a smaller classroom (<10,000 cubic feet) should be 0.6 seconds or less and for a larger classroom <0.7 seconds.

☐ Classroom observations should be performed to examine acoustics, teacher presentation (rate, language, volume), teaching methods, and organization of material. This can be informal or use forms such as the Classroom Observation Checklist and Classroom-at-a-Glance Checklist (Deconde Johnson & Seaton, 2021).

□ Teacher, parent, and child questionnaires can be used to determine functional performance in the classroom. Some that are used include:

- Children's Auditory Performance Scale: C.H.A.P.S. (http://www.edaud.org) has 36 questions on a 6-point scale, with six listening conditions (Noise, Quiet, Ideal, Multiple Inputs, Auditory Memory Sequencing, Auditory Attention Span). The child's performance is rated by parents or teachers in these areas as compared to their same-aged peers.

- Screening Instrument for Targeting Educational Risk: SIFTER (http://successforkidswithhearingloss.com) has 15 questions on a 5-point scale, in five areas (academics, attention, communication, classroom participation, behavior). The child's performance is rated by parents or teachers in these areas as compared to same-aged peers. Preschool, Elementary, and Secondary versions are available.

- Listening Inventory for Education: LIFE (http://successforkidswithhearingloss.com) has two versions, one for the child (10 questions) and one for the teacher (15 questions). Questions relate to commonly encountered educational listening environments and has the child/teacher rate on a scale from always easy to always difficult for the child or no challenge to almost always challenged for the teacher's choices.

■ The audiologist will also be responsible for assessing the performance of the child's amplification equipment. This includes verification and validation measures to confirm equipment is functioning properly. The educational audiologist also needs to assess how the child is performing functionally in the classroom and determine if a HATS is beneficial; an FLE can be used for this assessment (Deconde Johnson & VonAlmen, 1993, updated 2013).

□ An FLE compares a child's listening ability in a variety of situations to identify effects of noise, distance, and visual cues. Testing can also be performed with HATS.

□ An FLE can be used to estimate a child's listening performance in different listening situations, provide evidence for benefits of HATS, and make decisions about what components of HATS meet a child's needs.

□ Performing an FLE

- For an evaluation of functional performance, sentences should be used to be more representative of conversational speech encountered in the classroom. Some sentence lists include Blair, Pediatric Az Bio, CID Everyday Sentences, BKB Sin, WIPI Sentences, and HINT Sentences.

- Signal can be provided via live voice (monitored through a sound level meter) or recorded (with video for visual cue condition).

- Presentation level should be an average 65 dB A at the student's ear when the examiner/ recording is 3 ft away.

- Recorded noise that is representative of the child's listening environment (e.g., multitalker babble, cafeteria noise, Child's Noise CD from Auditec) presented at an average 60 dB A at the student's ear, when the noise is 3 ft from the child's ear. Noise should come from the direction that is typical of the child's environment. Figure 6–5 shows the setup of the noise and signal used in FLE testing.

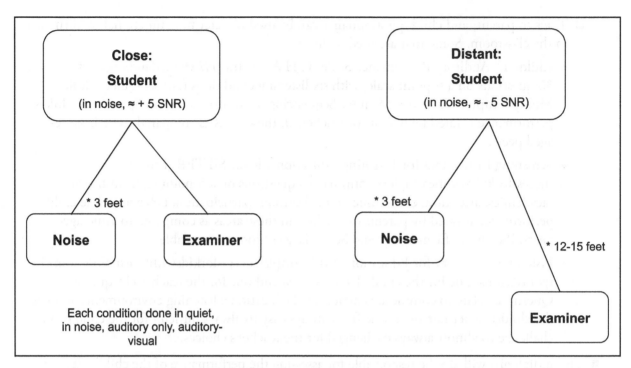

FIGURE 6–5. Functional listening evaluation setup diagram.

Q & A

Figure 6–6 is adapted from Deconde Johnson and VonAlmen (1993, updated in 2013) and shows scoring for a child's FLE evaluation.

On this form are a few sample readings. For this case, examine the child's scores in quiet in the functional listening scorebox. The score for the auditory-only condition is 88% (Box 2). Next, examine the scores in noise for this condition (Box 4), which shows 72% correct.

Question: What does that tell you about the child's speech understanding in noise?

Answer: Noise has a negative effect on the child's speech recognition performance.

Any area with a diagonal line can be performed both with and without a HATS system. Scores above the line show performance without the HATS system. Scores below the line represent findings using the HATS system. In this case, there is an example shown in the auditory, distant condition, in noise (shown in Box 6).

Question: What does the change from 46% to 92% correct suggest?

Answer: The child's performance improves significantly with the use of HATS.

INTERPRETATION MATRIX

Noise

	quiet	noise
close-aud	[2] 88	[4] 72
close-aud/vis	[1] 92	[3] 76
distant-aud	[7] 60	[6] 46
distant-aud/vis	[8] 64	[5] 50

Distance

	close	distant
quiet-aud	[2] 88	[7] 60
quiet-aud/vis	[1] 92	[8] 64
noise-aud	[4] 72	[6] 46
quiet-aud/vis	[3] 76	[5] 50

Visual Input

	aud/vis	aud
close-quiet	[1] 92	[2] 88
close-noise	[3] 76	[4] 72
distant-noise	[5] 50	[6] 46
distant-quiet	[8] 64	[7] 60

Average of above scores: 76 % 61 %
quiet noise

82 % 55 %
close distant

70.5 % 66.5 %
aud/vis aud

With Hearing Assistance Technology:

Average of above scores: ___ % ___ %
quiet noise

___ % ___ %
close distant

___ % ___ %
aud/vis aud

INTERPRETATION AND RECOMMENDATIONS

AUDIOMETRIC RESULTS

Hearing Sensitivity: Pure Tone Ave: Right Ear ___ dB Left Ear ___ dB
PTA used: ☐ 500, 1K, 2K ☐ 1K, 2K, 4K

Word Recognition: Right Ear ___ % @ ___ dBHL Left Ear ___ % @ ___ dBHL
Sound Field: Aided ☐ Unaided ☐
Quiet ___ % @ ___ dBHL
Noise ___ % @ ___ dBHL @ ___ S/N

FUNCTIONAL LISTENING EVALUATION CONDITIONS

Amplification: ☐ None ☐ Hearing Aids ☐ Cochlear Implants ☐ Baha
Hearing Assistance Technology: ☐ FM ☐ Classroom Other ___
Classroom Noise Level: Unoccupied ___ dBA SPL Occupied ___ dBA SPL
Assessment Material: ___
Distance (distant condition): ___ ft
Noise Stimulus: ☐ Multitalker ☐ Classroom ☐ Other ___
Speech level @ listener's ear: ___ dBA SPL @ 1 ft from examiner: ___ dBA SPL
Noise level @ listener's ear: ___ dBA SPL
Approximate speech to noise levels: close + ___ dB distant - ___ dB
Modifications in protocol: ___

FUNCTIONAL LISTENING SCOREBOX

	close/quiet	close/noise	distant/quiet	distant/noise
auditory-visual	[1] 92	[3] 76	[8] 64	[5] 50
auditory	[2] 88	[4] 72	[7] 60	[6] 46

FIGURE 6–6. Sample FLE form. Adapted from Deconde Johnson, C., & VonAlmen, P. (1993 updated in 2013) with permission.

- Presentation of the signals is presented with the child wearing their daily amplification configuration.
- Sentences (or other signals) presented in different conditions: auditory only (A) versus auditory with visual cues (A/V), close versus distant (12–15 feet), and in quiet versus noise, creating eight conditions that are then repeated with HATS in place

- Interpretation and recommendations of the FLE
  - □ Describe the effects of different listening conditions to describe what situations enhance or decrease auditory function
  - □ Identify best listening environment as far as visual cues and distance
  - □ Recommend HATS and components that improve hearing in noise
  - □ Recommend other accommodations that would reduce noise (e.g., reduce reverberation) or increase visual cues (e.g., have the teacher face the child)

- Another issue related to a student's equipment is equipment transparency. With the addition of another device (receiver) to a child's hearing aid, there is the possibility that the frequency response (output) is affected. Transparency addresses whether addition of the receiver impacts the frequency response of a hearing aid.
  - □ Measures are used to determine if a change in the frequency response occurs. If the hearing aid is transparent, there is not a significant change to electroacoustic output in the speech frequencies when testing through the hearing aid microphone versus the output when presented through the HATS transmitter.
  - □ Testing performed with the hearing aid inside the test box at 65 dB SPL and the output for 750, 1000, and 2000 Hz is noted.
  - □ The hearing aid is then placed outside the test box but still connected to the 2- cc coupler. Because it is outside the test box and the hearing aid microphone is still active, testing must be conducted in a quiet setting.
  - □ The HATS microphone is placed inside the test box. Then testing is performed again, noting the output for the three primary frequencies.
  - □ The results with hearing aid alone are subtracted from the results through the HAT transmitter and then averaged.
  - □ Transparent systems will show no more than ± 2 dB as the average.
  - □ If the system is transparent, then you know that the system is not significantly changing the frequency response.
  - □ If there is a significant difference, then the HATS should be adjusted.
  - □ Testing setup varies based on the hearing aid companies and requires some specific setting or verification mode. Instructions for specific companies need to be downloaded and used.
    - Phonak Offset Protocol (POP) (Phonak, 2021)
    - EduMic Verification Guide (Oticon, n.d.)

- Assessment of social skills, self-advocacy, and auditory fatigue are other areas that an audiologist will provide input on during assessment. Using various scales and observations, the audiologist can determine the impact of the hearing loss on these areas. This information will be helpful to the psychologist or counselor in examining the impact of hearing loss.

☐ Hearing loss impacts how a child learns to interact with others by impacting ToM, pragmatic language, and social skills. Checklists such as The Pragmatic Checklist or Summary of Social Interaction can give an idea of areas of difficulty.

☐ Self-advocacy is often an area of concern for children with hearing loss. Use of equipment and communication strategies is important to help the child show they have taken ownership of their hearing loss. The Student Expectations for Advocacy and Monitoring Hearing Technology questionnaire monitors a child's understanding of and advocacy for hearing aid use. Self-advocacy in different listening situations is also covered in the LIFE, which has Before-LIFE and After-LIFE sections where students discuss how they would handle different situations and is designed to be a pre- and postmeasure of training.

☐ Fatigue due to the additional load of processing the auditory signal may be experienced by the child with a hearing loss. This can be examined informally or with tests such as the Vanderbilt Fatigue Scale–Child (VFS-C; Hornsby et al., 2022).

■ Scales and questionnaires mentioned in this chapter section are samples of available test materials. For more options, check resources.

☐ Educational Audiology Handbook (Deconde Johnson & Seaton, 2021)

☐ Building Skills for Success in the Fast-Paced Classroom: Optimizing Achievement for Students with Hearing Loss (Anderson & Arnoldi, 2011). This resource also comes with supplemental files, including assessments.

Management by Educational Audiologists

Recommendations related to management of hearing loss include monitoring the hearing status and providing the school information about the child's ongoing performance and progress. The student who is DHH should have regular hearing evaluations to monitor any progression of hearing loss, examine changes that would affect the aided audibility, and make referrals/recommendations if there are changes in hearing status. Providing information to the school should extend beyond presenting the standard audiogram. Audibility information using the Count-the-Dot Audiogram or a measure of the audibility index (AI) to provide insight into aided audibility is important to the management process. Aural habilitation for speech perception and auditory skills is addressed as a multidisciplinary team along with the speech-language pathologist and teacher of the deaf. More information about aural habilitation can be found in Chapter 4.

■ Managing the educational environment by the audiologist includes addressing the classroom SNR issues, providing HATS, and implementing recommendations based on FLE results.

☐ Classroom participation and observation data will provide information to assist with facilitating access to communication in the classroom, leading to management strategies such as controlling other students and classroom noise; modifying teacher presentation level, rate, and vocabulary; and facilitating reception of signals from other media (e.g., HATS for computer, closed captioning).

Theory of Mind

Theory of Mind (ToM) is the ability to understand and consider the mental state (beliefs, intents, desires, emotions) of others and understand these states may be different from our own. It includes using what is known about other people to understand a situation, as well as predicting what others are thinking by what we know of them. Children with hearing loss experience difficulties with ToM and are often delayed and need assessment in the educational setting.

- Impact of hearing loss on ToM
  - Research has shown that children with hearing loss act much like children with autism on ToM tasks and struggle with pragmatic issues (Westby, 2017).
  - Research indicates that children with hearing loss are around 3 years behind peers with normal hearing (Lundy, 2002).
  - Children who sign and are from a home environment rich in sign (e.g., Deaf parents who sign) have ToM development similar to typical development.
  - Difficulties developing ToM are associated with limited incidental conversational access.
  - Language skills were found to be related to the child's vocabulary and ability to comprehend syntactic complements.
- Table 6–8 provides a description of the subdivisions and expected development of ToM.

TABLE 6–8. Development of Cognitive and Affective Theory of Mind

	COGNITIVE THEORY OF MIND	AFFECTIVE THEORY OF MIND
AGE	**SKILL**	**SKILL**
Birth–6 months		• Responds to emotional reactions of others • Imitates expressions
6–8 months	• Has joint attention	• Displays joy, sadness, disgust, and anger
8–12 months	• Follows line of regard • Regulates behavior to initiate request • Initiates joint attention of objects	• Uses expressions of others as social reference for approach/avoidance • Displays happy, mad, sad, surprised, disgusted, afraid
13–17 months	• Understands line of sight and its impact on behavior	• Tries to change how others feel by direct contact • Coordinates interactions
18 months–2 years	• Develops sense of self • Engages in pretend • Understands different people like different things	• Recognizes distress of others • Develops altruistic behaviors to comfort others • Uses words "happy," "mad," "sad," and "scared"

TABLE 6–8. *continued*

AGE	COGNITIVE THEORY OF MIND SKILL	AFFECTIVE THEORY OF MIND SKILL
3 years	• Knows imaginary objects are different than real • Knows actions dictates desires, intentions, and thoughts • Knows perceptual activity is connected to knowing • Uses words such as "remember," "know," and "think" • Realizes different people see things differently	• Identifies happy, sad, mad, and afraid in photos • Matches primary emotions to situations in pictures • Develops schematic facial recognition • Discusses causes and outcomes of emotions • Works with object and a friend to change affect • Evidences self-conscious emotions such as pride and guilt
4–5 years	• Can pass false content and false beliefs tasks • Predicts person's action based on false beliefs • Understands how something someone sees appears to them • Knows people access information by casually hearing/seeing • Understands beliefs cause people to act in a particular way	• Identifies what another may be feeling based on whether wishes are fulfilled • Predicts what people should be feeling • Describes a situation where they were sad, mad, happy, surprised, or scared • Understands emotions can be caused by what someone thinks, even if what they think conflicts with reality • Has sense of self in the moment and in the future
6–8 years	• Develops an opinion on what one person may be thinking about what another person thinks • Judges situations based on what a person knows, remembers, forgets, or guesses	• Describes what they believe another feels • Identifies situations that cause complex emotion • Recognizes a person can have first one and then another emotion to situations • Uses words like proud, jealous, worried • Uses strategies to regulate emotions
8–10 years	• Uses strategies to hide/detect deceit and recognizes lies • Understands figurative language • Facilitates comprehension by using metacognitive strategies	• Understands someone can have two opposite emotions at the same time to a situation • Recognizes, understands, and uses sarcasm • Identifies social faux pas • Hides emotions • Understands and can perform polite lies • Begins to use words such as relieve and disappointed

Source: Adapted from Westby, C., & Robinson. L. (2014). A developmental perspective for promoting theory of mind. *Topics in Language Disorders, 34*(4), 362–382.

- ToM is often assessed using a false-belief task where the child is presented with a specific situation. Then, something changes in the situation that would be known to only one of the individuals from the example situation (thus creating conflict between what the two individuals from the story would be thinking). The person in the situation now has a false belief that the situation is still the same as when they left it. An example of a false-belief task is provided in the upcoming Audiology Nugget.

  □ Example false-belief tasks: Sally-Anne Story, Mark Story, Theory of Mind Test (Anderson & Arnoldi, 2014)

 AUDIOLOGY NUGGET: SALLY-ANNE STORY

The child is presented with a puppet show or toys to act out the situation. You will need two characters, a small ball, a yellow box, and a green box.

Story: This is Sally. Sally places a ball into the yellow box. Then she leaves to go to ballet class. This is Anne, Sally's friend. While Sally is gone at ballet, Anne takes the ball from the yellow box and places it in the green box. Then Anne goes outside to play. Sally comes home from ballet class. She wants to play with her ball.

Question for the child:

    Where will Sally look for her ball first? The answer should be the yellow box.

The second two questions are to help problem-solve if the child misses the first question and reports the green box.

    Where was the ball when Sally went out?

    Where is the ball now?

A child should be able to correctly answer the first question at approximately 4 years of age (Anderson & Arnoldi, 2014). If the child reports the ball to be in the yellow box because Sally was not there when the ball was moved to the green box by Anne, this demonstrates that the child understands that Sally and Anne have two different perspectives of where the ball should be located.

Recommended Readings

Anderson, K. L., & Arnoldi, K. A. (2011). *Building skills for success in the fast-paced classroom: Optimizing achievement for students with hearing loss.* Butte Publications.

Bagatto, M. P., Moodie, S. T., Seewald, R. C., Bartlett, D. J., & Scollie, S. D. (2011). A critical review of audiological outcome measures for infants and children. *Trends in Amplification, 15*(1–2), 23–33. http://doi.org/10.1177/1084713811412056

Chermak, G. D., & Musiek, F. E. (2014). *Handbook of central auditory processing: Comprehensive intervention* (Vol. 2). Plural Publishing.

Deconde Johnson, C., & Seaton, J. B. (2021). *Educational audiology handbook* (3rd ed.). Plural Publishing.

Diefendorf, A. O., & Tharpe, A. M. (2017). Behavioral audiometry in infants and children. In A. M. Tharpe & R. C. Seewald (Eds.), *Comprehensive handbook of pediatric audiology* (2nd ed., pp. 591–607). Plural Publishing.

Hill, M. (2017). Hearing development: Embryology of the ear. In A. M. Tharpe & R. C. Seewald (Eds.), *Comprehensive handbook of pediatric audiology* (2nd ed., pp. 3–22). Plural Publishing.

Interacoustics Academy. (n.d.). https://www.interacoustics.com/academy.

Korczak, P., Smart, J., Delgado, R., Strobel, T. M., & Bradford, C. (2012). Tutorial: Auditory steady-state response. *Journal of the American Academy of Audiology, 23,* 146–170.

Peck, J. E. (2017). Pseudohypacusis: False and exaggerated hearing loss. In A. M. Tharpe & R. C. Seewald (Eds.), *Comprehensive handbook of pediatric audiology* (2nd ed., pp. 295–306). Plural Publishing.

Rawool, V.W. (2016). *Auditory processing deficits.* Thieme Publishers.

Sinninger, Y. S., Hunter, L. L., Roush, P. A., Windmill, S., Hayes, D., & Uhler, K. M. (2020). Protocol for rapid, accurate, electrophysiologic, auditory assessment of infants and toddlers. *Journal of the American Academy of Audiology, 31,* 455–468.

Thibodeau, L. M. (2007). Speech audiometry. In R. Roeser, M. Valente, & H. Hosford-Dunn (Eds.), *Audiology diagnosis* (2nd ed., pp. 300–301). Thieme Publishers.

Westby, C., & Robinson, L. (2014). A developmental perspective for promoting theory of mind. *Topics in Language Disorders, 34*(4), 362–382. https://doi.org/10.1097/TLD.0000000000000035

References

Abdala, C., Winter, M., & Shera, C. A. (2017). Otoacoustic emissions in infants and children: An updated approach. In A. M. Tharpe & R. C. Seewald (Eds.), *Comprehensive handbook of pediatric audiology* (2nd ed., p. 489). Plural Publishing.

American Academy of Audiology. (2010, August). *Diagnosis, treatment and management of children and adults with central auditory processing disorder* [Clinical practice guidelines]. https://audiology-web.s3.amazonaws.com/migrated/CAPD%20Guidelines%208-2010.pdf_539952af956c79.73897613.pdf

American Speech-Language-Hearing Association. (1997). *Guidelines for audiological screening* [Guidelines]. http://www.asha.org/policy

American Speech-Language-Hearing Association. (2004). *Guidelines for the audiological assessment of children from birth to 5 years of age* [Guidelines]. http://www.asha.org/policy

American Speech-Language-Hearing Association. (2005). *(Central) auditory processing disorders* [Technical Report]. http://www.asha.org/docs/html/TR2005 00043.html

American Speech-Language-Hearing Association. (n.d.). *Sound field measurement tutorial.* https://www.cdc.gov/ncbddd/actearly/milestones/index.html

Anderson, K. L., & Arnoldi, K. A. (2014). *Documenting skills for success: Data-gathering resources—Informal assessments from building success in the fast-paces classroom.* Supporting Success for Children with Hearing Loss.

Anderson, K. L., & Smaldino, J. J. (2000, redesigned 2011). *CHILD Children's Home Inventory for Listening Difficulties.* http://www.kandersonaudconsulting.com

Bagatto, M. P., Moodie, S. T., Seewald, R. C., Bartlett, D. J., & Scollie, S. D. (2011). A critical review of audiological outcome measures for infants and children. *Trends in Amplification, 15*(1–2), 23–33. https://doi.org/10.1177/1084713811412056

Beck, D. L., Speidel, D. P., & Petrak, M. (2007). Auditory steady-state response (ASSR): A beginner's guide. *The Hearing Review.* https://hearingreview.com/hearing-products/accessories/components/auditory-steady-state-response-assr-a-beginners-guide

Berlin, C., Hood, L. J., Morlet, T., Wilensky, D., St. John, P., Montgomery, E., & Thibodaux, M. (2005). Absent or elevated middle ear muscle reflexes in the presence of normal otoacoustic emissions: A universal finding in 136 cases of auditory neuropathy/dys-synchrony. *Journal of the American Academy of Audiology, 16*(8), 546–553. https://doi.org/10.3766/jaaa.16.8.3

Bleile, K. M. (2015). *The manual of speech sound disorders: A book for students and clinicians* (3rd ed.). Cengage Learning.

Cacace, A. T., & McFarland, D. J. (2015). Middle-latency auditory evoked potentials. In J. Katz (Ed.), *Handbook of clinical audiology* (7th ed., pp. 315–336). Wolters Kluwer.

Centers for Disease Control and Prevention. (n.d.). *CDC's developmental milestones*. https://www.cdc.gov/ncbddd/actearly/milestones/index.html

Chermak, G. D. (2014). Central resources training: Cognitive, metacognitive, and metalinguistics skills and strategies. In G. D. Chermak & F. E. Musiek (Eds.), *Handbook of central auditory processing: Comprehensive intervention* (Vol. 2, pp. 243–309). Plural Publishing.

Chermak, G. D., Pederson, C. M., & Bendel, R. B. (1984). Equivalent forms and split-half reliability of the NU-CHIPS administered in noise. *Journal of Speech and Hearing Disorders, 49*, 196–201.

Cobb, K. M., & Stuart, A. (2016). Neonate auditory brainstem responses to CE-chirp and CE-chirp octave band stimuli I: Versus click and tone burst stimuli. *Ear and Hearing, 37*(6), 710–723.

Deconde Johnson, C., & Seaton, J. B. (2021). *Educational audiology handbook* (3rd ed.). Plural Publishing.

Deconde Johnson, C., & VonAlmen, P. (1993, updated in 2013). *The Functional Listening Evaluation*. http://www.ADEvantage.com

Dhar, S., & Hall, J. W., III. (2018). *Otoacoustic emissions: Principles, procedures, and protocols* (2nd ed.). Plural Publishing.

Diefendorf, A. O., & Tharpe, A. M. (2017). Behavioral audiometry in infants and children. In A. M. Tharpe & R. C. Seewald (Eds.), *Comprehensive handbook of pediatric audiology* (2nd ed., pp. 591–607). Plural Publishing.

Eder, K., Schuster, M. E., Polterauer, D., Neuling, M., Hoster, E., Hempel, J.-M., & Semmelbauer, S. (2020). Comparison of ABR and ASSR using NB-chirp-stimuli in children with severe and profound hearing loss. *International Journal of Pediatric Otorhinolaryngology, 131*, 1–6.

English, K. (2001). Assessing auditory processing problems in the school setting. *Journal of Educational Audiology, 9*, 42–46.

Farinetti, A., Raji, A., Wu, H., Wanna, B., & Vincent, C. (2018). International consensus (ICON) on audiological assessment of hearing loss in children. *European Annals of Otorhinolaryngology, Head and Neck Diseases, 135*(1), S41–S48.

Feldman, A. S. (1976). Tympanometry: Application and interpretation. *Annals of Otology, Rhinology, & Laryngology, 85*(2, Suppl.), 202–208.

Geers, A. E., & Moog, J. S. (2012). *CID ESP: Early Speech Perception Test*. CID.

Gustafson, T. J. S., & Keith, R. (2005). Relationship of auditory processing categories as determined by the Staggered Spondaic Word Test (SSW) to Speech-Language and Other Auditory Processing Test Results. *Journal of Educational Audiology, 12*, 49–58.

Hicks, C. B., & Tharpe, A. M. (2002). Listening effort and fatigue in school-age children with and without hearing loss. *Journal of Speech, Language, and Hearing Research, 45*(3), 573–584.

Hicks, C. B., Tharpe, A. M., & Ashmead, D. H. (2000). Behavioral auditory assessment of young infants: Methodological limitations or lack of auditory responsiveness? *American Journal of Audiology, 9*(2), 124–130.

Hill, M. (2017). Hearing development: Embryology of the ear. In A. M. Tharpe & R. C. Seewald (Eds.), *Comprehensive handbook of pediatric audiology* (2nd ed., pp. 3–22). Plural Publishing.

Hoffmann, A., Deuster, D., Rosslau, K., Knief, A., am Zehnhoff-Dinnesen, A., & Schmidt, C. M. (2013). Feasibility of 1000 Hz tympanometry in infants: Tympanometric trace classification and choice of probe tone in relation to age. *International Journal of Pediatric Otorhinolaryngology, 77*(7), 1198-1203.

Hornsby, B. W. Y., Camarata, S., Cho, S.-J., Davis, H., McGarrigle, R., & Bess, F. H. (2022). Development and evaluation of pediatric versions of the Vanderbilt Fatigue Scale for children with hearing loss. *Journal of Speech, Language, and Hearing Research, 65*(6), 2343–2363.

Hunter, L. L., & Blankenship, C. M. (2017). Middle ear measurement. In A. M. Tharpe & R. C. Seewald (Eds.), *Comprehensive handbook of pediatric audiology* (2nd ed., pp. 449–473). Plural Publishing.

Jackler, R. K., Luxford, W. M., & House, W. F. (1987). Congenital malformations of the inner ear: A classification based on embryogenesis. *Laryngoscope, 3*(2, Suppl. 40), 2–14. https://doi.org/10.1002/lary.5540971301

Jerger, J. (1970). Clinical experience with impedance audiometry. *Archives of Otolaryngology, 92*(4), 311–324.

Joint Committee on Infant Hearing. (2019). Year 2019 position statement: Principles and guidelines for early hearing detection and intervention programs. *Journal of Early Hearing Detection and Intervention, 4*(2), 1–44. https://doi.org/10.15142/fptk-b748

Jutras, B., Loubert, M., Dupuis, J. L., Marcoux, C., Dumont, V., & Baril, M. (2007). Applicability of central auditory processing disorder models. *American Journal of Audiology, 16*(2), 100–106. https://doi.org/10.1044/1059-0889(2007/014)

Korczak, P., Smart, J., Delgado, R., Strobel, T. M., & Bradford, C. (2012). Tutorial: Auditory steady-state response. *Journal of the American Academy of Audiology, 23*, 146–170.

Krishnan, A. (2023). *Auditory brainstem evoked potentials: Clinical and research applications.* Plural Publishing.

Liberman, M. C., & Guinan, J. J., Jr. (1998). Feedback control of the auditory periphery: Anti-masking effects of the middle ear muscles vs. olivocochlear efferents. *Journal of Communication Disorders. 31*, 471-483.

Lundy, J. E. B. (2002). Age and language skills of deaf children in relation to theory of mind development. *The Journal of Deaf Studies and Deaf Education, 7*(1), 41–56. https://doi.org/10.1093/deafed/7.1.41

Martin, F. N., & Clark, J. G. (2006). *Introduction to audiology* (9th ed.). Allyn & Bacon.

McCreery, R. W., & Walker, E. A. (2017). Diagnosis of hearing loss: A foundation for pediatric amplification. In *Pediatric amplification: Enhancing auditory access* (pp. 23–50). Plural Publishing.

Moncrieff, D., & Wertz, D. (2008). Auditory rehabilitation for interaural asymmetry: Preliminary evidence of improved dichotic listening performance following intensive training. *International Journal of Audiology, 47*, 84–97.

Moore, J. M., Wilson, W. R., & Thompson, M. (1977). Visual reinforcement of head-turn responses in infants under 12 months of age. *Journal of Speech and Hearing Disorders, 42*, 328–334.

Musiek, F. E., & Baran, J. A. (2020). *The Auditory System.* Plural Publishing.

Musiek, F. E., Chermak, G. D., & Weihing, J. (2014). Auditory training. In G. D. Chermak & F. E. Musiek (Eds.), *Handbook of central auditory processing: Comprehensive intervention* (Vol. 2, pp. 157–200). Plural Publishing.

Nightengale, E. E., Wolter-Warmerdam, K., Yoon, P. J., Daniels, D., & Hickey, F. (2020). Behavioral audi-

ology procedures in children with Down syndrome. *American Journal of Audiology, 29*(3), 356–364.

Norrix, L. W., & Velenovsky, D. S. (2014). Auditory neuropathy spectrum disorder: A review. *Journal of Speech, Language, and Hearing Research, 57*, 1564–1576.

Northern, J. L. (2014). *Hearing in children* (6th ed., pp. 535–583). Plural Publishing.

Northern, J. L., & Downs, M. P. (2002). *Hearing in children* (5th ed.). Lippincott, Williams, & Wilkins.

Oticon. (n.d.). *EduMic Verification Guide: Verifit1 and Verifit2.* https://wdh02.azureedge.net/-/media/oticon-us/main/download-center---myoticon--product-literature/edumic/pi/15555-9922---verification-guide.pdf?rev=B3E6&la=en

Peck, J. E. (2017). Pseudohypacusis: False and exaggerated hearing loss. In A. M. Tharpe & R. C. Seewald (Eds.), *Comprehensive handbook of pediatric audiology* (2nd ed., pp. 295–306). Plural Publishing.

Phonak. (2021). *Phonak Roger verification guide.* https://www.phonakpro.com/content/dam/phonakpro/gc_us/en/training_sessions/ec/roger/documents/POP_verification_protocol.pdf

Rawool, V.W. (2016). *Auditory processing deficits.* Thieme Publishers.

Rosenfeld, R. M., Tunkel, D. E., Schwartz, S. R., Anne, S., Bishop, C. E., Chelius, D. C., . . . Monjur, T. M. (2022). Clinical practice guideline: Tympanostomy tubes in children (update). *Otolaryngology-Head and Neck Surgery, 166*(1S), S1–S55. https://doi.org/10.1177/01945998211065662

Roush, J., & Corbin, N. E. (2017). Screening for hearing loss and middle ear disorders: Beyond the newborn period. In A. M. Tharpe & R. C. Seewald (Eds.), *Comprehensive handbook of pediatric audiology* (2nd ed., pp. 383–411). Plural Publishing.

Sanderson-Leepa, M. E., & Rintelmann, W. F. (1976). Articulation functions and test-retest performance of normal-hearing children on three speech discrimination tests: WIPI, PBK-50, and NU Auditory Test No. 6. *Journal of Speech and Hearing Disorders, 41*(4), 503–519.

Shahnaz, N., Aithal, S., & Bargen, G. A. (2023). Wideband acoustic immittance in children. *Seminars in Hearing, 44*(1), 46–64. https://doi.org/10.1055/s-0043-1763294

Sinninger, Y. S., Hunter, L. L., Roush, P. A., Windmill, S., Hayes, D., & Uhler, K. M. (2020). Protocol for rapid, accurate, electrophysiologic, auditory assessment of infants and toddlers. *Journal of the American Academy of Audiology, 31,* 455–468.

Skoe, E., & Kraus, N. (2010). Auditory brain stem response to complex sounds: A tutorial. *Ear and Hearing, 31*(3), 302–324. https://doi.org/10.1097/AUD.0b013e3181cdb272

Small, S. A., & Stapells, S. R. (2017). Threshold assessment in infants using the frequency-specific auditory brainstem response and auditory steady-state response. In A. M. Tharpe & R. C. Seewald (Eds.), *Comprehensive handbook of pediatric audiology* (2nd ed., pp. 506–507). Plural Publishing.

Stout, G. G., & Windle, J. V. E. (1986). *A developmental approach to successful listening: DASL.* Developmental Approach to Successful Listening.

Tremblay, K., & Clinard, C. (2015). Cortical auditory-evoked potentials. In J. Katz (Ed.), *Handbook of clinical audiology* (7th ed., pp. 337–357). Wolters Kluwer.

Uhler, K., Warner-Czyz, A., Gifford, R., & PMSTB Working Group. (2017). Pediatric minimum speech test battery. *Journal of the American Academy of Audiology, 28,* 232–247.

Westby, C. (2017). Keep this theory in mind. *The ASHA Leader, 22*(4). https://doi.org/10.1044/leader.AEA.22042017.18

Wilkes, E. M. (2001). *Cottage Acquisition Scales for Listening, Language & Speech* (2nd ed.). Sunshine Cottage Educational Products.

Winiger, A. M., Alexander, J. M., & Diefendorf, A. O. (2016). Minimal hearing loss: From a failure based approach to evidence-based practice. *American Journal of Audiology, 25,* 232–245.

Practice Questions

1. Jason is having difficulty in Spanish class perceiving the rolled or trilled "r" but does not have any difficulty with the single "r." The audiologist called and spoke to the Spanish teacher, who indicated that the only difference between the two speech sounds is the speed at which they are produced. If auditory processing difficulties are the reason for his issue correctly perceiving the rolled "r," which area of auditory processing is most likely affected?

   a. Auditory figure-ground

   b. Temporal processing

   c. Discrimination

   d. Dichotic listening

Explanation: The correct answer is temporal processing as it refers to the effectiveness of processing auditory information over time, and the Spanish instructor indicated that the difference between the two sounds is a difference in production speed. Figure-ground is related to hearing in noise. Discrimination is related to a person knowing two sounds are different from one another. Dichotic listening applies when there are two different signals presented, one to each ear. Therefore, the correct answer is b.

2. Which anatomical location is attributed to the initial stage for processing of the natural speech signal?

   a. Medial geniculate body

   b. Dorsal cochlear nucleus

   c. Lateral superior olivary complex

   d. Auditory cortex

Explanation: The medial geniculate body, which is located within the thalamus (a site known for integration of multiple neural pathways), is the site believed to be responsible for the initial processing of speech. The perception of speech requires the integration of several spectral and temporal cues provided by various lower auditory regions and integrated in the MGB of the thalamus. The cochlear nucleus has the role of transmitting precise timing patterns, whereas the superior olivary complex relates to interaural timing and regulates the efferent systems. The auditory cortex is responsible for processing the suprasegmental cues and then transferring the information to the left side to assign meaning to the signal via the corpus callosum. Thus, the answer is a.

3. Jillian has a mild to moderate hearing loss, bilaterally. The audiologist wishes to examine her performance in an academic setting. Which of the following is/are teacher checklist(s)/rating scales that can be used to determine how a student with hearing loss is functioning in the classroom:

   a. Functional Listening Evaluation

   b. Categorical Individual Performance Profile

   c. Screening Instrument for Targeting Educational Risk

   d. Beliefs About Deafness Scale

Explanation: The SIFTER is a checklist that examines a child's performance on different functional aspects needed for educational success (e.g., academics, participation). A functional listening evaluation examines a child's performance in various listening conditions to determine the impact of noise, distance, and visual cues on sentence repetition. It is used to measure amplification and HATS benefits. The BADS is a scale to examine how the patient versus other significant people in the life feel about hearing loss. It is more often used for adults. Therefore, the answer is c.

4. Johnny is experiencing difficulty hearing at school, and he failed his hearing screening at 4000 Hz. His pure-tone audiogram indicated a high-frequency conductive loss; however, his tympanogram was a typical Type A tympanogram. You performed the G tympanogram below at resonant frequency and obtained these results.

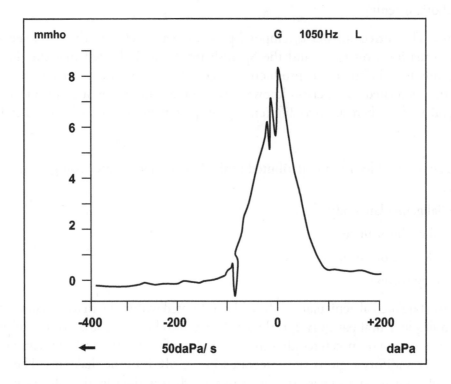

How would you interpret these findings?

a. This is a normal pattern for a G tympanogram, suggesting that there is no explanation for the conductive component.

b. There are too few peaks to be on a G tympanogram, and explains the conductive component.

c. There are too many peaks for the G tympanogram, and explains the conductive component.

d. Abnormal G tympanograms have no bearing on the function of the middle ear system.

Explanation: The G is representative of the conduction of the middle ear system. This pattern is abnormal because there should never be more than three extrema on a G tympanogram. This suggests a middle ear problem that has changed the friction of the middle ear. Therefore, the answer is c.

5. Sylvia, a 5-year-old, is being evaluated. By case history report, Sylvia started kindergarten this year. She is in the process of having her speech and language evaluated by the school speech-language pathologist. According to her parent, they can understand approximately half of Sylvia's speech. The parents feel she understands them when they talk to her. You find a mild bilateral sensorineural hearing loss. You now want to test word recognition for Sylvia. Which of the following is the best option:

   a. PBK words

   b. NU-6 words

   c. Spondee words

   d. WIPI words

Explanation: Given the difficulties in understanding Sylvia's speech, a picture-pointing task such as the WIPI would be appropriate. The PBK words would be appropriate age-wise, but interpretation/scoring would be impacted by Sylvia's articulation difficulties. The NU-6 words are an adult word list; spondee words are typically used for speech threshold testing, not word recognition. Therefore, the answer is d.

Example Case (Questions 6–10)

A 5-month-old (George) is scheduled for a hearing evaluation. His mother noted that she was sick in the first trimester of her pregnancy with a fever, sore throat, and fatigue, but she did not seek medical care at that time. The mother reports that George was born at 27 weeks gestational age and was in the NICU for 8 weeks. During that time, George received oxygen due to underdeveloped lungs. His mother also noted that George did not show any other symptoms of sickness at birth and that George passed his ABR newborn hearing screening in the NICU. George has had approximately four ear infections in the past 3 months, which have been treated with antibiotics. His most recent ear infection was last week. At this time, George's pediatrician is talking to his family about getting PE tubes for George. On the test date, George showed normal movement of the tympanic membranes and absent otoacoustic emissions. You are scheduling additional testing for this child to estimate hearing ability.

6. How would you estimate hearing ability in this patient?

   a. Soundfield VRA thresholds

   b. BO results

   c. Air- and bone-conduction ABR thresholds

   d. VRA thresholds under headphones

Explanation: This child was born 13 weeks prematurely; even though the child is 5 months chronological age, he is approximately 2 to 3 months developmentally. You must base the choice of behavioral testing on developmental age rather than chronological age. Because the child is developmentally 2 to 3 months of age, VRA is not appropriate. Responses to sound could be seen via BO, but such responses cannot be used to estimate hearing sensitivity. As such, air- and bone-conduction ABR should be utilized to estimate hearing sensitivity of this child. Thus, the answer is c.

7. Related to embryological development of the ear, which risk factor is of most significant concern?

   a. Mother's sickness in first trimester

   b. George's premature birth

   c. Oxygen given to George after birth

   d. George's history of ear infections

Explanation: The largest risk for the ear development is in the first trimester, which is when the mom's sickness occurred. This is the time when the major portions of the ear are developing. While there is maturation in the third trimester, it would not be the biggest concern (ruling out the premature birth). The oxygen after birth and the ear infections are not in utero, and as such would not constitute an embryologic concern. Therefore, the answer is a.

8. Your additional test results indicate a moderately severe sensorineural hearing loss of a progressive nature. Based on case history, what would be the most likely cause of the hearing loss?

    a. Loss due to ear infections

    b. Common cavity deformity

    c. Cytomegalovirus

    d. Michel's aplasia

Explanation: Cytomegalovirus impacts the ear during development and is associated with a progressive hearing loss. This is why the child may have passed the hearing screening at birth. A loss due to ear infections is typically associated with a temporary conductive hearing loss. Both the common cavity deformity and Michel's aplasia would be associated with significant hearing loss at birth (leading to a failed newborn hearing screening). Thus, the answer is c.

9. If you could obtain only one piece of information, which of the following would be best for fitting amplification on this child?

    a. Behavioral results

    b. Click-evoked ABR

    c. Tone-burst ABR

    d. OAEs

Explanation: Tone-burst ABR results would provide frequency and ear-specific results that can be used to fit amplification. With the infant being too young developmentally for VRA, you would only be able to see behavioral responses to sound using BO, which is not appropriate for diagnosing a hearing loss or programming hearing aids. The OAEs do not provide threshold estimates, and the click-evoked ABR results are not frequency specific. Thus, the answer is c.

10. Because of the history of possible middle ear dysfunction, you want to perform immittance testing. How would you perform immittance testing on this child?

    a. Utilize a lower-frequency probe Hz for tympanometry and acoustic reflexes

    b. Utilize a higher-frequency probe Hz for tympanometry and acoustic reflexes

    c. Perform tympanometry and reflexes in same manner as for older children/adults

    d. You cannot perform tympanometry or acoustic reflexes on children of this age

Explanation: Higher-frequency probe frequency, such as 1000 Hz, is recommended for children under 6 to 9 months of age. The lower-frequency probe tone does not provide reliable results in young infants/toddlers, and the older children/adults are tested typically with the lower-frequency probe tone. Therefore, the answer is b.

Appendix 6–A

Abnormal Auditory Electrophysiological Findings

ELECTROPHYSIOLOGIC MEASURE	DIAGNOSTIC OUTCOME	AUDITORY STATUS
ABR	Absent waveforms	Presentation level below auditory threshold
		Alternating polarity: possible ANSD
	Delayed wave V	Presentation level close to auditory threshold
		Brainstem lesion depending on other findings
	"Kissing" or reversing waveforms with condensing and rarefacting polarities	ANSD
	Present wave I, absent or delayed waves III and V	Vestibular schwannoma/acoustic neuroma; pontine lesions
	Normal latency I, delayed III with normal III-V interpeak	Lesion at the CN/SOC
	Normal latency waves I & III with normal I-III interpeak, delayed wave V	Lesion at the LL/IC
	Abnormal prolongations to high repetition rates (>0.1 ms shift per decade (10) increase in stimulus rate)	Demyelinating disease (e.g., multiple sclerosis)
ABR Latency/Intensity Functions	Delayed wave V at all intensities; higher threshold than normal	Conductive hearing loss
	Normal wave V latency at high intensities, delayed at lower intensities with higher threshold than normal	Cochlear hearing loss
	Delayed wave V with any pattern of latency shift; higher threshold than normal	Neural hearing loss
MLR	Absent waveforms	Abnormal transmission of neural signals through the thalamocortical tract
	Abnormal amplitude differences between ears	
	Abnormal amplitude differences between electrodes	

continues

APPENDIX 6–A. *continued*

ELECTROPHYSIOLOGIC MEASURE	DIAGNOSTIC OUTCOME	AUDITORY STATUS
LLR	Abnormal P1/N1/P2 amplitudes	Abnormal maturation or function of the auditory cortex
	Absent P300 response	Abnormality in top-down (decision making) or bottom-up (difference detection) processing; often seen with cortical lesions or delayed auditory development

Chapter 7

Vestibular Assessment and Differential Diagnosis

Jamie M. Bogle

Introduction

The vestibular system is a set of sensory end organs that detect angular and linear acceleration. This information is transmitted through various reflex pathways to maintain appropriate balance and visual stability. Vestibular assessments use these pathways to identify weaknesses and to suggest possible diagnoses.

Vestibular System Anatomy and Physiology

Vestibular system end organs are housed within the inner ear. The membranous labyrinth is located within the otic capsule and is filled with endolymph, a fluid with high potassium concentration (Smith et al., 1965). There are five vestibular end organs: three semicircular canals (SCCs) and two otolith organs (Figure 7–1). Each end organ contains its own sensory epithelium, the crista ampullaris for the semicircular canals and the maculae for the otolith organs. The hair cells within the sensory epithelium transmit mechanical energy into neural impulses encoding acceleration information. The superior vestibular nerve branch of cranial nerve VIII (CN VIII) innervates the horizontal and superior semicircular canals and utricle, while the inferior vestibular nerve branch innervates the posterior canal and saccule.

Semicircular Canals (SCCs)

SCCs detect angular acceleration, meaning that they encode rotational movements. They are labeled based on their orientation as the horizontal (or lateral), anterior (or superior), and posterior (or inferior) SCC. Each SCC detects angular acceleration in a specific plane to create a three-dimensional model of head movement.

- Each SCC has a sensory epithelium at one end with the other open to the common vestibule. The ampulla houses the sensory epithelium, called the crista ampullaris, and the cupula. The cupula is a gelatinous structure that extends across the SCC to create a fluid-tight seal (Lysakowski et al., 1998). Think of the cupula as a sail, deflecting when the head turns to trigger the underlying sensory epithelium. The cupula only responds to angular acceleration

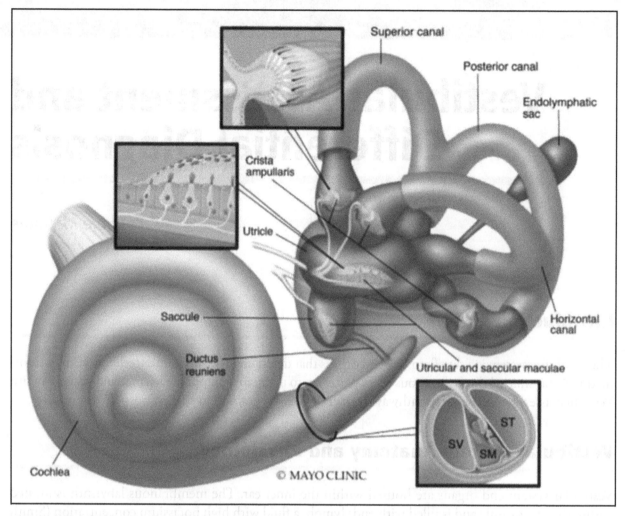

Superior canal

Posterior canal

Endolymphatic
sac

Crista
ampullaris

Utricle

Horizontal
canal

Saccule

Ductus
reuniens

Utricular and saccular maculae

Cochlea

ST

SV

SM

© MAYO CLINIC

FIGURE 7–1. Anatomy of the peripheral vestibular labyrinth. *Source:* From Lane JI, Witte RJ, Bolster B, Bernstein MA, Johnson K & Morris J. *AJNR Am J Neuroradiol.* 2008 Sep;*29*(8):1436–1440; used with permission of Mayo Foundation for Medical Education and Research, all rights reserved.

 AUDIOLOGY NUGGET

The SCCs work together between ears as a pair—described as a co-planar or push-pull mechanism. The horizontal SCCs form a pair. For example, as you turn your head to the right, the right horizontal SCC experiences ampullopetal flow (excitatory), while the left experiences ampullofugal flow (inhibitory). Each anterior SCC is paired with the contralateral posterior SCC to describe the RALP (right anterior/left posterior) and LARP (left anterior/right posterior) planes. This co-planar relationship is vital to vestibular system performance because each head movement transmits both excitatory and inhibitory information to encode a range of accelerations.

because it has the same specific gravity as the surrounding endolymph. This also means that it does not respond to linear acceleration.

■ For the horizontal SCC, as the head turns, endolymph lags and pushes on the cupula to depolarize (i.e., excite) the sensory hair cells. This type of endolymph flow is called ampullopetal. Conversely, a head turn in the opposite direction will hyperpolarize (i.e., inhibit) these same sensory hair cells. This type of endolymph flow is called ampullofugal. The anterior and posterior SCCs are oriented differently—ampullopetal flow inhibits, ampullofugal flow excites (Lysakowski et al., 1998).

Otolith Organs

The utricle and saccule are collectively known as the otolith organs. They are housed in the vestibular labyrinth (see Figure 7–1). These end organs are responsible for detecting linear acceleration, including gravity. The utricle generally encodes horizontal acceleration while the saccule encodes vertical acceleration.

■ Each otolith organ contains a sensory epithelium called the otolithic membrane. This structure is embedded with calcium carbonate crystals called otoconia or otoliths (Lundberg et al., 2006). The otoconia increase the specific weight of the otolithic membrane, causing it to pull toward gravity or to lag during linear acceleration, thus triggering the underlying sensory hair cells.

Vestibular Nerve

Cranial nerve VIII (CN VIII) innervates both the cochlea and vestibular system. The vestibular portion further divides into two branches. The superior vestibular nerve branch innervates the horizontal SCC, anterior SCC, and utricle. The inferior vestibular nerve innervates the posterior SCC and saccule (Naito et al., 1995).

■ Both vestibular nerve branches travel from the peripheral vestibular system through the internal auditory canal and cerebellar pontine angle to synapse at various vestibular nuclei in the brainstem.

■ The vestibular nerve has a high spontaneous firing rate ranging from 70 to 100 spikes per second (Goldberg & Férnandez, 1971; Lysakowski et al., 1995). When excited, the vestibular nerve can fire up to 400 spikes per second (Uchino et al., 1982). Because of the high resting neural firing rate, inhibition can be encoded, providing the mechanism for co-planar stimulation.

Blood Supply

The labyrinthine artery supplies blood to the vestibular system. This artery typically arises from the anterior inferior cerebellar artery (AICA) (Baloh & Honrubia, 2001). One branch (superior vestibular artery) supplies the horizontal SCC, anterior SCC, and utricle, while the other (common cochlear artery) supplies the posterior SCC, saccule, and cochlea. The blood supply to vestibular structures in the brainstem and cerebellum is provided from various branches of the vertebrobasilar artery.

Central Vestibular System

Once information from the vestibular end organs enters the brainstem, it synapses within the vestibular nuclei (VN). The VN contains several substructures, including the superior VN, medial VN, lateral VN, and inferior VN. Each of these substructures transmits specific end-organ information to the appropriate reflex pathways.

- Cerebellum: the superior VN and lateral VN are highly connected to the cerebellum, with predominant information transmitted from the otolith organs (Carpenter & Sutin, 1983; Pansky et al., 1988; Watson, 1991). The cerebellum transmits this information to the reticulospinal tract, lateral vestibulospinal tract, and reticular formation (Pansky et al., 1988). Information from the cerebellum is heavily used for motor control.

- Reticular formation: the reticular formation uses information primarily from the otolith organs and descends the length of the spinal cord (Fetter & Dichgans, 1996; Honrubia & Hoffman, 1997). Vestibular system activation along this pathway may trigger sweating, nausea, and vomiting (Pansky et al., 1988).

- Thalamocortical projections: information from the VN ascends to the thalamus, further projecting to the parietoinsular vestibular cortex (PIVC). The PIVC serves as a major integration site for vestibular, visual, and motor system information. Thalamocortical projections are also traced to the hippocampus, where they influence spatial perception and cognition (Bigelow et al., 2016; Brandt et al., 2005; Semenov et al., 2016) and descend to the VN/brainstem (Berthoz, 1996) to contribute to the efferent vestibular system.

- Autonomic system: vestibular system information also influences autonomic system function. The autonomic system controls various sympathetic and parasympathetic responses. The otolith organs specifically contribute to blood pressure regulation during movement and postural change (Goldberg et al., 2012; Yates et al., 2014).

Vestibular Reflexes

Reflex pathways are used to evaluate vestibular system performance. There are several basic vestibular system reflexes.

- Vestibulo-ocular reflex (VOR): enables visual stability during motion. The VOR is a reflex pathway from the SCCs to specific extra ocular muscles to produce equal and opposite eye movements in response to a head turn. If the VOR is not working properly, the patient may experience oscillopsia—the perception of oscillating movement in the environment during motion. Figure 7–2 provides the horizontal SCC VOR pathway. All SCCs provide information to the VOR, but the horizontal SCC is the most evaluated pathway (e.g., caloric testing, rotational chair testing, head impulse testing). The utricle also provides a translational VOR (e.g., ocular vestibular evoked myogenic potentials).

- Vestibulo-collic reflex (VCR): enables the head to remain still during movement (Hain & Helminski, 2014). The proposed pathway for the VCR includes the saccule, inferior vestibular nerve branch of CN VIII, medial VN, CN XI (spinal accessory), and ending in the trapezius and sternocleidomastoid (SCM) muscles.

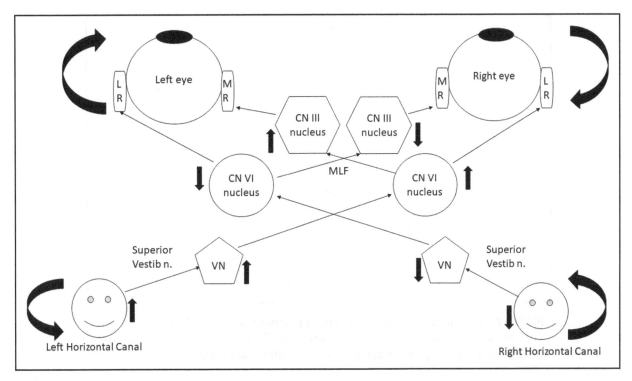

FIGURE 7–2. The vestibulo-ocular reflex (VOR) pathway includes the vestibular nuclei (VN), cranial nerve VI (CN VI), cranial nerve III (CN III), the medial longitudinal fasciculus (MLF), lateral rectus muscle (LR), and medial rectus muscle (MR). *Source:* From *Balance Function Assessment and Management, Third Edition* (pp. 1–717) by Jacobson, G. P., Shepard, N. T., Barin, K., Burkard, R. F., Janky, K., & McCaslin, D. L. Copyright © 2021 Plural Publishing, Inc. All rights reserved.

- Vestibulo-spinal reflex (VSR): triggers upper and lower limb responses to changes in balance (Schubert & Shepard, 2016). Patients with damage to the vestibular system may demonstrate imbalance acutely but should recover as vestibular compensation occurs. The VSR can be evaluated using a range of bedside (e.g., Romberg test) and forceplate measures (e.g., computerized dynamic posturography).

Vestibular Nystagmus

Most vestibular diagnostic testing measures nystagmus—rapid, involuntary eye movements. Nystagmus allows the clinician to (1) evaluate a possible site of lesion in those with spontaneous nystagmus and (2) define peripheral vestibular system performance as measured in induced nystagmus. Nystagmus represents the VOR (Figure 7–3). The slow phase component corresponds to vestibular system information, while the fast phase is a reset saccade initiated to bring the eyes back to midline. Nystagmus is named by the fast phase for most analyses and is measured by the velocity (°/second) of the slow phase.

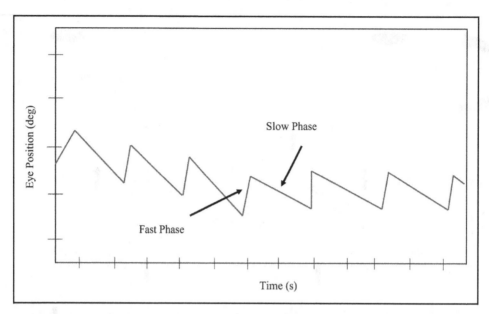

FIGURE 7–3. Vestibular nystagmus. In this example, the eyes drift slowly to the left (slow phase; downward on the graph) and quickly reset to the right (fast phase; upward on the graph). This tracing describes right-beating nystagmus.

 KNOWLEDGE CHECKPOINT

Peripheral vestibular nystagmus follows Ewald's laws (Ewald, 1882). These laws describe how endolymph flow reliably influences the VOR to create predictable nystagmus.

1. The axis of nystagmus parallels the axis of the SCC that generated it.

2. Ampullopetal endolymph flow produces a stronger response than ampullofugal flow in the horizontal SCCs.

3. Ampullofugal endolymph flow produces a stronger response than ampullopetal flow in the anterior and posterior SCCs.

Vestibular Case History and Questionnaires

The case history is one of the most important components of the vestibular assessment. A thorough case history should include:

- Temporal features of dizziness symptoms: timing, triggers

- Dizziness characteristics: spinning, rocking, imbalance, lightheadedness, drunk feeling, spacey, and so on

- Additional symptoms: hearing loss, tinnitus, headache, nausea/vomiting, unsteadiness, other neurological concerns

- Vascular risk factors: for example, cardiac syncope, atherosclerosis, heart disease, vertebrobasilar artery insufficiency

- Neurological risk factors: for example, migraine, stroke, transient ischemic attack (TIA), concussion, multiple sclerosis

- Medications (Table 7–1)

  □ Some medications may cause vestibulotoxicity and many others cause dizziness/imbalance.

  □ Many patients use multiple medications to manage various conditions. Polypharmacy—the simultaneous use of >4 medications (Masnoon et al., 2017)—is a common cause of dizziness. Nearly 70% of patients presenting with dizziness and polypharmacy most often have diagnoses including diabetes, hypertension, other cardiovascular abnormalities, and depression (Jeong et al., 2022).

Questionnaires are useful tools to identify the patient's self-perceived symptoms as well as how symptoms impact quality of life. There are many questionnaires available, with commonly used options provided in Table 7–2.

TABLE 7–1. Medications Associated With Vestibulotoxicity, Dizziness, and Imbalance

Classes of Vestibulotoxic Medications	Antibiotics (e.g., gentamicin)
	Platinum-based chemotherapeutics
	Loop diuretics
	Antimalarial drugs
	Nonsteroidal anti-inflammatory drugs (NSAIDs)
	Acetylsalicylic acid
Classes of Medications Associated With Dizziness/ Imbalance	Antispasmodics used for intestinal mobility disorders
	Diuretics
	Beta-blockers
	Hypertension medications
	Antihistamines
	Hypnotic/anxiolytic medications
	First-generation antipsychotics
	Tricyclic antidepressants
	Analgesics
	Migraine medications
	Antiepileptic medications
	Parkinson medications
	Antibiotics
	HIV medications
	Corticosteroids
	Hormone therapies

Source: Altissimi et al. (2020).

TABLE 7–2. Commonly Used Questionnaires to Evaluate Patients With Dizziness/Imbalance

QUESTIONNAIRE	PURPOSE
General Scales	
Hospital Anxiety and Depression Scale (HADS) (Zigmond & Snaith, 1983)	Determine levels of anxiety and depression in an outpatient setting
Generalized Anxiety Disorder–7 (GAD-7) (Spitzer et al., 2006)	Screen for generalized anxiety disorder
Patient Health Questionnaire–9 (PHQ-9) (Kroenke et al., 2001)	Screen for depression
Dizziness Scales	
Dizziness Handicap Inventory (DHI) (Jacobson & Newman, 1990)	Evaluate self-perceived handicap due to dizziness
Activities-Specific Balance Confidence Scale (ABC) (Powell & Myers, 1994)	Assess balance confidence and determine fall risk
Visual Vertigo Analog Scale (VVAS) (Dannenbaum et al., 2011)	Quantify dizziness symptoms to visually provoking situations
Dizziness Symptom Profile (DSP) (Jacobson et al., 2019)	Assist in identifying common vestibular disorders

Bedside Evaluation

Patients presenting for audiometric testing may also report dizziness/imbalance. Bedside testing provides clues to identify patients who may be experiencing vestibular system dysfunction (Table 7–3).

Electronystagmography/Videonystagmography (ENG/VNG)

The most common vestibular diagnostic battery is the ENG/VNG. The name of the test describes the recording method; however, the subtests are the same for both.

ENG

ENG recording takes advantage of the corneoretinal potential (CP). Electrodes are placed on the inner canthi, outer canthi, and above and below the eyes to record electrical activity. Measuring the changes in electrical activity identifies nystagmus and other oculomotor movements. Most clinicians use bitemporal electrode placement, with the horizontal electrodes placed on the outer canthus of each eye (Figure 7–4). With this montage, the electrical activity between the eyes is averaged and the tracing cannot identify disconjugate eye movements. Monocular (i.e., recording each eye individually) can also be completed. ENG is rarely completed today due to advances in video recording technology.

TABLE 7–3. Bedside Evaluation Options Summary

TEST	PURPOSE	TECHNIQUE	INTERPRETATION
Spontaneous vestibular nystagmus	Identify a static imbalance between right and left peripheral vestibular systems	Observe the patient's eyes for nystagmus in vision and vision-denied conditions.	Normal: no nystagmus Abnormal: nystagmus; determine if it follows Alexander's law
Head impulse test	Identify VOR dysfunction	Examiner moves the patient's head in low-amplitude, high-velocity head turns; observe the patient's eyes for loss of visual fixation.	Normal: no loss of fixation Abnormal: loss of fixation; patient demonstrates a "catch-up" saccade to regain fixation
Head shake nystagmus	Identify asymmetrical neural integration of VOR; measure of compensation	Patient oscillates the head for 25 cycles at 2 Hz; vision denied.	Normal: <3 beats of post-headshake nystagmus Abnormal: > 3 beats of post-headshake nystagmus; fast phase typically beats toward the better ear
Dynamic visual acuity test	Identify oscillopsia with head movement	Patient reads to the lowest level on an eye chart with the head stable and with the head oscillating at 2 Hz.	Normal: ≤2 lines of change on the eye chart Abnormal: > 2 lines of change on the eye chart
Valsalva-induced nystagmus	Identify the effect of intracranial pressure change on nystagmus	Patient increases intracranial pressure by performing Valsalva maneuver for 10–15 seconds.	Normal: no dizziness or nystagmus Abnormal: conjugate eye movement toward the contralesional ear; nystagmus, dizziness
Modified Clinical Test of Sensory Interaction on Balance (mCTSIB)	Measure postural control under various conditions	Patient maintains balance for 30 seconds in four conditions: (1) eyes open, firm surface; (2) eyes closed, firm surface; (3) eyes open, foam surface; (4) eyes closed, foam surface.	Normal: ability to maintain balance in all conditions for 30 seconds Abnormal: inability to maintain balance in all conditions for 30 seconds Results may also be compared to age-specific normative values using forceplate analyses.
Romberg Test	Measure postural control under various conditions	Patient maintains balance for 30 seconds in two conditions: (1) eyes open, firm surface and (2) eyes closed, firm surface.	Normal: ability to maintain balance in all conditions for 30 seconds Abnormal: inability to maintain balance in all conditions for 30 seconds

continues

TABLE 7–3. *continued*

TEST	PURPOSE	TECHNIQUE	INTERPRETATION
Gait Speed	Measure functional mobility	Patient walks at comfortable and fast speeds for 3–10 meters.	Gait speed = distance/time Normal values vary by age, gender, use of assistive device, and walking speed.
Timed Up-and-Go (TUG)	Measure functional mobility	Patient transitions from seated to standing, walks a 3-meter line, turns around, and sits down.	Normal: ≤13.5 seconds Abnormal: >13.5 seconds
Dynamic Gait Index (DGI)	Measure of balance in dynamic conditions	Patient completes a series of balance tasks: (1) gait on level surface, (2) change in gait speed, (3) gait with horizontal head turns, (4) gait with vertical head turns, (5) gait and pivot turn, (6) step over obstacle, (7) step around obstacle, and (8) steps. The examiner scores the patient's ability using a rubric.	Normal: ≥22/24 Abnormal: <19/24

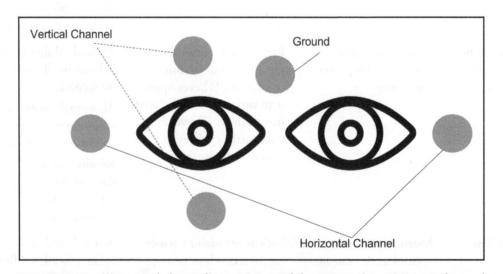

FIGURE 7–4. Bitemporal electrode montage and the connections to a two-channel differential amplifier (i.e., two channels permit the recording of horizontal and vertical eye deviations). *Source:* From *Balance Function Assessment and Management, Third Edition* (pp. 1–717) by Jacobson, G. P., Shepard, N. T., Barin, K., Burkard, R. F., Janky, K., & McCaslin, D. L. Copyright © 2021 Plural Publishing, Inc. All rights reserved.

VNG

VNG recording uses pupil localizing technology to calculate the pupil's position and gaze angle. Most systems are fit with infrared diodes, reflexive glass mirrors, and small cameras.

- The remaining discussion will use VNG as the default terminology. VNG testing includes three major components (Table 7–4): oculomotor assessment, positional/positioning assessment, and caloric assessment.

Gaze Testing

Gaze testing evaluates the patient's ability to maintain gaze on a target in primary gaze (gaze center) and in eccentric positions (right, left, up, down) in both vision/fixation and vision-denied conditions (i.e., 10 conditions total). Abnormalities in gaze testing can occur from peripheral or central vestibular system disorders. Look for nystagmus in primary and eccentric positions for vision and vision-denied conditions.

   If nystagmus is observed, document the velocity, direction, and in which condition(s) it occurs. Peripheral vestibular nystagmus should be horizontal or a combination of horizontal and torsional—it should follow Alexander's law. The following criteria are used to identify significant nystagmus:

- Nystagmus present in any gaze position with velocity >5°/second
- Nystagmus present in four or more conditions with velocity <6°/second
- Nystagmus present sporadically in all gaze positions with velocity <6°/second
- Direction-changing nystagmus noted within any gaze position

TABLE 7–4. Key Components of Videonystagmography (VNG) Testing

COMPONENT	SUBTEST	FUNCTION
Oculomotor Assessment	Gaze with/without fixation	Hold an image stable when the head is still
	Saccades	Quickly move the eyes to fixate on an object of interest
	Smooth pursuit	Hold/track a moving object with the eyes
	Optokinetic nystagmus (OKN)	Maintain clear vision when the head or target is in constant motion
Positional/Positioning Assessment	Static positional recording in four to six conditions: supine, head right, head left, lateral right, lateral left, caloric test position	Evaluate the effects of head orientation and neck position on spontaneous nystagmus
	Dix-Hallpike test	Evaluate for BPPV
	Lateral head roll test	
Caloric Assessment		Assess peripheral VOR performance; gold standard for identifying unilateral peripheral weakness

Note. BPPV: benign paroxysmal positional vertigo; VOR: vestibulo-ocular reflex.

KNOWLEDGE CHECKPOINT: ALEXANDER'S LAW

Alexander's law is associated with gaze-evoked nystagmus that occurs after an acute unilateral vestibular loss. It was originally described to explain how the vestibular system, specifically the VOR, responds to the injury. Alexander's law includes three components:

1. Spontaneous nystagmus after peripheral vestibular insult has the fast phase directed toward the healthy ear.

2. Spontaneous nystagmus (a) is greatest when gaze is directed toward the fast phase, (b) is attenuated in center gaze, and (c) may be absent when directed toward the slow phase.

3. Spontaneous nystagmus is reduced with fixation and enhanced with vision-denied.

Spontaneous nystagmus is defined by the number of gaze positions. For example, if nystagmus is only observed in gaze left, it is considered first-degree gaze-evoked nystagmus. Nystagmus present in gaze left and center gaze is described as second-degree nystagmus, and third-degree gaze-evoked nystagmus occurs with nystagmus in all three positions (Figure 7–5). Importantly, peripheral vestibular nystagmus does not change direction or present with up-beating or down-beating nystagmus—these presentations relate to central vestibular pathology.

Degree	Gaze Left	Gaze Center	Gaze Right	Definition
First	← ← ←			Nystagmus present in lateral gaze <u>only</u> in the direction of the fast phase.
Second	← ← ←	← ← ←		Nystagmus present in lateral gaze in the direction of the fast phase and in center gaze
Third	← ← ←	← ← ←	← ← ←	Nystagmus present in all three positions; greatest in the direction of the fast phase and least in the direction of the slow phase

FIGURE 7–5. Gaze evoked nystagmus is defined by the presence of nystagmus in one, two, or three gaze positions. Peripheral vestibular nystagmus follows Alexander's law.

Saccades

Saccades are conjugate eye movements that reposition the fovea on the target of interest. Saccades are the fastest type of eye movements and can be evaluated using numerous protocols. Most clinical protocols use a random saccade paradigm, meaning that the saccade location, intrasaccadic interval, and fixation duration are random. Saccade abnormalities are not related to peripheral vestibular system performance. Random saccade performance uses the frontal eye fields, brainstem, midbrain, superior colliculus, cerebellum, frontal lobe, posterior parietal cortex, basal ganglia, and thalamus. It is important to record each eye individually to identify disconjugate (i.e., eyes not moving together) eye movements. There are three primary parameters for saccade analysis (Figure 7–6; Table 7–5).

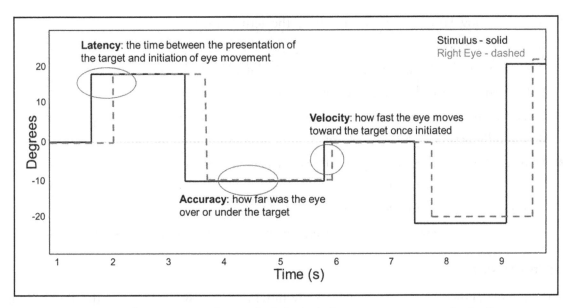

FIGURE 7–6. Saccade parameters for analysis include latency, accuracy, and velocity.

TABLE 7–5. Summary of Saccadic Eye Movement Abnormalities

PARAMETER	ABNORMALITY
Velocity	Reduced velocity, both eyes • Fatigue, medications • Abnormal performance of reticular formation, MLF, cerebral hemispheres, superior colliculus, cerebellum Reduced velocity, one eye or restricted direction • Abnormal performance of reticular formation, MLF; question INO Enhanced velocity • Calibration error • Restrictive syndromes, late myasthenia gravis
Accuracy	Hypometria • Fatigue, medications • Bidirectional: cerebellar dorsal vermis • Unidirectional: ipsilateral cerebellum/brainstem Hypermetria • Cerebellum
Latency	Both eyes, all directions • Fatigue, medications • Superior colliculus, reticular formation

Note. MLF: medial longitudinal fasciculus; INO: intranuclear ophthalmoplegia.

- Accuracy: how far is the eye position from the actual target
  - □ Measured in percent (%)
  - □ Hypometria/undershooting: eyes are significantly short of reaching the target
  - □ Hypermetria/overshooting: eyes are significantly over the target
- Latency: time between initiation of target movement to the initiation of eye movement
  - □ Typically between 150 and 200 ms
- Velocity: how fast the eyes move to the target once movement begins
  - □ Measured as peak velocity
  - □ Ranges from 300° to 700°/second
  - □ The farther the target from the current eye position, the higher the expected peak velocity.

Smooth Pursuit

Smooth pursuit allows the eyes to hold a slow-moving target of interest on the fovea. This eye movement performs most optimally below 70°/second. The underlying neural pathways include the pons, cerebellum, VN, and pontine reticular formation. It is critical to use age-specific normative data to interpret smooth pursuit, especially for advancing age. Smooth pursuit is the most sensitive oculomotor subtest for cerebellar dysfunction and should correlate with other metrics of cerebellar function. Figure 7–7 provides an example of abnormal smooth pursuit. Note the stair step or saccadic quality to this tracing. Gain for all test stimuli was significantly reduced. Additional oculomotor performance was abnormal with down-beating nystagmus noted throughout gaze testing, prolonged saccade latencies,

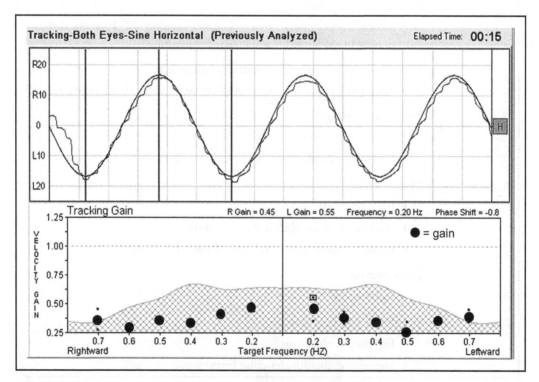

FIGURE 7–7. Smooth pursuit tracing at 0.2 Hz for a 65-year-old male presenting with onset of unsteadiness over the last 6 months.

and reduced optokinetic nystagmus. VOR performance as measured by caloric testing and sinusoidal harmonic acceleration (SHA) was within normal limits; however, the patient demonstrated inability to appropriately fixate (VOR-Fixation). This patient presentation is highly suspicious for central vestibular system pathology, specifically involving the cerebellum. Smooth pursuit is evaluated with the following parameters:

- Velocity gain = peak eye velocity/peak target velocity
  - □ Abnormal performance may be associated with increased saccadic movements and could relate to (a) acute peripheral vestibulopathy with active spontaneous nystagmus or (b) brainstem or cerebellar lesion.
  - □ Asymmetrically reduced performance may relate to involvement of the ipsilateral cerebellum, brainstem, or parieto-occipital region.
- Asymmetry: difference in velocity gain between rightward and leftward eye movements; results given in percent (%)
- Phase angle: how much the eyes are ahead of (leading) or behind (lagging) the target
- Saccadic component: how much the patient uses saccades instead of smooth pursuit to follow the target; results given in percent (%)

Optokinetic Nystagmus (OKN)

OKN testing is a measure of both smooth pursuit and another neural substrate that encodes moving visual stimuli. As the visual stimuli move, the eyes should generate a nystagmus response comparable to the velocity of the visual field. To truly measure this response, the visual stimuli must fill >90% of the visual field and generally requires testing within an enclosure. OKN paradigms that use a lightbar are not true OKN measures and can only be used to describe the smooth pursuit pathway. OKN is the least sensitive oculomotor measure for central pathology. OKN is evaluated with the following parameter:

- Velocity gain = peak eye velocity/peak target velocity
- OKN is generally reported as normal or abnormal; velocity gain should be >0.5 of the target velocity for an appropriate response.

Positional Assessment

The positional assessment evaluates the presence of nystagmus in various head positions in relation to gravity. Nystagmus may occur with or without dizziness when the patient is in these static positions. Observed nystagmus may relate to impaired SCC(s), otolith organ(s), or central vestibular pathways. By changing the head position, the orientation of the inner ear toward gravity changes, thus altering the underlying neural firing that represents the specific head position. In general, positional nystagmus should relate to asymmetrical peripheral or central vestibular system performance. Positional nystagmus is also commonly observed with alcohol consumption and some medication use. Most clinicians evaluate the following positions:

- Supine, head center
- Supine, head right
- Supine, head left

- Caloric test position (30° recumbent), head center
- Optional positions may be included if nystagmus is observed in the above conditions or if a specific condition is known to provoke dizziness.
  - Lateral, body right
  - Lateral, body left
  - Head hanging, center
  - Head hanging, right
  - Head hanging, left

The following criteria are used to determine if any visualized nystagmus is significant. Note that these criteria are the same as those used for evaluating spontaneous nystagmus in gaze testing.

- Nystagmus present in any position with velocity >5°/second
- Nystagmus present in four or more positions with velocity <6°/second
- Nystagmus present sporadically in all positions with velocity <6°/second
- Direction-changing nystagmus noted within any position

If the nystagmus noted in positional testing is the same velocity and direction as that observed in gaze testing, it is not a significant/novel finding (i.e., it is consistent with the underlying spontaneous nystagmus).

- Nystagmus will be either direction-fixed (only one direction of nystagmus noted in all positions) or will change direction depending on head position. In this case, nystagmus is described as geotropic (toward the ground) or ageotropic (away from the ground). This is NOT direction-changing nystagmus. Geotropic/ageotropic nystagmus changes direction with different head positions but is consistent within the same head position. This presentation relates to the altered interactions between the otolith organs and SCCs in acute peripheral vestibular loss; however, central vestibular pathology may also present with this finding, and the site of lesion is determined by evaluating the patient's entire presentation and case history. In either case, the patient is generally asymptomatic. If the patient becomes dizzy with these changes in head position, consider benign paroxysmal positional vertigo (BPPV) as a possible diagnosis.

Positioning Assessment/Dix-Hallpike Test

Positionally provoked dizziness is the most common type of peripheral vestibular system pathology. It can be easily tested for in isolation or as part of the VNG protocol. See sections below on BPPV for testing, clinical presentation, and management.

Caloric Assessment

The caloric assessment is the most common measure of peripheral vestibular system integrity. Abnormal findings are associated with a peripheral lesion involving the horizontal SCC and/or superior branch of the vestibular nerve on the side with the weaker response. This test can be completed with water or air as a stimulus, but specific temperatures and irrigation characteristics must be used. Water irrigations are considered more reliable than air irrigations because there is less room for technical/user error. Further, water provides a more robust stimulus and therefore requires a shorter irrigation time. Water irrigations cannot be used in cases of eardrum perforations due to increased risk of infection. Air irrigations should be used in these situations.

The nystagmus response to caloric stimulation follows an expected pattern due to the ampullopetal (excitatory) flow induced by warm irrigations and ampullofugal (inhibitory) flow induced by cool irrigations. To remember the expected response, think "COWS"—cool opposite, warm same.

During the irrigation, the patient may experience a sense of dizziness or vertigo. This typically begins about halfway through the irrigation and peaks by 30 seconds after the irrigation is complete (i.e., 60 seconds for water, 90 seconds for air). At this point, it is important to provide a fixation target to document the patient's ability to suppress the caloric response (fixation suppression/fixation index).

Q & A

Question: What specific irrigation temperatures, durations, and volumes are needed for water and air caloric stimuli?

Answer: The irrigation parameters recommended by the British Society of Audiology (BSA, 2010) are provided in Table 7–6.

Question: What nystagmus response do you expect for each ear following each irrigation temperature?

Answer: You should expect the following caloric responses based on the test ear and irrigation temperature (Table 7–7).

TABLE 7–6. Caloric Stimulus Parameters

STIMULUS	TEMPERATURE	DURATION	VOLUME
Water	Warm: 44 degrees Celsius Cool: 30 degrees Celsius	30 seconds	250 ± 10 ml
Air	Warm: 50 degrees Celsius Cool: 24 degrees Celsius	60 seconds	8 ± 0.5 liters

TABLE 7–7. Expected Caloric Responses by Ear and Temperature

TEMPERATURE	EAR	RESULT
Warm	Right	Right-beating nystagmus
	Left	Left-beating nystagmus
Cool	Right	Left-beating nystagmus
	Left	Right-beating nystagmus

The fixation target should be visible for approximately 10 seconds before returning to the vision-denied condition to document the increase in nystagmus velocity (Figure 7–8). This ensures that any decline in nystagmus velocity is related to the patient's fixation ability and not simply due to the natural decline in velocity. Nystagmus should be reduced by at least 60% with fixation.

To interpret the caloric response, identify the peak nystagmus velocity for each irrigation and evaluate for the following:

- Unilateral weakness
  - Also known as canal paresis (CP)
  - Calculate the difference between ears using Jongkees's formula:

$$CP = \frac{[(\text{right warm} + \text{right cool}) - (\text{left warm} + \text{left cool})]}{(\text{right warm} + \text{right cool} + \text{left warm} + \text{left cool})}$$

  - Abnormal CP >25%
  - Almost always due to peripheral vestibulopathy
  - Rule out technical error: poor irrigation, cerumen blocking the ear canal, surgical ear, ear drum perforation
- Bilateral weakness
  - Also known as bilateral areflexia or hypofunction
  - Calculate the total eye speed (TES) for each ear:

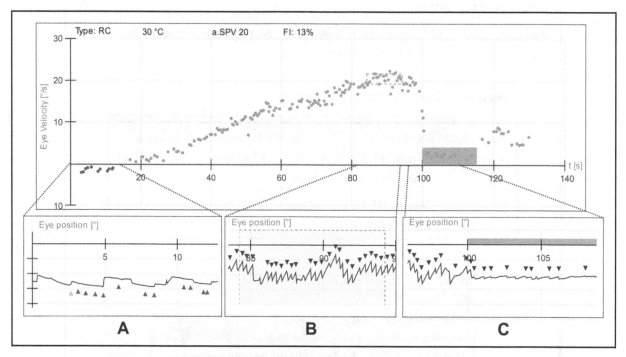

FIGURE 7–8. Analysis of caloric nystagmus in three time intervals: A. Around 10 to 15 seconds after the onset of the irrigation to determine the baseline shift. B. Around 60 to 90 seconds after the onset of the irrigation to determine the peak caloric response. C. Around 5 seconds before and 10 seconds after visual fixation (identified by gray timeline) to determine fixation suppression of caloric nystagmus. *Source:* From *Balance Function Assessment and Management, Third Edition* (pp. 1–717) by Jacobson, G. P., Shepard, N. T., Barin, K., Burkard, R. F., Janky, K., & McCaslin, D. L. Copyright © 2021 Plural Publishing, Inc. All rights reserved.

- Right TES = right warm + right cool
- Left TES = left warm + left cool

□ Bilateral weakness is defined when each ear's TES is <12°/second.

□ May occur due to bilateral peripheral vestibulopathy (e.g., ototoxicity) or central vestibulopathy (e.g., cerebellar degeneration)

□ Rule out technical error: poor irrigation, cerumen blocking the ear canal, surgical ear, use of vestibular suppressant medications (e.g., meclizine)

□ Confirm with additional VOR metrics such as rotational chair, video head impulse testing (vHIT), DVAT, mCTSIB/balance testing, and/or ice water caloric irrigations

- Hyperactive responses

  □ Calculate the TES for each ear as above

  □ Caloric hyperfunction is defined when each ear's TES is >140°/second

  □ Rule out technical error: perforated eardrum, altered mastoid

  □ May be associated with loss of VOR inhibition in the vestibular nuclei or cerebellum (Baloh et al., 1975)

- Directional preponderance

  □ Comparison of right-beating versus left-beating nystagmus

  □ Calculate TES for each nystagmus direction

  - Right-beating TES: right warm + left cool
  - Left-beating TES: left warm + right cool

  □ Calculate directional preponderance (DP)

$$DP = \frac{[(\text{right warm} + \text{left cool}) - (\text{left warm} + \text{right cool})]}{(\text{right warm} + \text{right cool} + \text{left warm} + \text{left cool})}$$

  □ Abnormal DP >30%

  □ Most commonly abnormal in patients with underlying spontaneous nystagmus. If present in a case with no spontaneous nystagmus, consider technical error or nonlocalizing finding.

- Fixation index

  □ Also known as fixation suppression

  □ Comparison of peak nystagmus velocity to nystagmus velocity during fixation

  □ Abnormal fixation index <60%

  □ Abnormal fixation index suggests cerebellar involvement. Confirm with other measures of cerebellar performance (e.g., smooth pursuit)

- Monothermal irrigations

  □ Some laboratories use monothermal irrigations to screen patients. Either warm or cool irrigations are used.

  □ Calculate CP using a modified Jongkees's formula:

$$CP = \frac{\text{right} - \text{left}}{\text{right} + \text{left}}$$

- ☐ Monothermal irrigations should only be used if:
  - Right ear and left ear responses are both >11°/second
  - There are no additional abnormalities noted in oculomotor testing
  - CP is <10% to 15%
  - If these conditions are not met, bithermal irrigations are indicated.

Caloric testing is the most common VOR task completed in everyday clinical practice. There are some additional considerations to remember when completing this protocol.

- ■ Alerting tasks
  - ☐ Any vestibular test completed without fixation requires alerting tasks. This keeps the patient alert and allows for consistent nystagmus generation. Tasks vary but should involve interaction between the patient and examiner. This may include having the patient recall things from memory (e.g., city/state names) and should be moderately challenging to the patient. Using topics of patient interest is also helpful.
  - ☐ If the patient is not sufficiently alert, the VOR response will likely be reduced and may not appropriately represent inner ear performance.
- ■ Order effect
  - ☐ ANSI (2009) and BSA (2010) standards recommend beginning with warm irrigations.
  - ☐ ANSI standard (ANSI, 2009) recommends beginning with the right ear, while the BSA standard (BSA, 2010) does not specify.
- ■ Waiting time between irrigations
  - ☐ 3 to 5 minutes is recommended between irrigations to ensure that any residual temperature effect will not influence the next caloric irrigation (ANSI, 2009).
- ■ Caloric testing is generally not recommended for children <6 years of age due to poor tolerance of the procedure.

Rotational Chair Assessment

Rotational chair assessment provides another measure of horizontal SCC and superior vestibular nerve function. There are several subtests, but most laboratories complete sinusoidal harmonic acceleration (SHA) testing. For this task, the patient is secured in the examination chair and fit with infrared goggles like those used in VNG testing. SHA testing must be done with vision denied. The patient is oscillated across a range of frequencies (0.01–0.64 Hz) at a set maximum chair velocity (typically 50° or 60°/second). Nystagmus is calculated and compared to normative values for the following measures (Figure 7–9).

- ■ Gain: ratio of recorded nystagmus velocity to the set maximum chair velocity
  - ☐ Normative values vary depending on the stimulus frequency.
  - ☐ Gain is measured to identify the presence of bilateral peripheral or central hypofunction or an acute unilateral lesion.
  - ☐ Gain for bilateral hypofunction remains reduced over time; acute lesions will demonstrate increased gain as compensation occurs.

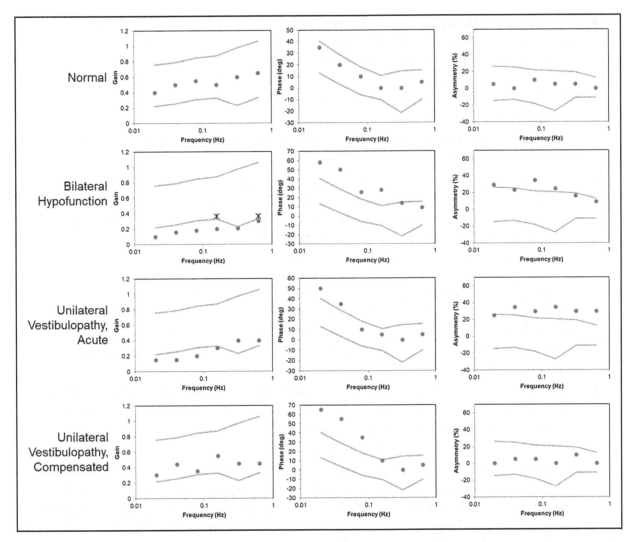

FIGURE 7–9. Comparison of sinusoidal harmonic acceleration (SHA) responses across frequencies for normal and various abnormal presentations.

- Phase: timing relationship between chair movement and eye movement
  - □ Phase describes the central processing of horizontal SCC information.
  - □ Normative values depend on the stimulus frequency.
  - □ Abnormal phase can occur due to peripheral or central vestibular system dysfunction.
  - □ Abnormal low-frequency phase lead is the most common abnormality and suggests history of peripheral or central vestibulopathy.
  - □ Phase abnormalities do not change with compensation.
- Symmetry: comparison of right-beating versus left-beating nystagmus
  - □ Comparable to directional preponderance as described in caloric testing.
  - □ Asymmetry generally occurs with present spontaneous nystagmus.

Besides SHA testing, there are several other subtests that may be completed, depending on patient presentation.

- VOR fixation/VOR suppression testing is completed to determine the patient's ability to suppress the VOR response. A fixation point is provided to the patient and repeated SHA oscillations are completed, commonly at 0.08 or 0.16 Hz. The nystagmus velocity during the fixation condition is compared to the vision-denied condition to determine the fixation index (%). VOR fixation in this paradigm should be between 75% and 90% (Barber & Stockwell, 1980).

  □ Abnormal fixation index suggests cerebellar involvement. Confirm with other measures of cerebellar performance (e.g., smooth pursuit).

- Visually enhanced VOR (VVOR) testing evaluates the interaction between the visual and vestibular systems. It is key to identifying the site of lesion for bilateral hypofunction, that is, is the bilateral loss related to central or peripheral system dysfunction? In this subtest, the patient is oscillated as described in SHA testing; however, the OKN stimulus is projected onto the walls of the enclosure. The nystagmus recorded during this trial is a summation of VOR and smooth pursuit systems and should result in gain between 0.7 and 1.1. Patients with bilateral hypofunction associated with peripheral vestibulopathy (e.g., ototoxicity) will demonstrate increased gain and generally fall within normal limits. Those with bilateral hypofunction associated with central vestibulopathy (e.g., cerebellar degeneration) will not. These patients should also demonstrate other central signs such as poor smooth pursuit and reduced fixation suppression ability.

- Trapezoidal acceleration/step testing may be completed with either a low- or high-velocity paradigm. Low-velocity testing (60°/second) is used to measure the rate of nystagmus decay in response to abrupt accelerations. High-velocity testing (240°/second) is used to support the diagnosis of unilateral peripheral vestibulopathy.

  □ In both protocols, the patient is abruptly accelerated to the maximum velocity (either 60° or 240°/second) and maintained at this velocity until the observed nystagmus is 37% of its peak value (Stockwell & Bojrab, 1997). The time it takes to reach this point is called the time constant or decay time. Typical responses for 60°/second stimuli should be between 10 and 30 seconds (Goulson et al., 2016).

    - Time constants <10 seconds are associated with abnormal performance of the peripheral vestibular system, vestibular nerve, and/or vestibular nuclei.

    - Time constants >30 seconds suggest abnormal central vestibular system processing.

    - Time decay is typically only evaluated for low-velocity trials (60°/second).

  □ Gain is also evaluated as the peak slow-phase velocity response divided by the target velocity. Gain is typically only calculated for high-velocity trials (240°/second). At this velocity, the lagging ear is inhibited to the point that there is minimal contribution to the VOR, allowing for the comparison of right versus left VOR performance.

Video Head Impulse Test (vHIT)

VHIT provides another method of evaluating the horizontal SCC and superior vestibular nerve. Most systems also evaluate RALP and LARP planes, allowing for a clinically accessible method of evaluating these pathways. Importantly, vHIT provides a measure of high-frequency performance not captured by other VOR measures. It is not equivalent to other VOR measures but is complementary.

Video goggles are typically used for this test, and most evaluations can be completed in a few minutes. Some systems use remote cameras, especially when testing young children. The patient focuses on a target while the examiner moves the head abruptly to stimulate the appropriate SCC plane. Trials should be done at >150°/second for consistent results. The infrared camera records the eye movements as the patient attempts to maintain visual fixation. VHIT systems document the following (Figure 7–10):

- Gain: ratio of eye velocity to head velocity

  □ Appropriate gain >0.7

  □ Gain may improve over time with central compensation

- Corrective saccades occur in patients with reduced peripheral system performance to reposition the eyes on the target.

  □ These eye movements are part of the central compensation mechanism and adapt for a deficient VOR. At the initial insult, these saccades occur randomly, but over time become more time locked as compensation occurs. There are two types of corrective saccades.

  - Overt saccades: eye movements that occur after the head stops moving; often seen on bedside head thrust testing (see Table 7–3).

  - Covert saccades: eye movements that occur during the head movement; cannot be seen on bedside head thrust testing.

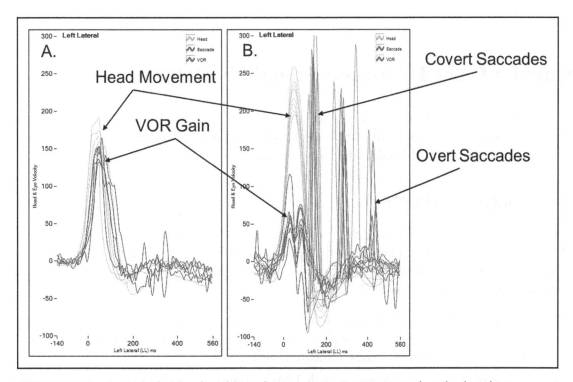

FIGURE 7–10. A. Typical video head impulse response (vHIT). Note that the head movement and VOR are overlaid for easy visualization of gain abnormalities. Head movement is noted in light gray; VOR performance is in dark gray. **B.** Abnormal vHIT is characterized by reduced gain and the presence of covert and/or overt saccades.

AUDIOLOGY NUGGET

There are numerous options for evaluating horizontal SCC performance (Table 7–8). Consider which test protocols are most appropriate for your patient to obtain the information needed for appropriate management.

TABLE 7–8. Comparison of Common Vestibulo-Ocular Reflex (VOR) Tests

	CALORIC	SHA	vHIT
Objective?	Yes	Yes	Yes
Independent SCC assessment?	Yes	No	Yes
Frequency (Hz)	Low	Low-mid	High
Tasking effect?	Yes	Yes	No
Cost	Less expensive	Expensive	Less expensive
Tolerated?	Yes	Yes	Yes
Minimum age	>6 years	>6 months	>3 months

Note. SHA: sinusoidal harmonic acceleration; vHIT: video head impulse test.

Vestibular Evoked Myogenic Potentials (VEMPs)

Until VEMPs, there was no clinically available method to evaluate the otolith organs. These tests have expanded the understanding of vestibular system function. VEMPs use surface electrodes to record the underlying electromyogram (EMG) of the target muscle.

Cervical VEMPs (cVEMPs)

The cVEMP reflex pathway includes the saccule, inferior branch of CN VIII, CN XI, and sterno-cleidomastoid (SCM) muscle. The recorded response is inhibitory, meaning that the SCM must be contracted to record the response. Most clinicians use air-conducted stimuli, but bone conduction and bone-tapping devices may also be used (Table 7–9).

- After electrodes and earphones are placed, the patient is instructed to contract the SCM during the stimulus. This is commonly done by asking the patient to raise the head from a reclined position and turn to the contralateral side.

- Current evoked potential systems provide EMG monitoring to allow the patient to maintain a consistent level of muscle contraction during the test. This is important—cVEMP response amplitude will increase with increased muscle contraction (McCaslin et al., 2014).

TABLE 7–9. Common Recording Parameters for cVEMPs and oVEMPs

	cVEMP	oVEMP
Electrode montage	Noninverting: upper half of SCM Inverting: sternoclavicular junction Ground: forehead	Noninverting: infraorbital midline Inverting: inner canthus Ground: forehead
Electrode impedance	<10 kOhms	<10 kOhms; interelectrode differences ≤2 kOhms
Channels	1 channel	1 or 2 channels
Amplification (gain)	× 5,000	× 30,000–50,000
Artifact rejection	Disabled	Enabled
Filter	10–1000 Hz	1–1000 Hz
Window/epoch	100 ms (20 ms prestimulus)	100 ms (20 ms prestimulus)
Number of sweeps	~100	100–200
Number of averages	2	2
Stimulus	500 Hz tonebursts Rarefaction 120 dB pSPL 5 Hz repetition rate Blackman gating 2-ms rise/fall, 0-ms plateau	500 Hz tonebursts Rarefaction 120 dB pSPL 5 Hz repetition rate Blackman gating 2-ms rise/fall, 0-ms plateau

- To reduce the risk of response asymmetry due to asymmetric muscle contraction, systems can apply EMG limiting (i.e., only accepting sweeps within a set EMG range) and/or response normalization. Response normalization adjusts the response amplitude by the amount of prestimulus EMG activity (Figure 7–11).

The recorded cVEMP response is evaluated in terms of peak latency, response amplitude, and amplitude asymmetry ratio. Absolute cVEMP amplitude demonstrates considerable variability and is therefore not as clinically meaningful. Table 7–10 provides basic interpretation for cVEMP responses.

- Peak latency
  - p1: 13 ms; abnormal >21 ms
  - n1: 23 ms; abnormal >26 ms
  - Significantly prolonged latencies are associated with retrolabyrinthine involvement.
  - Note: SCM muscle fatigue may also lead to prolonged n1 latencies.

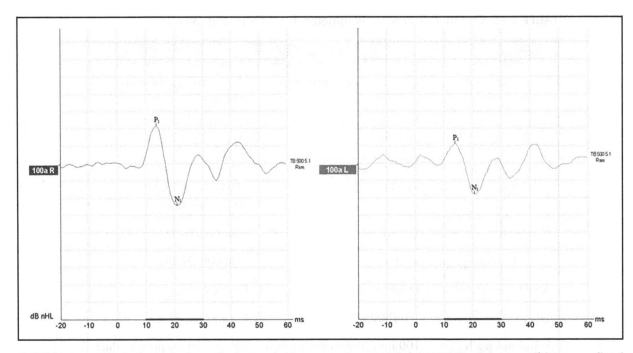

FIGURE 7–11. Typical cervical vestibular evoked myogenic potential (cVEMP) response. This normalized response demonstrates typical cVEMP presentation. For the right ear (*left side*), p1 and n1 occur at 14.00 and 20.67 ms, respectively, and p1-n1 normalized amplitude is 1.164. For the left ear (*right side*), p1 and n1 occur at 13.67 and 21.00 ms, respectively, and p1-n1 normalized amplitude is 1.833. Amplitude asymmetry is 22%.

TABLE 7–10. Basic VEMP Interpretation

FINDING	INTERPRETATION
Absent responses bilaterally	• Consider technical error, especially in younger patients • Bilateral peripheral or central otolith reflex pathway involvement • Common in vestibular migraine, advancing age
Absent response unilaterally; asymmetrical response amplitude	• Unilateral peripheral or central otolith reflex pathway involvement • Common in peripheral lesions, vestibular migraine
Significantly enhanced amplitude	• Consider third window disorder
Significantly reduced threshold	• Consider third window disorder
Present response at 4000 Hz	• Consider third window disorder
Prolonged latencies	• Central otolith reflex pathway involvement (e.g., multiple sclerosis) • Consider SCM fatigue for cVEMP

- Response threshold: lowest intensity with repeatable cVEMP responses
  - Normal thresholds >75 dB nHL
  - Thresholds <75 dB nHL suggest third window disorder (Zuniga et al., 2013).
- Amplitude asymmetry: comparison of right and left ear responses

$$\text{Amplitude asymmetry (\%)} = \frac{\text{right ear amplitude} - \text{left ear amplitude}}{\text{right ear amplitude} + \text{left ear amplitude}}$$

  - Normal: 20% to 45% (McCaslin et al., 2013; Welgampola & Colebatch, 2005)

 Q & A

Question: What are the differences between cervical versus ocular VEMPs?

Answer: Cervical VEMPs measure an inhibitory pathway describing the saccule, inferior vestibular nerve, and descending vestibulo-spinal pathway to the SCM. This pathway is a vestibulo-collic reflex. Ocular VEMPs measure an excitatory pathway describing the utricle, superior vestibular nerve, and ascending vestibulo-ocular reflex. These two pathways are different and cannot be used interchangeably.

Ocular VEMPs (oVEMPs)

The oVEMP reflex pathway includes the utricle, superior branch of CN VIII, CN III, and the contralateral inferior oblique muscle. The oVEMP is an excitatory contralateral reflex, meaning that right ear stimulation is recorded from the left inferior oblique. This reflex pathway describes a translational VOR—a specific otolith-ocular reflex pathway that encodes linear acceleration.

Once electrodes are placed, the patient is instructed to gaze upward by approximately 30°. The change in gaze position leads to increased oVEMP amplitude due to (1) reduced distance from the muscle to the recording electrode and/or (2) increased underlying EMG activity (Rosengren et al., 2013). The recorded oVEMP is evaluated in terms of peak latency, response threshold, response amplitude/n1-p1 amplitude, and amplitude asymmetry ratio (Figure 7–12). Table 7–10 provides basic interpretation for oVEMP responses.

- Peak latency
  - n1: 12 ms; abnormal >15 ms
  - p1: 17 ms; abnormal >21 ms
  - Significantly prolonged latencies are rare; generally associated with central pathology.
- Threshold: lowest intensity with repeatable oVEMP responses
  - Normal thresholds >85 dB nHL
  - Thresholds <85 dB nHL suggest third window disorder (Zuniga et al., 2013)
- Response amplitude/n1-p1 amplitude
  - There is less variability in raw oVEMP amplitude compared to raw cVEMP amplitude.
  - Electrode montage significantly impacts response amplitude.

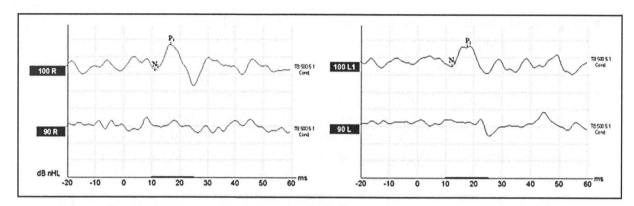

FIGURE 7–12. Typical ocular vestibular evoked myogenic potential (oVEMP) response. This response demonstrates typical oVEMP presentation. For the right ear (*left side*), n1 and p1 occur at 11.00 and 16.67 ms, respectively, and n1-p1 amplitude is 3.017 µV. For the left ear (*right side*), n1 and p1 occur at 12.00 and 17.67 ms, respectively, and n1-p1 amplitude is 2.281 µV. Amplitude asymmetry is 14%. There is no repeatable response noted at 90 dB nHL.

□ Using the electrode montage provided in Table 7–10 should provide mean (standard deviation) amplitude of 5.67 ± 3.42 µV (Sandhu et al., 2013).

■ Amplitude asymmetry: comparison of right ear versus left ear responses

$$\text{Amplitude asymmetry (\%)} = \frac{\text{right ear amplitude} - \text{left ear amplitude}}{\text{right ear amplitude} + \text{left ear amplitude}}$$

□ Normal: <40% (Piker et al., 2011; Zaleski et al., 2015)

Electrocochleography (ECochG)

ECochG is an evoked potential describing the cochlear microphonic, summating potential (SP), and whole nerve action potential (AP) generated by CN VIII. See Chapter 5 for recording parameters and specific considerations for ECochG. Remember that the SP/AP ratio is the reported outcome measure, with ratios >0.4 considered abnormal depending on the electrodes used (Kileny & McCaslin, 2021).

■ Some clinics use ECochG as part of the vestibular test battery, especially in cases of suspected Ménière disease or third window disorder, because this test may be sensitive to altered hydrodynamic forces within the inner ear. In these cases, the SP/AP ratio may be abnormally elevated (Aso et al., 1991; Kileny & McCaslin, 2021).

■ Remember that electrode placement is extremely important for reliable ECochG recordings—transtympanic electrode placement will produce better results than those obtained from tympanic membrane electrodes.

Functional Assessment

Identifying the functional impact of an underlying vestibular disorder allows for appropriate understanding of the impact on the patient's daily activities as well as provides guidance for rehabilitation recommendations.

Balance Testing

Poor balance is often the primary concern for a patient coming in for vestibular evaluation. There are numerous options for balance testing. Some may be done at bedside as described in Table 7–3. Other options are computerized and use additional technology. The most common computerized balance test is called computerized dynamic posturography (CDP). CDP is typically available in larger vestibular laboratories and physical therapy practices. This system allows for evaluation of the patient's ability to use visual, vestibular, and somatosensory information in maintaining appropriate balance. There are three main subtests:

- Sensory organization test (SOT) evaluates six conditions to identify which system(s) contributes to reduced balance (Figure 7–13). The conditions are:

    1. Eyes open/firm surface

    2. Eyes closed/firm surface

    3. Eyes open/firm surface/sway-referenced visual surround

    4. Eyes open/sway-referenced surface

    5. Eyes closed/sway-referenced surface

    6. Eyes open/sway-referenced surface/sway-referenced visual surround

    □ Balance performance is measured by calculating the center of gravity sway angle over the course of each 20-second trial.

    □ An equilibrium score is provided for each trial, defined as a percentage that compares the patient's peak amplitude of anterior-posterior sway with the theoretical anterior-posterior limits of stability. Scores closer to 100% suggest very little sway and those closer to 0% suggest significant sway and that the patient is reaching/exceeding the limits of stability.

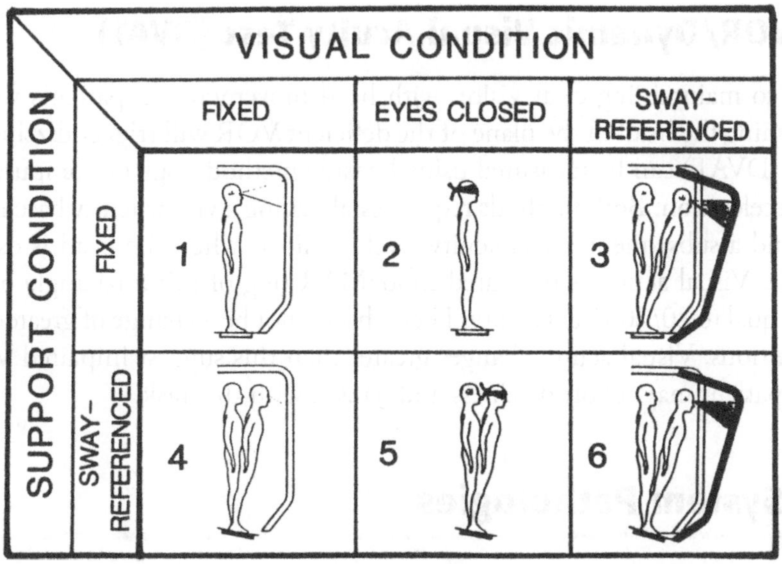

FIGURE 7–13. The SOT protocol showing the six sensory test conditions. *Source:* From *Handbook of Balance Function Testing.* Jacobson et al., 1997.

TABLE 7–11. Sensory Analysis Interpretation

RATIO NAME	CALCULATION	SIGNIFICANCE OF ABNORMAL PERFORMANCE
Somatosensory	Condition 2/Condition 1	Poor use of somatosensory cues
Visual	Condition 4/Condition 1	Poor use of visual cues
Vestibular	Condition 5/Condition 1	Poor use of vestibular cues
Visual Preference	Conditions 3 + 6/ Conditions 2 + 5	Overreliance on visual cues, even when inaccurate

☐ The composite score provides an overview of balance performance. This is a weighted average considering Conditions 3 to 6 more heavily than Conditions 1 and 2.

☐ Sensory analysis provides an understanding of which sensory system(s) may be contributing to abnormal balance performance (Table 7–11).

■ Motor control test (MCT) evaluates the automatic postural reflexes elicited by abrupt horizontal translations of the support surface. Patients are slid backward and forward in three translational sizes (small, medium, large). The outcome measures are the active force latency (ms), active force strength, and weight asymmetry.

■ Adaptation test (ADT) evaluates the adaptation of the automatic postural control system by tilting the support surface toes up or toes down. Five identical trials of 8° rotations are completed to evaluate the patient's ability to adapt to this rotation. The outcome measure is a sway energy score, defined as the magnitude of center of gravity sway immediately after a forceplate rotation.

Functional VOR/Dynamic Visual Acuity Test (DVAT)

The VOR is key to maintaining clear vision with head movement. In patients with VOR pathway abnormalities, turning the head in the plane of the deficient VOR will trigger dizziness and oscillopsia. Functional VOR (DVAT) can be measured using bedside methodology or computerized systems that document head acceleration. Both methods require establishing a visual acuity baseline measured when the head is still and a subsequent visual acuity level obtained when the head is oscillating ±20° at a frequency of 2 Hz. Visual acuity is measured in logMAR (log of minimal angle of resolution), with logMAR of 0.00 equal to 20/20 visual acuity. There should not be a change of greater than 0.2 logMAR between the conditions. Visual acuity changes greater than this suggest impaired VOR performance. Additionally, the patient may report dizziness and nausea with this task.

Vestibular System Pathologies

There are innumerable underlying causes for dizziness and patient self-reported symptom characteristics are not always reliable for identifying the problem. Consider the case history and temporal (timing) features of the patient's symptoms to better identify possible etiologies (Table 7–12).

TABLE 7–12. Approach for Identifying Vestibular System Pathology Using Temporal Features

CATEGORY	PERIPHERAL ETIOLOGY	CENTRAL ETIOLOGY
Acute vestibular syndrome	Vestibular neuritis	Brainstem, cerebellar infarct
Recurrent vertigo	Ménière disease	Vestibular migraine
	Superior semicircular canal dehiscence (SSCD)	Transient ischemic attack (TIA)
Positional vertigo	Benign paroxysmal positional vertigo (BPPV)	Cerebellar disorder
		Vestibular migraine
Chronic dizziness, unsteadiness	Bilateral vestibulopathy	Persistent postural-perceptual dizziness (PPPD)
	Vestibular schwannoma	

Vestibular Neuritis

Vestibular neuritis occurs with an infection/inflammation of the vestibular nerve, most often involving the superior branch. It is suspected in cases presenting with acute onset of vertigo, nausea/vomiting, and generalized imbalance. The acute phase can last for hours to days, but imbalance may linger for weeks after. There is no hearing loss or tinnitus associated with vestibular neuritis.

Consider this case example of suspected vestibular neuritis.

Patient was a 61-year-old male who reported waking up to rotational vertigo 2 months before testing. He described rotational vertigo lasting for hours, with continued imbalance, lightheadedness, and nausea with quick head movements. He denied other otologic symptoms.

VNG testing was abnormal. Gaze testing in neutral gaze without fixation demonstrated right-beating nystagmus averaging 2°/second (Figure 7–14). This was not significant but likely consistent with the remaining VNG battery and suggested a recent VOR insult. The remaining oculomotor battery was within normal limits.

Caloric testing demonstrated significantly reduced responses in the left ear, with CP of 63%. TES for the left ear was 5°/second, suggesting minimal VOR performance in this ear. There was no significant directional preponderance (Figure 7–15).

SHA testing demonstrated significantly reduced gain from 0.02 to 0.16 Hz, with significant phase lead from 0.02 to 0.04 Hz. Asymmetry was abnormal across all frequencies (0.02–0.64 Hz), consistent with the underlying spontaneous nystagmus (Figure 7–16).

CVEMP responses were within expected limits for the right ear, with questionable left ear response presence (Figure 7–17). These results are consistent with left peripheral loss.

Functional measures suggested that the patient had not yet compensated for his recent vestibular loss. DVAT demonstrated a significant loss of visual acuity (logMAR loss = 0.6) with leftward head movement. Rightward head movement was unimpaired. SOT results were consistent with poor use of vestibular system information, with reduced performance noted on Conditions 2, 5, and 6 (Figure 7–18).

Overall findings suggested that the patient was experiencing uncompensated vestibular symptoms associated with his vertigo episode 2 months prior. Medical consultation suggested vestibular neuritis was the likely cause of his symptoms. He was referred to vestibular rehabilitation to facilitate compensation.

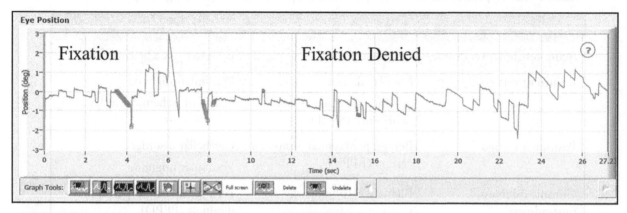

FIGURE 7–14. Case example: vestibular neuritis; spontaneous nystagmus noted in neutral gaze without fixation demonstrated right-beating nystagmus averaging 2°/second.

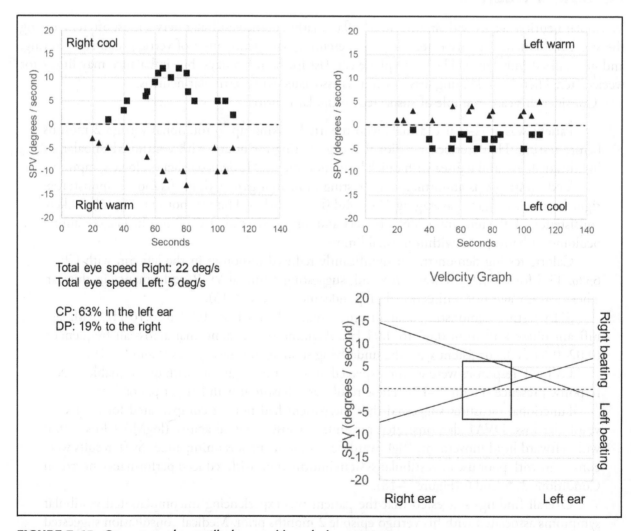

FIGURE 7–15. Case example: vestibular neuritis; caloric responses.

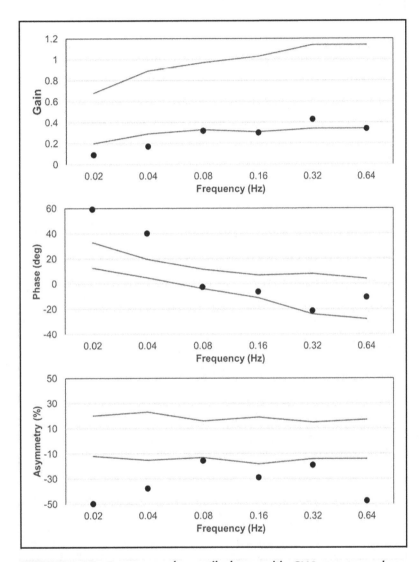

FIGURE 7–16. Case example: vestibular neuritis; SHA responses demonstrated low gain from 0.02 to 0.64 Hz, significant low-frequency phase lead from 0.02 to 0.04 Hz, and significant asymmetry from 0.02 to 0.64 Hz.

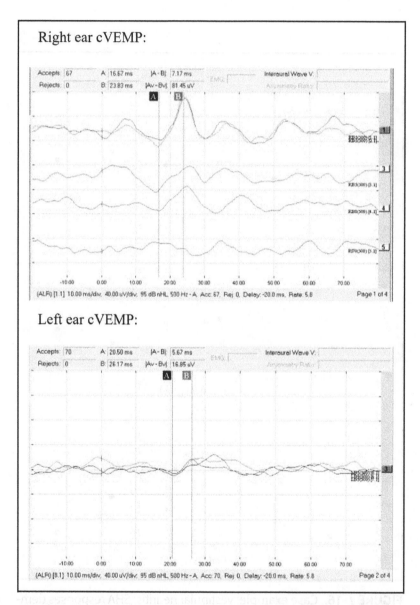

FIGURE 7–17. Case example: vestibular neuritis; cVEMPs. Note that waveforms are inverted (p1 is negatively deflected). The left cVEMP response is significantly reduced (16.85 μV), with poor repeatability. There is a significant amplitude asymmetry when compared to the right cVEMP response (81.45 μV; 66% asymmetry to the left).

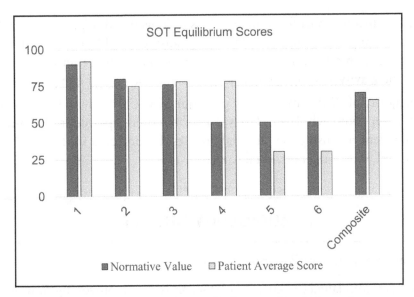

FIGURE 7–18. Case example: vestibular neuritis; SOT results.

Labyrinthitis

The clinical presentation of labyrinthitis is similar to vestibular neuritis, except that the patient will also report concurrent sudden hearing loss and tinnitus. The hearing loss and vertigo may occur simultaneously or within a few days of each other. Labyrinthitis occurs due to inflammation of the inner ear and/or CN VIII.

Vestibulotoxicity

Various medications and chemicals cause vestibular hair cell death, leading to imbalance and oscillopsia. Common pharmaceutical agents include aminoglycosides (e.g., streptomycin, gentamicin) and chemotherapeutics (e.g., cisplatin). Industrial or occupational exposure to chemical agents (e.g., xylene, toluene) can also occur. Because both ears are typically impacted, patients rarely report vertigo. Not all individuals exposed to these agents will experience vestibular dysfunction, and modern dosing methods for pharmaceuticals have aimed to reduce overall toxicity.

- Clinical presentation of vestibulotoxicity
  - Bilaterally reduced VOR performance ranging from mild to areflexia
  - Reduced otolith reflex pathway responses
  - Reported oscillopsia, imbalance
  - May or may not present with bilateral hearing loss/tinnitus

Benign Paroxysmal Positional Vertigo (BPPV)

BPPV is the most common peripheral vestibular disorder. It occurs more often in women and has been associated with advancing age, hormone changes, and head injury, and it may occur with other inner ear disorders (e.g., labyrinthitis, vestibular neuritis) (Chen et al., 2021).

- BPPV occurs when otoconia from the utricle is dislodged and migrates to a SCC (Figure 7–19). The otoconia change the function of the SCC, causing it to become sensitive to gravity. When the patient makes an offending head movement, such as rolling over in bed or tipping the head back, the gravity-sensitive SCC is triggered and the patient experiences vertigo.

- The vast majority of BPPV involves the posterior SCC (90%), with horizontal SCC BPPV diagnosed in approximately 10%. Rarely, BPPV has been reported in the anterior SCC. BPPV can be easily identified using the Dix-Hallpike test for otoconia in the vertical canals and the lateral head roll test for the horizontal canal.

AUDIOLOGY NUGGET

Clinical Presentation of Posterior SCC BPPV

- Symptom latency occurs 1 to 10 seconds after a provoking movement, such as rolling over in bed.

- Symptom duration <1 minute

- Torsional up-beating nystagmus beats toward the underneath ear, changes direction when the patient sits up

- Nystagmus and symptoms fatigue with repeated evaluation or repositioning

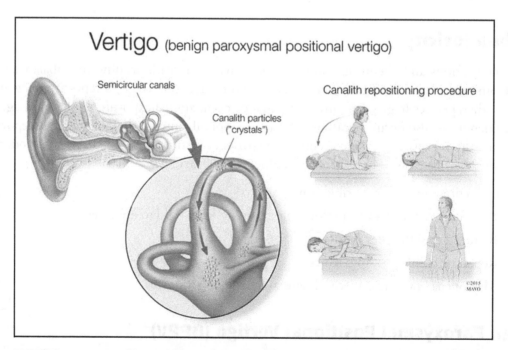

FIGURE 7–19. Benign paroxysmal positional vertigo (BPPV). BPPV occurs when otoconia are displaced and migrate into a semicircular canal, triggering vertigo with position changes. This condition can be resolved with canalith repositioning. *Source:* Used with permission of Mayo Foundation for Medical Education and Research, all rights reserved.

TABLE 7–13. Nystagmus Associated With BPPV by Involved SCC

INVOLVED SCC	RIGHT EAR	LEFT EAR
Posterior SCC	Up-beating	Up-beating
	Right-torsion	Left-torsion
Anterior SCC	Down-beating	Down-beating
	Right-torsion	Left-torsion
Horizontal SCCª	Geotropic/ageotropic	Geotropic/ageotropic

Note. ªCanalithiasis will present with geotropic nystagmus; cupulothiasis will present with ageotropic nystagmus; nystagmus will generally occur bilaterally, with the side with the larger velocity likely the suspect ear.

☐ Dix-Hallpike testing is a positioning test that evaluates for vertical canal BPPV. To complete the test, the patient turns the head 45° to the right or left depending on the ear in question. The patient is then laid back onto the examination table with the head hanging 30° below horizontal off the table. The examiner holds the patient's head in the appropriate position and observes for nystagmus. The Dix-Hallpike test should be held for 30 to 60 seconds.

■ Because otoconia can migrate to any SCC, knowing the presenting nystagmus pattern will help to identify the appropriate canal for management (Table 7–13).

Endolymphatic Hydrops/Ménière Disease

Endolymphatic hydrops includes any disorder associated with abnormal fluctuations in endolymph. The most commonly discussed is Ménière disease. Ménière disease is an idiopathic disorder of the inner ear that occurs when endolymph production or reabsorption is altered. Recent hypotheses suggest that vertigo attacks may occur when endolymph either drains too quickly or overfills the labyrinth (Gibson, 2010).

 Q & A

Question: What are the diagnostic criteria for Ménière disease?

Answer: Patients must meet the following criteria to be diagnosed with Ménière disease (Basura et al., 2020).

■ Two or more spontaneous episodes of vertigo each lasting 20 minutes to 12 hours

■ Audiometrically documented low- to mid-frequency sensorineural hearing loss in one ear, defining the affected ear, on at least one occasion before, during, or after one of the episodes of vertigo

■ Fluctuating aural symptoms (hearing loss, tinnitus, fullness) in the affected ear

■ Not better accounted for by another vestibular diagnosis

- Over time, damage to the underlying hair cells and support structures is more apparent. Eventually, the ear may "burn out," meaning that little hearing and/or vestibular function remains. In these later stages, the patient may experience Tumarkin otolithic crises or "drop attacks." These episodes are described as a sudden perception of being pushed or knocked to the ground and can lead to serious injury.

Consider this case of suspected Ménière disease.

Patient was a 64-year-old female reporting onset of hearing loss, tinnitus, aural fullness, rotational vertigo, nausea, and vomiting 3 years ago. Episodes lasted several hours. She reported that hearing loss in the left ear gets worse before her vertigo episodes but has not recovered as well as it has before. The patient reported that her last episode was 4 months before testing.

Audiometric findings demonstrated normal hearing sensitivity sloping to moderate sensorineural hearing loss in the right ear and mild sloping to moderate sensorineural hearing loss in the left ear (Figure 7–20).

Vestibular testing demonstrated findings consistent with significant left peripheral vestibulopathy. Caloric testing demonstrated a 55% CP in the left ear, with left ear TES of 11°/second (Figure 7–21).

SHA testing demonstrated appropriate gain for 0.02 to 0.64 Hz stimuli. A significant phase lead was noted for 0.02 to 0.04 Hz, consistent with the documented left peripheral vestibulopathy (Figure 7–22).

The remaining VNG was within normal limits, with no evidence of acute vestibulopathy. The overall clinical presentation is consistent with left peripheral vestibulopathy. The lesion has compensated over the 4-month interval between her last vertigo episode and presentation for testing. She continued to establish a management strategy with her ENT provider. She was counseled regarding reducing salt intake and the possible use of a diuretic.

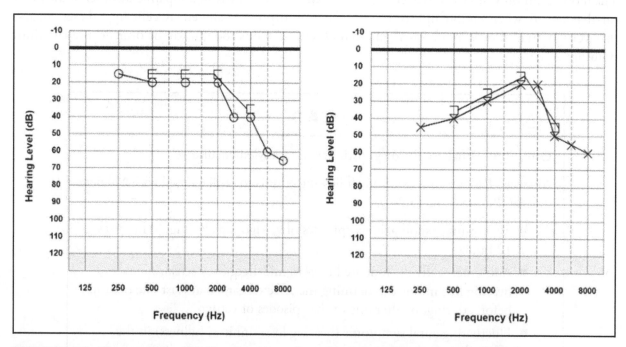

FIGURE 7–20. Case example: Ménière disease; audiometric presentation. Note the significant low-frequency sensorineural hearing loss in the left ear consistent with Ménière disease presentation.

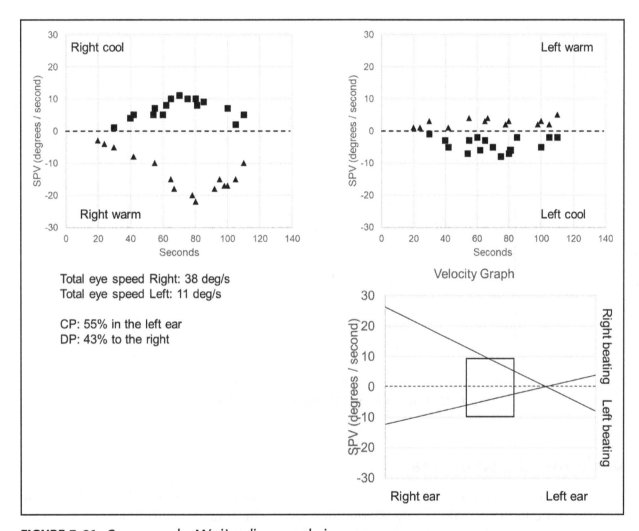

FIGURE 7–21. Case example: Ménière disease; caloric responses.

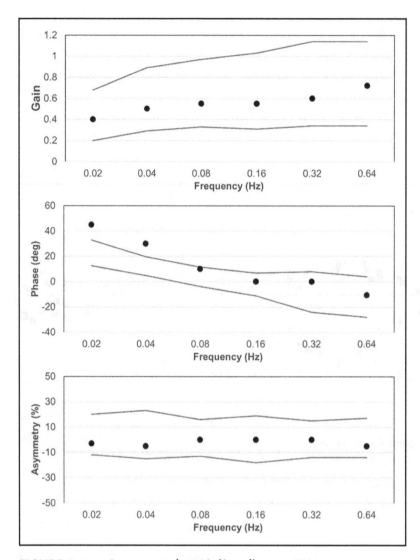

FIGURE 7–22. Case example: Ménière disease; SHA responses.

Vestibular Schwannoma

Vestibular schwannomae (or acoustic neuromae) are slow-growing, benign neoplasms arising from the Schwann cells of CN VIII. Nearly all arise from the vestibular nerve branch (Figure 7–23). Unilateral cases are generally sporadic and may be found incidentally. Bilateral cases are associated with neurofibromatosis type 2 (NF2), a rare genetic disorder that leads to the formation of benign tumors, commonly along CN VIII.

- Most cases of vestibular schwannoma present with asymmetrical hearing loss and unilateral tinnitus. Dizziness and vertigo are not reported as often due to the slow growth of the tumor, allowing the vestibular system time to compensate for the gradual decline in function.

  □ Patients may also present with facial weakness or numbness, suggesting that CN VII may also be impaired.

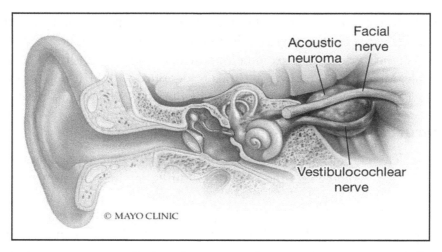

FIGURE 7–23. A vestibular schwannoma (or acoustic neuroma) typically arises from the superior branch of CN VIII, increasing pressure on and displacement of the surrounding structures over time. *Source:* Used with permission of Mayo Foundation for Medical Education and Research, all rights reserved.

□ Many patients remain under observation to determine if/when intervention is warranted. If the tumor is allowed to grow too large or within sensitive areas, it could lead to significant brainstem compression and subsequent complications, including death.

■ In most cases, the tumor itself is not overly problematic in terms of dizziness or balance performance, and most do not require specific management. Treatments for vestibular schwannoma, such as surgical removal or radiation therapy (e.g., gamma knife), however, may lead to abrupt vestibular system asymmetry.

□ In these cases, the patient may experience acute onset of vertigo and/or hearing loss. Vertigo symptoms reduce over time with compensation.

Third Window Disorders

Perilymph fistula, superior semicircular canal dehiscence (SSCD), and enlarged vestibular aqueduct syndrome (EVAS) are considered third window disorders. They act effectively as an additional "window" into the inner ear.

Perilymph Fistula

Perilymph fistula is a disorder that occurs when perilymph leaks from the labyrinth into the middle ear space following a tear in the round or oval window. This is most often associated with head trauma, barotrauma, or straining but can occur idiopathically. There are no universally accepted criteria for perilymph fistula diagnosis.

■ Symptoms include sudden unilateral hearing loss, tinnitus, aural fullness, and imbalance. Patients with diagnosed perilymph fistula also describe acute episodes of lightheadedness, imbalance, and motion intolerance that can be triggered by internal or external pressure changes.

■ Clinically, the fistula test has been used to identify a possible perilymph fistula. A positive fistula test is the presence of nystagmus when negative pressure is applied to the external auditory canal, such as with a tympanometer. Unfortunately, the sensitivity of the fistula test is variable. Most often, a perilymph fistula is identified with high-resolution computed tomography (CT) and magnetic resonance imaging (MRI) (Sarna et al., 2020).

Superior Semicircular Canal Dehiscence Syndrome (SSCD)

SSCD occurs with deterioration of the bony labyrinth covering the superior (anterior) SCC. The dehiscence acts as a third window into the labyrinth, leading to altered transmission of sound and pressure through the inner ear (Figure 7–24).

Patients with SSCD may describe unique symptoms, such as hearing their eyes move or experiencing vertigo in response to loud sounds (e.g., a dog bark). Overall symptoms are variable but may include:

■ Autophony

■ Dizziness, vertigo, disequilibrium—consider Tullio phenomenon, Hennebert phenomenon, dizziness triggered by internal/external pressure changes

■ Pulse-synchronized oscillopsia

■ Hyperacusis

■ Aural fullness

■ Pulsatile tinnitus

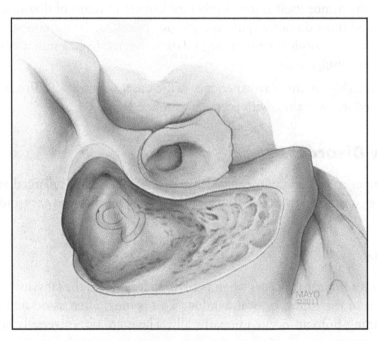

FIGURE 7–24. Superior semicircular canal dehiscence syndrome (SSCD) occurs when the bone overlying the superior SSC deteriorates and creates an additional opening into the inner ear. This can be repaired by plugging or capping the superior SCC. *Source:* Used with permission of Mayo Foundation for Medical Education and Research, all rights reserved.

■ Brain fog

■ Fatigue

■ Clinical signs include Tullio-/Hennebert-evoked nystagmus, exceptionally enhanced (or augmented) VEMPs, and paradoxical (or pseudo) conductive hearing loss with present middle ear muscle reflexes. Tullio phenomenon is defined as vertigo, dizziness, and eye movement induced by loud sounds (think Tullio = "too loud"). Hennebert sign is nystagmus evoked by internal or external pressure changes.

Consider this case of suspected SSCD.

The patient was a 52-year-old female reporting chronic imbalance and dizziness for several years. She noted that she experienced aural fullness, pulsatile tinnitus, and autophony (hearing her heartbeat, eye movements) in her right ear. She demonstrated a positive Hennebert sign, consistent with her noted increased dizziness with barometric pressure changes.

Audiometric testing was abnormal for low-frequency conductive hearing loss at 250 and 500 Hz only. Note the significantly low bone-conduction threshold (<0 dB HL) (Figure 7–25). Type A tympanograms and present ipsilateral and contralateral middle ear reflexes from 500 to 2000 Hz were documented bilaterally.

Cervical and ocular VEMPs were completed. CVEMPs were within normal limits bilaterally, with no enhancement noted. OVEMPs were significantly abnormal for the right ear, most apparent with 89.88 μV interpeak amplitude noted (Figure 7–26)—remember that average oVEMP amplitude is ~5 μV. Her remaining vestibular evaluation was within normal limits.

Management strategies were discussed. She was referred to ENT due to suspicion of third window disorder in the right ear. She was counseled to expect dizziness when in significant noise and to consider wearing an earplug in these situations. She also discussed plugging the superior SCC as a future option with the managing otologist.

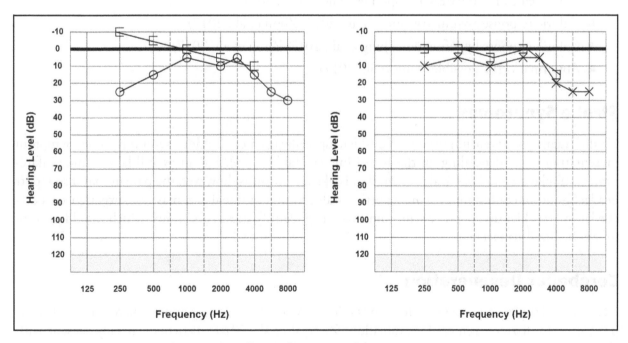

FIGURE 7–25. Case example: SSCD; audiometric presentation.

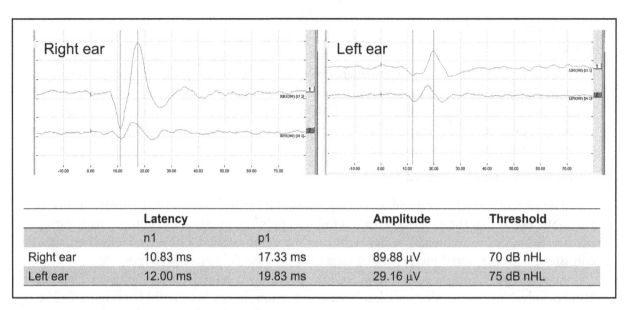

	Latency		Amplitude	Threshold
	n1	p1		
Right ear	10.83 ms	17.33 ms	89.88 µV	70 dB nHL
Left ear	12.00 ms	19.83 ms	29.16 µV	75 dB nHL

FIGURE 7-26. Case example: SSCD; oVEMPs.

Enlarged Vestibular Aqueduct Syndrome (EVAS)

EVAS—sometimes called large vestibular aqueduct syndrome (LVAS)—is a genetic condition associated with progressive hearing loss. EVAS can occur alone or with other conditions such as Pendred syndrome or brachio-oto-renal (BOR) syndrome. While progressive hearing loss is a known concern for patients with EVAS, the vestibular system may be involved in up to 70% (Berrettini et al., 2005). It is likely that vestibular dysfunction also occurs in a progressive manner. Clinical signs of vestibular dysfunction in patients with EVAS include:

- Enhanced cVEMP/oVEMP responses (Zhou et al., 2017)
- Caloric response asymmetry (Jung et al., 2017; Zhou et al., 2017)
- Caloric response hypofunction (Jung et al., 2017; Zhou et al., 2017)
- Abnormal vHIT possible (Jung et al., 2017)

Stroke Syndromes

Cardiovascular events are important to consider, especially in cases of sudden symptom onset. Symptom presentation varies depending on the site of infarct (Table 7–14). For an overall labyrinthine infarction, vestibular and audiological presentation is like labyrinthitis; however, the patient may also report headache and/or confusion. Patients reporting sudden onset of imbalance may have experienced a cerebellar infarct. Identifying other symptoms may help identify these conditions, which should prompt urgent medical management.

Cerebellar Degeneration

Cerebellar dizziness may occur with various etiologies and accounts for approximately 10% of those presenting to dizziness centers for evaluation (Zwergal et al., 2020). Patients generally present with chronic, progressive signs of cerebellar involvement such as ataxia, abnormal oculomotor performance, and down-beating nystagmus (Table 7–15).

TABLE 7–14. Presentation of Labyrinthine and Cerebellar Infarcts

	LABYRINTHINE INFARCT	CEREBELLAR INFARCT
Timing	Sudden Symptoms last hours to days Vertigo common	Sudden imbalance Spontaneous nystagmus >24 hours Vertigo rare
Trigger	Reduced blood flow to all or part of the labyrinth	Transient ischemic attack (TIA) in the cerebellar artery
Other symptoms	Sudden sensorineural hearing loss Headache Disorientation Diagnosed AICA stroke	Lateropulsion Decreased coordination Hiccoughs Ataxia

TABLE 7–15. Etiologies Associated With Cerebellar Dizziness

TIMING	CATEGORY	DIAGNOSIS
Chronic	Degenerative	Idiopathic late-onset cerebellar ataxia Cerebellar ataxia Downbeat nystagmus syndrome CANVAS
	Genetic/hereditary	Spinocerebellar ataxias Episodic ataxias
	Acquired	Paraneoplastic syndrome Autoimmune disorders Toxicities (e.g., alcohol) Vitamin deficiencies (e.g., B1, B12, E)
	Infection	Acute cerebellitis Postinfection cerebellar syndrome Chronic cerebellar infection
Recurrent		Episodic ataxias Vestibular migraine
Acute	Cerebellar stoke	PICA most common
	Inflammation	Multiple sclerosis Sarcoidosis

Source: Zwergal et al. (2020).

Cerebellar Ataxia With Neuropathy and Vestibular Areflexia Syndrome (CANVAS)

CANVAS is a recently described disorder that illustrates the clinical presentation possible with cerebellar degeneration. Patients with CANVAS experience slowly progressive symptoms and many have a family history positive for similar symptoms. Findings consistent with CANVAS include (Szmulewicz et al., 2016):

- Bilateral vestibulopathy
  - □ Decreased VOR performance: reduced caloric function, reduced SHA gain, present saccades/low gain on vHIT
  - □ Impaired VVOR testing
  - □ Poor fixation suppression
- Cerebellar involvement
  - □ Cerebellar atrophy specifically involving the vermis
  - □ Cerebellar dysarthria
  - □ Truncal ataxia
  - □ Dysphasia
  - □ Oculomotor abnormalities: saccadic smooth pursuit, gaze-evoked/direction-changing nystagmus, dysmetric saccades, rebound nystagmus
- Somatosensory impairment—neuronopathy
- There is no significant effect on the cochlea or cochlear branch of CN VIII.

Consider this case of suspected CANVAS.

Patient was a 67-year-old female presenting for >10-year history of imbalance. She reported neuronopathy in her hands and feet, as well as chronic throat spasms, chronic cough, and dysarthria. MRI noted mild atrophy of the vermis. The patient reported significant family history of similar symptoms, including in her brother, mother, maternal grandmother, and maternal aunt.

Oculomotor testing was significantly abnormal. Saccade testing demonstrated significantly prolonged latencies and reduced peak velocity. Optokinetic nystagmus was absent. Smooth pursuit was significantly saccadic (Figure 7–27).

VOR testing was consistent with significant vestibular dysfunction. She demonstrated bilateral caloric areflexia (TES = 0°/second). VHIT responses demonstrated significantly reduced gain bilaterally with significant overt and covert saccades (Figure 7–28).

SHA testing demonstrated significantly reduced gain from 0.02 to 0.32 Hz. Phase and asymmetry could not be calculated due to the low gain. VVOR response (*) at 0.16 Hz remained reduced, consistent with central bilateral vestibulopathy (Figure 7–29).

The patient demonstrated significant functional impairment. She was unable to complete SOT Conditions 3 to 6 without falling, suggesting a severe balance impairment and high fall risk. DVAT was attempted but could not be completed at the maximum logMAR level with head movement, suggesting severe deficits in the VOR pathway. These results were consistent with the significant vestibular impairment documented on testing.

The patient returned to her managing neurologist and was subsequently diagnosed with CANVAS. Unfortunately, CANVAS is a slowly progressive disorder with no noted therapies. She was encouraged to continue balance therapy to develop strategies for reducing fall risk.

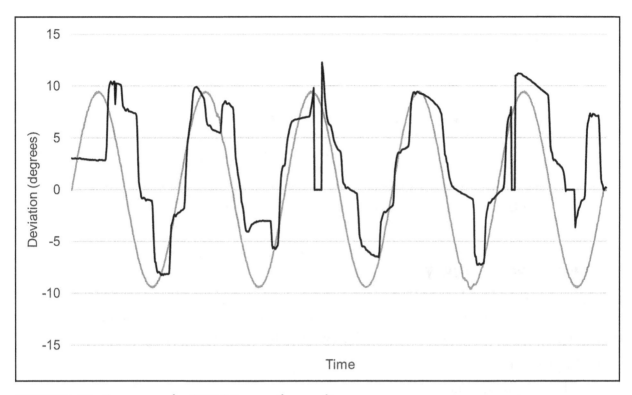

FIGURE 7–27. Case example: CANVAS; smooth pursuit.

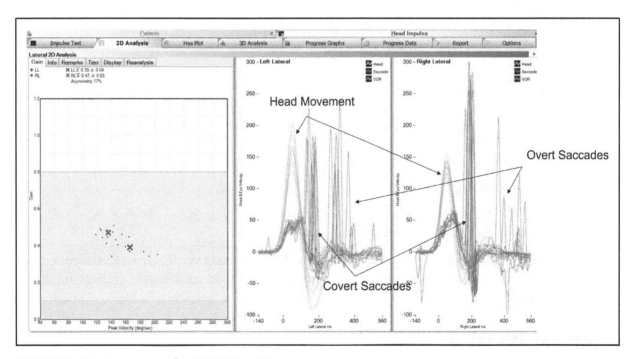

FIGURE 7–28. Case example: CANVAS; vHIT.

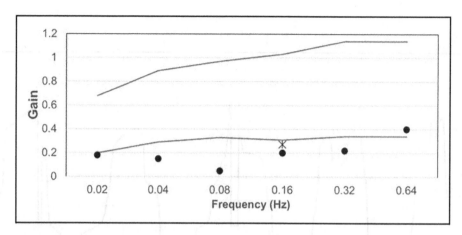

FIGURE 7–29. Case example: CANVAS; SHA responses.

Traumatic Brain Injury

Posttraumatic dizziness and imbalance are common. Patients may demonstrate increased motion sensitivity, imbalance, and dizziness with head movements and when in busy visual environments. Various underlying conditions may be associated with posttraumatic dizziness:

- Peripheral etiologies
  - Direct end-organ injury
  - BPPV
  - Labyrinthine concussion
  - Posttraumatic endolymphatic hydrops
  - SSCD
  - Otolith dysfunction
  - Medication side effects
- Central etiologies
  - Concomitant injury
  - Diffuse axonal injury
  - Postconcussion migraine
  - Cervical dizziness
  - Vestibulo-autonomic reflex impairment

Clinical presentation for acute posttraumatic dizziness should include vestibular and balance testing. These metrics can be used to direct rehabilitation strategies and monitor recovery (Ellis et al., 2017; Zhou & Brodsky, 2015).

Vestibular Migraine

Vestibular migraine is one of the most common disorders associated with dizziness. Most associate migraine with headache, but other sensory integration abnormalities, such as vision distortions, hypersensitivity to sensory stimuli, and paresthesias, are common. Patients with vestibular migraine describe a range of dizziness and balance concerns, and often report current or childhood history of motion sensitivity. There is no specific migraine test and laboratory findings vary. Vestibular migraine is diagnosed using International Headache Society classification criteria (IHS, 2018):

- At least five episodes of vestibular symptoms of moderate or severe intensity, lasting between 5 minutes and 72 hours
- Current or previous history of migraine with or without aura
- One or more migraine features with at least 50% of vestibular episodes
  - □ Headache with at least two of the following characteristics: unilateral location, pulsating quality, moderate or severe intensity, aggravated by routine physical activity
  - □ Photophobia, phonophobia
  - □ Visual aura
- Not better accounted for by another vestibular or headache diagnosis

Consider this case of suspected vestibular migraine.

The patient was a 37-year-old male presenting with 1 month of dizziness symptoms. He described a sense of "rocking" as if he were "on a boat." Dizziness symptoms increased in busy visual environments and with quick head movement. The patient noted longstanding motion sensitivity and migraine diagnosis at 18 years old. He reported no other otologic concerns.

VNG testing was within normal limits for all subtests. Balance performance was well within normal limits (SOT composite score = 89). Otolith reflexes were abnormal. CVEMP responses were present, but not as robust as expected (Figure 7–30), and oVEMP responses were absent bilaterally (Figure 7–31).

Functional VOR performance was significantly abnormal. The patient demonstrated 0.32 logMAR loss for leftward and 0.48 logMAR loss for rightward head movements. Atypical functional VOR presentation has been reported in those with vestibular migraine (Baker et al., 2013a, 2013b) and may prove to be a useful tool in describing the clinical presentation of this cohort.

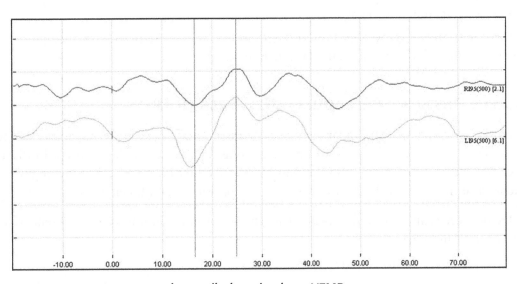

FIGURE 7–30. Case example: vestibular migraine; cVEMPs.

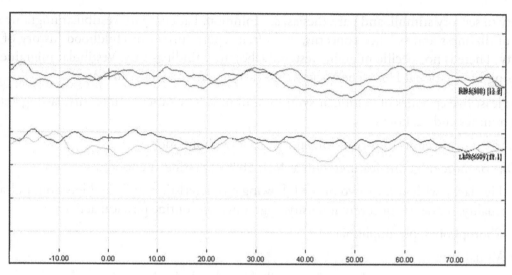

FIGURE 7–31. Case example: vestibular migraine; oVEMPs.

Psychiatric Aspects of Dizziness

There is an established relationship between dizziness and psychiatric disorders. Many patients with chronic dizziness also experience anxiety, depression, and panic attacks; conversely, those with these psychiatric conditions are at increased risk of developing dizziness. The relationship has a neurological basis as the limbic, autonomic, and vestibular centers have significant interconnections (Rajagopalan et al., 2017).

A patient's psychiatric condition may be the sole reason for dizziness symptoms, while another patient may experience a psychiatric response to a physical condition. Dizziness characteristics in psychiatric conditions include:

- Constant imbalance
- Dizziness triggered by movement, visual stimulation, specific situations
- Dizziness lasts minutes to days
- Symptoms rarely improve without intervention (e.g., cognitive behavioral therapy, pharmacological treatment, vestibular rehabilitation)

Persistent Postural-Perceptual Dizziness (PPPD)

PPPD is a chronic functional vestibular disorder, not a structural or psychiatric condition. Most often, patients develop PPPD after an acute vestibular episode, such as vestibular neuritis. PPPD management includes education about the disorder, vestibular rehabilitation, cognitive behavioral therapy, and pharmacological treatment. PPPD is diagnosed using specific criteria (Staab et al., 2017):

- One or more symptoms of dizziness, unsteadiness, or nonspinning vertigo present on most days for >3 months
  - □ Symptoms last hours but may wax and wane.

    ☐ Symptoms need not be present through the entire day.

- Persistent symptoms occur without provocation but are exacerbated by:

    ☐ Upright posture

    ☐ Active/passive motion without regard to direction or position

    ☐ Exposure to moving or complex visual environments

- Precipitated by conditions that cause vertigo, unsteadiness, problems with balance, including acute, episodic, or chronic vestibular syndromes, other neurological/medical issues, or psychological distress

- Symptoms cause significant distress or functional impairment.

- Symptoms are not better accounted for by another disease or diagnosis.

Vestibular Rehabilitation

Most vestibular rehabilitation is completed by physical therapists or audiologists with specialized training. There is a range of rehabilitation options available and will vary depending on the needs of the patient. Candidates for vestibular rehabilitation include those with:

- Acute vestibular impairment, including BPPV

- Chronic dizziness/oscillopsia

- Chronic imbalance/fall risk

- Central vestibular impairments, including vestibular migraine and concussion

BPPV

BPPV is the most common peripheral vestibular disorder, most often involving the posterior SCC. This can be easily identified with the Dix-Hallpike test. At this point, many clinicians will continue through the Epley maneuver (Figure 7–32) to reposition the displaced otoconia into the vestibule. This is sometimes called "canalith repositioning." Patients may need to go through the maneuver several times to alleviate symptoms, but 90% have symptom resolution in one to two treatments. Patients with recurrent symptoms may learn to treat themselves at home.

- For those with symptoms suggesting BPPV but who have negative Dix-Hallpike findings, the clinician should complete supine roll/lateral head roll testing to evaluate the patient for horizontal SCC BPPV. In positive cases, the patient will demonstrate nystagmus in both head right and head left conditions. The position with the strongest nystagmus and dizziness is the positive side.

- Most patients demonstrate geotropic nystagmus, meaning that in the head right position, nystagmus will beat toward the right ear and switch direction in the head left position. The side with the larger nystagmus velocity is the involved ear. Ageotropic nystagmus may occur in rare cases when otoconia adheres to the cupula. The side with the smaller nystagmus velocity is the involved ear. For those with identified horizontal SCC BPPV, they can be treated using the Lempert/barbecue roll maneuver or the Gufoni maneuver.

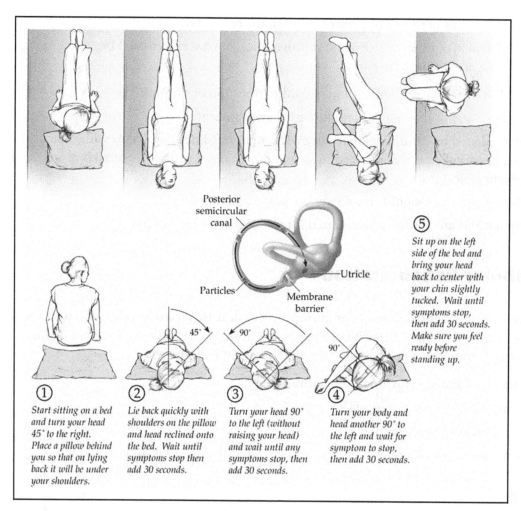

FIGURE 7–32. Steps for performing right posterior semicircular canal canalith repositioning (Epley maneuver) for BPPV. *Source:* From Mayo Clinic Patient Education. *Benign Paroxysmal Positional Vertigo* (BPPV) [MC6727]. Rochester, MN: Mayo Clinic, 2010, p. 4; used with permission of Mayo Foundation for Medical Education and Research, all rights reserved.

Vestibular Rehabilitation Therapy (VRT)

VRT is a significant component of dizziness rehabilitation and management. It has been well studied in those with peripheral vestibulopathy. VRT is designed to assist in vestibular compensation and uses treatment strategies focused on adaptation, habituation, and/or substitution. There are some known limitations to vestibular compensation, but it is expected to occur within 4 to 12 weeks (Whitney & Furman, 2021). There are three main components to VRT:

- Adaptation: ability to make long-term changes in the neural response to head movement, specifically focused on the functional VOR

- Habituation: repeated exposure to an offending stimulus to gradually inhibit the patient's response to that stimulus

■ Substitution: use of an intact sensory system to replace lost sensory system function; most often done in cases of bilateral vestibular hypofunction

AUDIOLOGY NUGGET

Some patients may be at risk for prolonged/incomplete vestibular compensation due to patient-specific characteristics.

- Cerebellar disorders
- Visual impairment
- Head injury
- Use of vestibular suppressants
- Movement restrictions/limitations
- Migraine
- Anxiety/depression

The initial VRT evaluation will include:

■ Case history, questionnaires
■ Physical examination
  □ Strength, range of motion, sensation
  □ Oculomotor performance: gaze, smooth pursuit, saccades, vergence
  □ Dix-Hallpike test
  □ Post-headshake nystagmus
  □ Head impulse test
  □ Dynamic visual acuity test
  □ Balance performance
■ Development of VRT program

Patients with vestibular deficits will begin with vestibular stimulation exercises called VORx1. To complete this task, the patient will tape a card with a small letter printed on it to the wall. The patient stands/sits about an arm's-length away so that the letter is readable. From here, the patient rotates the head side-to-side as quickly as possible while keeping the letter in focus for 1 to 2 minutes. This is repeated approximately three times per day. If the patient loses focus, they are instructed to reduce head speed, but to work on increasing the speed over time. Additional options make VORx1 more challenging:

■ Perform this exercise while sitting.
■ Perform this exercise while standing; progress to tandem stance, gait.
■ Repeat this exercise moving the head up and down.

- Perform this exercise with a larger letter placed 8 to 10 feet away.
- Perform this exercise with a letter placed on a patterned background.

Once VORx1 is mastered, many patients proceed to VORx2. For this task, the patient holds the card. The head and card are moved side-to-side, but in opposite directions for 1 to 2 minutes. This is repeated approximately three times per day. Again, the patient must keep the letter in focus. The additional options above can also make VORx2 more challenging.

KNOWLEDGE CHECKPOINT

VRT is used to assist in vestibular system compensation. Monitoring progress is important to document improvement and to know when modifications should be made in the VRT program. Some examples of monitoring include:

- Questionnaires
  - Dizziness Handicap Inventory (Jacobson & Newman, 1990)
  - Activities-Specific Balance Confidence Scale (Powell & Myers, 1994)
- Balance measures (see Table 7–3)
  - Bedside measures: Romberg, tandem, single-leg stance
  - Posturography: foam (modified Clinical Test of Sensory Integration and Balance—mCTSIB); computerized (sensory organization test—SOT)
  - Gait: gait speed, timed up-and-go (TUG), Dynamic Gait Index (DGI)

Central Vestibulopathy Considerations

VRT has been greatly successful in patients with central vestibulopathy but may take longer to reduce symptoms. Appropriate vestibular system compensation relies on stable central function. In some cases, there are fluctuations in performance, reducing the patient's ability to appropriately compensate.

- Common etiologies at risk for prolonged recovery include vestibular migraine, concussion, and autonomic impairment. It is key that the underlying disorder is appropriately managed as much as possible to facilitate compensation. For example, a patient with dizziness due to vestibular migraine may not see symptom improvement/resolution until the underlying migraine condition is managed or more stable.

Pediatric Rehabilitation Considerations

VRT is increasingly utilized for pediatric patients, especially those with concurrent sensorineural hearing loss, sensory integration disorders, and concussion. There is little understanding of the prevalence of congenital vestibulopathy; however, at least 14% of those with significant hearing loss demonstrate concurrent vestibular impairment (Martens et al., 2022) and may be at risk for significantly delayed gross motor skill development (Dhondt et al., 2022).

- Pediatric evaluations begin with similar bedside evaluations as noted above and rehabilitation planning focuses on the same underlying principles of adaptation, habituation, and substitution. Modifications, such as using toys or games, are needed to ensure that activities are engaging and age appropriate.

Aging and Rehabilitation Considerations

Dizziness and imbalance are more likely with age; 33% of those over 70 years and >50% of those over 80 years of age report difficulties (Jonsson et al., 2004). The most common type of dizziness in older adults is (1) presyncope (i.e., state of lightheadedness, muscle weakness, blurred vision, and feeling faint), followed by (2) medication side effects and (3) vestibular pathology (Meldrum & Hall, 2021).

- BPPV is nearly seven times more common in those >60 years of age than in younger adults (von Brevern et al., 2007). Patients over 60 years of age also demonstrate more severe imbalance and prolonged recovery when compared to younger patients (Scheltinga et al., 2016).

Recommended Readings

Barin, K. (2016). Interpretation and usefulness of caloric testing. In G. P. Jacobson & N. T. Shepard (Eds.), *Balance function assessment and management* (pp. 319–345). Plural Publishing.

Leigh, J., & Zee, D. (2006). *The neurology of eye movements* (4th ed.). Oxford University Press.

McCaslin, D., & Jacobson, G. (2021). Vestibular-evoked myogenic potentials (VEMPs). In G. Jacobson, N. Shepard, K. Barin, R. Burkard, K. Janky, & D. McCaslin (Eds.), *Balance function assessment and management* (pp. 399–438). Plural Publishing.

Welgampola, M., & Colebatch, J. (2005). Characteristics and clinical applications of vestibular-evoked myogenic potentials. *Neurology, 64*, 1682–1688. https://doi.org/10.1212/01.WNL.0000161876.20552.AA

Whitney, S., & Furman, J. (2021). Vestibular rehabilitation. In G. Jacobson, N. Shepard, K. Barin, R. Burkard, K. Janky, & D. McCaslin (Eds.), *Balance function assessment and management* (pp. 549–576). Plural Publishing.

Zuniga, M., Janky, K., Nguyen, K., Welgampola, M., & Carey, J. (2013). Ocular versus cervical VEMPs in the diagnosis of superior semicircular canal dehiscence syndrome. *Otology & Neurotology, 34*, 121–126. https://doi.org/10.1097/MAO.0b013e31827136b0

Zwergal, A., Feil, K., Schniepp, R., & Strupp, M. (2020). Cerebellar dizziness and vertigo: Etiologies, diagnostic assessment, and treatment. *Seminars in Neurology, 40*(1), 87–96. https://doi.org/10.1055/s-0039-3400315

References

Altissimi, G., Colizza, A., Cianfrone, G., de Vincentiis, M., Greco, A., Taurone, S., . . . Ralli, M. (2020). Drugs inducing hearing loss, tinnitus, dizziness, and vertigo: An updated guide. *European Review for Medical and Pharmacological Sciences, 24*(15), 7946–7952. https://doi.org/10.26355/eurrev_202008_22477

ANSI. (2009). *Procedure for testing basic vestibular function* (S3.45-2009). Acoustical Society of America.

Aso, S., Watanabe, Y., & Mizukoshi, K. (1991). A clinical study of electrocochleography in Meniere's disease. *Acta Oto-Laryngologica, 111*(1), 44–52. https://doi.org/10.3109/00016489109137353

Baker, B., Curtis, A., Trueblood, P., & Vangsnes, E. (2013a). Vestibular function and migraine: Comparing those with and without vertigo to a normal population. *Journal of Laryngology & Otology, 127*, 1169–1176. https://doi.org/10.1017/S0022215113002302

Baker, B., Curtis, A., Trueblood, P., & Vangsnes, E. (2013b). Vestibular function and migraine: Pilot study comparing those with and without vertigo.

Journal of Laryngology & Otology, 127, 1056–1064. https://doi.org/10.1017/S0022215113002296

Baloh, R., & Honrubia, V. (2001). *Clinical neurophysiology of the vestibular system* (3rd ed.). F. A. Davis.

Baloh, R., Konrad, H., & Honrubia, V. (1975). Vestibulo-ocular function in patients with cerebellar atrophy. *Neurology, 25*(2), 160–168. https://doi.org/10.1212/wnl.25.2.160

Barber, H.O., & Stockwell, C.W. (1980). *Manual of electronystagmography.* Mosby.

Basura, G., Adams, M., Monfared, A., Schwartz, S., Antonelli, P., Burkard, R., . . . Buchanan, E. (2020). Clinical practice guideline: Ménière disease. *Otolaryngology-Head & Neck Surgery, 162*, S1–S55. https://doi.org/10.1177/0194599820909438

Berrettini, S., Forli, F., Bogazzi, F., Neri, E., Salvatori, L., Casani, A., & Franceschini, S. (2005). Large vestibular aqueduct syndrome: Audiological, radiological, clinical, and genetic features. *American Journal of Otolaryngology, 26*(6), 363–371. https://doi.org/10.1016/j.amjoto.2005.02.013

Berthoz, A. (1996). How does the cerebral cortex process and utilize vestibular signals? In R. Baloh & G. Halmagyi (Eds.), *Disorders of the vestibular system* (pp. 113–126). Oxford University Press.

Bigelow, R., Semenov, V., du Lac, S., Hoffman, H., & Agrawal, Y. (2016). Vestibular vertigo and comorbid cognitive and psychiatric impairment: The 2008 national health interview survey. *Journal of Neurology, Neurosurgery & Psychiatry, 87*(4), 367–372. https://doi.org/10.1136/jnnp-2005-310319

Brandt, T., Schautzer, F., Hamilton, D., Bruning, R., Markowitsch, H., Kalla, R., . . . Strupp, M. (2005). Vestibular loss causes hippocampal atrophy and impaired spatial memory in humans. *Brain, 128*(Pt 11), 2732–2741. https://doi.org/10.1093/brain/awh617

British Society of Audiology (BSA). (2010). *Recommended procedure: The caloric test.*

Carpenter, M., & Sutin, J. (1983). *Human neuroanatomy* (8th ed.). Williams & Wilkins.

Chen, J., Zhang, S., Cui, K., & Liu, C. (2021). Risk factors for benign paroxysmal positional vertigo recurrence: A systematic review and meta-analysis. *Journal of Neurology, 268*(11), 4117–4127. https://doi.org/10.1007/s00415-020-10175-0

Dannenbaum, E., Chilingaryan, G., & Fung, J. (2011). Visual vertigo analogue scale: An assessment questionnaire for visual vertigo. *Journal of Vestibular Research, 21*(3), 153–159. https://doi.org/10.3233/VES-2011-0412

Dhondt, C., Maes, L., Martens, S., Vanaudenaerde, S., Rombaut, L., Sucaet, M., . . . Dhooge, I. (2022). Predicting early vestibular and motor function in congenital cytomegalovirus infection. *Laryngoscope, 133*(7), 1757–1765. https://doi.org/10.1002/lary.30375

Ellis, M., Cordingley, D., Vis, S., Reimer, K., Leiter, J., & Russell, K. (2017). Clinical predictors of vestibulo-ocular dysfunction in pediatric sports-related concussion. *Journal of Neurosurgery: Pediatrics, 19*(1), 38–45. https://doi.org/10.3171/2016.7.PEDS16310

Ewald, J. (1882). *Physiologische Untersuchungen uber das Endorgan des Nervus Octavus.* Bergman.

Fetter, M., & Dichgans, J. (1996). How do the vestibulo-spinal reflexes work? In R. Baloh & G. Halmagyi (Eds.), *Disorders of the vestibular system* (pp. 105–112). Oxford University Press.

Gibson, W. (2010). Hypothetical mechanism for vertigo in Meniere's disease. *Otolaryngology Clinics of North America, 43*(5), 1019–1027.

Goldberg, J., & Férnandez, C. (1971). Physiology of peripheral neurons innervating semicircular canals of the squirrel monkey. I. Resting discharge and response to constant angular accelerations. *Journal of Neurophysiology, 34*, 635–660.

Goldberg, J., Wilson, V., Cullen, K., Angelaki, D., Broussard, D., Buttner-Ennever, J., . . . Minor, L. (2012). *The vestibular system: A sixth sense.* Oxford University Press.

Goulson, A., McPherson, J., & Shepard, N. (2016). Background and introduction to whole-body rotational testing. In G. Jacobson & N. Shepard (Eds.), *Balance function assessment and management* (pp. 347–364). Plural Publishing.

Hain, T., & Helminski, J. (2014). Anatomy and physiology of the normal vestibular system. In S. Herdman & R. Clendaniel (Eds.), *Vestibular rehabilitation* (4th ed., pp. 2–19). F. A. Davis.

Honrubia, V., & Hoffman, L. (1997). Practical anatomy and physiology of the vestibular system. In G. Jacobson, C. Newman, & J. Kartush (Eds.), *Handbook of balance function testing* (pp. 9–52). Delmar Cengage Learning.

International Headache Society (IHS). (2018). The international classification of headache disorders (3rd ed.). *Cephalalgia, 38*(1), 1–211.

Jacobson, G., Calder, J., Shepard, V., Rupp, K., & Newman, C. (1995). Reappraisal of the monothermal warm caloric screening test. *Annals of Otology, Rhinology, and Laryngology, 104*(12), 942–945.

Jacobson, G., & Newman, C. (1990). The development of the dizziness handicap inventory. *Archives of Otolaryngology Head & Neck Surgery, 116,* 424–427.

Jacobson, G., Piker, E., Hatton, K., Watford, K., Trone, T., McCaslin, D., . . . Roberts, R. (2019). Development and preliminary findings of the dizziness symptom profile. *Ear and Hearing, 40*(3), 568–576.

Jeong, S., Chen, T., Timor, T., Busch, A., Meyer, T., Nguyen, S., & Rizk, H. (2022). Prevalence of polypharmacy in patients with vestibular and balance complaints. *Ear and Hearing, 44*(3), 506–517. https://doi.org/10.1097/AUD.000000000000 1292

Jonsson, R., Sixt, E., Landahl, S., & Rosenhall, U. (2004). Prevalence of dizziness and vertigo in an urban elderly population. *Journal of Vestibular Research, 14*(1), 47–52.

Jung, J., Suh, M., & Kim, S. (2017). Discrepancies between video head impulse and caloric tests in patients with enlarged vestibular aqueduct. *Laryngoscope, 127*(4), 921–926.

Kileny, P., & McCaslin, D. (2021). Electrocochleography (ECochG). In G. Jacobson, N. Shepard, K. Barin, R. Burkard, K. Janky, & D. McCaslin (Eds.), *Balance function assessment and management* (3rd ed.). Plural Publishing.

Kroenke, K., Spitzer, R., & Williams, K. (2001). The PHQ-9: Validity of a brief depression severity measure. *Journal of General Internal Medicine, 16*(9), 606–613.

Lundberg, Y., Zhao, X., & Yamoah, E. (2006). Assembly of the otoconia complex to the macular sensory epithelium of the vestibule. *Brain Research, 1091*(1), 47–57.

Lysakowski, A., McCrea, R., & Tomlinson, R. (Eds.). (1998). *Anatomy of vestibular end organs and neural pathways* (3rd ed.). Mosby.

Lysakowski, A., Minor, L., Fernandez, C., & Goldberg, J. (1995). Physiological identification of morphologically distinct afferent classes innervating the cristae ampullares of the squirrel monkey. *Journal of Neurophysiology, 73,* 1270–1281.

Martens, S., Dhooge, I., Dhondt, C., Vanaudenaerde, S., Sucaet, M., Van Hoecke, H., . . . Maes, L. (2022). Three years of vestibular infant screening in infants with sensorineural hearing loss. *Pediatrics, 150*(1), e2021055340.

Masnoon, N., Shakib, S., Kalisch-Ellett, L., & Caughey, G. (2017). What is polypharmacy? A systematic review of definitions. *BMC Geriatrics, 17*(1), 1–10.

McCaslin, D., Flowler, A., & Jacobson, G. (2014). Amplitude normalization reduces cervical vestibular evoked myogenic potential (cVEMP) amplitude asymmetries in normal subjects: Proof of concept. *Journal of the American Academy of Audiology, 36*(3), 268–277.

McCaslin, D., & Jacobson, G. (2021). Vestibular-evoked myogenic potentials (VEMPs). In G. Jacobson, N. Shepard, K. Barin, R. Burkard, K. Janky, & D. McCaslin (Eds.), *Balance function assessment and management* (3rd ed., pp. 399–438). Plural Publishing.

McCaslin, D., Jacobson, G., Hatton, K., Fowler, A., & DeLong, A. (2013). The effects of amplitude normalization and EMG targets on cVEMP interaural amplitude asymmetry. *Ear and Hearing, 34*(4), 482–490.

Meldrum, D., & Hall, C. (2021). The aging vestibular system: Implications for rehabilitation. In G. Jacobson, N. Shepard, K. Barin, R. Burkard, K. Janky, & D. McCaslin (Eds.), *Balance function assessment and management* (3rd ed., pp. 577–596). Plural Publishing.

Naito, Y., Newman, A., Lee, W., Beykirch, K., & Honrubia, V. (1995). Projections of the individual vestibular end-organs in the brain stem of the squirrel monkey. *Hearing Research, 87,* 141–155.

Pansky, B., Allen, D., & Budd, G. (1988). *Review of neuroscience* (2nd ed.). Macmillan.

Piker, E., Jacobson, G., McCaslin, D., & Hood, L. (2011). Normal characteristics of the ocular vestibular evoked myogenic potential. *Journal of the American Academy of Audiology, 22,* 222–230.

Powell, L., & Myers, A. (1994). The activities-specific balance confidence (ABC) scale. *Journals of Gerontology. Series A, Biological Sciences and Medical Sciences, 50A*(1), M28–M34.

Rajagopalan, A., Jinu, K., Sailesh, K., Mishra, S., Reddy, U., & Mukkadan, J. (2017). Understanding the links between vestibular and limbic systems regulating emotions. *Journal of Natural Science, Biology and Medicine, 8*(1), 11–15.

Rosengren, S., Colebatch, J., Straumann, D., & Weber, P. (2013). Why do oVEMPs become larger when you look up? Explaining the effect of gaze elevation on the ocular vestibular evoked myogenic potential. *Clinical Neurophysiology, 124,* 785–791.

Sandhu, J., George, S., & Rea, P. (2013). The effect of electrode positioning on the ocular vestibular evoked myogenic potential to air-conducted sound. *Clinical Neurophysiology, 124*(6), 1232–1236.

Sarna, B., Abouzari, M., Merna, C., Jamshidi, S., Saber, T., & Djalilian, H. (2020). Perilymphatic fistula: A review of classification, etiology, diagnosis, and treatment. *Frontiers in Neurology, 11,* 1046.

Scheltinga, A., Honegger, F., Timmermans, D., & Allum, J. (2016). The effect of age on improvements in vestibulo-ocular reflexes and balance control after acute unilateral peripheral vestibular loss. *Frontiers in Neurology, 7,* 18.

Schubert, M., & Shepard, N. (2016). Practical anatomy and physiology of the vestibular system. In G. Jacobson & N. Shepard (Eds.), *Balance function assessment and management* (2nd ed., pp. 1–16). Plural Publishing.

Semenov, V., Bigelow, R., Xue, Q., du Lac, S., & Agrawal, Y. (2016). Association between vestibular and cognitive function in U.S. adults: Data from the national health and nutrition examination study. *Journal of Gerontology Series A, Biological Sciences and Medical Sciences, 71*(2), 243–250.

Smith, C., Lowry, O., & Wu, M. (1965). The electrolytes of the labyrinthine fluids. *Laryngoscope, 64,* 141–153.

Spitzer, R., Kroenke, K., Williams, J., & Lowe, B. (2006). A brief measure for assessing generalized anxiety disorder: The GAD-7. *Archives of Internal Medicine, 166*(10), 1092–1097.

Staab, J., Eckhardt-Henn, A., Horii, A., Jacob, R., Strupp, M., Brandt, T., & Bronstein, A. (2017). Diagnostic criteria for persistent postural-perceptual dizziness (PPPD): Consensus document of the committee for the classification of vestibular disorders of the Barany Society. *Journal of Vestibular Research, 27*(4), 191–208.

Stockwell, C., & Bojrab, D. (1997). Background and technique of rotational testing. In G. Jacobson, C. Newman, & J. Kartush (Eds.), *Handbook of balance function testing* (pp. 249–258). Singular Publishing.

Szmulewicz, D., Roberts, L., McLean, C., MacDougall, H., Halmagyi, G., & Storey, E. (2016). Proposed diagnostic criteria for cerebellar ataxia with neurop-

athy and vestibular areflexia syndrome (CANVAS). *Neurology Clinical Practice, 6*(1), PMC4753833.

Uchino, Y., Hirai, N., & Suzuki, S. (1982). Branching pattern and properties of vertical- and horizontal-related excitatory vestibuloocular neurons in the cat. *Journal of Neurophysiology, 48,* 891–903.

von Brevern, M., Radtke, A., Lezius, F., Feldmann, M., Ziese, T., Lempert, T., & Neuhauser, H. (2007). Epidemiology of benign paroxysmal positional vertigo: A population-based study. *Journal of Neurology, Neurosurgery & Psychiatry, 78*(7), 710–715.

Watson, C. (1991). *Basic human neuroanatomy. An introductory atlas* (4th ed.). Little, Brown.

Welgampola, M., & Colebatch, J. (2005). Characteristics and clinical applications of vestibular-evoked myogenic potentials. *Neurology, 64,* 1682–1688.

Whitney, S., & Furman, J. (2021). Vestibular rehabilitation. In G. Jacobson, N. Shepard, K. Barin, R. Burkard, K. Janky, & D. McCaslin (Eds.), *Balance function assessment and management* (3rd ed., pp. 549–576). Plural Publishing.

Yates, B., Bolton, P., & Macefield, V. (2014). Vestibulo-sympathetic responses. *Comprehensive Physiology, 4*(2), 851–887.

Zaleski, A., Bogle, J., Starling, A., Zapala, D., Davis, L., Wester, M., & Cevette, M. (2015). Vestibular evoked myogenic potentials in patients with vestibular migraine. *Otology & Neurotology, 36,* 295–302.

Zhou, G., & Brodsky, J. (2015). Objective vestibular testing of children with dizziness and balance complaints following sports-related concussions. *Otolaryngology Head & Neck Surgery, 152*(6), 1133–1139.

Zhou, Y., Wu, Y., Cong, N., Yu, J., Gu, J., Wang, J., & Chi, F. (2017). Contrasting results of tests of peripheral vestibular function in patients with bilateral large vestibular aqueduct syndrome. *Clinical Neurophysiology, 128*(8), 1513–1518.

Zigmond, A., & Snaith, R. (1983). The hospital anxiety and depression scale. *Acta Psychiatrica Scandinavica, 67*(6), 361–370.

Zuniga, M., Janky, K., Nguyen, K., Welgampola, M., & Carey, J. (2013). Ocular versus cervical VEMPs in the diagnosis of superior semicircular canal dehiscence syndrome. *Otology & Neurotology, 34,* 121–126.

Zwergal, A., Feil, K., Schniepp, R., & Strupp, M. (2020). Cerebellar dizziness and vertigo: Etiologies, diagnostic assessment, and treatment. *Seminars in Neurology, 40*(1), 87–96.

Practice Questions

Use the passage below to answer Questions 1–4.

> The patient is a 55-year-old male reporting sudden onset of left ear hearing loss, tinnitus, and vertigo 2 weeks ago. He reports that he experienced rotational vertigo for a few hours, which gradually reduced to a consistent feeling of unsteadiness. The patient reports no change in hearing and tinnitus in his left ear. VNG testing demonstrates 7°/second right-beating nystagmus in gaze center and gaze right with vision denied. Remaining oculomotor testing is within normal limits. Dix-Hallpike testing is negative bilaterally. Static positional testing demonstrates 7° second geotropic nystagmus in head right and head left positions. Caloric responses are as follows: right warm = right beating, 15°/second; right cool = left beating, 12°/second; left warm = left beating, 4°/second; left warm = right beating, 3°/second. Fixation suppression is appropriate.

1. What disorder do you suspect with this clinical presentation?
   a. Vestibular neuritis
   b. Superior semicircular canal dehiscence syndrome
   c. Benign paroxysmal positional vertigo
   d. Labyrinthitis

Explanation: While vestibular neuritis, benign paroxysmal positional vertigo, and labyrinthitis present with acute onset vertigo, only labyrinthitis presents with concurrent unilateral hearing loss. Therefore, d is the correct answer.

2. What is the canal paresis for the above case?
   a. 59%
   b. 6%
   c. 100%
   d. 74%

Explanation: Use Jongkees's formula to calculate the canal paresis. Total eye speed is 27°/second for the right ear and 7°/second for the left ear. Canal paresis is calculated as: [(27 − 7)/(27 + 7)]. Therefore, canal paresis is (a) 59%.

3. What degree of nystagmus is noted in gaze testing?
   a. First degree
   b. Second degree
   c. Third degree
   d. Fourth degree

Explanation: Significant gaze-evoked nystagmus is noted in gaze center and gaze right. Since nystagmus is noted in two conditions, it is considered (b) second-degree nystagmus.

4. You complete sinusoidal harmonic acceleration testing. What are your expected results?
   a. Normal gain, phase, asymmetry
   b. Normal gain, low-frequency phase lead, normal asymmetry
   c. Reduced gain, low-frequency phase lead, significant asymmetry
   d. Reduced gain, normal phase, normal asymmetry

Explanation: Acute vestibulopathy most often presents with reduced gain, low-frequency phase lead, and significant asymmetry. Therefore, c is the correct answer.

5. VEMP responses are expected to be abnormal in cases of SSCD. What is NOT an expected abnormality?
   a. Absent response in the affected ear
   b. Enhance amplitude in the affected ear
   c. Present response at 4 kHz
   d. Reduced threshold in the affected ear

Explanation: SSCD provides an unexpected "third window" into the inner ear, enhancing sound pressure conduction. VEMP responses are expected to demonstrate enhanced amplitude, reduced threshold, and present responses at unexpected frequencies. Therefore, a is the correct answer.

6. What is an expected characteristic of peripheral nystagmus?
   a. Down-beating nystagmus noted in gaze center
   b. Nystagmus follows Ewald's law
   c. Nystagmus is enhanced with fixation
   d. Nystagmus changes direction in eccentric gaze

Explanation: Peripheral nystagmus follows specific expectations outlined by (b) Ewald's law. Vertical nystagmus, nystagmus that enhances with fixation, and nystagmus that changes direction are characteristics of central nystagmus.

7. What stimulus frequency is most commonly used for VEMP testing?
   a. 125 Hz
   b. 250 Hz
   c. 500 Hz
   d. 750 Hz

Explanation: VEMP responses are influenced by the frequency tuning characteristics of the otolith organs. Responses are most reliably recorded using (c) 500 Hz stimuli.

8. In a patient with acute vestibulopathy, what SOT conditions are expected to be abnormal?

     a. Conditions 1–6

     b. Conditions 3, 6

     c. Condition 5

     d. Conditions 4–6

Explanation: SOT condition patterns relate to underlying balance dysfunction. An acute vestibulopathy most often presents with (c) abnormal 5. Balance performance in this condition relies on appropriate vestibular system performance.

9. Which aspect of vestibular rehabilitation is used for a patient with bilateral vestibular areflexia?

     a. Habituation

     b. Substitution

     c. Adaptation

     d. Rehabilitation

Explanation: A patient with bilateral vestibular areflexia does not have adequate VOR performance. Therefore, the patient must use (b) substitution for maintaining appropriate balance performance.

10. Which measure of VOR performance is most appropriate for evaluating a 4-month-old child?

     a. vHIT

     b. oVEMP

     c. SHA

     d. Caloric testing

Explanation: The most effective method for evaluating children <6 months of age is (a) vHIT. For these young children, vHIT is usually done with a remote camera system. Due to tolerance, the remaining options are not typically attempted until 6 months for SHA, 3 years for oVEMP, and 6 years for caloric testing.

Section IV

Prevention, Identification, and Treatment

Chapter 8

Screening and Hearing Conservation

Leigh Ann Reel

Introduction

Audiologists provide services designed to prevent, identify, diagnose, and treat hearing, balance, and related disorders in children and adults. Screening measures can be useful in preventing and identifying hearing loss, as well as balance, speech-language, and cognitive disorders. By identifying at-risk individuals, appropriate steps can be taken to prevent further decline and/or improve function in a particular area. For hearing loss, prevention primarily focuses on using hearing conservation efforts to prevent noise-induced hearing loss (NIHL). This chapter will review important topics related to screening for hearing and balance disorders and preventing NIHL through hearing conservation services for children and adults. Concepts relevant to evaluating speech and language and screening for cognitive disorders are covered in Chapter 4 and Chapter 5, respectively.

Screening Measures for Auditory and Balance Disorders

Undetected hearing and balance disorders can have a negative impact on many areas of life for children and adults. Screening measures can identify individuals who are at risk and may need more comprehensive testing, preventative measures, and/or intervention. As a result, appropriate screening may lead to better outcomes and improved quality of life. This section will focus on hearing and balance screening measures for children and adults.

Newborn Hearing Screening

Hearing screening for children includes newborn hearing screening (NBHS), early childhood screening, and school-age screening. Early Hearing Detection and Intervention (EHDI) guidelines (American Speech-Language-Hearing Association [ASHA], n.d.-d) include completing the NBHS by 1 month of age, diagnosis of any hearing loss by 3 months of age, hearing aid selection and fitting within 1 month of confirmation of hearing loss, and initiation of early intervention services by 6 months of age. Otoacoustic emissions (OAEs) and/or auditory brainstem response (ABR) testing may be used for NBHS.

- ABR: Screening with ABR can be conducted using nonautomated (i.e., diagnostic) or automated ABR (i.e., AABR) equipment. AABR equipment includes internal stopping rule criteria based on comparison to a template or statistical algorithms. Click stimuli are presented at 35 dB nHL at a rate of 30 to 37 clicks/second. Screening with ABR is less sensitive to outer ear debris and allows for detection of both neural and cochlear hearing losses. A drawback of only screening with the ABR is that it often misses minimal to mild hearing losses. The Joint Committee on Infant Hearing (JCIH, 2007) recommends ABR screening for newborns who stay more than 5 days in the NICU due to increased risk of neural hearing loss/auditory neuropathy spectrum disorder (ANSD).

- OAE: In well-baby nurseries, NBHS can also be performed using transient-evoked (TEOAE) or distortion product (DPOAE) otoacoustic emissions. Typically, results are considered to be passing when OAEs are present at 2000, 3000, and 4000 Hz at signal-to-noise ratios (SNRs) of at least 6 dB. OAEs are absent in cases of outer or middle ear problems, resulting in a higher false-positive rate than ABR due to the incidence of outer ear debris and/or middle ear fluid in newborns. OAEs are also not sensitive to disorders central to the outer hair cells (e.g., ANSD). As a result, screening with OAEs is only recommended for newborns in well-baby nurseries.

- Two-tier screening: Some locations use a combination of OAE and ABR screening. In two-tier screening, an OAE screening is completed in both ears first. If the OAE screening is not passed in both ears, an ABR screening is performed in the same session. If the newborn does not pass the ABR screening in one or both ears, he or she is referred for outpatient diagnostic testing.

Early Childhood and School-Age Hearing Screening

Failure to detect and appropriately manage hearing loss in children can lead to deficits in speech-language, academic, psychosocial, and emotional development. This can be true for even a minimal degree of hearing loss (thresholds of 15–25 dB HL). Screening all children will help identify any who failed the NBHS but were lost to follow-up or those with hearing loss that developed after birth (ASHA, n.d.-b).

- Early childhood: In early childhood, this includes ongoing hearing screening for children after the newborn period, required screening of hearing, vision, and overall development within 45 days of entering into Early Head Start and Head Start programs, monitoring children identified as high-risk of delayed-onset hearing loss by JCIH (2007) criteria, screening when a parent/caregiver/teacher/service provider raises concerns, and screening as part of any comprehensive speech-language evaluation.

- School-age: For school-age children, screening should be performed when a child first enters a school or transfers to a new school and every year in Grades K–3, 7, and 11 (ASHA, n.d.-b). In addition, hearing screening should be included as part of monitoring for children who are homeschooled or in private school. Hearing screening for school-age children should also be performed when a parent/caregiver/teacher/service provider raises concerns and should be included as part of any comprehensive speech-language evaluation.

- Screening protocols
  - Otoscopy/visual inspection: Otoscopy/visual inspection of the outer ear allows for visualization of the pinna, external auditory canal, and tympanic membrane. Any redness, drainage, foreign bodies, cerumen, or other abnormalities should be noted. Otoscopic

results are important in interpreting failed hearing screening results and determining the need for medical referral.

☐ Pure-tone screening: Screening with pure tones should be performed at 1000, 2000, and 4000 Hz in each ear at 20 dB HL. Programs should consider including 6000 and 8000 Hz to help identify early NIHL in children. Pure-tone hearing screening results are considered to be passing when responses are present at each frequency in each ear. Rooms used for school hearing screenings should be free of distractions. If a child has thresholds at 0 dB HL, the allowable ambient noise levels would be: 1000 Hz = 50 dB SPL, 2000 Hz = 58 dB SPL, and 4000 Hz = 76 dB SPL (ANSI 2003, as cited in ASHA, n.d.-b). If a sound level meter (SLM) with octave band filters is not available, a biologic check can be performed in which a person with known normal hearing is tested to ensure that thresholds can be obtained at least 10 dB below the screening level at all frequencies.

☐ OAE screening: Use of OAEs may be appropriate for children who cannot be tested with pure-tone screening. It can also be helpful in identifying early NIHL. However, there are currently no ANSI standards for the screening environment when OAEs are used.

☐ Tympanometry: Tympanometry can be added to a pure-tone or OAE screening protocol to measure movement of the tympanic membrane. Tympanometric results are useful in identifying conditions that require medical referral, such as Eustachian tube dysfunction, otitis media, perforation of the tympanic membrane, or other middle ear disorders.

■ Referral and rescreening: When the hearing screening is failed, a rescreen should be performed within 6 to 8 weeks based on the expected timeline for spontaneous recovery from middle ear effusion. Some schools may choose a timeframe of 2 to 4 weeks, which may result in over referral of children with resolving middle ear effusion.

Adult Hearing Screening

Without appropriate treatment, hearing loss in adults can result in higher risk of depression, anxiety, and dementia (e.g., Lin et al., 2011). Routine hearing screenings may help reduce the negative impact of hearing loss by reducing the likelihood of undiagnosed and untreated hearing loss. Adult hearing screenings can be performed at primary care visits, residential facilities, speech-language pathology visits, and health fairs, as well as through occupational hearing screening programs and via remote methods (e.g., phone, online) (ASHA, n.d.-a). Adult hearing screening consists of screening for disorder (health condition), impairment (body structure and function), and disability (activities and participation).

■ Screening for disorder is accomplished through case history and otoscopy.

■ Screening for impairment involves pure-tone screening. ASHA (n.d.-a) recommends screening at 1000, 2000, and 4000 Hz in each ear at 25 dB HL. In order to pass, responses must be present at each frequency in each ear. The screening environment should be free of distractions. Noise levels can exceed recommended maximum permissible ambient noise levels (MPANLs) for audiometric test rooms but must be low enough to allow accurate screening. If an SLM with octave band filters is not available, a biologic check can be performed in which a person with known normal hearingis tested to ensure that thresholds can be obtained at least 10 dB below the screening level at all frequencies.

■ Screening for disability can be performed using self-report questionnaires, such as the Hearing Handicap Inventory for the Elderly–Screening Version (HHIE-S; Ventry & Weinstein, 1983); the Speech, Spatial and Qualities of Hearing Scale (SSQ; Gatehouse & Noble, 2004);

Self-Assessment of Communication (SAC; Schow & Nerbonne, 1982); and Significant Other Assessment of Communication (SOAC; Schow & Nerbonne, 1982).

Vestibular Screening

Vestibular screening can help identify individuals with dizziness/imbalance symptoms who need more in-depth diagnostic testing or evaluation by a physician who specializes in vestibular disorders. Screening for vestibular disorders can include case history, questionnaires, and functional screenings.

- Case history questions should gather information on the person's symptoms and any factors that point to a possible cause of the symptoms. Symptoms of balance problems may include dizziness, vertigo (sensation of the room spinning), lightheadedness, motion sickness, unsteadiness, falling, trouble walking, and blurry vision (ASHA, n.d.-c). It is important to note the duration, frequency, onset, and pattern of the symptoms, as well as any aggravating (e.g., motion, position, diet) and alleviating factors. Causes of dizziness/imbalance problems include inner ear disorders, sudden hearing loss, tumors on the auditory nerve, viruses/infections, medications, injury to the ear or vestibular system, or cochlear implant placement.

- Questionnaires may be used to screen for vestibular problems in children and adults.
  - Dizziness Handicap Inventory for Children (DHI-C): The DHI-C consists of 25 items typically completed by the child's caregiver (McCaslin et al., 2015). The items are essentially the same as the adult version of the questionnaire (see below).
  - Pediatric Vestibular System Questionnaire (PVSQ): The PVSQ consists of 10 items that identify and quantify the severity of the child's vestibular symptoms (Pavlou et al., 2016). There is also an 11th item that asks if the child's symptoms prevent participation in activities.
  - Pediatric Visually Induced Dizziness Questionnaire (PVID): The PVID includes 11 items that quantify the severity of visually induced dizziness (e.g., crowds, scrolling computer screens) (Pavlou et al., 2017).
  - Dizziness Handicap Inventory (DHI): Validated in adults, the DHI consists of 25 items divided into three subscales: emotional, functional, and physical (Jacobson & Newman, 1990).
  - The Activities-Specific Balance Confidence (ABC) Scale: The ABC scale consists of 16 items validated for adults 65 years and older (Powell & Myers, 1995). The purpose is to identify senior citizens at risk of falling.

- Functional screenings can also provide information helpful in determining when a full vestibular evaluation should be performed. Examples include:
  - Clinical Test of Sensory Integration of Balance (CTSIB): The CTSIB consists of six conditions (Shumway-Cook & Horak, 1986). The patient stands on a flat firm surface and on a compliant foam surface in three visual conditions: eyes open, eyes closed, and while wearing a sensory conflict dome with no shoes and the feet together. Results are used to evaluate the patient's use of visual, vestibular, and proprioceptive sensory information for posture.
  - Timed "Up and Go" (TUG) Test: The TUG was developed for use with elderly adults. The patient is asked to get up from a chair, walk for 3 minutes, turn around, walk back to the

chair, and sit down (Podsiadlo & Richardson, 1991). Research has shown the TUG to be useful in assessing fall risk in individuals with vestibular disorders.

☐ 5 Times Sit to Stand Test (FTSST): The FTSST measures how long it takes a patient to move from sitting to standing five times in a row. Results can be helpful in assessing postural control, risk of falling, lower-extremity strength, proprioception, and disability (Whitney et al., 2005).

☐ Beside Dynamic Visual Acuity (DVA) Test: The bedside DVA test assesses how well the retina can focus on an object while the head is moving (i.e., the vestibulo-ocular reflex) (Barber, 1984). Patients with vestibular hypofunction (unilateral or bilateral) will experience oscillopsia (i.e., blurring or bouncing of visual objects with movement of the head). As a bedside screening, the test is performed with the patient using their best-corrected vision. An Early Treatment Diabetic Retinopathy Study (ETDRS) eye chart is placed at a specific distance, and the examiner moves the patient's head back and forth (less than 20 degrees) at a frequency of 2 Hz while the patient reads the lines on the chart.

☐ Beside Head Impulse Test (HIT): The beside HIT uses the oculocephalic response (i.e., doll's eye reflex) to screen for unilateral and bilateral peripheral vestibular disorders (Halmagyi & Curthoys, 1988). It is performed by having the examiner gently grasp the patient's head, tilt it forward 30 degrees (i.e., to position the lateral semicircular canal coplanar to the ground), and passively turn the head 10 degrees from center. The patient is asked to fixate on the examiner's nose. The examiner then rapidly moves the patient's head 15 to 20 degrees to midline. The test is repeated on the other side. If peripheral vestibular function is normal, the rapid head turn to each side will elicit a compensatory eye movement that is close to 180 degrees out-of-phase from the movement of the head. Left side peripheral vestibular damage will result in a catchup saccade to the right when the head is rapidly turned to the left, with normal results when the head is turned to the right. This pattern of results will be reversed when there is damage to the peripheral vestibular system on the right side.

☐ Single-Leg Standing: In single-leg standing, the patient is asked to stand on one leg. The other leg cannot touch the weightbearing leg (e.g., Horak et al., 1992). The patient is asked to not move the weightbearing leg or the arms from the start position. The amount of time the patient can maintain this position is timed, and changes are tracked over the course of rehabilitation.

Hearing Conservation

Hearing conservation is an essential "preventive medicine service provided by all audiologists, regardless of their work setting" (Beamer, 2008, para. 1). Audiologists can provide a variety of different hearing conservation services, including:

- Measuring noise levels
- Assessing the risk of developing NIHL
- Providing and supervising audiometric monitoring
- Reviewing problem audiograms to determine need for further evaluation or management

- Recognizing administrative and engineering controls that can reduce noise exposure
- Recommending and fitting hearing protection devices (HPDs)
- Evaluating the effectiveness of HPDs
- Providing education to help children and adults protect their hearing
- Monitoring hearing conservation programs to ensure compliance with occupational noise regulations
- Advocating for effective hearing loss prevention

Through these services, audiologists work to prevent NIHL in children and adults.

Overview of NIHL

NIHL develops when the sensitive structures of the inner ear are damaged by exposure to high noise levels for extended periods of time or to intense impulsive sounds. Although exposure to noise in the workplace is a common cause of NIHL, many nonoccupational activities can also produce noise levels high enough to damage hearing. As a result, NIHL is seen in people of all different ages and backgrounds.

Effects of Noise Exposure

Exposure to loud noise can damage the auditory system and cause other nonauditory problems. Some of these problems may appear during or immediately after the noise exposure, while others can develop slowly over time with repeated exposure to loud noise. In some cases, the symptoms improve over time after the noise exposure ceases. However, in other cases, the damage is permanent.

- Temporary threshold shift (TTS): Exposure to high noise levels can cause temporary metabolic changes to the cochlea, including swelling of the hair cells and auditory nerve terminals. As a result, a listener may experience decreased hearing, tinnitus, perception of speech sounding dull or muffled, and aural fullness. These symptoms typically last less than 1 hour to several hours or days. In some cases, the symptoms may completely resolve (indicating complete recovery), but in other cases, there may be effects that persist long term (indicating incomplete recovery).
- Permanent threshold shift (PTS): When the effects of a TTS do not completely resolve, the effect on hearing is considered to be a PTS (i.e., permanent NIHL). A PTS occurs when noise exposure causes the hair cells to swell to the point of rupturing. Because human hair cells do not regenerate, the damaged hair cells are replaced by scar tissue. The stereocilia on the tops of the hair cells can become fused together, thus interfering with the hair cell transduction process. Over time, the auditory nerve terminals connected to the damaged hair cells will degenerate. Although NIHL can be prevented by avoiding exposure to loud noise or wearing effective hearing protection, there is no treatment to reverse the damage once it occurs.
  - □ The classic presentation of a PTS includes permanent bilateral sensorineural hearing loss, with a "noise notch" in the high frequencies. In adults, a noise notch presents as decreased hearing sensitivity at 3000, 4000, or 6000 Hz, with better hearing at lower and higher frequencies. In children, the noise notch typically occurs at 6000 Hz (Niskar et al., 2001). NIHL is often symmetrical between ears for most types of industrial noise exposure,

whereas musicians and hunters/shooters typically have asymmetrical hearing loss (i.e., primarily for those who shoot rifles and shotguns).

☐ In addition to hearing loss, those with permanent NIHL also often experience tinnitus and hyperacusis.

■ Acoustic trauma: Exposure to impulse noise greater than 140 dB SPL can cause instant, permanent hearing damage called acoustic trauma. At this level, the pressure wave traveling through the auditory system is so intense that it can cause mechanical damage. The tympanic membrane may rupture. The ossicles can disarticulate, and the delicate structures of the cochlea may be torn. The resulting hearing loss is typically severe to profound and permanent.

■ Nonauditory effects: Exposure to loud noise can also cause various nonauditory problems, such as increased stress, anxiety, depression, distractibility, and annoyance, as well as increased risk of high blood pressure and heart disease (Basner et al., 2014; Dzhambov & Dimitrova, 2016). Communicating in high-noise environments can also cause vocal strain due to the need to talk over the noise. Working in a high-noise environment can decrease job performance, especially when the task is complicated or involves multitasking. As a result, a higher incidence of accidents is seen in high-noise work environments (e.g., Neitzel et al., 2017; Picard et al., 2008).

 AUDIOLOGY NUGGET

Noise exposure resulting in a TTS can cause cochlear synaptopathy, which is permanent damage to the synapses between the inner hair cells of the cochlea and the auditory nerve fibers (e.g., Kujawa & Liberman, 2009). Some studies have found a significant correlation between cochlear synaptopathy (indirectly measured by evoked auditory potentials) and hearing in noise performance in patients with behavioral hearing thresholds that fall within normal limits for 250 to 8000 Hz on the pure-tone audiogram (e.g., Grant et al., 2020). Difficulty understanding speech in background noise when audiometric thresholds are clinically normal has been termed "hidden hearing loss." Cochlear synaptopathy following noise exposure has been documented in various animal species, with some species showing spontaneous synaptic recovery (Kauer et al., 2019) while others do not (Kujawa & Liberman, 2009; Liu et al., 2012). However, much remains unknown about cochlear synaptopathy in humans because human studies must rely on indirect electrophysiological measures due to inability to directly measure cochlear synaptopathy in vivo (i.e., within a living organism). Human studies have reported inconsistent results, with some finding evidence of permanent cochlear synaptopathy in listeners with a history of noise exposure and clinically normal audiometric thresholds (Bramhall et al., 2017) and others finding no synaptic deficits in similar groups of adults (Grinn & Le Prell, 2022).

Causes of NIHL

As a general rule, exposure to any noise 85 dBA or greater has the potential to damage hearing, depending on the length of exposure. For occupational noise exposure, mining, manufacturing, construction, farming, military, law enforcement, and forestry are associated with the highest noise levels and highest prevalence of NIHL (Masterson et al., 2013). Power tools, guns, and music are among the most common sources of hazardous nonoccupational noise exposure. In most cases, occupational and nonoccupational noise sources cause gradual onset of NIHL, with repeated TTSs that eventually progress to permanent NIHL. However, immediate permanent NIHL is possible with exposure to a single loud impulse noise, such as a gunshot. Bomb blasts, jet engines, firecrackers detonating near the ear, and airbag deployment can also generate noise levels above 140 dB SPL, thus creating the potential for acoustic trauma.

Prevalence of NIHL

NIHL can begin at any age and affects millions of children and adults in the United States. It is ranked as the second most common cause of sensorineural hearing loss, with presbycusis being the most common cause (Rabinowitz, 2000). Approximately 24% of adults in the United States have audiometric notches, but more than 50% of adults with NIHL do not have noisy jobs (Carroll et al., 2017). Among the general population, an estimated 12.5% of children 6 to 19 years of age have NIHL (Niskar et al., 2001). Older children (12–19 years) have a higher prevalence at 17.1%. A significantly higher prevalence has been reported among rural children, with 22.5% of children 6 to 19 years of age and 26.5% of children 12 to 19 years of age having NIHL (Renick et al., 2009). Together, these findings highlight the need for hearing conservation efforts, not only for workers in high-noise job settings but also for children and adults exposed to nonoccupational noise.

Industrial Audiology

Most recommendations regarding safe versus hazardous noise exposures, when hearing protection should be worn, and when a hearing conservation program should be implemented come from consensus noise standards developed for occupational safety based on basic and applied research. These recommendations are often also applied to nonoccupational noise exposure due to the lack of specific recommendations related to prevention of nonoccupational NIHL.

OSHA Noise Regulation/Standard

The Occupational Safety and Health Administration (OSHA) Noise Regulation 29 CFR 1910.95 (last revised in 1983) includes OSHA's requirements for hearing conservation programs. OSHA (2022, December 6) covers most, but not all, private-sector workers and employers. It is worth noting that although some sources (e.g., Bruce et al., 2014) differentiate between a "standard" and a "regulation, OSHA (2023, May 24) uses the terms interchangeably, defining both as "a regulatory requirement established and published by the agency to serve as criteria for measuring whether employers are in compliance with the OSH Act laws" ("What Is a Standard/Regulation?" section).

- Purpose: OSHA creates and enforces the federal noise regulation/standard and issues citations when there are violations (Bruce et al., 2014). OSHA takes into consideration the economic effects of the noise regulations/standards issued.

- Exchange rate: Also known as the time-intensity tradeoff or doubling rate, the exchange rate refers to the relationship between noise levels and their allowable exposure times. Stated differently, the allowed exposure time is cut in half for every increase in exposure level of

5 dBA or doubled for every decrease in exposure level of 5 dBA. OSHA (1983) uses a 5-dB exchange rate. Therefore, exposure to 90 dBA for 8 hours is expected to cause the same amount of auditory damage as exposure to 85 dBA for 16 hours or to 95 dBA for 4 hours.

- Action level (AL): Workers must be enrolled in a hearing conservation program, and HPDs must be made available when noise exposure is an 8-hour time-weighted average (TWA) of 85 dBA or greater (or the equivalent). A TWA combines all of the sound levels measured during a work shift into one integrated overall exposure value.

- Permissible exposure level (PEL): Workers exposed to an 8-hour TWA of 90 dBA or greater (or the equivalent) must be enrolled in a hearing conservation program, and feasible administrative or engineering controls must be used. If these controls fail to reduce noise exposure to the PEL or less, HPDs must be worn.

NIOSH Criteria for a Recommended Standard

The National Institute for Occupational Safety and Health (NIOSH) makes noise standard recommendations (last revised in 1998) to protect workers from developing occupational NIHL.

- Purpose: NIOSH conducts research and makes recommendations for best practice based on current research, without factoring in economic considerations (Themann et al., 2013). NIOSH recommendations for noise exposure and hearing conservation are generally more conservative (i.e., offer greater protection) than the OSHA standard.

- Exchange rate: NIOSH (1998) uses a 3-dB exchange rate. As such, every 3-dB increase in the noise exposure level results in a halving of the allowable exposure time, and every 3-dB decrease in the noise level results in a doubling of the allowable exposure time.

- Recommended exposure level (REL): Workers exposed to an 8-hour TWA of 85 dBA or greater (or the equivalent) must be enrolled in a hearing conservation program, and feasible administrative and engineering controls must be used to reduce noise exposure below the REL. If these controls fail to reduce noise exposure below the REL, HPDs must be worn.

See Appendix 8–A for a summary of key components of the OSHA regulation/standard and NIOSH noise recommendations.

MSHA Regulations

The purpose of the Mining Safety and Health Administration (MSHA, 2000) Noise Regulation 30 CFR Part 62 is to prevent NIHL among workers in the underground and surface mining industry.

- Exchange rate: MSHA uses a 5-dB exchange rate.
- Action level (AL): Miners must be enrolled in a hearing conservation program, and HPDs must be made available when noise exposure is an 8-hour TWA of 85 dBA or greater (or the equivalent).
- PEL: Miners exposed to an 8-hour TWA greater than 90 dBA (or the equivalent) must be enrolled in a hearing conservation program, and all feasible engineering and administrative controls must be used to reduce noise exposure to the PEL. If the noise exposure cannot be reduced below the PEL using all feasible engineering and administrative controls, the miner must wear hearing protection.

Other Noise Regulations

Other U.S. agencies and organizations have their own noise regulations for workers. Examples include:

- Federal Railroad Association: Applies to employees exposed to noise in the locomotive cab (U.S. Department of Transportation, 2006)
- Department of Defense: Applies to U.S. military personnel and civilian personnel exposed to hazardous occupational and operational noise (U.S. Department of Defense, 2019)
- Department of Transportation: Applies to truck and bus drivers through the Federal Motor Carrier Safety Administration (1994)

 AUDIOLOGY NUGGET

The OSHA maximum PEL and the NIOSH REL are not designed to protect all workers from any degree of NIHL (Johnson, 2018; Neitzel, 2008; NIOSH, 1998). Excess risk is the "percentage of people in a noise-exposed population who develop a material hearing impairment (as defined by OSHA or NIOSH) above and beyond the percentage of people in a non-noise-exposed population who develop a material hearing impairment" (Johnson, 2018, p. 5). Calculation of excess risk is based on an 8-hour workday, 5 days per week, over a 40-year working lifetime. Using the NIOSH definition of material hearing impairment (1000, 2000, 3000, and 4000 Hz), an average exposure level of 90 dBA over a working lifetime will result in an estimated 25% excess risk of developing hearing loss, compared to an excess risk of only 8% if the average exposure is 85 dBA (NIOSH, 1998). While neither limit protects all workers from all hearing loss, the NIOSH REL of 85 dBA is more protective and results in fewer workers developing significant hearing loss. In order to protect the most sensitive individuals, NIOSH recommends hearing protection be worn any time noise exposure exceeds 85 dBA for any duration (Kardous et al., 2016).

Noise Measurement and Exposure Analysis

In occupational settings, measurement of noise levels can serve different purposes (Moritz, 2014). While audiologists may perform basic noise measurements, industries typically engage the services of industrial hygienists to measure and identify noise exposures as part of comprehensive assessment of worksite health and safety risks. The results of noise monitoring can be used to:

- Identify workers with exposures that exceed occupational standards who must therefore be enrolled in a hearing conservation program
- Determine if administrative and/or engineering controls are needed
- Decide how much attenuation is needed from HPDs
- Educate and motivate workers to protect their hearing

- Predict if a worker's hearing loss could be caused by their noise exposure in workers' compensation cases
- Determine if ambient noise levels in rooms where audiometric testing is performed meet recommended standards

Equipment Used for Noise Measurement

Noise levels are measured using a SLM or a noise dosimeter. SLMs can be held by the user or attached to a stand/tripod and are used mainly for area noise monitoring to determine if noise levels in specific work locations could be potentially hazardous to hearing. The SLM should be calibrated before and after each use by placing the acoustic calibrator on top of the microphone. SLMs must meet the American National Standards Institute Specification for Sound Level Meters (ANSI S1.4, 1983, as cited in Gelfand, 2009) if used for measuring noise for compliance with occupational noise requirements. There are several types of SLMs (ANSI, 2006, as cited in Gelfand, 2009):

- Type 0: Also called a laboratory standard SLM, a Type 0 SLM has an accuracy of ± 0.7 dB.
- Type 1: Known as a precision SLM, a Type 1 SLM has an accuracy of ± 1 dB.
- Type 2: Considered a general-purpose SLM, a Type 2 SLM has an accuracy of ± 2 dB. This is the minimum required by OSHA and NIOSH for occupational noise measurements.
- Type S (Special purpose): A Type S SLM has limited capabilities/settings and is not used for occupational noise measurements.
- Integrating: An integrating SLM has the same functions as a Type 1 or Type 2 SLM, but it averages the measured noise levels over a period of time.

A noise dosimeter is a small, integrating SLM that can be worn for extended periods of time (i.e., a work shift) to determine a worker's noise exposure. The noise dosimeter is typically clipped to the listener's shirt at the shoulder to be closer to ear level. Since SLMs are rather unwieldly for measuring the noise exposure of individual workers who change locations and tasks during their work shift, noise dosimeters are preferred for such scenarios. Noise dosimeters can be set to measure according to different occupational noise standards, with some capable of measuring using different settings simultaneously (e.g., measuring using the OSHA and NIOSH settings at the same time). Noise dosimeters should be calibrated before and after each use, and they must meet the American National Standards Specification for Personal Noise Dosimeters (ANSI S1.25, as cited in Moritz, 2014) if used for measuring noise for compliance with occupational noise standards.

Settings and Features

SLMs and noise dosimeters have various settings and features that can be changed depending on the purpose of the noise measurement. For occupational noise measurement, it is important that these settings comply with recommendations or regulations specified by the governing safety organization. Examples of the most common settings include:

- Threshold: The threshold represents the lowest sound level to be measured by an integrating SLM/noise dosimeter. OSHA requires that occupational noise measurements include all continuous, intermittent, and impulse noise levels between 80 dBA and 130 dBA. NIOSH recommends including all continuous, intermittent, and impulse noise levels between 80 dBA and 140 dBA.

■ Criterion: The criterion level is the maximum allowable "safe" noise level. For OSHA, the maximum PEL of 90 dBA is considered the criterion. In contrast, NIOSH recommends 85 dBA as the REL or criterion.

■ Exchange rate: Based on the equal energy principle, the exchange rate represents the relationship between the permissible exposure time and different noise levels. OSHA uses a 5-dB exchange rate, and NIOSH uses a 3-dB exchange rate.

■ Response time: The response time refers to the amount of time needed for the SLM/noise dosimeter to reach 63% of its maximum reading (Gelfand, 2009). OSHA and NIOSH require use of a slow response time, which has a time constant of 1 second, allowing sound level fluctuations to be averaged out. A fast response time has a time constant of 0.125 seconds, which is more appropriate for measuring variability in noise levels.

■ Frequency weighting scales: The weighting given to the frequencies measured by a SLM/noise dosimeter can be changed by selecting different weighting scales (Figure 8–1). A linear scale applies no weighting and measures the overall SPL for all sound detected by the microphone (Gelfand, 2009).

  □ The dBA scale deemphasizes the low frequencies considerably below 1000 Hz and thus mimics the ear's response to low-intensity sounds (i.e., less sensitivity to low frequencies). The dBA scale is required by OSHA and NIOSH for occupational noise exposure measurements to assess hearing damage risk.

  □ The dBB scale deemphasizes the low frequencies but not as much as the dBA scale, thus mimicking the ear's response to moderate-intensity sounds. This scale is rarely used.

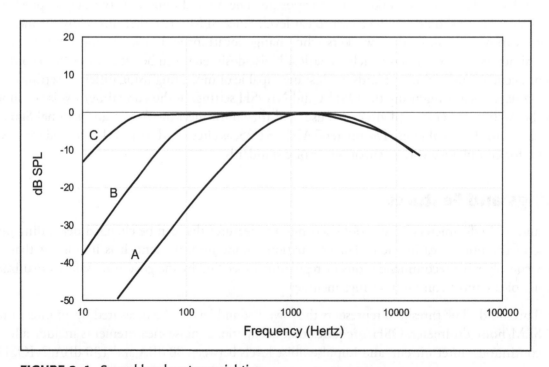

FIGURE 8–1. Sound level meter weighting.

- □ Very similar to the linear response, the dBC scale only slightly deemphasizes very low and very high frequencies. The dBC scale is designed to mimic the ear's response to high-intensity sounds, so it is used when assessing peak sound pressures from very loud impulsive sources.

- □ Finally, newer SLMs and noise dosimeters include the dBZ scale as an option. The dBZ scale provides a flat frequency response (±1.5 dB) for 10 Hz to 20,000 Hz. This replaces the older "linear" response (which did not define the frequency range over which the meter would be linear) (NoiseMeters Inc., 2022).

- ■ Octave and one-third octave band analysis: Some SLMs and noise dosimeters have octave-band or one-third octave band filters that allow measurement of noise in specific frequency ranges/bands. Octave band filters span one octave (e.g., 2800 to 5600 Hz with a center frequency of 4000 Hz), whereas one-third octave band filters span one-third of an octave (e.g., 450 to 560 Hz with a center frequency of 500 Hz). These features are necessary when noise must be measured in specific frequency bands, such as when determining if background noise levels meet requirements for audiometric test rooms (ANSI, S3.1–1999, as cited in Frank, 2000; OSHA, 1983) or when acoustical engineers consider options for effective noise controls.

Q & A

Question: Why do OSHA and NIOSH require use of the dBA scale?

Answer: The human ear is not equally sensitive to all frequencies. Sensitivity is best at about 4000 Hz and poorest in the low frequencies. SLMs can be set to different frequency weighting scales that represent responses of the human ear at different intensity levels. The dBA scale mimics the human ear's response to moderate sound levels. OSHA and NIOSH require use of the dBA scale for noise measurements because it most closely correlates with the risk of developing NIHL.

Quantification of Noise Exposure

SLMs and noise dosimeters provide a variety of numerical values that can help quantify a person's noise exposure and subsequent risk of NIHL. Fortunately, current integrating SLMs and noise dosimeters can calculate these values automatically. However, the same values can be calculated manually if an integrating SLM or noise dosimeter is not available. Some of the most commonly used values include:

- ■ Peak level: The peak level is the highest instantaneous sound level that the SLM/noise dosimeter measures without using a frequency weighting scale or response time.

- ■ Maximum level: The maximum level is the highest sound level measured using the selected frequency weighting scale and response time.

- ■ Lavg (or LAVG): The Lavg represents the logarithmic average sound level measured, but when a threshold is set, the Lavg does not include any sound at levels below the threshold.

- Leq: The Leq represents the true equivalent sound level. The Leq is equivalent to the Lavg, but it is only used when the exchange rate is 3 dB and the threshold is 0 dB.

- Time-weighted average (TWA): The TWA represents a constant sound level lasting 8 hours that would result in the same amount of sound energy as the noise that was measured. The TWA is less than the Lavg for a duration less than 8 hours and is equal to the Lavg at 8 hours.

  □ Using OSHA's (1983) 90 dBA exposure limit and a 5-dB exchange rate, the TWA is calculated as:

$$TWA = 16.61 \times \log(D/100) + 90$$

Where: D = dose

  □ Using NIOSH's (1998) 85 dBA exposure limit and a 3-dB exchange rate, the TWA is calculated as:

$$TWA = 10.0 \times \log(D/100) + 85$$

Where: D = dose

- Noise dose: The noise dose describes the amount of actual noise exposure relative to the amount of allowable exposure, where 100% and above represents noise-hazardous exposures (NIOSH, 1998). Table 8–1 shows OSHA's (1983) maximum PELs and NIOSH's (1998) RELs expressed as an 8-hour TWA and a noise dose. The noise dose is calculated as:

$$D = [C1/T1 + C2/T2 + Cn/Tn] \times 100$$

Where:
Cn = total time of exposure at a specified noise level
Tn = exposure time at which noise for this level becomes hazardous

The total time of exposure at each noise level and the exposure time at which noise at that level becomes hazardous can be reported in hours or minutes as long as the same unit is used for each noise level in the calculation.

TABLE 8–1. OSHA's (1983) Maximum Permissible Exposure Levels (PELs) and NIOSH's (1999) Recommended Exposure Levels (RELs) Expressed as an 8-Hour Time-Weighted Average (TWA) and a Noise Dose

DOSE	OSHA 8-HOUR TWA	NIOSH 8-HOUR TWA
25%	80 dBA	79 dBA
50%	85 dBA	82 dBA
100%	90 dBA	85 dBA
200%	95 dBA	88 dBA
400%	100 dBA	91 dBA
800%	105 dBA	94 dBA

CASE EXAMPLE

A worker is exposed to the following noise levels during his 8-hour work shift:

- 94 dBA for 3 hours
- 88 dBA for 2 hours
- 97 dBA for 3 hours

One can use the formulae described above to determine the worker's noise dose and his 8-hour TWA using the NIOSH recommendations. First calculate the noise dose. Remember each numerator (i.e., the top number in each fraction) represents how long the worker was exposed at a specific noise level. The denominator (i.e., the bottom number in each fraction) represents how long the worker can safely be exposed at that level using the NIOSH recommendations. These values can be reported in hours or minutes as long as the same unit is used for all of the fractions. In this example, the length of time the worker can safely be exposed at each level can be determined either by using the table provided in the NIOSH noise standard recommendations or by using the quick rule of decreasing the exposure time by half for every 3-dB increase in noise level, with an exposure of 85 dBA for 8 hours as the reference point.

$$D = [180 \text{ minutes}/60 \text{ minutes} + 120 \text{ minutes}/240 \text{ minutes} + 180 \text{ minutes}/30 \text{ minutes}] \times 100$$
$$= 950\%$$

Therefore, the worker is exposed to a daily noise dose of 950%, which is well above the maximum allowable 100% dose. To calculate the 8-hour TWA associated with a 950% dose, simply use the following NIOSH formula:

$$TWA = 10.0 \times \log (950/100) + 85$$
$$= 94.78 \text{ dBA}$$

The worker is exposed to an 8-hour TWA of 94.78 dBA. This is above the NIOSH REL of 85 dBA. As a result, the worker would need to wear HPDs at work, have an annual audiometric evaluation, and participate in a hearing conservation program.

Noise Control

Results of noise monitoring can be used to determine the most appropriate options for reducing workers' noise exposure. Noise can be controlled at the source, the path, and/or the receiver.

- Source: Reducing noise at the source involves implementing engineering controls. Examples include replacing older equipment with newer, quieter equipment or modifying existing equipment to be quieter. This is the best long-term option for noise control, but it can be expensive.

- Path: Reducing noise levels along the path involves using sound-absorbing materials to reduce noise as it travels from the source to the listener. Examples include adding sound-absorbing materials to the room surfaces (e.g., ceiling, walls), building barriers around noisy areas, installing noise-reducing curtains, and enclosing the worker in a sound-treated room/booth.

- Receiver: Controlling noise at the receiver involves reducing the noise at the listener's ear. Examples include using HPDs and using administrative controls to modify work schedules to limit workers' noise exposure.

Types of Hearing Protection

Reducing noise levels at the source or along the path can be expensive. Therefore, use of HPDs is the most common method for reducing noise exposure. There are many types and styles of HPDs available. The primary styles are earplugs, earmuffs, and banded earplugs, but special protectors with additional features are available within these categories. The main types of HPDs include user-molded foam earplugs, premolded earplugs, push-to-fit (hybrid) earplugs, banded earplugs (semi-inserts or canal caps), passive earmuffs, flat (uniform) attenuation earplugs, nonlinear-level dependent (amplitude-sensitive) devices, devices with amplification (earplugs or earmuffs), noise-isolating entertainment devices, and communication headsets. Table 8–2 describes advantages and disadvantages of each type of HPD.

AUDIOLOGY NUGGET

Traditional earplugs and earmuffs attenuate high frequencies more than mid and low frequencies (Chasin, 2009). This can interfere with speech under-standing and music perception. Flat attenuation earplugs and earmuffs (also called uniform attenuation, high fidelity, or musician plugs) are designed to provide approximately even attenuation across the frequency range, thus pre-serving the natural balance between the low-frequency fundamental energy and the high-frequency harmonic energy. Therefore, flat attenuation earplugs can be beneficial, not only for music listening but also for situations where speech understanding is important.

HPD Fitting, Care, and Cleaning

HPDs must be properly worn and cared for in order to achieve the desired noise reduction/attenuation. The fit of an HPD can be checked visually or acoustically.

- Visual check: When earplugs with stems are fit properly, only the stem should be visible when looking at the wearer from the front. Earplugs without stems should not be visible when viewed from the front. Earmuffs should be worn with the ear cushions surrounding the ears, pressing tightly against the head.

- Acoustic check: The fit of earplugs can be checked by having the wearer insert the earplugs and then cover the ears with his or her hands. If the earplugs are properly inserted, this should

TABLE 8–2. Advantages and Disadvantages of Different Types of Hearing Protection Devices

TYPE	ADVANTAGES	DISADVANTAGES
Nonelectronic		
User-Molded Foam Earplugs	Inexpensive Comfortable for longer wearing times Cooler than earmuffs in hot weather Range of sizes Can provide good attenuation if properly worn	Not reusable Easier to lose Inconvenient for intermittent use Must wash hands before reinserting Can be difficult to properly insert Attenuation varies depending on fit
Premolded Earplugs	Reusable/washable Comfortable for longer wearing times Cooler than earmuffs in hot weather Range of sizes and shapes Stem or tab for easier insertion and removal	Slightly more expensive than user-molded foam earplugs Must be cleaned after each use May have to reinsert/adjust fit after talking/chewing Attenuation varies depending on fit
Push-to-Fit (Hybrid) Earplugs	Easy to insert Hygienic to remove/reinsert when hands are dirty	Slightly more expensive than user-molded foam earplugs Attenuation varies depending on fit
Custom Earplugs	More comfortable Better fit Can be easier to insert Reusable—Designed to last an extended period of time Can be made for attachment to noise-isolating entertainment and communication headsets	More expensive Attenuation depends on quality of the impression and manufacturing
Banded Earplugs (Semi-Inserts or Canal Caps)	Easy to insert and remove Convenient for intermittent use	More expensive than user-molded foam earplugs Greater occlusion effect Causes an annoying sound when the band is bumped or hit Less attenuation than most other types of earplugs
Passive Earmuffs	Easier to fit than earplugs Comfortable in cold temperatures Less variability in attenuation Convenient for intermittent noise Easier to monitor use because of high visibility Special types available for wearing with other personal protective equipment (e.g., back-band earmuffs with welding helmets, earmuff–hard hat combinations, face shields, etc.)	Higher cost than earplugs (except custom-molded) Can be uncomfortable over long periods of time Uncomfortable in hot temperatures Reduced comfort and attenuation when worn with safety glasses

continues

not cause any significant change in the subjective noise level perceived by the wearer. The fit of earmuffs and earplugs can be generally checked by determining if loud sounds become softer and if the wearer's voice sounds muffled or hollow.

HPDs must also be appropriately maintained and cleaned. It is important to follow the recommendations specific to each type of HPD.

TABLE 8–2. *continued*

TYPE	ADVANTAGES	DISADVANTAGES
Flat (Uniform) Attenuation Earplugs	Equal attenuation for low- and high-frequency noise, creating more natural sound Allows for better speech understanding and music appreciation Good for environments with moderate noise levels Beneficial for workers with hearing loss Available in noncustom and custom options	Slightly higher cost than other earplugs Less attenuation than other types of earplugs
Non-Linear Level Dependent (Amplitude-Sensitive) Devices	Good for intermittent noise Allow the wearer to hear soft speech and warning sounds while attenuating loud noise Available in passive (nonelectronic) or active (electronic) options	More expensive than other earplugs Only appropriate for specific environments (e.g., gunfire)
Electronic		
Devices with Amplification (Earplugs or Earmuffs)	Allows for better speech understanding and situational awareness by amplifying soft sounds and attenuating loud sounds Especially helpful for impulse noise May be beneficial for workers with hearing loss	More expensive than nonelectronic devices May not be waterproof Batteries must be replaced
Noise-Isolating Entertainment Devices	Appropriate for environments with low noise levels May result in greater acceptance and wear time	More expensive than nonelectronic devices Not appropriate for all noise environments May interfere with situational awareness/cause safety risks
Communication Headsets	Allows for radio communication and noise attenuation Improves situational awareness/safety	More expensive than nonelectronic devices

- Foam earplugs: Foam earplugs can only be used two to three times before replacing and should not be washed. They should be replaced when they do not return to their original shape.

- Premolded earplugs: Premolded earplugs can be washed using warm water and mild soap and used for days to weeks. They should be replaced when the flanges are damaged or are no longer soft.

- Push-to-fit (hybrid) earplugs: Push-to-fit earplugs can only be used two to three times before replacing and should not be washed. They should be replaced when the foam does not return to its original shape.

- Custom earplugs: Custom earplugs can be washed using warm water and mild soap and used for years. However, they can shrink and harden over time. The fit can also change due to the listener's weight gain or loss.

- Earmuffs: The earmuff manufacturer's specific instructions should be followed. The outside of the earmuff can be cleaned with soap and water. Solvents should not be used, and earmuffs should not be stored at high temperatures. Earmuffs should be inspected for cracked or hardened earcup seals and to confirm that headband tension is adequate to maintain adequate noise reduction.

HPD Attenuation

To reduce the risk of developing NIHL, HPDs must provide an appropriate amount of noise reduction/attenuation. The amount of noise reduction/attenuation provided by a person's HPDs can be estimated using formulae that incorporate the noise reduction rating (NRR) or directly measured using different types of field attenuation-estimation systems (FAESs), colloquially referred to as "fit-test" systems (Voix et al., 2022).

Methods of Estimating HPD Attenuation

The NRR is a single number designed to estimate the amount of attenuation provided by a particular HPD. In the United States, the Environmental Protection Agency (EPA, 1979) requires the NRR to be included on HPD packages. The NRR for a particular type of HPD is derived from experiments where the hearing protector is fit by the experimenter. Open ear and occluded thresholds are obtained in soundfield using one-third octave band noise. The difference between the occluded and unoccluded thresholds is the rear ear attenuation at threshold (REAT). Data from at least 10 subjects are collected, and the NRR is calculated using a formula that involves mean attenuation and standard deviation across different frequencies. Refer to Rawool (2012) for the NRR formula and an example showing its calculation.

The NRR can be used in various ways to estimate a person's noise exposure when wearing a particular type of HPD. According to the EPA, the adequacy of hearing protection is estimated by subtracting the NRR of the hearing protector from the worker's C-weighted TWA noise exposure. However, OSHA (1983) and NIOSH (1998) require workers' noise exposure to be measured in dBA. To account for possible differences between the A-weighted and C-weighted noise exposure values, OSHA and NIOSH specify that 7 dB should be subtracted from the NRR when it is used with A-weighted noise exposure values (as shown in the formulae below). OSHA (1983) described both a required method and a recommended method of estimating HPD attenuation. OSHA (1983) requires using the following methods of estimating HPD attenuation.

Q & A

Question: Does the NRR accurately estimate the amount of attenuation workers receive when wearing hearing protection in the real world?

Answer: No. Research shows that the attenuation workers receive when wearing hearing protection in the real world is much less than the labeled NRR (Schulz & Madison, 2014). On average, the actual attenuation was about one third to one half of the labeled NRR. Much greater variability across workers is also seen, with standard deviations being two to three times greater in the real world. Lower attenuation and greater variability may be seen in the real world because:

- Workers in real-world settings tend to not fit earplugs as deeply in the ear canal as when experimenters fit the earplugs for NRR calculation studies.

- Earplugs may work themselves loose during a typical work shift as a worker chews and talks.

- Earmuffs may not fit as tightly and therefore may provide less attenuation when worn with safety glasses, goggles, or other personal protective equipment.

- When the TWA is measured in dBC: Estimated protected exposure (in dBA) = Unprotected TWA (in dBC) – NRR

- When the TWA is measured in dBA: Estimated protected exposure (in dBA) = Unprotected TWA (in dBA) – (NRR – 7)

However, OSHA (1983) recommends (but does not require) using a more conservative method in which the NRR is derated to more accurately estimate real-world attenuation.

- When the TWA is measured in dBC: Estimated protected exposure (in dBA) = Unprotected TWA (in dBC) – [NRR × 50%]

- When the TWA is measured in dBA: Estimated protected exposure (in dBA) = Unprotected TWA (in dBA) – [(NRR – 7) × 50%]

NIOSH (1998) specifies its own recommendations designed to prevent the overestimation of noise attenuation that can occur when using the NRR. When possible, NIOSH recommends using subject fit (instead of experimenter fit) data. If subject fit data are not available, NIOSH recommends using the following deratings of the NRR. Different derating values are recommended for different types of hearing protection.

- Foam earplugs
    - When the TWA is measured in dBC: Estimated protected exposure (in dBA) = Unprotected TWA (in dBC) – (NRR × 50%)
    - When the TWA is measured in dBA: Estimated protected exposure (in dBA) = Unprotected TWA (in dBA) – [(NRR – 7) × 50%]

- Other types of earplugs
  - □ When the TWA is measured in dBC: Estimated protected exposure (in dBA) = Unprotected TWA (in dBC) – (NRR × 30%)
  - □ When the TWA is measured in dBA: Estimated protected exposure (in dBA) = Unprotected TWA (in dBA) – [(NRR – 7) × 30%]
- Earmuffs
  - □ When the TWA is measured in dBC: Estimated protected exposure (in dBA) = Unprotected TWA (in dBC) – (NRR × 75%)
  - □ When the TWA is measured in dBA: Estimated protected exposure (in dBA) = Unprotected TWA (in dBA) – [(NRR – 7) × 75%]

In some situations, noise levels can be so high that wearing one type of HPD is not enough to attenuate the noise to a safe level. Wearing double (dual) hearing protection (e.g., wearing earplugs and earmuffs simultaneously) is one possible solution. Different organizations have different recommendations for when double hearing protection should be used.

- **OSHA:** The OSHA (1983) noise regulation states that employers can require double hearing protection if there is evidence of progressive NIHL.
- **MSHA:** For workers in the mining industry, MSHA requires double hearing protection when exposure is equal to or greater than a TWA of 105 dBA.
- **NIOSH:** To best protect hearing, NIOSH (1998) recommends using double hearing protection when noise exposure is equal to or greater than a TWA of 100 dBA.
- **Military:** The U.S. Marine Corps (n.d.) requires all personnel to wear double hearing protection when noise exposure exceeds an 8-hour TWA of 100 dBA. The U.S. Army (2015) requires double hearing protection for those exposed to greater than an 8-hour TWA of 103 dBA, whereas the U.S. Navy (2020) requires use of double hearing protection when noise reaches 104 dBA or greater.

Wearing double hearing protection typically only adds 5 to 10 dB to the maximum attenuation provided by a single hearing protector. OSHA recommends that to estimate a worker's noise exposure when wearing double hearing protection, the previously described formulae are used, but 5 dB is added

---

Q & A

Question: Does OSHA require employees with hearing loss to wear hearing protection?

Answer: Although not addressed in OSHA's (1983) Occupational Noise Standard 29 CRF 1910.95, OSHA provided clarification on this issue through an interpretation letter (Fairfax, 2004). The letter states that the noise regulation applies to all employees, with no exception for those with hearing loss. Hearing aids worn in the OFF position cannot satisfy the requirement for wearing hearing protection. OSHA states that employees with hearing loss should wear their hearing aids with earmuffs that provide sufficient attenuation to reduce workplace noise to below 85 dBA.

to the NRR of the HPD with the higher NRR. Therefore, if earmuffs with an NRR of 30 dB and foam earplugs with an NRR of 20 dB are worn simultaneously, dual protection will provide an estimated 35 dB of attenuation if both are worn properly. An NRR of 35 dB could then be used in the previously described equations to more accurately estimate real-world attenuation.

Measuring the Personal Attenuation Rating (PAR)

When HPD attenuation is estimated, the amount of attenuation a particular person experiences may be overestimated or underestimated. To best protect hearing, individuals should undergo individual fit testing to measure the PAR, the amount of attenuation actually provided by an individual's HPDs as they are wearing them. The calculated PAR is a more realistic estimate of attenuation provided to an individual in "real-world" use, rather than predicting attenuation from laboratory data as derived using the NRR. Results of HPD fit testing can be used to train employees on proper HPD fit, teach people how to train employees on proper HPD fit, help ensure HPDs are providing enough attenuation, provide documentation of HPD attenuation, and help with selection of appropriate HPDs.

Different types of HPD fit testing are available (Hager, 2011). Some test methods allow the individual to wear their own HPDs, and others require the individual to wear HPDs that are specifically designed to be used with the fit test equipment.

- REAT: This method involves measuring thresholds in soundfield with and without the listener wearing their HPDs. One-third octave bands of noise are typically used as the stimulus signal. The amount of attenuation provided by the HPDs is calculated as the difference between the thresholds obtained with and without the HPDs. REAT is considered the gold standard for HPD fit testing, and it can be performed using any type of earplug or earmuff. However, REAT can be more time-consuming than the other methods of HPD fit testing.

- Field microphone-in-the-ear (F-MIRE): For F-MIRE testing, a probe microphone is placed in the ear canal, and real ear insertion gain is measured in the unoccluded condition (i.e., without hearing protection) and the occluded condition (i.e., with hearing protection). Attenuation is represented by negative deviation from 0 dB. One disadvantage of commercially available F-MIRE systems is that they require use of special earplugs with the probe built in, which are not available for many earplug models.

- Loudness balance systems: With loudness balance systems, the listener wears headphones and adjusts the volume until the sound is of equal loudness in both ears. This process is completed in the unoccluded condition (i.e., without hearing protection), in the occluded right ear condition (i.e., with hearing protection only worn in the right ear), and in the occluded left ear condition (i.e., with hearing protection only worn in the left ear). The amount the level had to be increased in the occluded ear to be perceived as equally loud to the unoccluded ear is the calculated PAR, which estimates the attenuation provided to the individual being tested. Some disadvantages of loudness balance fit testing include that it can only be used with earplugs and can be difficult for workers with hearing loss to perform.

Audiometric Monitoring

The purpose of audiometric monitoring is to identify signs of NIHL early so that steps can be taken to prevent the hearing loss from progressing. For nonoccupational noise exposure, hearing screening is often recommended for children and adults. However, it is possible to pass a hearing screening and still have permanent NIHL. For example, in the early stages of NIHL, hearing thresholds can still be within normal limits, despite having a noticeable "noise notch" that would only be seen if a threshold pure-tone evaluation is performed. In other cases, the noise notch may occur at a frequency not included in a typical hearing screening (e.g., 3000 or 6000 Hz). Therefore, best practice is to recommend an annual audiological evaluation for any child or adult exposed to high noise levels to monitor their hearing sensitivity.

For occupational noise exposure, different organizations have different regulations/recommendations related to audiometric monitoring. OSHA (1983) and NIOSH (1998) both state that audiometric monitoring should:

- Be available for/provided to all employees exposed to an 8-hour TWA of 85 dBA or greater
- Be performed by a licensed audiologist, a physician, or a technician certified by the Council for Accreditation in Occupational Hearing Conservation (CAOHC), working under the supervision of an audiologist or physician
- Include air-conduction, pure-tone audiometry at 500, 1000, 2000, 3000, 4000, and 6000 Hz

There are some differences between the OSHA (1983) and NIOSH (1998) audiometric monitoring requirements/recommendations. For example, while OSHA will allow someone without training to use a microprocessor audiometer, NIOSH has strongly recommended against this practice. In addition, OSHA does not require testing 8000 Hz, but NIOSH considers inclusion of 8000 Hz to be a best practice option since it is a useful source of information about the etiology of a hearing loss (i.e., the presence of "noise notches" at 6000 Hz) for audiologists and physicians in their review of audiograms for determination of NIHL and work-related hearing loss.

Test Environment and Equipment

Occupational standards do not require that audiometric monitoring be performed in a sound booth. However, in order to help ensure valid results, background noise levels in rooms where audiometric testing is performed must not exceed specified limits. As shown in Table 8–3, OSHA (1983) allows higher levels of ambient background noise than those allowed by ANSI S3.1–1999 (as cited in Frank, 2000). Previous research has shown that in audiometric test rooms where ambient noise levels are at the OSHA MPANLs, hearing thresholds cannot be accurately measured down to 0 dB HL (e.g., Berger & Killion, 1989, as cited in Frank & Williams, 1994).

OSHA and NIOSH also require that audiometers (whether manual or microprocessor) meet certain requirements (Danielson, 2014). OSHA requires that the operation of the audiometer be checked before each day's use with a daily (biological or bioacoustic) calibration check and functional

TABLE 8–3. Maximum Permissible Ambient Noise Levels (Measured in dB SPL) in Audiometric Test Rooms Allowed by OSHA (1983) and ANSI (S3.1–1999)

	125 Hz	250 Hz	500 Hz	1000 Hz	2000 Hz	4000 Hz	8000 Hz
OSHA (1983)			40	40	47	57	62
ANSI (S3.1–1999)	49	35	21	26	34	37	37
Difference			19	14	13	20	25

(listening) check. The audiometer must also meet ANSI S3.6–1969 requirements for calibration, which includes an annual acoustical check and an exhaustive calibration every 2 years. NIOSH recommends that audiometers meet ANSI S3.6–1996. Calibration should include a daily functional check, an acoustical check when the daily check shows a threshold difference greater than 10 dB in either headphone at any frequency, and an exhaustive calibration every year or when the acoustic check indicates the need.

Baseline and Annual Audiograms

The baseline audiogram is meant to document a worker's hearing thresholds prior to being exposed to noise at a particular job. These baseline thresholds are used in comparisons with results of subsequent periodic audiograms.

■ OSHA (1983) requires that the baseline audiogram be performed within 6 months of exposure at or above a TWA of 85 dBA or within 1 year if testing is conducted using a mobile test van. The baseline audiogram must be preceded by at least 14 hours without workplace noise exposure (i.e., noise-free period), but if this is not feasible, the worker can wear hearing protection instead.

■ NIOSH (1999) recommends that the baseline audiogram be performed before employment or within 30 days of employment for workers exposed to a TWA of 85 dBA or greater. The baseline audiogram must be preceded by at least 12 hours of quiet, and use of hearing protection cannot be substituted.

Each year the annual audiogram is compared to the baseline audiogram to determine if the worker has experienced a decline in hearing that could be due to occupational noise exposure.

■ OSHA (1983) requires that annual audiometric testing be performed for all employees with noise exposure at or above a TWA of 85 dBA. The annual audiogram can be obtained any time during the work shift, but testing at the end of the work shift to account for the exposure is encouraged.

■ NIOSH (1998) recommends that the annual audiogram (i.e., the monitoring audiogram) be performed for all employees with noise exposure at or above a TWA of 85 dBA. The test should be scheduled at the end of or late in the work shift to detect any TTSs.

Threshold Shift

A worker's baseline audiogram is compared to the annual audiogram to determine if a significant change in hearing has occurred. Although there are some similarities, OSHA (1983) and NIOSH (1998) differ in some of the specific requirements/recommendations for determining whether a significant change in hearing has occurred and what the subsequent actions should be.

■ OSHA (1983) refers to a significant change in hearing as a standard threshold shift (STS). An STS is defined as an average change of 10 dB or more at 2000, 3000, and 4000 Hz in either ear when compared to the baseline audiogram. The results must be reviewed by an audiologist or physician, and a retest can be performed within 30 days. If the annual audiogram showing an STS is determined to be valid, it becomes the worker's new baseline. An employee who is identified as having an STS must be notified in writing of the test results within 21 days. OSHA permits use of age corrections when determining if an STS has occurred (i.e., a portion of the change in hearing is attributed to age and subtracted from the STS calculation).

☐ If an STS is identified, the following actions are required: fit, train, and require HPD use; refit and retrain employees who have previously worn hearing protection; refer for evaluation by an audiologist or otolaryngologist if a medical pathology of the ear is suspected; and notify employees when an otologic exam is needed for an ear problem that is nonwork related.

☐ OSHA requires that a hearing loss be recorded in the OSHA 300 Log of Work-Related Injuries and Illnesses when an STS is present (age corrections are allowed); the current audiogram shows hearing thresholds of an average of 25 dB HL or greater at 2000, 3000, and 4000 Hz (in the same ear that showed the STS); and the shift in hearing is related to occupational noise exposure (Wells, 2014).

■ NIOSH (1998) refers to a significant change in hearing as a significant threshold shift, defined as a change of 15 dB or more in either ear at any of the following frequencies: 500, 1000, 2000, 3000, 4000, or 6000 Hz. The results must be reviewed by an audiologist or physician, and a retest can be performed immediately or within 30 days. The annual audiogram with the significant threshold shift becomes the new baseline. If a significant threshold shift is identified, the employee must be notified within 30 days. NIOSH recommends that age corrections not be used when calculating a significant threshold shift.

☐ If a significant threshold shift is identified, a minimum of the following actions is recommended: reinstruct and refit hearing protection, retrain on worker responsibilities for hearing conservation, and/or reassign the worker to work in a quieter area.

Threshold Shift Case Example

A 40-year-old male has worked at a tire manufacturing plant for 15 years. At his current annual audiometric evaluation, a change in hearing is seen in both ears. The first two lines of Table 8–4 show the worker's right ear thresholds at the baseline and current audiometric evaluations. The first two lines of Table 8–5 show his left ear thresholds for the baseline and current audiometric evaluations. OSHA (1983) defines an STS as an average change of 10 dB or more at 2000, 3000, and 4000 Hz in either ear compared to the baseline audiogram. As shown below, the change in hearing in each ear meets the criteria for an STS.

■ Right ear
  ☐ Baseline average of 2000, 3000, and 4000 Hz = 11.67 dB
  ☐ Current average of 2000, 3000, and 4000 Hz = 25 dB
  ☐ Shift = 13.33 dB
■ Left ear
  ☐ Baseline average of 2000, 3000, and 4000 Hz = 13.33 dB
  ☐ Current average of 2000, 3000, and 4000 Hz = 25 dB
  ☐ Shift = 11.67 dB

Given that the shift in the average of 2000, 3000, and 4000 Hz is at least 10 dB in each ear, the employee would be considered to have had an STS. However, OSHA (1983) allows use of age correction

TABLE 8–4. Age Correction Case Study Results—Right Ear

	AUDIOMETRIC TEST FREQUENCY (Hz)					
	500	**1000**	**2000**	**3000**	**4000**	**6000**
Baseline (Age = 25 Years)	5	5	10	10	15	5
Current (Age = 40 Years)	5	10	20	20	35	25
Average Change in Thresholds (2000, 3000, and 4000 Hz)	Baseline Average = 11.67 Current Average = 25 Average Change in Thresholds = 13.33					STS
Age Correction Values at 25 Years			3	5	7	
Age Correction Values at 40 Years			6	10	14	
Difference in Age Correction Values			3	5	7	
Age-Corrected Current Thresholds			17	15	28	
Age-Corrected Average Change in Thresholds (2000, 3000, and 4000 Hz)	Baseline Average = 11.67 Age-Corrected Current Average = 20 Age-Corrected Average Change in Thresholds = 8.33					No Age-Corrected STS

TABLE 8–5. Age Correction Case Study Results—Left Ear

	AUDIOMETRIC TEST FREQUENCY (Hz)					
	500	**1000**	**2000**	**3000**	**4000**	**6000**
Baseline (Age = 25 Years)	5	5	10	15	15	10
Current (Age = 40 Years)	10	10	10	25	40	20
Average Change in Thresholds (2000, 3000, and 4000 Hz)	Baseline Average = 13.33 Current Average = 25 Average Change in Thresholds = 11.67					STS
Age Correction Values at 25 Years			3	5	7	
Age Correction Values at 40 Years			6	10	14	
Difference in Age Correction Values			3	5	7	
Age-Corrected Current Thresholds			7	20	33	
Age-Corrected Average Change in Thresholds (2000, 3000, and 4000 Hz)	Baseline Average = 13.33 Age-Corrected Current Average = 20 Age-Corrected Average Change in Thresholds = 6.67					No Age-Corrected STS

factors in determining whether an STS has occurred. To apply age correction factors, the following steps are used:

- Use Tables F–1 (for males) and F–2 (for females) from the OSHA (1983) noise standard to find the age correction values for each frequency for the employee's age at the baseline (25 years) and the current evaluation (40 years). These values are shown in the fourth and fifth lines of Table 8–4 (right ear) and Table 8–5 (left ear).

- At each frequency, calculate the difference between the age correction factors for the employee's current age compared to his age at the baseline (i.e., subtract the baseline values from the current age values). These difference values represent the amount of hearing loss that may be attributed to aging between the baseline and the current audiogram.

- For each frequency, the difference value is subtracted from the threshold obtained at the current annual audiometric evaluation. Table 8–4 (right ear) and Table 8–5 (left ear) show the baseline thresholds and the age-corrected thresholds for the current audiogram in each ear.

Using the age-corrected current thresholds, the employee's change in hearing no longer meets the criteria for an STS in either ear.

- Right ear
  - Baseline average of 2000, 3000, and 4000 Hz = 11.67 dB
  - Current average of 2000, 3000, and 4000 Hz using age corrections = 20 dB
  - Shift = 8.33 dB
- Left ear
  - Baseline average of 2000, 3000, and 4000 Hz = 13.33 dB
  - Current average of 2000, 3000, and 4000 Hz using age corrections = 20 dB
  - Shift = 6.67 dB

OSHA (2001) requires that a hearing loss be recorded in the OSHA 300 Log of Work-Related Injuries and Illnesses when an STS is present (age corrections are allowed); the current audiogram shows hearing thresholds of an average of 25 dB HL or greater at 2000, 3000, and 4000 Hz; and the shift in hearing is related to occupational noise exposure (Wells, 2014). If age correction factors are not applied, this employee's hearing loss would be recorded in the OSHA Log, and his current annual audiogram would become his new baseline audiogram. If age correction factors are applied, the employee's hearing loss would not be recorded in the OSHA Log; therefore, his hearing test results obtained at 25 years of age would continue to be used as his baseline audiogram.

Referral Criteria

The American Academy of Otolaryngology-Head and Neck Surgery (1997) has published the *Otological Referral Criteria for Occupational Hearing Conservation Programs*. Although not required by OSHA or NIOSH, the criteria are helpful in determining when changes in hearing or abnormal conditions likely require medical evaluation. Medical referral should be made if:

- The baseline audiogram shows an average hearing threshold of 25 dB HL at 500, 1000, 2000, and 3000 Hz in either ear or if the difference in the average hearing threshold between ears is more than 15 dB at 500, 1000, and 2000 Hz or more than 30 dB at 3000, 4000, and 6000 Hz.

- The annual audiogram shows a decline in the average hearing threshold in either ear of 15 dB at 500, 1000, and 2000 Hz or more than 20 dB at 3000, 4000, and 6000 Hz compared to the baseline audiogram.
- There is a history of ear signs or symptoms, such as ear pain, drainage, dizziness, severe and persistent tinnitus, sudden fluctuating or rapidly progressing hearing loss, or fullness/discomfort in either ear in the last year.
- There is cerumen obstructing the ear canal.

Hearing Conservation Education and Training

Numerous studies have shown that the majority of children (e.g., Reel et al., 2022) and adults (e.g., Carroll et al., 2017) seldom or never wear hearing protection around loud noise. Hearing conservation programs for children and adults aim to educate and motivate participants to protect their hearing. The OSHA (1983) noise regulation requires that occupational hearing conservation programs include five key components:

1. Effects of noise on hearing
2. Purpose of hearing protectors
3. Advantages, disadvantages, and attenuation of different types of hearing protectors
4. Instructions on selection, fitting, use, and care of hearing protectors
5. Purpose of audiometric testing and explanation of the test procedures

Other hearing conservation programs for children and adults address similar topics, with the common goal being to prevent NIHL.

Recommended Readings

Hutchison, T. L., & Schulz, T. Y. (Eds.). (2014). *Hearing conservation manual* (5th ed.). Council for the Accreditation in Occupational Hearing Conservation.

Meinke, D. K., Berger E. H., Neitzel R. L., Driscoll, D. P., & Bright, K. (Eds.). (2022). *The noise manual* (6th ed.). American Industrial Hygiene Association.

Occupational Safety and Health Administration. (1983). Occupational noise exposure: Hearing conservation amendment; Final rule (Standard No. 29CFR 1910.95). *Federal Register, 48*(46), 97429772.

Rawool, V. W. (2012). *Hearing conservation in occupational, recreational, educational, and home settings.* Thieme Publishing.

References

American Academy of Otolaryngology-Head and Neck Surgery. (1997). *Otologic referral criteria for occupational hearing conservation programs* [Pamphlet].

American Speech-Language-Hearing Association. (n.d.-a). *Adult hearing screening* [Practice portal]. https://www.asha.org/Practice-Portal/Professional-Issues/Adult-Hearing-Screening/

American Speech-Language-Hearing Association. (n.d.-b). *Childhood hearing screening* [Practice portal]. https://www.asha.org/Practice-Portal/Profes sional-Issues/Childhood-Hearing-Screening/

American Speech-Language-Hearing Association. (n.d.-c). *Dizziness and balance.* https://www.asha .org/public/hearing/dizziness-and-balance/

American Speech-Language-Hearing Association. (n.d.-d). *Newborn hearing screening* [Practice portal]. https://www.asha.org/Practice-Portal/Professional-Issues/Newborn-Hearing-Screening/

Barber, H. O. (1984). Vestibular neurophysiology. *Otolaryngology-Head and Neck Surgery, 92*, 151–157. https://doi.org/10.1177/019459988409200112

Basner, M., Babisch, W., Davis, A., Brink, M., Clark, C., Janssen, S., & Stansfeld, S. (2014). Auditory and non-auditory effects of noise on health. *The Lancet, 383*, 1325–1332. https://doi.org/10.1016/s0140-6736(13)61613-x

Beamer, S. L. (2008). *Hearing conservation*. American Speech-Language-Hearing Association. https://www.asha.org/Articles/Hearing-Conservation/

Bramhall, N. F., Konrad-Martin, D., McMillan, G. P., & Griest, S. E. (2017). Auditory brainstem response altered in humans with noise exposure despite normal outer hair cell function. *Ear and Hearing, 38*, e1–e12. https://doi.org/10.1097/AUD. 0000000000000370

Bruce, R., Hart, N., & Arellano, J. (2014). Standards and regulations. In T. L. Hutchison & T. Y. Schulz (Eds.), *Hearing conservation manual* (5th ed., pp. 35–46). Council for the Accreditation in Occupational Hearing Conservation.

Carroll, Y. I., Eichwald, J., Scinicariello, F., Hoffman, H. J., Deitchman, S., Radke, M. S., . . . Breysse, P. (2017). Vital signs: Noise-induced hearing loss among adults—United States 2011–2012. *Morbidity and Mortality Weekly Report, 66*(5), 139–144. https://doi.org/10.15585/mmwr.mm6605e3

Chasin, M. (2009). *Hearing loss in musicians: Prevention and management*. Plural Publishing.

Danielson, R. W. (2014). Planning the audiometric monitoring program. In T. L. Hutchison & T. Y. Schulz (Eds.), *Hearing conservation manual* (5th ed., pp. 79–90). Council for the Accreditation in Occupational Hearing Conservation.

Dzhambov, A. M., & Dimitrova, D. D. (2016). Occupational noise and ischemic heart disease: A systematic review. *Noise & Health, 18*(83), 167–177. https://doi.org/10.4103/1463-1741.189241

Environmental Protection Agency. (1979). Noise labeling requirements for hearing protectors. *Federal Register, 44*(190), 130–135.

Fairfax, R. E. (2004, August 3). *Application of the occupational noise standard to employees who are deaf or have a diminished capacity to hear*. Occupational Safety and Health Administration. https://www.osha.gov/laws-regs/standardinterpretations/2004-08-03-0

Federal Motor Carrier Safety Administration. (1994). *Qualifications of drivers and longer combination vehicle (LCV) driver instructors* (49 CFR Part 391). https://www.ecfr.gov/current/title-49/subtitle-B/chapter-III/subchapter-B/part-391

Frank, T. (2000). ANSI update: Maximum permissible ambient noise levels for audiometric test rooms. *American Journal of Audiology, 9*, 3–8. https://doi.org/10.1044/1059-0889(2000/003)

Frank, T., & Williams, D. L. (1994). Ambient noise levels in industrial audiometric test rooms. *American Industrial Hygiene Association Journal, 55*(5), 433–443. https://doi.org/10.1080 /15428119491018871

Gatehouse, S., & Noble, W. (2004). The Speech, Spatial, and Qualities of Hearing Scale (SSQ). *International Journal of Audiology, 43*(2), 85–99. https://doi.org/10.1080/14992020400050014

Gelfand, S. A. (2009). *Essentials of audiology* (3rd ed.). Thieme Publishing.

Grant, K. J., Mepani, A. M., Wu, P., Hancock, K. E., de Gruttola, V., Liberman, M. C., & Maison, S. F. (2020). Electrophysiological markers of cochlear function correlate with hearing-in-noise performance among audiometrically normal subjects. *Journal of Neurophysiology, 124*, 418–431. https://doi.org/10.1152/jn.00016.2020

Grinn, S. K., & Le Prell, C. G. (2022) Evaluation of hidden hearing loss in normal-hearing firearm users. *Frontiers in Neuroscience, 16*, 1–17. https://doi.org/10.3389/fnins.2022.1005148

Hager, L. D. (2011). Fit-testing hearing protectors: An idea whose time has come. *Noise & Health, 13*(51), 147–151. https://doi.org/10.4103/1463-1741.77217

Halmagyi, G. M., & Curthoys, I. S. (1988). A clinical sign of canal paresis. *Archives of Neurology, 45*, 737–739. https://doi.org/10.1001/archneur.1988.00520310043015

Horak, F. B., Jones-Rycewicz, C., Black, F. O., & Shumway-Cook, A. (1992). Effects of vestibular rehabilitation on dizziness and imbalance. *Otolaryngology-Head and Neck Surgery, 106*(2), 175–180.

Jacobson, G. P., & Newman, C. W. (1990). The development of the Dizziness Handicap Inventory. *Archives of Otolaryngology, Head, and Neck Surgery,*

116, 424–427. https://doi.org/10.1001/archotol.1990.01870040046011

Johnson, P. T. (2018). *Noise exposure: Explanation of OSHA and NIOSH safe-exposure limits and the importance of noise dosimetry* (Report No. ER078114-B). Etymotic Research. https://thedoctorsearplugs.com/wp-content/uploads/2018/03/White-Paper-PTJ.pdf

Joint Committee on Infant Hearing (JCIH). (2007). Year 2007 position statement: Principles and guidelines for early hearing detection and intervention programs. *Pediatrics, 120*, 898– 921. https://doi.org/10.1542/peds.2007-2333

Kardous, C., Themann, C. L., Morata, T. C., & Lotz, W. G. (2016). *Understanding noise exposure limits: Occupational vs. general environmental noise.* Centers for Disease Control and Prevention. https://blogs.cdc.gov/niosh-science-blog/2016/02/08/noise/

Kauer, T., Clayman, A. C., Nash, A. J., Schrader, A. D., Warchol, M. E., & Ohlemiller, K. K. (2019). Lack of fractalkine receptor on macrophages impairs spontaneous recovery of ribbon synapses after moderate noise trauma in C57BL/6 mice. *Frontiers in Neuroscience, 13*, 620. https://doi.org/10.3389/fnins.2019.00620

Kujawa, S. G., & Liberman, M. C. (2009). Adding insult to injury: Cochlear nerve degeneration after "temporary" noise-induced hearing loss. *Journal of Neuroscience, 29*, 14077–14085. https://doi.org/10.1523%2FJNEUROSCI.2845-09.2009

Lin, F. R., Metter, J., O'Brien, R. J., Resnick, S. M., Zonderman, A. B., & Ferrucci, L. (2011). Hearing loss and incident dementia. *Archives of Neurology, 68*, 214–220. https://doi.org/10.1001/archneurol.2010.362

Liu, L., Wang, H., Shi, L., Almuklass, A., He, T., Aiken, S., . . . Wang. J. (2012). Silent damage of noise on cochlear afferent innervation in guinea pigs and the impact on temporal processing. *PLoS ONE, 7*, e49550. https://doi.org/10.1371/journal.pone.0049550

Masterson, E. A., Tak, S., Themann, C. L., Wall, D. K., Groenewold, M. R., Deddens, J. A., & Calvert, G. M. (2013). Prevalence of hearing loss in the United States by industry. *American Journal of Industrial Medicine, 56*(6), 670–681. https://doi.org/10.1002/ajim.22082

McCaslin, D. L., Jacobson, G. P., Lambert, W., English, L. N., & Kemph, A. J. (2015). The development of the Vanderbilt Pediatric Dizziness Handicap Inventory for Patient Caregivers (DHI-PC). *International Journal of Pediatric Otorhinolaryngology, 79*(10), 1662–1666. https://doi.org/10.1016/j.ijporl.2015.07.017

Mining Safety and Health Administration. (2000). *Occupational noise exposure: Noise regulation* (30 CFR Part 62). https://www.govinfo.gov/content/pkg/CFR-2020-title30-vol1/pdf/CFR-2020-title30-vol1-chapI.pdf

Moritz, C. (2014). Noise measurement and control. In T. L. Hutchison & T. Y. Schulz (Eds.), *Hearing conservation manual* (5th ed., pp. 47–54). Council for the Accreditation in Occupational Hearing Conservation.

National Institute for Occupational Safety and Health. (1998). *Occupational noise exposure: Revised criteria 1998* (DHHS Pub. No. 98–126). http://www.cdc.gov/niosh/docs/98-126/pdfs/98-126.pdf

Neitzel, R. (2008, September 29). *NIOSH and OSHA permissible noise exposure limits.* Audiology Online. https://www.audiologyonline.com/ask-the-experts/niosh-and-osha-permissible-noise-247

Neitzel, R. L., Swinburn, T. K., Hammer, M. S., & Eisenberg, D. (2017). Economic impact of hearing loss and reduction of noise-induced hearing loss in the United States. *Journal of Speech, Language, and Hearing Research, 60*(1), 182–189. https://doi.org/10.1044/2016_JSLHR-H-15-0365

Niskar, A. S., Kieszak, S. M., Holmes, A. E., Esteban, E., Rubin, C., & Brody, D. J. (2001). Estimated prevalence of noise induced hearing threshold shifts among children 6 to 19 years of age: The third national health and nutritional examination survey, 1988–1994, United States. *Pediatrics, 108*, 40–43. https://doi.org/10.1542/peds.108.1.40

NoiseMeters Inc. (2022, December 6). *Frequency weightings—A-weighted, C-weighted, or Z-weighted?* https://noisemeters.com/help/faq/frequency-weighting/

Occupational Safety and Health Administration. (1983). *Occupational safety and health standards: Occupational health and environmental control* (Standard No. 19 CFR 1910.95). https://www.osha.gov/laws-regs/regulations/standardnumber/1910/1910.95

Occupational Safety and Health Administration. (2001). Occupational injury and illness recording and reporting requirements (Standard No. 29 CFR Part 1904). *Federal Register, 66*(198), 52031–52034.

Occupational Safety and Health Administration. (2022, December 6). *OSHA worker rights and protections—Am I covered by OSHA?* https://www.osha.gov/workers

Occupational Safety and Health Administration. (2023, May 24). *Laws and regulations—What is a standard/regulation?* https://www.osha.gov/laws-regs

Pavlou, M., Whitney, S., Alkathiry, A. A., Huett, M., Luxon, L. M., Raglan, . . . Eva-Bamiou, D. (2016). The Pediatric Vestibular Symptom Questionnaire: A validation study. *The Journal of Pediatrics, 168,* 171–177. https://doi.org/10.1016/j.jpeds.2015.09.075

Pavlou, M., Whitney, S., Alkathiry, A. A., Huett, M., Luxon, L. M., Raglan, E., . . . Eva-Bamiou, D. (2017). Visually induced dizziness in children and the validation of the Pediatric Visually Induced Dizziness Questionnaire. *Frontiers in Neurology, 8,* Article 656. https://doi.org/10.3389/fneur.2017.00656

Picard, M., Girard, S.A., Simard, M., Larocque, R., Leroux, T., & Turcotte, F. (2008). Association of work-related accidents with noise exposure in the workplace and noise-induced hearing loss based on the experience of some 240,000 person-years of observation. *Accident Analysis & Prevention, 40*(5), 1644–1652. https://doi.org/10.1016/j.aap.2008.05.013

Podsiadlo, D., & Richardson, S. (1991). The timed "Up & Go": A test of basic functional mobility for frail elderly persons. *Journal of the American Geriatric Society, 39*(2), 142–148. https://doi.org/10.1111/j.1532-5415.1991.tb01616.x

Powell, L. E., & Myers, A. M. (1995). The Activities-specific balance confidence (ABC) scale. *Journal of Gerontology Medical Sciences, 50*(1), M28–M34. https://doi.org/10.1093/gerona/50a.1.m28

Rabinowitz, P. M. (2000). Noise-induced hearing loss. *American Family Physician, 61,* 2749–2756, 2759–2760.

Rawool, V. W. (2012). *Hearing conservation in occupational, recreational, educational, and home settings.* Thieme.

Reel, L. A., Hicks, C. B., & Arnold, C. (2022). Noise exposure and use of hearing protection among adolescents in rural areas. *American Journal of Audiology, 31*(1), 32–44. https://doi.org/10.1044/2021_AJA-20-00196

Renick, K. M., Crawford, J. M., & Wilkins, J. R. (2009). Hearing loss among Ohio farm youth: A comparison to a national sample. *American Journal of Industrial Medicine, 52,* 233–239. https://doi.org/10.1002/ajim.20668

Schow, R. L., & Nerbonne, M. A. (1982). Communication screening profile: Use with elderly clients. *Ear and Hearing, 3*(3), 135–147. https://doi.org/10.1097/00003446-198205000-00007

Schulz, T., & Madison, T. (2014). Hearing protection devices. In T. L. Hutchison & T. Y. Schulz (Eds.), *Hearing conservation manual* (5th ed., pp. 107–118). Council for the Accreditation in Occupational Hearing Conservation.

Shumway-Cook, A., & Horak, F. B. (1986). Assessing the influence of sensory interaction on balance. *Physical Therapy, 66,* 1548–1550. https://doi.org/10.1093/ptj/66.10.1548

Themann, C., Suter, A. H., & Stephenson, M. R. (2013). National research agenda for the prevention of occupational hearing loss—Part 1. *Seminars in Hearing, 34*(3), 145–207. https://doi.org/10.1055/s-0033-1349352

U.S. Army. (2015). *Army hearing program* (Department of the Army Pamphlet 40-501). https://armypubs.army.mil/epubs/DR_pubs/DR_a/pdf/web/p40_501.pdf

U.S. Department of Defense. (2019). *Hearing conservation program (HCP)* (DoD Instruction 6055.12). https://www.esd.whs.mil/Portals/54/Documents/DD/issuances/dodi/605512p.pdf?ver=2017-10-25-110159-777

U.S. Department of Transportation. (2006). *Occupational noise exposure* (49 CFR Chapter 11, Part 227). https://www.govinfo.gov/content/pkg/CFR-2011-title49-vol4/xml/CFR-2011-title49-vol4-part227.xml

U.S. Marine Corps. (n.d.). *Hearing conservation.* https://www.safety.marines.mil/OnDuty/Hearing-Conservation/

U.S. Navy. (2020). *Navy medicine hearing conservation program technical manual* (NMCPHC TM-6260.51.99-3). https://www.med.navy.mil/Portals/62/Documents/NMFA/NMCPHC/root/Documents/oem/NMCPHC_TM_6260.51.99-3-NavyMedicine_HCP_TM_July_2020.pdf?ver=X8bwy910DCdrxsXuZ_ppUw%3D%3D

Ventry, I. M., & Weinstein, B. E. (1983). Identification of elderly people with hearing problems. *ASHA, 25*(7), 37–42.

Voix, J., Smith, P., & Berger, E. (2022). Field fit-testing and attenuation-estimation procedures. In

D. K. Meinke, E. H. Berger, D. P. Driscoll, R. L. Neitzel, & K. Bright (Eds.), *The noise manual* (6th ed., pp. 309–328). American Industrial Hygiene Association.

Wells, L. (2014). The "problem audiogram," the occupational hearing conservationist and the professional supervisor. In T. L. Hutchison & T. Y. Schulz (Eds.), *Hearing conservation manual* (5th ed., pp. 91–105). Council for the Accreditation in Occupational Hearing Conservation.

Whitney, S. L., Wrisley, D. M., Marchetti, G. F., Gee, M. A., Redfern, M. S., & Furman, J. M. (2005). Clinical measurement of sit-to-stand performance in people with balance disorders: Validity of data for the Five-Times-Sit-to-Stand Test. *Physical Therapy*, 85(10), 1034–1045.

Practice Questions

1. An audiologist is performing annual audiometric testing for a company that manufactures oil field pipelines. According to requirements of the Occupational Safety and Health Administration (OSHA), which of the following criteria must be used to determine if each employee has had a standard threshold shift compared to their baseline audiogram?

   a. Hearing thresholds have changed by an average of 15 dB or more at 1000, 2000, and 4000 Hz in either ear.

   b. Hearing thresholds have changed by 10 dB or more in either ear at any of the following frequencies: 1000, 2000, or 4000 Hz.

   c. Hearing thresholds have changed by 15 dB or more in either ear at any of the following frequencies: 500, 1000, 2000, or 4000 Hz.

   d. Hearing thresholds have changed by an average of 10 dB or more at 2000, 3000, and 4000 Hz in either ear.

Explanation: OSHA (1983) defines a standard threshold shift (STS) as an average change of 10 dB or more at 2000, 3000, and 4000 Hz in either ear compared to the baseline audiogram. NIOSH (1998) defines a standard threshold shift as a change of 15 dB or more in either ear at any of the following frequencies: 500, 1000, 2000, 3000, 4000, or 6000 Hz. Therefore, d is the correct answer.

2. An adult who works in very high-intensity noise wears "double" hearing protection: foam earplugs with a noise reduction rating (NRR) of 32 dB and protective earmuffs with a noise reduction rating of 25 dB. According to OSHA regulations, wearing the earplugs and earmuffs simultaneously should provide approximately how much noise reduction (attenuation)?

   a. 30 dB

   b. 37 dB

   c. 47 dB

   d. 57 dB

Explanation: According to OSHA (1983), employers can require double hearing protection if there is evidence of progressive NIHL. Wearing the second hearing protection device is assumed to provide an increase of 5 dB over the attenuation of the HPD with the higher NRR. In the example, the higher NRR is 32, so adding a second HPD would provide approximately 37 dB of attenuation. Therefore, b is the correct answer.

3. A 50-year-old adult wears earmuffs over his baseball cap and safety glasses at work. Which of the following types of individual fit testing would be most appropriate for the audiologist to use to measure the amount of noise reduction (attenuation) the worker actually receives when wearing his hearing protection at work?

   a. Real ear attenuation at threshold

   b. Loudness balance

   c. Field microphone in-the-ear

   d. OSHA correction factor

Explanation: Real ear attenuation at threshold (REAT) is the gold standard for fit testing. It can be performed in a sound booth and involves measuring the patient's thresholds with and without hearing protection. This will allow the patient to wear his own earmuffs over his baseball cap and safety glasses as he normally would at work. F-MIRE systems typically come with special earplugs with the probe built in, which means the patient could not be tested while wearing his own earmuffs. Loudness balance systems require the patient to wear headphones over earplugs. The OSHA correction factor is only applied to the NRR reported for a particular type of hearing protection. It allows for estimation of the attenuation provided by different types of hearing protection and does not involve actually measuring the attenuation. Therefore, a is the correct answer.

4. A 41-year-old male works in a tire factory. His job involves working in two different areas of the factory, one inside and one outside. Noise measurement results reveal 97 dB LAeq at his indoor work location and 88 dB LAeq at his outdoor location. On average, he spends 6 hours at the indoor location and 2 hours at the outdoor location each day. Which of the following is closest to the worker's daily noise dose using recommendations from the National Institute for Occupational Safety and Health (NIOSH)?

   a. 200%

   b. 1,250%

   c. 1,600%

   d. 1,800%

Explanation: According to NIOSH (1998), a person can be exposed to 97 dBA safely for 0.5 hours and 88 dBA for 4 hours. Using these values and the equation for dose shown below, the worker's daily dose would be approximately 1,250%. Therefore, b is the correct answer.

$$D = [C1/T1 + C2/T2 + Cn/Tn] \times 100$$
$$D = [6/0.5 + 2/4] \times 100$$
$$D = [12 + 0.5] \times 100$$
$$D = 1250\%$$

Where:
Cn = total time of exposure at a specified noise level
Tn = exposure time at which noise for this level becomes hazardous

5. In order to comply with the Occupational Safety and Health Administration's (OSHA) noise regulation, which of the following workers would not be required to wear hearing protection devices?

   a. A worker who is exposed to an 8-hour time-weighted average (TWA) of 92 dBA

   b. A worker who is exposed to an 8-hour time-weighted average (TWA) of 85 dBA who has not experienced a standard threshold shift (STS)

   c. A worker who is exposed to an 8-hour time-weighted average (TWA) of 88 dBA and has experienced a standard threshold shift (STS)

   d. A worker who started working at the company 8 months ago and is exposed to an 8- hour time-weighted average (TWA) of 89 dBA but has not received their baseline audiogram yet

Explanation: According to the OSHA (1983) noise regulation, hearing protection must be worn by employees when:

- Exposure is 90 dBA TWA or greater
- Exposure is 85 dBA TWA or greater if:
  - No baseline audiogram has been obtained after 6 months of exposure at or above 85 dBA TWA
  - An STS has occurred

Therefore, b is the correct answer.

6. A child with noise-induced hearing loss is most likely to show a noise notch at which of the following frequencies?
   a. 2000 Hz
   b. 3000 Hz
   c. 4000 Hz
   d. 6000 Hz

Explanation: Research shows that for children with noise-induced hearing loss, the noise notch typically occurs at 6000 Hz (Niskar et al., 2001). Therefore, d is the correct answer.

7. A 56-year-old male works around heavy machinery in a factory, but he does not consistently wear hearing protection because he feels that he cannot hear speech when he wears them. Which of the following types of hearing protection would be most appropriate to protect the worker's hearing while still addressing his concerns regarding hearing speech?
   a. Custom earplugs (no filters)
   b. Semi-insert earplugs with a band that goes behind his head
   c. Flat attenuation (high-fidelity) earplugs (custom or noncustom)
   d. Traditional earmuffs

Explanation: Traditional earplugs and earmuffs typically attenuate high frequencies more than mid and low frequencies. Flat attenuation earplugs and earmuffs (also called uniform attenuation, high fidelity, or musicians plugs) are designed to provide approximately even attenuation across the frequency range, thus preserving the natural balance between the low-frequency fundamental energy and the high-frequency harmonic energy. This can be beneficial for music listening and speech understanding. Therefore, c is the correct answer.

8. An audiology practice has contracts with several large companies to conduct their employees' annual audiological evaluations. In order to comply with OSHA regulations, which of the following lists all the frequencies that are required to be tested?
   a. 250, 500, 1000, 2000, 3000, and 4000 Hz
   b. 500, 1000, 2000, 3000, 4000, and 6000 Hz
   c. 250, 500, 1000, 2000, 4000, and 8000 Hz
   d. 500, 1000, 2000, 3000, 4000, and 8000 Hz

Explanation: OSHA (1983) and NIOSH (1999) both require that the baseline and annual audiometric evaluations include measuring pure-tone air conduction thresholds at 500, 1000, 2000, 3000, 4000, and 6000 Hz. Neither organization requires testing at 250 or 8000 Hz. Therefore, b is the correct answer.

9. A newborn has been in the neonatal intensive care unit (NICU) for 7 days. Which of the following would be the most appropriate hearing screening method to use based on Early Hearing Detection and Intervention (EHDI) guidelines?
   a. Otoacoustic emissions for the initial screening and any rescreening
   b. Otoacoustic emissions for the initial screening and automated auditory brainstem response (AABR) for rescreening
   c. Automated auditory brainstem response (AABR) for the initial screening and otoacoustic emissions for rescreening
   d. Automated auditory brainstem response (AABR) for the initial screening and any rescreening

Explanation: The Joint Committee on Infant Hearing (JCIH, 2007) recommends use of an automated auditory brainstem response (AABR) screening for newborns who stay more than 5 days in the NICU due to increased risk of neural hearing loss. Use of the AABR allows for detection of auditory neuropathy. Therefore, d is the correct answer.

10. A 7-month-old baby is seen for a diagnostic ABR test. Parents report the baby failed the newborn hearing screening performed 7 days after birth and the rescreening performed 2 weeks later. A diagnostic ABR was recommended, but the family was unable to attend the appointment because the family moved to a different state for the father's job. Due to challenges in establishing a new pediatrician and obtaining a referral to a local audiologist, the child is now being seen for his first diagnostic ABR. Results reveal a bilateral moderate flat sensorineural hearing loss. The child is subsequently fit with bilateral behind-the-ear hearing aids at 8 months of age. Based on Early Hearing Detection and Intervention (EHDI) guidelines, which of the following statements is true regarding identification of the child's hearing loss?
    a. The initial newborn hearing screening should have been performed within 48 hours of the child's birth.
    b. The newborn hearing rescreening should have been performed within 7 days of the initial failed screening.
    c. Because the child failed the newborn hearing screening and rescreening, the audiological evaluation to confirm his hearing should have been completed by 5 months of age.
    d. Since a hearing loss was identified, early intervention services (including fitting with amplification) should have begun no later than 6 months of age.

Explanation: Early Hearing Detection and Intervention (EHDI) guidelines (ASHA, 2022) recommend a minimum of 1-3-6 goals. This includes:
- hearing screening completion by 1 month of age,
- diagnosis of any hearing loss by 3 months of age,
- hearing aid selection and fitting within 1 month of confirmation of hearing loss, and
- starting early intervention services by 6 months of age.

For programs able to meet the 1-3-6 goal, EHDI guidelines suggest programs consider a new target of 1-2-3. Therefore, d is the correct answer.

Appendix 8–A

Comparison of the OSHA Noise Standard and the NIOSH Noise Recommendations

	OSHA	NIOSH
Noise Exposure Limits	Maximum permissible exposure level (PEL) = 90 dBA as an 8-hour time-weighted average (TWA)	Recommended exposure level (REL) = 85 dBA as an 8-hour TWA
Exchange Rate	5 dB	3 dB
Hazardous Exposure	Above the PEL (or the equivalent)	At or above the REL (or the equivalent)
Protections	Feasible administrative or engineering controls shall be used for employees exceeding the PEL. If these controls fail to reduce noise exposure to the PEL or less, hearing protection devices (HPDs) must be worn.	Feasible administrative and engineering controls shall be used to reduce noise exposures below the REL. Employees must wear HPDs if their noise exposure equals or exceeds the REL.
Ceiling	Impact or impulse noise exposure should not be greater than a peak sound pressure level (SPL) of 140 dB.	No noise (continuous, varying, intermittent, or impulse) should exceed 140 dBA.
Action Level	8-hour TWA of 85 dBA or a dose of 50%	
Noise Exposure Monitoring	Conducted for employees with noise exposure of 85 dBA TWA or greater	Conducted for employees with noise exposure of 85 dBA TWA or greater
Noise Monitoring Strategy	Use representative personal noise sampling when workers move around, noise levels vary significantly, or impulse noise is present.	Can use a task-based exposure monitoring strategy when workers move around and/or noise levels vary
Types of Noise Included	All continuous, intermittent, and impulse noise from 80 to 130 dBA	All continuous, varying, intermittent, and impulse noise from 80 to 140 dBA
Instrumentation	Calibrated sound level meter or dosimeter set to slow and dBA	Calibrated sound level meter (Type 2 or better) set to slow and dBA
Repeat Noise Measurements	If there is a significant increase in noise exposure	At least every 2 years for workers with an 8-hour TWA of 85 dBA or greater
Audiometric Testing	Available for all employees exposed to 85 dBA TWA or greater	Provided for all employees exposed to 85 dBA TWA or greater
Audiometric Test Personnel	Audiologist, a physician, a technician certified by the Council for Accreditation in Occupational Hearing Conservation (CAOHC), or an individual with equivalent training	Audiologist, a physician, a technician certified by the Council for Accreditation in Occupational Hearing Conservation (CAOHC), or an individual with equivalent training

continues

	OSHA	NIOSH
Test Frequencies	Air-conduction, pure-tone audiometry at 500, 1000, 2000, 3000, 4000, and 6000 Hz	Air-conduction, pure-tone audiometry at 500, 1000, 2000, 3000, 4000, and 6000 Hz
Audiometric Equipment	Audiometers must meet ANSI S3.6–1969.	Audiometers must meet ANSI S3.6–1996.
Calibration	Daily functional check, annual acoustical check, and exhaustive calibration every 2 years	Daily functional check, acoustical check when the daily check shows a threshold difference greater than 10 dB in either headphone at any frequency, and exhaustive calibration every year or when the acoustic check indicates the need
Test Environment	Test rooms must not have noise levels (in dB SPL) greater than: • 500 Hz = 40 • 1000 Hz = 40 • 2000 Hz = 47 • 4000 Hz = 57 • 8000 Hz = 62 Measured using at least a Type 2 sound level meter (ANSI S1.4–1971)	Following ANSI S3.1–1991, test rooms must not have noise levels (in dB SPL) greater than: • 125 Hz = 49 • 250 Hz = 35 • 500 Hz = 21 • 1000 Hz = 26 • 2000 Hz = 34 • 4000 Hz = 37 • 8000 Hz = 37 Measured using at least a Type 1 sound level meter (ANSI S1.4–1983)
Baseline Audiogram	Within 6 months of exposure at or above 85 dBA TWA or 1 year if testing using a mobile test van Must be preceded by at least 14 hours without workplace noise exposure (can substitute use of hearing protection)	Before employment or within 30 days of employment for workers exposed to 85 dBA TWA or greater Must be preceded by at least 12 hours of quiet (cannot substitute use of hearing protection)
Annual Audiogram	Performed for all employees with noise exposure at or above 85 dBA TWA	Performed for all employees with noise exposure at or above 85 dBA TWA Referred to as the "monitoring audiogram"
Test Scheduling		Should be scheduled at the end of or late in the work shift to detect any temporary threshold shifts
Threshold Shift	Standard threshold shift (STS)—Average change of 10 dB or more at 2000, 3000, and 4000 Hz in either ear compared to the baseline audiogram	Significant threshold shift—Change of 15 dB or more in either ear at any of the following frequencies: 500, 1000, 2000, 3000, 4000, or 6000 Hz
Audiometric Retest	Can retest within 30 days	Can retest immediately but must retest within 30 days

	OSHA	NIOSH
Audiogram Review	Must be performed by an audiologist or physician	Must be performed by an audiologist or physician
Baseline Revision	Annual audiogram with the STS becomes the new baseline	Annual audiogram with the significant threshold shift becomes the new baseline
Notification	Employees must be notified in writing within 21 days if an STS is detected.	Employees must be notified within 30 days if a significant threshold shift is detected.
Actions After a Threshold Shift	Required actions: • Fit, train, and require the employee to use hearing protection • Refit and retrain employees who have previously worn hearing protection • Refer for evaluation by an audiologist or otolaryngologist if a medical pathology of the ear is suspected • Notify employees when an otologic exam is needed for an ear problem that is nonwork related	A minimum of the following appropriate actions: • Reinstruct and refit hearing protection • Retrain on worker responsibilities for hearing conservation • Reassign to work in a quieter area
Availability of Hearing Protection	Available to all employees exposed to 85 dBA TWA or greater at no cost to the employee Must be replaced as needed	
Use of Hearing Protection	Must be worn by employees when: • Exposure is 90 dBA TWA or greater • Exposure is 85 dBA TWA or greater if no baseline audiogram has been obtained after 6 months of exposure at or above 85 dBA TWA or an STS has occurred	Must be worn by employees when noise is 85 dBA TWA or greater Provided at no cost to the employee
Hearing Protection Selection	Must allow employees to select from a variety of appropriate options	Must train employees at least annually to select, fit, and use a variety of appropriate hearing protectors
Employee Training	Must train employees in care and use of hearing protection	
Hearing Protection Fitting	Must ensure appropriate initial fit and supervise correct use	
Hearing Protection Attenuation	Must attenuate to at least 90 dBA (85 dBA if the employee has had an STS)	Must attenuate to below 85 dBA TWA

continues

	OSHA	NIOSH
Hearing Protection Evaluation	Evaluation based on the NRR when using the dBC or the dBA scale for noise measurement:	Evaluation using correction factors applied to the NRR to estimate field attenuation:
	Estimated Exposure (dBA) = TWA (dBC) – NRR	Earmuffs—Subtract 25% from the NRR
	Estimated Exposure (dBA) = TWA (dBA) – (NRR – 7)	Formable earplugs—Subtract 50% from the NRR
	Strongly recommended correction factor for estimating field attenuation:	All other earplugs—Subtract 70% from the NRR
	Estimated Exposure (dBA) = TWA (dBC) – [NRR × 50%]	
	Estimated Exposure (dBA) = TWA (dBA) – [(NRR – 7) × 50%]	
Double Hearing Protection	*NRRh—Represents the higher NRR of the two types of protection	Should be worn by employees exposed to greater than 100 dBA TWA
	Estimated Exposure (dBA) = TWA (dBC) – (NRRh + 5)	
	Estimated Exposure (dBA) = TWA (dBA) – [(NRRh – 7) + 5]	
Employee Involvement	Reevaluate when employee noise exposure increases to the point that the current hearing protection may not provide sufficient attenuation	Train employees at least annually to select, fit, and use a variety of appropriate hearing protectors
Hearing Conservation Training Program	Provided to employees exposed to 85 dBA TWA or greater and must ensure participation	Provided to employees exposed to 85 dBA TWA or greater and must ensure participation
Hearing Conservation Training Program Topics	• Effects of noise on hearing • Purpose of HPDs, advantages, disadvantages, and attenuation of different types of HPDs • Instructions on selection, fitting, use, and care of HPDs • Explanation of audiometric testing	• Effects of noise and hearing loss • Selection, fitting, use, and care of HPDs • Audiometric testing • Roles and responsibilities of employers and employees in preventing NIHL
Hearing Conservation Training Timeframe	Repeated annually	Repeated annually
Recordkeeping	Store all noise exposure records for at least 2 years	Store all noise exposure records for 30 years
	Keep all audiometric test records for at least the duration of employment	Keep all audiometric test records for the duration of employment, plus 30 years
	Transfer all records to the next employer if the business is sold	

Chapter 9

Treatment: Topics in Amplification

Emily Jo Venskytis and Melanie Lutz

Introduction to Hearing Aids

Modern hearing aid (HA) technology has progressed from basic analog amplifiers to complex digital signal processing. Many HA styles are now available to accommodate a range of hearing loss severity, provide increased comfort, improve accessibility and connectivity with communication devices, and enhance cosmetic appeal. Within the casing of each HA, similar processing takes place at the fundamental level. Refer to Chapter 3 for a description and visual of digital signal processing (DSP) basics. The term HA used in this chapter will refer to prescription hearing aids (non-over-the-counter devices) unless otherwise noted.

Candidacy

HA candidacy is first determined by a comprehensive audiologic evaluation. If aidable hearing loss is identified, the audiologist may proceed with amplification or make a medical referral. All pediatric patients must be evaluated by a physician prior to a HA fitting. Requirements for when to refer adult patients to an otolaryngologist may vary by state. Clinical findings that warrant a referral prior to hearing aid fitting include but are not limited to:

- The patient has an outer-ear malformation.
- There is occluding cerumen and/or a foreign body identified in the external auditory canal (depending upon the audiologist's scope of practice defined by their state).
- The patient reports, or the audiologist identifies, active ear drainage in the last 90 days.
- There is a sudden onset of hearing loss, either unilateral or bilateral.
- The patient reports acute or chronic dizziness.
- The audiologic evaluation identifies significant air-bone gaps or a significant asymmetry between ears.

In addition to audiologic and otologic indicators, a patient-centered care approach supports the consideration of additional personal factors to guide amplification recommendations for each patient. These considerations include:

- The patient's identified needs and difficulties
- The patient's perspective of their activity limitations and participation restrictions
- The patient's level of motivation to obtain and consistently utilize amplification
- The patient's goals
- The patient's activities of daily living

HA candidacy decisions also include whether the patient should be fit monaurally (in one ear) or binaurally (in both ears). Patients with bilateral hearing loss should normally be fit binaurally. Benefits of binaural amplification include:

- Loudness summation: binaural amplification provides equal access to sound at each ear, which increases the perception of loudness.
- Reducing negative consequences of the head shadow effect: the intensity of a sound arriving from one side of the head is reduced when it reaches the other side of the head. High-frequency sounds arriving at one ear may be attenuated 10 to 15 dB at the contralateral ear. A monaural HA fitting on a patient with bilateral hearing loss may exacerbate this effect.
- Speech intelligibility in noise: an improvement in speech intelligibility in noise is expected when using binaural amplification compared to monaural amplification.
- Sound localization: localization relies on comparisons made between amplitude and time differences of sound reaching each ear. Monaural HA fittings on a patient with bilateral hearing loss will negatively impact their localization by distorting the interaural timing differences and interaural level differences between ears. Binaural HA fittings should result in improved sound localization compared to a monaural HA fitting.

 AUDIOLOGY NUGGET

Although binaural amplification is typically recommended for patients with bilateral hearing loss, some individuals may have poorer speech recognition associated with a binaural HA fitting compared to a monaural fitting. This phenomenon is known as binaural interference, and research suggests it is present in 16.7% of listeners (Mussoi & Bentler, 2017). Speech-in-noise tests such as the Hearing in Noise Test (HINT) as well as monaural (right and left tested separately) versus binaural aided word recognition testing may help the audiologist identify binaural interference in patients with a preference for one HA rather than two.

When individuals with hearing loss forgo the implementation of amplification, they may face negative effects on their health and well-being. Potential consequences of untreated hearing loss include:

- Exertion of additional effort to hear and understand speech compared to normal-hearing peers. This may result in stress, strain, and fatigue related to communication experiences throughout their day.

- Avoidance of the stress of communication difficulties by withdrawing from social activities. A withdrawal from community may lead to anxiety, loneliness, and/or depression.
- Poor job performance and reduced earning potential
- Decrease in alertness and environmental awareness may result in safety risks.
- Negative effects on memory and a frequently discussed relationship with cognitive decline

AUDIOLOGY NUGGET

Untreated hearing loss is associated with cognitive decline; however, research has yet to determine a causal link (i.e., cause-effect relationship) between the two. At this time, it is incorrect to state that untreated hearing loss causes cognitive decline. Additional factors related to untreated hearing loss, such as reduced communication and isolation, must also be considered. For additional information on this topic, please refer to Slade et al. (2020) or Yeo et al. (2022).

The timely diagnosis of hearing loss and administration of amplification is especially crucial for pediatric patients when the desired communication method is spoken language. The Joint Committee on Infant Hearing (JCIH) Position Statement 2007 dictates a goal for Early Hearing Detection and Intervention (EHDI) to maximize linguistic and literacy development for children who are deaf or hard of hearing. Guidelines were created and are referred to as the 1, 3, 6 rule. Per the 1, 3, 6 rule, infants should receive a newborn hearing screening by 1 month of age. If indicated, a comprehensive diagnostic evaluation should be completed by 3 months of age. For those who qualify, early intervention services and audiologic and/or otologic management should be initiated by 6 months of age. In 2019, EHDI updated these guidelines and now recommend that those states able to meet the 1, 3, 6 rule should now meet a 1-, 2-, and 3-month timeline.

KNOWLEDGE CHECKPOINT

A patient's chronological age is the age as determined by their date of birth. Not all children develop in line with their chronological age. Delayed physical, intellectual, and/or social development may place a child at a younger developmental age, compared to their chronological age. It is important to consider the patient's developmental age when anticipating their ability to participate in behavioral testing or meet auditory milestones.

Hearing Aid Technology

When compared to analog HAs of the past, modern HA technology has become increasingly smaller and electronically more sophisticated. The advent of DSP drastically improved the ability to manipulate HA settings and create a more comfortable fit with the potential for improved audibility without feedback.

Power Source

Energy is provided to HAs via disposable or rechargeable batteries.

- Disposable batteries are typically air-activated zinc batteries, available in a range of sizes coded by color and number. Larger batteries (i.e., 13 or 675) are used for HAs with more powerful output capabilities and will last longer compared to smaller batteries (i.e., 10 or 312).
  - Battery life will depend on several things, for example, daily length of use, battery size, and utilization of different functions in the HA (such as streaming). Battery size is also linked to the lifespan of the battery: Larger batteries (10–14 days) last longer than smaller batteries (4–10 days). More wireless (streaming) usage will reduce the battery life.
- Rechargeable HAs are typically equipped with lithium ion (Li-Ion) batteries. It is recommended that a rechargeable HA is placed on the manufacturer-specific charger each night to ensure a full day of HA use.

Transducers and Amplifiers

Regardless of HA style, the internal components remain relatively the same. Two essential internal components are transducers and amplifiers.

- A transducer converts one type of energy to a different type of energy. The pathway of sound traveling through a DSP HA requires multiple energy conversions.
- Transducers in modern HAs include the microphone, the receiver, and the telecoil.
  - The microphone converts acoustic signals to electric signals (i.e., analog to digital signals).
  - The telecoil converts electromagnetic signals to electric signals.
  - The receiver converts the electric signal to an acoustic signal.
- The amplifier provides gain to incoming acoustic signals. Electric input waveforms are digitized then converted back to analog.
  - Gain of a HA is sound or additional "volume" added to the incoming signal. ANSI (2014) defined gain as the difference between the output and input sound pressure level (SPL) in a coupler. This numerical value is expressed in decibels (dB).
  - Output of a HA is the total sound produced by the HA. This numerical value is expressed as dB SPL.

Gain and Amplitude Compression

HAs can operate in linear and nonlinear ways. The term linear refers to changes in output that coincide with equal changes in input (as input increases by 10 dB, output increases by 10 dB). Nonlinear refers to changes in output that do not coincide with equal changes in input (as input increases by 10 dB, output increases by 5 dB). In this case, there is a 2:1 relationship, which is referred to as the compression ratio (CR).

- This relationship can be viewed in Figure 9–1 wherein the dashed line shows an increase in input (along the x-axis) from 20 to 40 dB (change of 20) equaling a change in output (along the y-axis) from 60 to 80 dB (change of 20). This represents a linear input/output function. Now view the change in input from 40 to 60 dB (change in 20) and the corresponding

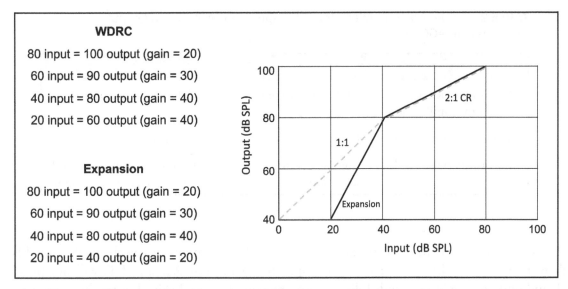

FIGURE 9–1. Graphical representation of compression and expansion. This image conceptualizes the input to output of compression and expansion as compared to a linear (1:1) input-output function.

change in output from 80 to 90 dB (change in 10). This is a nonlinear input/output function demonstrating nonlinearity or compression (specifically a CR of 2:1).

- The compression knee point (TK) is the point at which compression is activated (gain is reduced) and the input/output becomes nonlinear. Gain is linear below this point and nonlinear above this point (as shown in Figure 9–1). The TK is often described by being either high or low based on the specific compression application.

- A high TK is typically ≥85 dB SPL, meaning gain will not be reduced until the incoming signal reaches 85 dB SPL. The decision to implement a high TK may be made to maximize listening comfort by limiting the output of the HA but limiting the compression (gain reduction) of average conversational speech (approximately 65–70 dB SPL).

- A low TK describes a TK <50 dB SPL. A low TK may be used to increase the audibility of soft sounds but reduces gain for conversational speech levels, which can have deleterious consequences for speech recognition. In these cases, increasing the TK allows for more linear processing of conversational level speech and potential improvements in speech understanding.

HA compression can be categorized as input (AGC-I) or output compression (AGC-O). See Table 9–1 for distinctions between these types of compression. The time it takes for HA compression to activate and deactivate is also variable and directly impacts sound quality and signal integrity. These factors are known as the attack time (AT) and release time (RT).

- AT is the time elapsed between the onset of a sound at or above the TK and the adjustment to reduce gain.

- RT is the time between the cessation of the sound that activated compression (and reduced gain) and the return of HA gain to precompression levels.

Adaptive RTs reduce distortion by automatically changing the RT depending on the length of the compression activating signal. The use of fast ATs and RTs may be useful in providing improved

TABLE 9–1. Differences Between Input Compression (AGC-I) and Output Compression (AGC-O)

VARIABLE	AGC-O	AGC-I
AGC occurrence in relation to amplification	After volume control	Before volume control
Subject of compression	Output signal	Input signal
Role of volume control	Volume control can alter knee point	Change in volume control will not change knee point

audibility for low-level consonant sounds present after higher-intensity vowel signals, but this may result in temporal envelope distortion of the speech signal. Slow ATs and RTs will not provide as much audibility to low-level sounds following compression (reduced gain) but results in less temporal envelope distortion. Temporal envelope cues are important for listeners with poor frequency selectivity associated with increasing degrees of hearing loss. The choice of fast- or slow-acting compression should be made based on the individual patient. For more information including the advantages and disadvantages of compression speed, please review Moore (2008).

Frequency-specific manipulation of gain is made possible due to an increased number of compression channels and frequency bands.

- Compression channels are frequency regions that can be manipulated independently of each other across the frequency range. This allows for varying levels of compression characteristics at different frequencies.

- Frequency bands are regions where gain can be independently adjusted. An adjustment to one frequency band impacts gain for all levels of input within that frequency band.

- The ability to manipulate multiple compression channels and/or frequency bands enables the audiologist to program HAs for a wide array of audiometric configurations.

- The technology of multichannel compression allows the HA to more accurately respond to acoustic input comprising one frequency region, without impacting the entire frequency range. However, research also demonstrates that a higher number of compression channels may lead to distortion of temporal and spectral cues (Souza, 2002), and as such, care should be taken when adjusting compression parameters.

- Modern HAs also feature improved noise management because of multichannel compression.

An individual with hearing loss typically experiences reduced hearing sensitivity to soft sounds (due to OHC dysfunction and loss of the active mechanism of the cochlea). Meanwhile, the impact on audibility of moderate to loud sounds is more limited. The audiologist must place a vast number of environmental sounds that vary in intensity into the reduced dynamic range of the patient.

- Wide dynamic range compression (WDRC) enables modern HAs to be programmed in such a way that the user perceives soft sounds as soft yet audible, moderate sounds as comfortable, and loud sounds as loud but comfortable by adjusting the amount of gain for each input level (see Figure 9–1). See Table 9–2 for more information on WDRC. While WDRC is often the preferred choice for HA programming, potential drawbacks include the following:

☐ Background noise may be amplified in situations where the background noise is softer than the speech signal because of increased gain for lower-level inputs.

☐ The gain may not be adequate for someone with a severe-to-profound hearing loss who requires more gain for higher input level signals, sometimes near maximum power output (MPO).

☐ Patients may be bothered by soft sounds (e.g., refrigerator running, clocks ticking) that they are not used to hearing due to increased gain for low-level inputs (which may be reduced by expansion, which will be described).

In utilizing WDRC to make soft sounds audible, potentially bothersome, low-level sounds may also become noticeable. This includes machine noise from household appliances or even internal noises from the HA (referred to as equivalent input noise or EIN). Expansion is a strategy for low-level sound reduction that helps to ensure perceived quiet when the patient is in a quiet environment.

■ Expansion provides different amounts of gain depending on the incoming signal, similar to compression.

■ Unlike compression, expansion acts on inputs with intensity levels below the expansion knee point and <u>decreases gain as signal input level decreases</u> (as sounds become softer less gain is applied). This can be visualized in Figure 9–1.

■ While the reduced amplification of low-level sounds may increase comfort for some, it also has the potential to decrease audibility of low-level speech sounds when the expansion threshold is set at a high intensity (above approximately 40 dB SPL). Therefore, it is especially important to consider the impact of expansion on HA programming for pediatric patients who require audibility of soft speech sounds for speech and language development.

■ Another potential benefit of expansion is reducing EIN (commonly referred to as circuit noise) when listeners possess normal low-frequency hearing thresholds (typically below 10–15 dB HL).

TABLE 9–2. Wide Dynamic Range Compression

CHARACTERISTIC	WDRC	REASONING
Compression Type	Multichannel	Provides hearing aid programming flexibility needed for a variety of hearing loss configurations
Compression Knee Point	Low, typically 50 dB SPL or lower	Makes soft sounds audible
Input or Output Control	AGC-I	Better to achieve goal of audibility
Attack Time and Release Time	AT: <20 ms RT: 10–100 ms (short), >500 ms (long)	HA users with lower cognitive status may be negatively affected by fast release times, dependent on speech stimulus (Cox & Xu, 2010)
Compression Ratio	4:1 or less	Ratios greater than 4:1 may cause excessive distortion of the signal

AUDIOLOGY NUGGET

The advent of power DSP HAs (circa 2003–2004) presented an opportunity to introduce listeners with severe-to-profound sensorineural hearing loss (SNHL) to digital HAs. Anecdotally (according to the authors of the text, JD and KF, who are of a certain age and remember fitting these devices on patients), many of these patients reported low-level sounds to be too intense but conversational speech as unclear, mumbled, or garbled. These complaints were contrary to what was expected of this high-quality DSP aid, and most patients preferred the analog processing of their previous HAs.

So, why were these complaints likely occurring? If WDRC processing was implemented, the complaints were likely due to the fact that having a low TK increased gain for low-level input, to which they were not accustomed, and compression (gain reduction) of signals at conversation speech intensity (65–75 dB SPL), thus creating the situation where low-level sounds were too intense and conversational speech was being altered in a negative way through unwanted reductions in gain.

Noise Reduction

Digital noise reduction (DNR) is an additional tool available in modern HAs. Noise in this case is defined as undesirable background sounds and may include mechanical noise, multitalker babble, wind noise, and other common environmental sounds.

- The goal of DNR is to limit the amplification of noise compared to the speech signal, that is, improve the signal-to-noise ratio (SNR). DNR is accomplished primarily through gain reduction at affected bands but may also implement adaptive beam forming via directional microphones.

- The HA utilizes an environmental classification algorithm that continuously assesses temporal, spectral, and intensity of sound input. The HA will then determine if DNR is needed, how much is needed, and how fast to implement changes.

- DNR does not improve speech intelligibility for HA users, but it may improve comfort of listening in noise and reduce listening effort.

DNR in pediatric HA programming may limit chances for incidental language learning and is not always recommended but depending on the age of the child may be warranted. Several studies with school-aged children found that DNR did not impact word recognition and improved novel word learning in children ages 11 to 12 years, and therefore these technologies may be appropriate for older children who can effectively manage their use. Special consideration should be made for children with a greater degree of hearing loss. More severe hearing loss may result in poorer audibility in background noise and different outcomes with DNR (McCreery et al., 2012). For more information on DNR, please review Bentler and Chiou (2006).

Directional Microphones

Microphones can be directional or omnidirectional and have specific applications for various listening environments.

- A directional microphone is more sensitive to sounds arriving to the front of the listener and less sensitive to sounds arriving to the sides and back.

- An omnidirectional microphone does not include directional sensitivity and is equally sensitive to sounds arriving from all directions.

- Figure 9–2 includes the polar plots of various microphone sensitivity options. The polar plot is a 360° representation of microphone sensitivity to sounds arriving from different locations.

- Directionality is quantified using the Directivity Index (DI), which is a single-number indicator of directional performance (higher values providing more directionality). Typical first-order directional microphones (two microphone systems) provide for a DI value between approximately 3 and 4, with second-order microphones (three or more microphones) resulting in increased directionality. For a more detailed review of directional microphones, please review foundational information from Ricketts (2005) as well as a recent review on novel directional microphone technology by Zhang (2020).

- HA manufacturers are consistently updating the functionality of directional microphone systems and techniques used to improve speech recognition in noisy listening conditions, making it important to continually update one's knowledge of these systems.

Acoustic Feedback

Feedback reduction aims to suppress the signal components of HA output that escape from the receiver and are picked up by the microphone and reamplified (acoustic feedback loop). Two common methods of feedback reduction include adaptive gain reduction and feedback path cancellation (often referred to as phase cancellation).

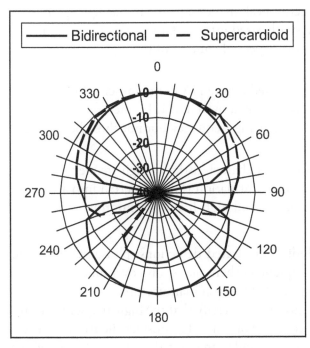
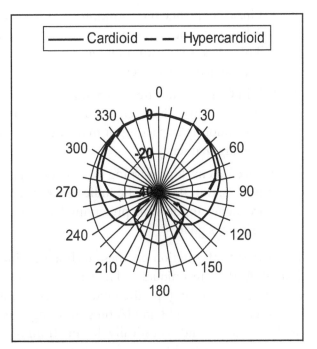

FIGURE 9–2. Polar plots for hearing aid microphone configurations. Microphone directionality as seen from a 360° graphic representation. *Source*: From *Essentials of Modern Hearing Aids: Selection, Fitting, and Verification* (pp. 1–888) by Ricketts, T. A., Bentler, R., & Mueller, H. G. Copyright © 2019 Plural Publishing, Inc. All rights reserved.

- Through adaptive gain reduction, the HA works to automatically reduce gain at a specific channel when feedback is detected.

- Feedback path cancellation (phase cancellation) creates an internal signal that is opposite in phase, thus reducing/eliminating the feedback. This method does not require significant gain reduction.

- Additional methods to prevent feedback include creating a well-fitting earmold, modifying venting parameters, and ensuring proper placement of the receiver or earmold in the ear canal.

- Limiting gain is typically considered a last resort for dealing with acoustic feedback.

Frequency Lowering

Although the use of modern HA features discussed above allows the audiologist to adequately fit a range of hearing loss configurations with expanded frequency ranges, high-frequency amplification continues to be variable above approximately 6000 Hz. For patients with high-frequency hearing loss, this often means certain high-frequency consonant sounds (e.g., /s/, /sh/, /th/) are left underamplified and inaudible. Frequency-lowering (FL) technology is implemented to deal with the limitations of high-frequency amplification for certain and more severe degrees of hearing loss. Four major FL techniques are utilized across different manufacturers, including linear frequency compression, linear frequency transposition, nonlinear frequency compression (NLFC), and spectral envelope warping (Alexander, 2013).

- Linear frequency compression uses a spectral balance detector to analyze the frequency components of incoming signals. If the energy of the signal is greater in the frequency region above 2500 Hz, compared to the region below 2500 Hz, frequency lowering will activate. If not, frequency lowering will not be implemented.

- Linear frequency transposition identifies a spectral peak in a designated frequency region. A band of input around the spectral peak is resynthesized into the target frequency region. This process is continuous when activated, but the spectral content of the input will determine what signals are impacted.

- NLFC uses a start frequency that may be manipulated by the HA programmer, which typically ranges between 1500 Hz and 6000 Hz. When activated, this FL method will continuously impact input frequencies above the starting frequency but not those below the starting frequency.

- Spectral envelope warping occurs as the HA looks for characteristics of high-frequency information that may be indicative of speech. This information is then inserted into a lower-frequency input while preserving harmonic structure and high-frequency information of the original signal.

For detailed information on these techniques, including illustrated depictions, please see Alexander (2013). As these techniques and how manufacturers implement them may evolve over time, the authors recommend reviewing specific (and current) details provided by each manufacturer.

When activating FL in HA programming, it is important to verify that the high-frequency sounds are both audible and acoustically distinct from one another. For example, consider the fricative speech sounds /s/ and /sh/. FL may place those sounds into an audible range for the patient, but they may not be distinguishable from one another and should be verified. Figures 9–3, 9–4, and 9–5 provide techniques by which FL is commonly verified.

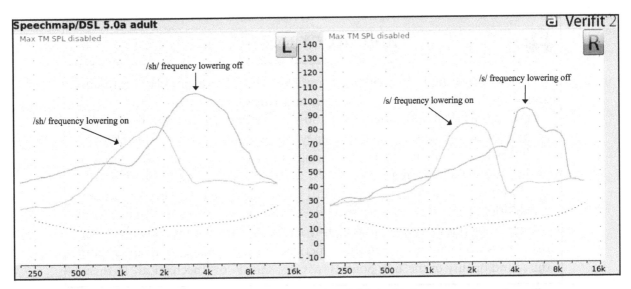

FIGURE 9–3. Difference in HA acoustic output for /s/ and /sh/ with frequency lowering off vs. on.

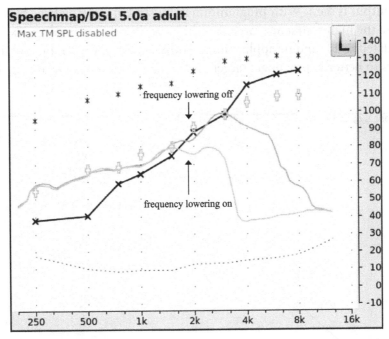

FIGURE 9–4. Speechmapping results with frequency lowering off vs. on.

- Figure 9–3 shows the acoustic output produced by a HA for the /sh/ and /s/ sound with frequency lowering off and on. Note the expected shift in peak energy to a lower frequency for both speech sounds.

- Figure 9–4 shows Speechmapping results for a steeply sloping audiogram with frequency lowering off and on. With frequency lowering off (the full bandwidth option), the high-frequency targets (4000 Hz and above) are not met. This is often the case with steeply sloping audiograms and highlights the difficulties amplifying significant high-frequency hearing loss

AUDIOLOGY NUGGET

Frequency lowering is especially important to the pediatric population. Infants and young children are learning speech and language and require access to all speech sounds (Stelmachowicz et al., 2004). HAs can be limited in their ability to provide access to soft high-frequency sounds (e.g., /s/, /z/, /sh/) through traditional gain. The use of FL technology in pediatric patients has proven to be beneficial to high-frequency speech detection and recognition (Glista et al., 2009). FL should be considered in HA fittings when the hearing loss and capabilities of HA output prevent the HA from meeting prescriptive targets in frequency regions that encompass high-frequency speech sounds. Note, however, that adults who have not previously experienced FL may have complaints about the sound quality of the aids: Sounds may be "slushy" or "mechanical" to them.

with traditional techniques. With FL on, the shift in peak energy and reduction of high-frequency output is seen. With programming adjustments, it may have been possible to better approximate the high-frequency targets in this case, but this example is used to illustrate concepts related to FL and its applications. Additionally, in the FL on condition, gain adjustments to better approximate targets at frequencies 1 to 4 kHz are needed.

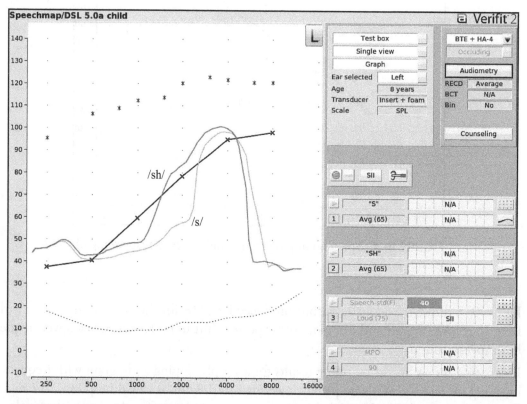

FIGURE 9–5. Example of Speechmapping verification of distinction between /s/ and /sh/ with frequency lowering on.

■ Another means of verifying FL is to evaluate whether the processed /s/ and /sh/ sounds are acoustically distinct, meaning the /s/ sound produces a HA output that is distinctly different from the /sh/ sound. This is shown in Figure 9–5, where the two sounds (both recorded with FL on) produce a distinctive acoustic output for the listener. This technique must be interpreted with the caveat that while the acoustic output of the HA produces two distinct tracings, it should not be assumed that this difference is perceptible to the listener and should be verified with behavioral discrimination.

Connectivity

Many HAs are equipped with short-range communication abilities. Depending on the manufacturer, this may connect via near-field magnetic induction (NFMI), 2.4 GHz (commonly referred to as Bluetooth technology), or 900 MHz communication. This allows for communication between a pair of HAs and communication to manufacturer-proprietary accessories.

■ Ear-to-ear communication between HAs allows for optimized signal processing such as speech-in-noise and advanced directionality features.

  □ NFMI is often used for this type of communication due to the short-range capabilities and relatively low battery drain.

■ Accessory devices such as basic remote microphones, television audio streaming devices, and remote controls also use short-range communication.

  □ 2.4 to 2.48 GHz or 900 MHz are often used for these functions due to the longer-range capabilities compared to NFMI.

An additional feature within HAs is the telecoil. The telecoil (T-coil) is a small copper wire within the HA casing that acts as a receiver. T-coils can be found in landline telephones or looped systems around venues. With the advent of Bluetooth compatibility, T-coil use has declined in the United States. Venues such as public theaters, community meeting rooms, and places of worship may be equipped with a looped system that patients may utilize.

■ The advent of Bluetooth compatibility for HAs allows users to wirelessly stream audio to their HAs from connected devices such as smartphones and tablets. This can include phone calls, music, video audio, and more. The specific Bluetooth capabilities of the device are dependent on the type of Bluetooth technology incorporated into the HA and varies by manufacturer. Additional uses for Bluetooth include:

  □ Wireless programming

  □ Identifying last known location of a lost HA

  □ Mobile app use for easily accessible program and/or volume adjustment

In addition to traditional HAs, remote microphone hearing assistive technology (RM-HAT) is commonly used. These include frequency modulation (FM) systems and digital modulation (DM) systems.

■ Both FM and DM systems can be utilized to improve the signal-to-noise ratio (SNR) with the primary differences being the transmission method.

■ RM-HAT systems consist of a remote microphone placed near the desired speech signal. That signal is transmitted to the users' HAs via a receiver, an ear-level nonamplifying device, or a speaker system.

- The benefits of RM-HAT are pervasive in the literature in support of using ear-level RM-HAT systems in children with hearing loss to improve SNR in the classroom (Anderson & Goldstein, 2004; Anderson et al., 2005).

- RM-HAT systems have also proven beneficial in normal-hearing patients with a central auditory processing disorder (Schafer et al., 2020).

- The recent advent of integrated RM-HAT receivers into HAs without an additional attached receiver component has increased ease and accessibility of system use.

 AUDIOLOGY NUGGET

Children require more favorable SNRs compared to adults because children are less able to utilize contextual cues and are still developing language and auditory processing skills. The ANSI Standards for classroom acoustics includes a SNR of at least +15 dB at the child's ears. Despite this, typical classrooms are regularly impacted by high reverberation times and background noise sources such heating and cooling systems. Rabelo et al. (2014) found average classroom SNRs at 54 to 74 dBA. As such, implementing RM-HAT systems can positively impact the SNR for children with hearing loss.

Additional Features

HA programming software allows the audiologist to create multiple programs for the patient to manually adjust situational HA function. Although modern HAs are able to make real-time changes in response to the environment, there are certain situations where the patient may benefit from manually switching to different predetermined settings. Examples of programs include:

- Noise program: a HA patient may consistently experience increased difficulty hearing in noise when entering a particular space. For example, a college student may have difficulty hearing friends when in the cafeteria. A noise program may be created by increasing directionality of the microphones and increasing noise reduction.

- Music program: for patients who enjoy listening to live music or playing an instrument, a music program is often recommended. Programming changes to this may include disabling features such as noise reduction, feedback management, and frequency lowering.

- Tinnitus program: patients with tinnitus may utilize customizable tinnitus maskers and tinnitus management activities within manufacturer apps aimed to distract the HA user from their tinnitus.

Datalogging is a feature in modern HAs that provides the audiologist with a numerical representation of HA wear time between programming sessions.

- Typically, this value is the number of hours worn divided by the number of days since the HA was last connected to the manufacturer software. This is provided as an average daily wear time.

- Programming software may also provide insight into how often the patient spends in each of their HA programs and how often they spend in various types of listening environments (e.g., quiet, noise, speech-in-noise).

- HA wear time can be a useful indicator of how well the patient is complying with HA use.

- Datalogging is especially useful when working with pediatric patients. If a pediatric patient is seen for a HA check and datalogging reveals an average daily wear time of 0.5 hours per day, additional counseling and goal setting with the patient and their family is warranted.

 Q & A

Question: What is the current status of over-the-counter (OTC) amplification devices and when is an OTC appropriate to recommend to a patient?

Answer: A relatively new factor to consider when assessing HA candidacy and counseling patients on audiologic intervention is OTC hearing devices. In an effort to increase accessibility of amplification to Americans with hearing loss, the United States Food and Drug Administration (FDA) released a final ruling on OTC HAs effective October 17, 2022. The ruling states that OTC HAs will be available for adults ages 18 years or older with a mild-to-moderate hearing loss. The devices may come ready to wear out of the box or may utilize technology for consumer self-fitting. Additionally, consumers interested in OTC HAs are not required to obtain an audiologic evaluation or prescription for the devices, nor will they be required to pursue any follow-up care from a licensed hearing healthcare professional. At this time, the exact features that will be available in OTC devices are not known.

Hearing Aid Types and Styles

HAs are available in a variety of styles offering a range of comfort, cosmetic appeal, power, and performance. Appendix 9–A displays a list of traditional HA styles and their characteristics.

- One additional HA style is the invisible in-the-canal (IIC) HA, which is smaller than a CIC. The HA manufacturer Phonak has created an IIC known as the Lyric™. This device is inserted into the external auditory canal by professionals who have received specific training with the device.
  □ The Lyric remains in the ear canal at all times and is not removed until the battery needs to be replaced. Phonak states that the Lyric™ can last a maximum of 120 days before it needs replacing.
  □ Other manufacturers create IICs that are removable by the patient.

Other HA options exist beyond the traditional HA types listed above. This includes the contralateral routing of signals (CROS) and bilateral contralateral routing of signals (BICROS).

- CROS, named for its function of contralateral routing of signal, is an amplification option recommended for patients with unilateral hearing loss when the poorer-hearing ear cannot benefit from a traditional HA due to the severity of the hearing loss and/or poor word recognition scores and the better-hearing ear has normal hearing.
  □ A patient with a CROS wears an ear-level device on each ear (a transmitter on the poorer ear and receiver on the normal-hearing ear). Recently, these are receiver-in-the-canal (RIC) devices with an open fitting.

- □ The CROS device (transmitter) is worn on the poorer-hearing ear. The CROS detects sounds arriving at the poorer ear and transmits to the receiver of the device worn on the normal-hearing ear, often utilizing NFMI ear-to-ear communication.

- □ No amplification is added to the signal delivered to the normal-hearing ear.

- A BICROS system is recommended for patients with an asymmetrical hearing loss where the poorer ear cannot benefit from traditional amplification and the better-hearing ear also requires amplification. Acoustic input reaching the poorer ear is routed to the better-hearing ear and presented along with the addition of gain prescribed for the loss in the better-hearing ear.

- Additional information about CROS and BICROS can be found in the comprehensive literature review by Stewart and Woodward (2021).

- A relatively new amplification option for those with asymmetrical hearing loss is AmpCROS. With an AmpCROS system, the signal arriving at the device worn on the poorer-hearing ear will be amplified and sent to both ears. The device on the better-hearing ear will deliver the amplified signal from the other HA, along with a signal picked up from that HA. As this amplification system is new to the market, additional research on its use and clinical value is needed.

Hearing Aid Coupling

Earmolds

Noncustom HAs like the behind-the-ear (BTE; traditional, RICs, and slim tubes) require a method of retention to channel sound from the HA into to the ear canal. The type of HA coupling selected must consider degree of hearing loss and gain requirements, risk of feedback, and patient preference. HA coupling can be a custom-made earmold or a non-custom modular fitting.

A modular fitting includes various sizes and shapes of small disposable domes. These can be used as coupling options for RIC HAs and BTE HAs fit with a slim tube. Dome-style options include closed dome, open dome, semi-open/tulip dome, and double/power dome.

- A nonoccluding dome allows for a more open fit that can reduce occlusion effect and improve patient comfort. The domes are easy and low cost to replace. Domes are also considered less visible and more cosmetically appealing. With a non-custom dome, sound is more likely to escape the ear canal, and therefore gain potential is limited.

- Unfortunately, as gain requirements increase, the greater the likelihood of feedback occurring when using a dome as compared to a more tightly fitting custom earmold option. Another drawback to modular fittings includes ease of insertion. A patient with limited dexterity may have more difficulty properly inserting a dome into the ear canal compared to a larger custom earmold.

- It should be noted that while modular fittings have the potential to reduce occlusion, certain dome styles such as power/double domes can create a seal similar to that of a closed fit. Therefore, the occlusion effect is still possible with a modular fitting depending on dome characteristics.

A custom earmold begins with the creation of an earmold impression. There are several earmold impression materials, including methyl methacrylate and silicone. Silicone, which is more commonly utilized, has a high viscosity and can result in a tighter-fitting earmold, which may be required for high-gain applications (those with severe or severe-to-profound hearing loss). For a comprehensive review of earmolds, their applications, acoustical properties, troubleshooting, and other pertinent information, please refer to the *Microsonic Custom Earmold Manual* (https://store.microsonic-inc.com/manual/earmolds_manual2.pdf).

 AUDIOLOGY NUGGET

Some patients with chronic middle ear disease or other otologic disorders require one or more otologic surgeries. These procedures may result in a change in the size and shape of the ear canal and/or external auditory meatus. Increased care and attention are needed when creating earmold impressions for this patient population due to the changes in ear canal shape, which may create difficulty in removing the impression material once it hardens. Collaboration with an otologist can be helpful to assist in packing the ear cavity prior to inserting impression material. This can improve the resulting earmold and prevent complications from earmold impressions.

The earmold may be created using a variety of materials, including acrylic, polyethylene, vinyl, and silicone. The selection of earmold material may depend on texture of the ear, degree of hearing loss, age of patient, and any known allergies to one of the earmold materials. See Table 9–3 for a list and

TABLE 9–3. Custom Earmold Styles

CUSTOM EARMOLD	DESCRIPTION
Full Shell	Accommodates more severe hearing losses due to maximal retention. Most common selection for infants and young children. May be slightly harder to insert due to large size.
Half Shell	Similar to full shell but top portion of canal is removed.
Skeleton	Can accommodate a range of hearing loss severity. More cosmetically appealing than full shell.
Canal	Best for a mild to moderate hearing loss. With a well-fitted earmold, accommodates more severe losses. May be easier to insert, but retention may not be as secure.
Custom Open	May be best for open fit BTE or CROS. Improved retention compared to a noncustom coupling option.
Canal Lock	Similar to a canal style with an added "lock" that lays posterior against the concha bowl.
Semi-Skeleton	An open-fitting custom option.

description of custom earmold styles. Special considerations for earmolds should be made for pediatric patients; these include:

- The frequency of remakes needed and the durability of the earmold material.
  - □ Infants and young children grow quickly and will require new earmolds frequently.
  - □ More durable material may be required for smaller earmolds due to the size of the tubing compared to the ear canal to prevent ripping with everyday use.
- The warranty on the earmolds and the cost per mold
- Color and design options
- Tamperproof options such as cemented tubing and tube locks

Venting

When selecting custom earmolds for HA coupling, the audiologist must also select venting options. Venting is used to manage the occlusion effect, increase comfort, and in some instances allow for low-frequency sounds to enter the ear canal naturally. There are a number of vent options, including parallel, diagonal, trench, select-a-vent (SAV), pressure, and acoustically optimized venting (AOV).

- The use of a vent impacts the low-frequency response more than high-frequency response. Specifically, the greater the vent diameter, the less low-frequency gain will reach the tympanic membrane due to low-frequency signals escaping the ear canal and a mixing of natural sound with processed sound.
- A reduction in the low-frequency response can increase patient comfort by reducing unwanted amplitude and occlusion. For many individuals with a downward-sloping high-frequency hearing loss, with normal hearing in the low-frequency region, a larger vent can enable low-frequency sounds to reach the ear more naturally. However, the greater the vent size, the greater the chance of feedback, as more HA output will escape the ear canal.
- Parallel venting (where the vent runs parallel to the sound bore) is typically preferred to diagonal venting (where the vent intersects the sound bore) due to the possibility of reducing the high-frequency output. Diagonal venting is often used with small ear sizes where parallel venting is not possible. Trench venting involves creating a groove or channel along the bottom of the HA or mold (near the bottom of the canal). Trenching a vent is typically a last resort when significant occlusion is reported and other solutions prove to be ineffective at reducing occlusion.
- Occlusion can exist because of the physical presence of the HA in the ear or due to acoustic features of HA programming. One way to quickly assess the source of occlusion is to have the patient speak while the HA is in their ear and turned off. If the patient continues to report the same concerns, the problem is physical occlusion. If the reported concerns are resolved, this is acoustic occlusion. Physical occlusion can be addressed by modifications to the HA like a different canal length or vent diameter. An acoustic occlusion may be addressed using frequency modifications, such as a decrease in low-frequency gain. For more information on dealing with occlusion and other related hearing aid sound quality troubleshooting, refer to *The Starkey Compression Handbook* available on their website (https://order.starkeypro.com/pdfs/The_Compression_Handbook.pdf).

■ Venting is not appropriate for all HA users, especially those with greater degrees of hearing loss. As a general rule, the greater severity of hearing gloss, the smaller the recommended vent size due to the need to amplify low-frequency input as well as reduce the possibility of feedback. A pressure vent is typically required for individuals with severe-to-profound losses if venting is desired. Many manufacturers and earmold companies offer the option of requesting what is often referred to as an AOV prescribed based on their experience and research. For additional details related venting and its applications, please refer to the *Microsonic Custom Earmold Manual* (https://store.microsonic-inc.com/manual/earmolds_manual2.pdf).

Ear Hooks

BTEs commonly utilize ear hooks, which aid in retention of the HA while also funneling sound from the HA to the tubing. It is important for pediatric and adult patients that the size of the ear hook is appropriate. Ear hooks may also be selected based on their acoustic characteristics, such as dampers.

■ Dampers are made of a screen-like material and are included in some ear hooks.

■ Damping is used to reduce resonant peaks in the mid-frequency region (approximately 1–3 kHz) of the HA frequency response.

■ Wavelength resonances contribute to resonant peaks and while modern HA technology can smooth peaks, the use of dampers provides additional smoothing.

■ The positioning of the dampers can also be manipulated for different acoustic effects. The closer the damper is in relation to the tubing, the greater the effect of the damper.

Tubing

HA coupling also includes tubing selection. The National Association of Earmold Laboratories created a naming convention for tubing based on tube diameter in 1979. The #13 tubing, also referred to as standard tubing, is the most common tubing diameter, especially for traditional BTE fittings.

■ A thin tube (0.90–0.95 mm internal diameter) may be used for mini-BTEs in place of an ear hook and traditional tubing configuration. Reducing the internal diameter of tubing will lower both the frequencies of resonant peaks and the magnitude of the peaks. Thin tubing will also create more roll-off (reduced frequency response) in the high-frequency region. Thus, a slim tube coupled with a BTE and custom earmold may not be an appropriate tubing option for a patient with a significant high-frequency hearing loss. Slim tubes may provide improved aesthetics over standard tubing and may be considered with mild-to-moderate hearing losses in the high-frequency region.

■ To naturally increase the high-frequency response (above 2–3 kHz), Libby Horns or belled bores (sound bores that increase in diameter) can be utilized. To naturally reduce the high-frequency response, reverse horns can be utilized. It should be noted that due to the advent of digital hearing aids and the ability to fine-tune the frequency response using programming software, the use of earmold coupling to modify frequency responses is often less utilized. However, modifying the acoustic coupling of a fitting to naturally alter the acoustic response should not be discounted as a means of improving the quality of the fitting.

Q & A

Question: Patient X is a 13-month-old with bilateral, moderately severe SNHL. She is fit with traditional behind-the-ear HAs and a full-shell silicone earmold with #13 tubing. Which venting selection would be best for this patient and why?

Answer: In this case, no venting should be added to the earmolds. This hearing loss requires a high level of gain across the frequency range. The introduction of a vent would allow some of that needed output power to escape out of the ear canal (particularly in the low-frequency region). A vent in this case would potentially create feedback. Additionally, venting should be used with caution in pediatric patients as it allows another point for sound to escape and can exacerbate feedback as the child outgrows their earmold. If this were an adult patient, one might consider a pressure vent depending on certain fitting and patient characteristics, but in the case of a child, venting is not advisable.

Hearing Aid Fitting

Programming

The means by which a HA is programmed related to gain and other signal processing considerations is determined by its prescriptive fitting method. Each prescriptive method configures the HA programming to provide amplification based on audiometric and patient characteristics. Prescriptive fitting methods can be divided into the following two categories:

- Proprietary fitting strategies: these prescriptive fitting methods are specific to a particular HA company and software. Each proprietary method uses algorithms developed based on research by the HA company to program the signal processing features and gain characteristics of the HA.

- Device-independent (universal) fitting strategies: the use of thresholds and/or loudness discomfort levels (LDLs) are used to calculate coupler or real ear targets. The targets can be applied to any programmable HA and are not derived from the HA manufacturer.

With the foundations of loudness equalization and loudness normalization, a variety of device-independent fitting strategies were developed. Device-independent fitting strategies include the following:

- NAL-NL2: created by National Acoustic Laboratories, this strategy is designed to maximize speech intelligibility while maintaining a comfortable level of loudness.
  - □ Loudness equalization, the method of amplifying speech so that all speech frequencies are perceived as equal in loudness, is at the foundation of this strategy.
  - □ Provides less low-frequency gain compared to other listed strategies
  - □ NAL-NL2 provides more high-frequency emphasis compared to other methods (except DSL).
  - □ Uses relatively low compression ratios.
  - □ When the entered age indicates a pediatric fitting, NAL-NL2 will increase the overall gain.

- DSL v5: created by faculty at the University of Western Ontario, this acronym in this strategy stands for "desired sensation level."

  - Loudness normalization (i.e., maintaining the natural amplitude differences across frequencies) is at the foundation of this strategy.

  - This strategy was initially developed for pediatric HA fittings and is typically the preferred fitting formula for pediatric HA fittings.

  - The goal of DSL v5 is to maximize speech information without creating discomfort.

  - Utilizes threshold data without needing LDL values.

  - There is a "pediatric" and "adult" version of the DSL v5, with the pediatric version prescribing more gain overall.

- IHAFF: the independent HA fitting formula is used to restore loudness perception across the entire frequency range.

  - Loudness normalization is the foundation of this strategy.

- FIG 6: The Figure 6 fitting strategy is used to calculate gain on a frequency-specific basis for three input levels (40, 65, 90 dB).

  - Loudness normalization is the foundation of this strategy.

  - This strategy is not recommended for hearing losses with thresholds greater than 70 dB HL.

 Q & A

Question: How do the amplification needs of children differ from those of adults? Do clinicians need to modify the characteristics of amplification and prescribed gain based on the patient's age?

Answer: Unlike adults with acquired hearing loss who have significant language experiences, children are actively developing speech and language. The success of this development relies on adequate auditory access to speech sounds across the frequency range. It is widely accepted that there is a greater importance of both high-frequency and soft speech information for children due to the speech spectra of their frequent communication partners (women and other children) and the need for and benefits of incidental language learning. According to the American Academy of Audiology (AAA, 2013) Pediatric Amplification Guidelines, "The primary goal of amplification is to provide, to the degree possible given the hearing loss and limitation of hearing aid amplification, audibility across the long-term average speech spectrum (LTASS), without delivering any signal that is of an intensity that would be either uncomfortable or unsafe" (p. 8). Additionally, children are at an increased risk for the adverse effects of noise on speech recognition and they require a more favorable SNR (McCreery et al., 2012). The American Speech-Language-Hearing Association's (ASHA) Working Group on Classroom Acoustics recommends a signal-to-noise ratio of at least +15 dB at ear level. The use of appropriately fit HAs as well as remote microphone technology in the classroom are both important to achieve this recommendation.

- CAM 2: the Cambridge fitting formula focuses on speech levels of 65 and 85 dB SPL.
  - □ Loudness equalization is the foundation of this strategy.

Hearing Aid Verification

HA verification refers to a process of using objective measurements to ensure appropriate HA programming for a particular patient. Verification can be performed while the patient wears the HA, using a probe microphone, or in a specialized test box using a coupler in place of the patient's ear cavity. The use of real ear (sometime referred to as probe microphone) or coupler measures to verify HAs is considered best practice for device fittings. The following are terminology related to HA verification, with expanded information provided for commonly utilized measurements.

- Frequency response: total output of the HA measured in dB SPL
- Gain: HA output level subtracted by HA input level
- Real ear unaided response (REUR): SPL as a function of frequency measured in an unaided and open ear canal
- Real ear aided response (REAR): SPL as a function of frequency in a person's ear canal with the HA inserted and turned on
- Real ear to coupler difference (RECD): difference between the output of a stimulus in the ear canal compared to the output of the same stimulus in a 2-cc coupler
  - □ This value will vary based on the individual's ear canal volume (the physical size of their ear canal) and is useful in creating an improved HA fitting by correcting for the individual's ear canal volume in the fitting software. These values can be measured or estimated by the verification equipment, with measured RECD values being the preferred method.
  - □ The use of RECD values is especially important in pediatric HA fittings as children's ear canal volumes will differ from a 2-cc coupler (and the estimated RECD values) more than in adults. Children's ear canal volumes are often smaller than the 2-cc coupler, and without measured RECD values, HA fittings may be inappropriate if calculated in the coupler and not using on-ear measures.
- Real ear unaided gain (REUG): Gain created from the individual's pinna and ear canal, as measured in the ear canal; provides information regarding natural resonance of the ear
- Real ear aided gain (REAG): HA gain measured in the ear canal
- Real ear insertion gain (REIG): gain created by insertion of the HA calculated by subtracting REUG from REAG
- Even if real ear verification utilizing on-ear measurements is not possible, for example, due to patient inability to sit still during the verification speech passage, the clinician should still strive to obtain RECD to verify HA output in conjunction with test box verification. Test box verification can be completed using HA couplers in conjunction with the patient's RECD to simulate the patient's ear canal as an alternative to completing the entire verification on ear. If RECD cannot be completed due to patient tolerance, ear drainage, occluding cerumen, or other clinical contraindication, an age-specific estimation of RECD may be used. See Table 9–4 for a brief overview of available coupler types.

Real ear measures enable the clinician to:

- Fine-tune and individualize HA output

TABLE 9–4. Coupler Types

COUPLER TYPE	DESCRIPTION
HA-2	2 cc. Measures acoustic pressure generated by behind the ear hearing aids. Hearing aid is connected to coupler via tubing.
HA-1	2cc. Measures acoustic pressure generated by ITE/ITC hearing aids. Putty material is used to hold hearing aid in place.
HA-3	2 cc. Designed to test faceplates before they have been fully assembled. Rarely used and difficult to acquire.
CIC	Small volume of 0.4 cc representative of ear canal volume associated with deeper insertion of CIC

- Verify the in-situ HA response is meeting prescribed targets
- Verify that in-situ performance is stable at annual evaluations
- Verify output of HA is not exceeding uncomfortable levels (UCLs/LDLs), which are manually entered or predicted based on the patient's hearing loss

The first step in completing HA verification using real ear measures is to achieve a proper probe tube placement in the ear canal. The tip of the probe tube should be placed within 5 mm of the tympanic membrane. If the probe tube is not sufficiently deep in the canal, reflective interference and radial waves can distort high-frequency measurements, leading to a reduced high-frequency response. Newer verification equipment can emit a broadband signal and provide the clinician with an indication as to when insertion depth is sufficient.

 Q & A

Question: A 2-month-old baby is identified with a moderate sensorineural hearing loss using auditory brainstem response (ABR) in both ears and hearing aids are recommended. How do you use the ABR data to program the hearing aids?

Answer: Hearing thresholds can be derived from ABR testing using tone-burst stimuli to estimate hearing levels; however, the unit of measure for an ABR (dB nHL) is different from behavioral hearing data (dB HL). These units differ for a few reasons. The first is that dB nHL was developed using different referent values from dB HL. Second, behavioral and electrophysiologic tests are not evaluating the same region of the auditory system. Third, the stimuli are different between tone-burst ABRs and behavioral measures. For these reasons, among others, a correction factor needs to be applied to convert dB nHL values to estimated hearing levels for hearing aid fittings, referred to as dB eHL. Correction factors vary by frequency and fitting formula. For more information on using correction factors for ABR thresholds, refer to Fuglholt (2010).

Electroacoustic measurements can be completed with a verification system by using the test box. These measurements include but are not limited to:

- OSPL90: output sound pressure level assesses the maximum output of a HA by measuring the response to a 90 dB SPL input stimulus.

- Harmonic distortion: harmonic distortion occurs when a single frequency is presented as input to the HA and the output contains the addition of an undesired frequency. The harmonic distortion test provided in the Verifit2 measures harmonic distortion at the second or third harmonics while varying input level and frequency.

- Directionality: the directionality of HA microphones may be assessed by presenting noise to the back microphone and speech stimuli to the front microphone. The intensity level of both types of stimuli can be manipulated while the SPL is recorded.

- Noise reduction: the output of the hearing aid is measured both before and during the presentation of a broadband noise stimulus. A comparison can be made between the noise and the hearing aid's response to the noise, which provides a noise reduction value measured in dB.

- Input/output: a curve displaying HA output created based on the input stimulus intensity and frequency.

- ANSI test: a sequence of tests performed to assess HA regulations designated by ANSI S3.22. The HA should be positioned in the test box as specifically directed by the verification equipment protocol.

- Battery drain test: measures the current of the battery while presenting varying inputs frequencies and amplitudes. Battery life is estimated based on those measurements.

For additional details on various topics related to verification, please refer to the *Audioscan Verifit2 Users Guide* (Audioscan, 2022).

 KNOWLEDGE CHECKPOINT

The speech intelligibility index (SII) is an electroacoustic measurement that uses a patient's audiometric thresholds and the HA output to calculate a number from 0.0 to 1.0, which is often converted to a percentage from 0% to 100%. This percentage is correlated with the amount of speech that will be audible (not intelligible) to the patient, with a higher obtained SII value equating to increased audibility and potential for intelligibility. For example, an SII value of .5 or 50% equates to 50% of average conversational speech being audible to the listener.

The SII is a value that may be used to counsel patients and their families. The aided SII value can be utilized to demonstrate how HAs improve speech audibility (Stiles et al., 2012). The unaided SII may also be used to indicate the need for amplification, as demonstrated by low unaided SII values. When assessing HA programming, SII data may assist the audiologist in determining if increasing gain levels to increase SII values (audibility) is required. For additional information on the SII, please review Hornsby and Mueller (2004).

CROS and BICROS Verification

Verification of a CROS or BICROS device is performed differently than traditional HAs. Probe microphone measures may be completed using a verification system to confirm that the CROS/BICROS is able to overcome the head shadow effect while worn by the patient without over- or underamplifying the better-hearing ear (i.e., does the system improve high-frequency output naturally reduced by the head and torso). Most manufacturers offering CROS and BICROS technology provide detailed guides to complete on-ear verification. Specific instructions for verification of CROS systems can be found in the Verifit2 manual listed in the references.

Hearing Aid Validation

HA validation includes functional outcomes of HA use and subjective measures of performance. Validation measures include the following:

- Aided threshold detection
  - □ This may be completed with the patient wearing their device(s) to respond to sounds via a soundfield speaker utilizing age-appropriate audiometric test techniques.
  - □ This technique may have limitations related to the negative interaction between automated HA systems such as compression, digital noise reduction, and expansion and the detection of tonal signals. Currently, there is debate regarding the utility and accuracy of aided threshold measurements.
  - □ For a comprehensive review of this topic, refer to Kuk and Ludvigsen (2003).
- Speech perception testing
  - □ Speech perception measures can help determine device benefit by comparing speech perception skill progression over time and the difference in speech perception with and without amplification. Speech perception testing can occur in a variety of settings including:
    - Testing with or without noise
    - Varying intensity levels (comparing soft speech to conversational speech intensities)
    - Closed-set testing versus open-set testing
  - □ Speech perception tests differ between adult and pediatric patients, and the patient's developmental status should be taken into consideration when choosing an assessment measure.
- Language outcomes
  - □ Language outcomes can be assessed in collaboration with a speech-language pathologist and should be monitored in the pediatric population.
- Quality of life outcomes
  - □ Assessing health-related quality of life (HRQOL) is a validation measure that can examine a patient's outcomes on a more global scale. HRQOL can include an individual's perception of their mental and physical health, as well as their social well-being (Yin et al., 2016).
  - □ A HRQOL outcome measure related to hearing loss and amplification is the Hearing Environments and Reflection on Quality of Life (HEAR QL). These questionnaires were

designed for children and adolescents who have hearing loss. The HEAR QL examines how the patient experiences their hearing loss and identifies potential areas of the patient's life that could use additional hearing support.

- Surveys assessing functional outcomes
  - □ Functional validation measures provide insight into everyday listening experiences and skill development. Input can be received by the patient as well as their communication partners. Some examples include International Outcome Inventory for Hearing Aids (IOI-HA), Client Oriented Scale of Improvement (COSI), and the Abbreviated Profile of Hearing Aid Benefit (APHAB). For the pediatric population, these measures can include feedback from parents and teachers.

Special Populations

Pediatric Minimal or Mild Hearing Loss

The recommendation of amplification as a means for auditory habilitation or rehabilitation is not always straightforward when one considers the degree of hearing loss. For patients with hearing loss severity ranging from moderate to severe, amplification is typically a standard recommendation. For those with a minimal or mild hearing loss, however, management plans vary. Prior to the implementation of universal newborn hearing screenings, a minimal or mild hearing loss may have easily been missed as its effects are often more subtle than that of a more severe hearing loss. Currently, minimal and mild hearing losses are identified more often and at earlier ages.

- Research shows children with a minimal degree of hearing loss are at risk for negative outcomes in areas including speech-language and education (McKay et al., 2008).
- Some individuals from this population may benefit from amplification.
- Current research supports using unaided SII when considering whether to recommend amplification for a minimal/mild hearing loss. Calculations of SII should always include real ear to coupler difference measures, when possible. If the child has an unaided SII <0.8 in the better ear, they should be considered for amplification (McCreery et al., 2020).
- All pediatric patients with minimal or mild hearing loss should be considered candidates for a RM-HAT system per the American Academy of Audiology Pediatric Amplification Protocol (2013).

Auditory Neuropathy Spectrum Disorder (ANSD)

HA candidacy in the ANSD population is another instance of complex decision-making.

- For children with ANSD, hearing sensitivity cannot be accurately determined using objective test techniques in the same way as children with SNHL. The ABR can predict hearing thresholds for SNHL, but the ABR is significantly abnormal or absent with ANSD and therefore cannot be used for threshold estimation.
- There is no current consensus on sufficient evidence for a hearing aid fitting protocol for children with ANSD. According to the AAA 2004 Pediatric Amplification Guidelines,

children with ANSD should begin a HA trial once behavioral audiologic testing indicates hearing sensitivity is not adequate for conversational speech audibility. If significant concerns exist regarding access to sounds in patients with ANSD, close behavioral observations of the child's responses to sounds can be used to guide hearing aid fitting prior to obtaining true behavioral thresholds (Walker et al., 2016).

- Unfortunately, even a complete audiologic evaluation is not always a reliable indicator for amplification performance due to fluctuations in hearing sensitivity associated with ANSD.

- The audiologist must determine if the patient's speech understanding improves with the addition of amplification.

- Regardless of hearing thresholds, patients with ANSD should always be considered for a RM-HAT system due to the poorer performance in noise than those with other types of sensorineural loss.

Unilateral Hearing Loss (UHL)

The management of patients with UHL is also considered a special case as there are several treatment options and the success of patients can vary significantly. An individual with unilateral hearing loss wherein the poorer ear presents with hearing loss from mild to severe and is therefore a candidate for traditional amplification may pursue the following options:

- Unilateral, conventional HA fitting
- No amplification
  - □ In this instance, environmental modifications may be discussed.
  - □ Close audiologic monitoring is recommended even when the patient does not pursue audiologic intervention.

For those cases of UHL in which the poorer-hearing ear is not aidable due to the severity of hearing loss and/or poor word recognition, the following options are available:

- CROS
- Bone-anchored hearing device for single-sided deafness (SSD)
- Unilateral cochlear implant (CI)
- No amplification

Conductive Hearing Loss

For patients with conductive or mixed hearing loss who have an intact ear canal, air-conduction HAs are an option. The managing audiologist should consider the following:

- Power level: when an air-bone gap is present, more gain than for sensorineural losses (to overcome the conductive component) with the same air-conduction thresholds is required.
  - □ Tables 9–5 and 9–6 review the target values for average (65 dB SPL) speech signal in the Verifit2® for a flat 60 dB HL hearing loss with average RECD. This compares (1) prescribed values for a SNHL with bone-conduction thresholds equivalent to air-conduction thresholds and (2) prescribed values for a conductive hearing loss with bone-conduction

TABLE 9–5. Comparison of Prescriptive Targets for NAL-NL2 With Sensorineural Versus Conductive Hearing Loss

	FREQUENCY (Hz)									
	250	500	750	1K	1.5K	2K	3K	4K	6K	8K
NAL-NL2 target outputs for average LTASS with a flat, 60 dB HL sensorineural hearing loss	56	66	66	66	69	73	75	72	66	62
NAL-NL2 target outputs for average LTASS with a flat, 60 dB HL conductive hearing loss	83	84	80	77	81	85	86	84	74	71
Difference (conductive-SNHL)	27	18	14	11	12	12	11	12	8	9

TABLE 9–6. Comparison of Prescriptive Targets for DSL v5 Pediatric for a Sensorineural Versus Conductive Hearing Loss

	FREQUENCY (Hz)									
	250	500	750	1K	1.5K	2K	3K	4K	6K	8K
DSL v5 pediatric target outputs for average LTASS with a flat, 60 dB HL sensorineural hearing loss	81	82	80	80	79	83	83	83	78	75
DSL v5 pediatric target outputs for average LTASS with a flat, 60 dB HL conductive hearing loss	85	86	84	84	82	87	87	87	81	77
Difference (conductive-SNHL)	4	4	4	4	3	4	4	4	3	2

thresholds at 10 dB HL. As shown for both NAL-NL2, in Table 9–5, and for DSL v5 pediatric, in Table 9–6, when there is an air-bone gap, additional gain is prescribed across the frequency range.

■ If gain requirements cannot be met with an air-conduction HA, a bone-conduction hearing device (BCHD) should be considered.

Introduction to Cochlear Implants

Some individuals do not receive benefit from traditional amplification, for example, those with more severe degrees of hearing loss and/or poor word recognition abilities. To provide better access to the auditory signal for this population, a cochlear implant (CI) may be required. All CIs comprise two general components, external and internal.

■ The CI uses an external component to take an acoustic signal, digitally filter it into components, and prepare it for electric stimulation. The external component is called the sound processor, which contains microphones and a digital signal processor, and an external coil and magnet with a transmitter

  □ The external coil and magnet may be separate from the processor when the processor is at ear level, or it may be contained within one unit and is all at the connection point on the head in an off-the-ear configuration.

- The information is then transmitted to the internal component, which provides the electrical stimulation to the cochlea via an electrode contact using biphasic electrical pulses (pulses containing both a positive and negative voltage). The internal component comprises a receiver-stimulator, which contains a communicating coil, a digital signal processor, a stimulatory device, and an electrode array.

- The CI is intended to communicate directly via the auditory nerve, specifically with the spiral ganglion cell bodies being the target of stimulation.

Candidacy

CIs undergo regulatory approval by the Food and Drug Administration (FDA) and are considered Class III medical devices that are subject to the most stringent approval and review process due to the risk level of the patient. The individual manufacturers carry the burden of presenting the quality and safety of their devices after extensive scientific testing. Because of the regulatory process, new CI components are typically only released every few years as compared to HAs, which are Class I devices and undergo less stringent review and therefore have more frequent releases.

- Labeled indications are the guidelines developed by the manufacturer and approved by the FDA that specify the patient profile for who is eligible for the device. The labeled indications specify the degree of hearing loss and word recognition score that makes a patient eligible for implantation with that device according to the FDA.

- This further supports the insurance company's approval or rejection of coverage of the device. FDA criteria differ by manufacturer and may change, so they should be reviewed at the time of evaluation.

  CI recipients may not meet the labeled indications on FDA criteria yet still undergo implantation. This is considered an off-label use of the device. Clinicians are typically granted the latitude to determine who is a CI candidate when the benefits are determined to be greater than the risks and their potential outcomes are greater than the best nonsurgical option. Evaluation of candidacy should address multiple questions.

 CASE EXAMPLE

A patient with ANSD presents with behavioral hearing thresholds from 50 to 60 dB HL across frequencies in each ear of a sensorineural nature; however, this patient has a word recognition score of 36% at 95 dB HL. With binaural HAs, the patient has a binaural word recognition score of 40% at 55 dB HL. In noise, the patient achieves 12% at a +10 dB SNR. Although this patient would not meet FDA-labeled degree of hearing loss requirement, they may be recommended for cochlear implantation in an off-label capacity due to the poor speech recognition abilities in both quiet and noise.

Of note, insurance companies may also have their own criteria for cochlear implantation, which may be more or less strict than FDA-labeled indications. When a potential recipient is undergoing candidacy evaluations, the clinician should take their insurance coverage into consideration and include that in information that is presented to the patient. If the patient is insured with Medicare, the CI team should follow the Centers for Medicare & Medicaid Services (CMS) indicated guidelines in addition to FDA indications. In 2022, the CMS guidelines were expanded and indicate a candidate is someone who meets the following criteria:

- Bilateral moderate-to-profound SNHL
- Limited benefit from HAs as indicated by less than or equal to 60% correct on aided, open-set tests of sentence recognition
- No medical contraindications to undergoing surgery
- Appropriate motivation and cognition to undergo rehabilitation

Cochlear Implant Team

CI candidacy is determined by a team approach. In adult candidacy evaluations, the CI team at a minimum should include the audiologist, the otolaryngologist or otologist, and the patient.

- Audiologist: responsible for determining audiologic components of candidacy and testing for FDA indications, setting appropriate expectations, and assisting in manufacturer and device selection based on the patient's motivation and lifestyle factors
- Otolaryngologist/otologist: responsible for medical evaluation and medical determinants of candidacy, which may include imaging studies and assessment of health regarding anesthesia
- Patient: the patient is a key team member. It is important for the patient to understand potential risks and benefits of undergoing cochlear implantation. They must also have significant motivation to commit to habilitation with the device.

In pediatric candidacy evaluations, the CI team should include the audiologist, otologist/neurotologist, patient and their family, and the speech-language pathologist. Other team members may include a neuropsychologist or social worker.

- Audiologist and otologist: serve similar roles for pediatric candidacy as for adult candidacy.
  □ Medical evaluation may be slightly different for the pediatric team as they may require different imaging, medical prevention of meningitis, and other medical evaluations based on the child's clinical presentation.
- Patient/guardian: depending on age, the patient may be a member of the team; however, the parent or guardian often assumes that key role. Guardian buy-in of the process and understanding of realistic expectations and workload for success with a CI are vital.
- Speech-language pathologist (SLP): SLPs can be certified as a Listening and Spoken Language Specialist (LSLS) and/or an Auditory Verbal Therapist (AVT). This is ideal for the CI team as the overwhelming majority (95%) of children born with hearing loss have parents with normal hearing. The SLP contributes important information regarding the child's speech and language progress that is utilized for FDA indications. They will evaluate

the child's speech and language skills compared to normative data for children their age and determine delays. They should also be involved for auditory verbal therapy post implantation for ideal outcomes.

- Social worker: can address disparities in access to services and transportation and improve overall outcomes.

- Psychologist/neuropsychologist: can evaluate the nonverbal IQ and help set realistic expectations as well as help the parents in the acceptance of the hearing loss.

Adult Audiologic Candidacy Evaluations

Adult audiologic CI candidacy measures should also be used to assess CI recipients postoperatively. Cochlear implantation is historically underrecommended in the field of audiology (Buchman et al., 2020). Expanding indications have made improved access to sound a possibility for many patients. Updated guidelines support the 60/60 rule, which states that patients should be referred for a CI candidacy evaluation if their unaided pure-tone average is poorer than 60 dB HL in the better-hearing ear and if their single-word score in at least one ear is poorer than 60% (Zwolan et al., 2020).

- Unaided evaluations: standard audiologic assessment with air- and bone-conduction assessment and immittance measures. An ideal assessment includes frequencies from 125 to 8000 Hz.
  - CI candidates should not have an air-bone gap and ideally are free from fluctuating middle ear issues.
  - Speech recognition may be included in the unaided evaluation but is not required for candidacy.
- Subjective measures: a complete candidacy evaluation will include subjective questionnaires. Some examples include:
  - Nijmegen Cochlear Implant Questionnaire (NCIQ): 60 questions, serves as a measure to assess quality of life. Comprehensive look at patient from the perspective of CI candidacy; however, may be unfamiliar to insurance companies and is not as commonly used with limited normative data and therefore interpretation can be more challenging.
  - Cochlear Implant Function Index (CIFI): evaluates performance with hearing in the candidate's day-to-day life. Looks at things such as need for visual cues and hearing in a variety of listening situations. The questionnaire has been found to correlate well to speech perception measures and patient performance after cochlear implantation. It is not widely used and therefore not as well known.
  - Other questionnaires may be used, for example, the Hearing Handicap Questionnaire, APHAB, COSI, and Speech, Spatial, and Quality of Hearing Scale (SSQ).
- Aided evaluations
  - All candidacy evaluations should be completed in the best-aided condition. It is essential that for candidacy evaluations, the recipient is in appropriately fitted HAs. All HAs should be evaluated using real ear (probe microphone) measures to determine if HAs match prescriptive settings for each individual's hearing loss. Refer to the real ear measures section of this chapter for guidance on programming HAs to prescriptive target.

◻ Aided evaluations must include sentence recognition measures as addressed in FDA guidelines. Individual word scores are not currently included in some manufacturer's FDA-labeled indications; however, studies are trending in support of using word scores for candidacy. Word scores also serve as an important baseline from which to compare implant performance. Both words and sentences should be used for pre- and postoperative evaluation of CI candidates.

◻ The Minimum Speech Test Battery (MSTB) is often utilized for both pre- and postoperative assessment. The MSTB utilizes the four following tasks:

- AZBio sentences in quiet (full 20-word list)
- AZBio sentences in noise (full 20-word list)
  - ○ Presented at +10 or –5 dB SNR
- CNC words in quiet (full 50-word list)
- BKB-SIN (16-sentence pair pre or 20-sentence pair post)

◻ The clinician should use the same assessment measures for pre- and postimplant testing. Postoperative testing should be completed for adults at 3 months postactivation and then at 6 and 12 months. Patients should then be evaluated every year thereafter.

◻ Test conditions

- 60 dBA presentation level
- Sound-treated room
- Soundfield speaker at 0 degrees azimuth 1 meter from the recipient
- Calibrated recorded materials

AUDIOLOGY NUGGET

HA recipients may not tolerate devices at their prescribed gain levels and therefore their day-to-day programming of the devices may be based on comfort rather than appropriate audibility. During candidacy evaluations, the patient's HAs may need to be reprogrammed to meet prescribed targets. If the potential recipient is not a CI candidate with appropriately fit HAs, this is an excellent counseling opportunity.

■ Candidacy evaluations should address the following:
  ◻ The patient's communication and listening goals
  ◻ Expected performance based on predictive measures
  ◻ Patient performance with their best nonsurgical treatment
  ◻ Patient's motivation and lifestyle

Pediatric Audiologic Candidacy Evaluations

Children undergoing cochlear implantation typically should strive to wear appropriately programmed HAs during all waking hours. This includes HAs fit using real ear probe microphone measures to prescriptive targets. If the child has been wearing appropriately fit amplification and are still unable to access soft speech sounds, they should undergo a candidacy evaluation for CIs. Due to the complexity of each child's speech/language skills and developmental differences, there is no common consensus of pediatric testing evaluations. As such, many of the evaluations are dictated by the child's abilities. Some general guidelines are provided here.

- Children require more access to sounds for development of speech and language and therefore off-label considerations are particularly important in the pediatric environment (Park et al., 2021). Additionally, greater outcomes are achieved with earlier implantation and implantation for children with better hearing than the most lenient current criteria.

- Unaided evaluations: standard audiologic assessment with air- and bone-conduction assessment and immittance measures.
  - For pediatric patients, testing may include otoacoustic emissions and ABR evaluation. Other behavioral electrophysiologic measures may be useful, for example, auditory steady-state response (ASSR) or cortical auditory evoked responses (CAER). For detailed information regarding these assessment measures, refer to Chapters 5 and 6.
  - Regardless of reliable objective information, an attempt at behavioral threshold assessment and speech perception should always be made in a potential pediatric CI recipient.
  - Speech recognition may be included in the unaided evaluation but is not required for candidacy.

- Subjective measures
  - Although these measures should be used with all children, these are required to be used when children cannot participate in behavioral testing and serve as a substitute for word recognition measures.
  - Subjective questionnaires may include the auditory skills checklist, LittlEars, and/or IT-MAIS. Certain questionnaires may be recommended by the insurance company for candidacy.

- Aided evaluations
  - Auditory access to speech sounds is of critical importance to pediatric patients. As soon as the child is developmentally appropriate for speech recognition testing, the clinician should obtain a baseline assessment. Frequent reevaluation of the child's speech recognition should occur during early childhood.
  - All candidacy evaluations should be completed in the best-aided condition.
  - The Pediatric Minimum Speech Test Battery (PMSTB) is a useful resource for developing a preoperative and postoperative protocol for audiologic assessment. According to the PMSTB, there are many options for evaluating speech perception when assessing implant candidacy. Descriptions of these tests and tips for success in pediatric CI candidates and recipients can be found in Table 9–7.
    - The test is chosen based on the patient developmental age and language abilities. Choose a test that corresponds with response ability of the child.
    - Closed-set versus open-set tasks are available.
    - Although the tests do have recommended age ranges in many cases, children with severe to profound hearing loss may not present with language abilities composite with their chronological age.

TABLE 9–7. Pediatric Speech Assessment Measures That Are Recommended for Cochlear Implant Candidacy Evaluations

TEST	OPEN/ CLOSED	STIMULI	CONDITION	ADVANTAGES	DISADVANTAGES
ESP	Closed	Words	Quiet	ESP Pattern: assess speech abilities with low verbal component ESP spondee and ESP monosyllable: assess higher verbal skills with large closed-set field	Complex to administer; toys may be distracting; multiple trials needed
PSI	Closed	Words, sentences	Quiet or noise	Different stimuli available	Few lists; may encounter learned practice effect
MLNT/ LNT	Open	Words	Quiet	Varying levels of difficulty; word and phoneme scoring	No normative data; may encounter learning effects
CNC	Open	Words	Quiet	Carrier phrase, adult test	Full 50-word list required, may be limited by child's attention
BKB	Open	Sentences	Quiet	Carrier phrase, single male talker	Not designed to be completed in quiet; norms for children >5 years
BKB-SIN	Open	Sentences	Noise	Carrier phrase, single male talker, variable SNR	Norms for children >5 years
Pediatric AzBio (BabyBio)	Open	Sentences	Quiet or noise	Normative data; equivalent lists; low context clues (more difficult)	Female talkers only

Note. Table is arranged in order of task difficulty with easier tasks at the top.

Source: Adapted from Uhler et al. (2017).

- o It is critically important to choose a developmentally appropriate test to get a best measure of the patient's performance.
- o If the child scores <25% on the task you attempt, consider floor effects and administer a less difficult test.
- o If the child scores from 25% to 79%, that test is currently appropriate and should be reassessed at follow-up.
- o If the child scores >80%, consider ceiling effects and administer a more difficult test.
- Test conditions vary based on test difficulty and patient ability. At a minimum, test conditions are as follows:
  - o Sound-treated room
  - o Soundfield speaker at 0 degrees azimuth 1 meter from the recipient

- ○ Ensure calibration of CD materials
- ■ Candidacy evaluations should address the following:
  - □ Family's communication and listening goals
  - □ Expected performance based on predictive measures
  - □ Patient performance with their best nonsurgical treatment
  - □ Family motivation and lifestyle
  - □ Family resources for access to services
    - • If the family does not have adequate access to services or resources to travel to appointments, other team members should be included to help the family access adequate services during the rehabilitation process.

Predicting Outcomes

Patient predictive factors are reviewed and assessed to help predict outcomes after cochlear implantation. An important thing to note about this section is that it refers to the relative overall word recognition score (i.e., sentence score) and performance in noise in comparison to other CI users. In general, even if the patient is likely to have poorer outcomes based on these predictive factors, candidates are still likely to have improved performance compared to their score with their best-fit nonsurgical amplification. Word and sentence recognition and quality of life can be improved with CIs, but audiologists can use these predictive factors to set expectations related to how the individual patient's performance will be compared to all CI recipients. Predictive factors for adult and pediatric patients are shown in Tables 9–8 and 9–9, respectively.

TABLE 9–8. Predictive Factors for Cochlear Implant Performance in Adults

PREDICTIVE FACTOR	BETTER OUTCOMES (RELATIVE)	POORER OUTCOMES (RELATIVE)	SPECIAL CONSIDERATIONS
Duration of hearing loss	Shorter duration	Longer duration	Full-time amplification use offsets duration
Age at implantation	Younger age	Older age	Duration of hearing loss linked to age; quality of life improvements with CI irrespective of age
Preoperative hearing status	Better residual hearing	Poorer residual hearing	Preoperative amplification offsets status
Etiology	Sudden idiopathic SNHL, Meniere's disease, genetic	Temporal bone fracture, acoustic neuroma, acquired ANSD	Bacterial meningitis: average performance; consider site of lesion for all patients
Cognition	Better performance with higher cognitive status	Potentially poorer performance with lower cognitive status	Dementia exacerbated with hearing loss, improving sound access prevents further cognitive decline; cognition may be improved with improved auditory signal access

Source: Key factors identified via Wolfe (2020).

TABLE 9–9. Predictive Factors for Cochlear Implant Performance in Pediatrics

PREDICTIVE FACTOR	BETTER OUTCOMES (RELATIVE)	POORER OUTCOMES (RELATIVE)	SPECIAL CONSIDERATIONS
Age of identification, management	Timely diagnosis and treatment	Delayed diagnosis and/or treatment	Most important factor. Critical for identification as soon as hearing changes, and management with amplification and appropriate intervention as soon as possible.
Mode of Communication	Listening and spoken language	Signed or manual communication	Influenced by child characteristics, family need, expected outcomes. Highest performers may be more likely to use listening and spoken language but may have initially used signed language.
Etiology	Genetic (particularly GJB2, SLC26A4, Usher syndrome)	Cochlear nerve aplasia or deficiency	Etiology-less influence on pediatric outcomes; congenital ANSD better performance than acquired ANSD
Family variables	Higher maternal education level and socioeconomic status (SES)	Lower maternal education level and SES	Greater financial flexibility allows for access to therapies and services
Child-specific factors	Quality of life, access to environmental sounds, ability to connect with family and peers		Childhood hearing loss may be the result of a syndrome or co-occur with a number of factors that can cause developmental delay. Comorbidities affect the outcomes of CI use.
Preoperative hearing	Residual hearing can be useful		Preoperative residual hearing not a necessity for children
Age of implantation (for prelingually deaf children)	Earliest is best; 9 to 12 months of age at implantation yields best outcomes	Later implantation exhibits poorer outcomes	Poorer outcomes if implanted after 2 to 3 years of age. Auditory maturation as measured by late evoked potentials cannot achieve normal latencies if implanted after age 7 (Sharma et al., 2005).

Source: Key factors identified via Wolfe (2020).

Surgery

A CI surgery completed by an experienced surgeon is considered a routine procedure. Adults are typically discharged the same day and children may undergo a 23-hour stay (23 hours to avoid charges for a full-day admission). The surgical procedure involves an incision behind the ear, the lifting of the skin flap, and drilling into the mastoid cavity. Ideally, the round window should then be identified by the surgeon. There are two primary surgical approaches: a cochleostomy, which involves drilling into the cochlea, and the round window approach, which has significantly less drilling. Regardless of surgical approach, the ideal placement of the electrode array is in the scala tympani (Finley et al., 2008).

Internal Devices

The electrode array is the component of the internal device that consists of the intracochlear electrode contacts and is typically housed in silicone. This is connected to the receiver-stimulator, which is the silicone and titanium device that receives the signal from the external sound processor and drives the electrode array.

- A perimodiolar electrode array is typically a precurved array that is designed to hug the internal wall of the scala tympani and position close to the modiolus. This type of array has the benefit of reduced current needed to elicit a response from the auditory nerve due to being closely and tightly placed to the modiolus. This can in turn provide greater battery life and more efficient loudness growth.
- A lateral wall electrode array is designed to lie against the lateral wall of the scala tympani. Theoretically, this better preserves the organ of Corti and scala media structures.

As there are advances in atraumatic surgical techniques and thinner electrode arrays, there is no current evidence to indicate that lateral wall or perimodiolar arrays are preferable for hearing preservation.

Post-Implantation and Device Management

Once the CI team approves a candidate and surgery is complete, the patient is considered a CI recipient. The device can be activated 2 to 4 weeks postsurgery, depending on recipient age and surgeon recommendation.

Cochlear Implant Signal Processing

CI signal processing is manufacturer specific and often proprietary. Table 9–10 identifies key features for the CI companies' signal processing strategies and internal devices. Please note, the list is not exhaustive but can be used as a guide to differentiate components of their internal devices and features. Note, some features are common between companies.

Programming

Programming CIs, also called mapping or MAPping, is completed by the audiologist. Programming will occur throughout a recipient's life, with the most substantial changes during the first year following implantation. After the initial activation period, substantial changes are seen during other times secondary to changes in the body such as puberty, pregnancy, hormone therapy, menopause, and aging. The clinician can evaluate and adjust a variety of parameters within a recipient's device. Appendix 9–B contains definitions of parameters that can be adjusted by the clinician and descriptions on their clinical implication when changes are made.

Goals of Device Programming

The goals of programming are dependent on the timing of the visit. The audiologist will have different goals whether it is during the initial stimulation period or during subsequent visits.

TABLE 9–10. Key Features of Manufacturer-Specific Cochlear Implant Internal Components and Signal Processing

PARAMETER	ADVANCED BIONICS	MED-EL	COCHLEAR
Number of electrodes	16	12	22
Numbering of electrodes	Apex to base	Apex to base	Base to apex
Electrode coupling	Monopolar	Monopolar	Monopolar
Electrode arrays	Lateral wall and perimodiolar	Longest available, all lateral wall; hybrid	Lateral wall and perimodiolar; hybrid
Current default strategy in U.S.	HiRes Optima	FS4-P	ACE
Signal analysis	Fast Fourier transform: splits signal into envelope and spectral peak information, frequency bands	Hilbert transform: separates slow moving envelope from fine temporal structure	Band-pass filters: breaks signal down into frequency bands
Method of electrode stimulation	Current steering; up to 120 virtual channels	Electrodes 6–12 (envelope information): virtual channels	No virtual channels or current steering
Channel selection and stimulation	HiResS: completely sequential; HiResP: partially simultaneous	Electrodes 1–5 (fine temporal structure): pulse packets with channel interaction compensation; allows stimulating two electrodes simultaneously	Stimulation of maxima (channels with the highest amplitude); continuously interleaved

- Goals of initial stimulation
  - □ Recipient will tolerate full-time use of the devices.
  - □ Recipient can detect auditory stimuli at a comfortable level.
- Goals of follow-up programming appointments

 KNOWLEDGE CHECKPOINT

The electrical dynamic range is different depending on the manufacturer of the device being programmed. Due to proprietary differences in current level and presentation method, the labeled electrical dynamic range will vary greatly. The clinician should refer to the manufacturer recommendation regarding preferred electrical dynamic range.

☐ Provide the recipient with an electrical dynamic range that the recipient finds comfortable and provides them access to soft sounds at a perceptually soft level and loud sounds at a perceptually loud level.

☐ Assess the recipient's performance with behavioral and objective measures.

Subjective Measures of Cochlear Implant Programming

At a fundamental level, changes are made to upper and lower stimulation levels by changing the amplitude of the current. Changes to pulse width can also affect recipient perception of loudness and may be used when the audiologist wants to change loudness percept without constraints of current level.

■ Measurement and considerations for threshold levels: threshold is the lowest amount of electrical signal that is transmitted to the recipient. The specific formula or specifications for which the threshold level is set are dependent on the CI manufacturer.

☐ Advanced bionics (AB): the recipient should be able to detect the threshold on 50% of presentations. It is labeled the T level. T level measurement is not required and may be set as a percentage of the upper stimulation level, typically between 5% and 10%.

☐ Cochlear: the recipient should be able to detect the threshold on 100% of presentations. It is labeled the T level. T levels are regularly measured by many audiologists who program cochlear devices. It can be programmed using the traditional audiologic Hughson-Westlake procedure. To ensure the recipient is hearing it at threshold level and to obtain that 100% mark, it may be obtained by having the recipient count the number of stimulation beeps they hear, often between two and five beeps.

☐ MED-EL: the threshold level should be just below the level of detection. It is labeled the THR level. THR-level measurement is not required and is set as a percentage of the upper stimulation level, automatically set at 0% to 10%.

■ Measurement and considerations for upper stimulation levels: upper stimulation level is the highest level of stimulation electrically provided to the recipient. The exact definition of the upper stimulation level and whether that level is the maximum electrical output is dependent on the manufacturer.

☐ Appropriate upper stimulation levels are essential for recipients and affect performance and acceptance.

☐ There are a variety of methods used to set upper stimulation levels, with psychophysical loudness scaling being the most common.

• Psychophysical loudness scaling is when the recipient reports when the sound is soft, medium, perfect, loud, uncomfortably loud, and so on.

☐ Despite its importance, behavioral setting of loudness by recipients is a skill that requires practice as the user adapts to electric stimulation.

☐ AB: upper stimulation levels are called M levels.

☐ Cochlear: upper stimulation levels are called C levels.

☐ MED-EL: upper stimulation levels are called MCL.

■ Loudness balancing: this measure is completed with the recipient's upper stimulation levels after they are set.

- Psychophysical loudness balancing is completed by playing upper stimulation levels at adjacent electrodes. The recipient then reports whether the two are equally loud. Adjustments should be made to ensure equal loudness across the electrode array. Upper stimulation levels that are equally loud result in better speech perception due to better transmission of the natural loudness relationships in the speech signal.

  - Recipients have difficulty adequately reporting loudness. Electrically evoked stapedial reflex threshold (ESRT), discussed below, is a more reliable measure to assess equal loudness and should be used when possible.

- Sweeping upper stimulation levels

  - This is a quick way to confirm equal loudness and appropriate pitch transitions. Each electrode is stimulated across the frequency range at the upper stimulation level. The recipient will then report unequal loudness or abnormal pitch transitions.

- Pitch scaling

  - It should also be confirmed that the recipient has appropriately ascending pitch. This can be done in a similar fashion to loudness balancing where two adjacent electrodes are played and the person confirms that the more basal electrode is higher in pitch. If the electrode is not higher in pitch or if it sounds like the same pitch, that electrode should be deactivated to ensure the auditory signal is transmitted optimally.

 Q & A

Question: Which programming parameter is the single most important for speech understanding and subjective sound quality?

Answer: Electrical dynamic range (threshold and upper stimulation levels). Specifically, optimal upper stimulation levels that are equally loud between channels allow for the natural transmission of loudness relationships that exist in the speech signal (Wolfe, 2020).

Objective Measures of Cochlear Implant Programming

There are a variety of options for objectively verifying stimulation levels for a recipient.

- ESRT

  - This is the only objective measure that demonstrates a strong correlation (0.79–0.92) to upper stimulation levels (e.g., Walkowiak et al., 2011; Wolfe, 2020).

  - This measure assesses the lowest level of electrical stimulation that elicits a stapedial reflex (middle ear muscle/acoustic reflex).

  - A reflex can be electrically stimulated in most recipients. Recipients with ANSD or nerve deficiency may not have measurable ESRT values.

  - ESRT is considered current best practice measure for objective assessment.

  - ESRT assists with programming upper stimulation at levels that are equally loud between channels.

KNOWLEDGE CHECKPOINT

Acoustic reflex measurements are a standard component of the audiologic test battery and are typically completed during immittance measures. ESRT activates the reflex pathway using electrical stimulation directly from the implant. For review on the reflex pathway, refer to Chapters 2 and 5.

□ Because recipients have a difficult time with loudness ratings, it is recommended to utilize this measure during programming sessions, even if the recipient can complete loudness scaling.

□ ESRT does not typically change over time. If the recipient cannot tolerate upper stimulation levels at their ESRT level, they may need time to acclimate to their device. Over time, upper stimulation levels should be near ESRT.

□ Upper stimulation levels should not be set over ESRT, as the stapedial reflex will be activated too frequently.

□ The number of clinical units below the ESRT to set the upper stimulation level varies by manufacturer. Consult with currently available research.

■ Measurement of ESRT

□ Measurement is obtained via a middle ear analyzer system. Some manufacturers have a dedicated ESRT setting, or the clinician may use reflex decay mode.

□ Tympanometry should be completed first to assess middle ear function in both ears.

□ ESRT cannot be measured in the presence of a PE tube, perforation, or middle ear dysfunction.

□ ESRT should be measured in the recipient's nonimplanted ear or the ear with the highest compensated acoustic admittance if both ears are implanted.

□ If ESRT cannot be measured with the traditional 226 Hz probe tone, a 678 or 1000 Hz probe tone may be utilized.

□ After the immittance probe is placed in the ear canal, the CI software is utilized to present three to four pulses at any one channel.

□ Any ESRT response is time-locked to the stimulus, similar to the traditional acoustic. The ESRT is the lowest stimulation that initiates a reflex response on two ascending trials.

■ Electrically evoked compound action potential (ECAP)

□ ECAP is a group of auditory nerve fibers exhibiting a synchronous response to a brief electrical pulse elicited from an intracochlear electrode. The response is recorded on a nearby intracochlear electrode.

□ This is another objective measure that can be utilized to confirm and set recipient electrical dynamic range.

• ECAP values more closely relate to upper stimulation levels, but the configuration is more reflective of threshold levels (Wolfe, 2020).

☐ ECAP has less objective utility than the ESRT and a weaker correlation (described as weak to poor) than ESRT to behaviorally measured stimulation levels (e.g., Wolfe, 2020; Zimmerling & Hochmair, 2002).

☐ The ECAP can be used to confirm that a response can be elicited from the auditory nerve via the recipient's CI. It can also be used to indicate that there is a synchronous auditory nerve response to electric stimulation. Most recipients have a recordable ECAP. ECAP may not be present with ANSD or cochlear nerve abnormalities.

☐ ECAP may be used intraoperatively to test auditory system response to the CI.

☐ Since ECAP measures do not significantly change over time, they also can be used as a reference of auditory system function that can be reassessed if concerns for performance or underlying physiologic function exist.

☐ Each CI manufacturer has a different name and recording mechanism for their ECAP measure.

  ● AB: neural response imaging (NRI)

  ● Cochlear: neural response telemetry (NRT)

  ● MED-EL: auditory response telemetry (ART)

■ Measurement of ECAP

☐ ECAP measurements are completed within the manufacturer software.

  ● The exact procedure varies by manufacturer, but it typically involves a series of increasing or decreasing electric stimuli with responses recorded on an amplitude growth function (AGF). The AGF is then used to derive the ECAP threshold.

  ● Some manufacturers offer the ability to manipulate some ECAP parameters such as pulse width if a response is not obtained via the default settings.

☐ The recipient can be in any state during measurement—moving, talking, asleep, under anesthesia, or awake.

CASE EXAMPLE

An 18-month-old with CHARGE syndrome presents with bilateral profound SNHL. After evaluation and approval by the CI team, the child undergoes implantation in one ear. Imaging reveals normal cochlear anatomy. Due to significant developmental delays, this child is unable to participate in behavioral programming methods but does exhibit changes in movement and eye gaze in response to stimulation. The child presents with an abnormal tympanogram in the implanted ear. In the contralateral ear, the child has a normal tympanogram. ESRT is therefore attempted as the acoustic reflex is a bilateral response. Unfortunately, the child exhibits too much movement, causing artifact in recording of the ESRT response. In this scenario, the next option is to utilize ECAP measures to estimate appropriate stimulation levels. This should be used with caution in combination with behavioral observation of the recipient's reactions to live speech. Over time, ESRT and behavioral assessments of loudness should be reattempted to achieve optimal programming levels.

- Electrical auditory brainstem response (EABR)
    - □ EABR is another assessment of the auditory neural pathway in response to the electric stimulus.
    - □ EABR may be utilized when ESRT or ECAP cannot be elicited, for example, when the person has an abnormal cochlea.
    - □ The setup and administration of EABR are comparable to the traditional ABR. The stimulus is elicited via a connection from the ABR system to the cochlear implant programming software.
    - □ As with traditional ABR, the recipient needs to be asleep or very still and calm with eyes closed for optimal recording.
    - □ EABR does not have a direct correlate to any one component of the electric dynamic range.

Considerations for Cochlear Implant Recipients

Facial Nerve Stimulation

Facial nerve stimulation is considered the most common side effect of cochlear implantation. This is when electrical stimulation of the auditory nerve causes additional stimulation of the facial nerve (due to close anatomical proximity). Facial nerve stimulation may present as any of the following during electric stimulation:

- Tingling sensation in the face
- Watering of the eye(s)
- Itching of the face or eye
- Facial spasm
- Pain in the face or at the eye

Facial stimulation can occur due to a wide array of factors that include proximity of the facial nerve to the cochlea, changes in the cochlea secondary to disease process, and the amount of electrical stimulation needed for individual loudness percepts. Abnormal cochlear and/or skull anatomy can also increase the likelihood of facial nerve stimulation. Facial nerve stimulation is abnormal and a recipient should never have active facial stimulation with CI use. The following process can be used to identify and eliminate facial nerve stimulation:

- Identify the electrode(s) that are exhibiting facial nerve stimulation.
    - □ Consider sweeping upper stimulation levels to identify the electrode or region that is causing facial nerve stimulation.
- Make changes to the recipient's map at the affected electrode(s).
    - □ If minimal reductions in upper stimulation levels eliminate facial stimulation, no further adjustments need to be made.
        - With AB devices, activate clipping, which restricts the maximal power output at that electrode, thereby preventing active stimulation at the level that causes facial nerve stimulation.
    - □ If changes of more than a few clinical units are required to eliminate facial nerve stimulation, increase the pulse width and remeasure upper and lower stimulation levels.

- Increasing pulse width allows for greater loudness percept with less energy.
  □ If facial nerve stimulation is confined to a small number of electrodes and programming adjustments will not yield an adequate loudness percept without stimulation, deactivate the affected electrodes.

Vestibular Considerations

Patients with SNHL are at greater risk for vestibular dysfunction before and after cochlear implantation.

- Vestibular testing may be completed before and after cochlear implantation and may be included as part of the candidacy evaluation. On studies of vestibular function of patients compared to baseline, Rasmussen et al. (2021) found that although recipients had significantly poorer overall scores on a vestibular battery 3 to 6 months after they underwent implantation, results of vestibular function continued to decline until 14 months after surgery. The authors noted that despite changes in testing scores, participants did not report significantly different scores of the Dizziness Handicap Inventory, which may have indicated little to no change in their subjective dizziness.

- A systematic review of studies that evaluated vestibular function before and after cochlear implantation, Hansel et al. (2018) found that <20% of recipients had new instances of vertigo after CI surgery, and <25% of recipients had vertigo prior to surgery with <8% resolving after surgery and <8% having no change postsurgery.
  □ Age was a significant factor; the older the patient was, the more likely they were to have postsurgery vertigo.
  □ In total, less than 10% of recipients have postsurgery vertigo. It is important to note that there are significant differences in studies, with some reporting higher incidence of subjective vertigo and others reporting fewer changes in subjective vertigo and more changes in postsurgical vestibular function testing.

- Overall, it is important to consider the potential impact of CI surgery on a recipient's vestibular system and to complete pre- and posttesting if possible. For concerns about a recipients' vestibular systems, referrals to a vestibular-specialized physical therapist are encouraged.

- Results of pediatric assessment are much more varied (Koyama et al., 2021) due to challenges with children appropriately participating in vestibular tasks and ability to follow directions. Again, if vestibular function is an area of concern, recipients should be referred to a specialized physical therapist to adequately address their needs. This is particularly important for young children to address areas such as late walking.

Preservation of Residual Hearing

Hearing preservation in cochlear implantation occurs when the patient has useable low-frequency (<1500 Hz) hearing thresholds prior to surgical placement of the electrode array and they still have measurable hearing on postoperative audiometric testing. Hearing preservation should be considered and attempted for recipients with low-frequency hearing thresholds in the moderately severe range or better.

- While preservation of preoperative hearing thresholds can be present across the entire frequency range, preservation is most clinically and functionally important in the lower frequency range (i.e., <1500 Hz).

■ Hearing preservation can be achieved with a shorter internal array, the Hybrid™ or electric-acoustic stimulation (EAS™) array, which is available with Cochlear or MED-EL, respectively, for recipients 18 years of age or older. Due to advances in technology and thinner, more flexible internal arrays, hearing preservation can also be achieved with full-length (traditional) electrode arrays. Figure 9–6 demonstrates the audiogram range when the CI team should consider a hybrid array or hearing preservation, based on the FDA criteria for Cochlear and MED-EL.

■ Recipients with residual hearing have better sound quality, better performance on speech-in-noise, and better music appreciation.

■ Some recipients with hearing preservation have low-frequency hearing that does not need amplification; for others, an acoustic component can be added to their processor to amplify the low frequencies, so they are hearing with electroacoustic stimulation.

AUDIOLOGY NUGGET

With advances in technology creating more flexible, atraumatic electrode arrays, and with greater surgeon experience, hearing preservation is possible with full-length electrode arrays (Dillon et al., 2020). Some surgeons are choosing to place full-length electrode arrays to accommodate the full length of the cochlea even when there is preservable hearing for natural or amplified acoustic or electric low-frequency hearing, should the hearing change postoperatively.

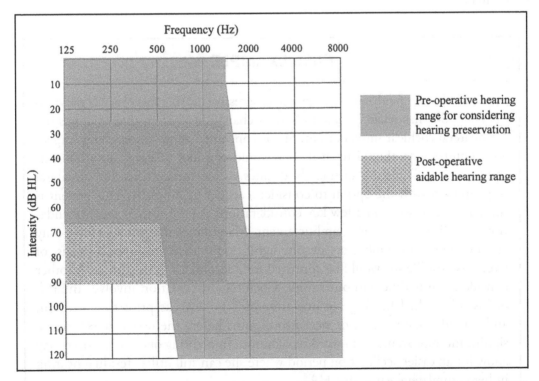

FIGURE 9–6. Audiogram representation of preservable hearing thresholds based on FDA criteria for Cochlear Hybrid™ and MED-EL EAS™ devices, with the least restrictive audiogram criteria being chosen.

■ Frequency allocation of the electric stimulation is adjusted based on the resulting audiogram of the recipient.

Better hearing preoperatively makes it more likely that the recipient will have hearing preservation. There can be some reduction of hearing thresholds post implantation.

Hearing Assistive Technology

Despite using advanced pre- and post-hoc signal processing (e.g., directional microphones, digital noise reduction) to improve speech-in-noise performance, CI recipients still experience poorer performance in noise than individuals with normal hearing. Adding hearing assistive technology (HAT) is particularly useful for recipients. With all CI orders, recipients can choose accessory devices. These can be waterproof options, additional wearing options, extra batteries, or HAT in the form of remote microphones and others such as television connectors.

Special Populations

Bilateral and Bimodal

When a user has one HA and one CI, it is referred to as bimodal. When a user has a CI on each ear, it is referred to as bilateral implantation.

■ If a patient is unilaterally implanted, better performance and satisfaction with hearing status can be achieved by adding a HA on the contralateral ear, regardless of degree of hearing loss. This is due to improved access to low-frequency sounds, which has a positive correlation with sound quality.

 CASE EXAMPLE

An adult HA user has been experiencing progressive hearing loss over the previous 10 years. She has recently had a bilateral change in hearing that qualifies her for bilateral cochlear implantation. She is concerned about undergoing surgery and inquires with the CI team if they would consider bilateral, simultaneous implantation. The team ultimately decides to recommend her for unilateral implantation with the option to consider a sequential implant. This patient is ultimately counseled on a few key considerations as part of their recommendation. The first is insurance reimbursement. Many insurance providers will only approve one CI for adult users, despite significant evidence to support the use of two. It is possible she would be approved for a second CI in the future. Another consideration is time without sound. Cochlear implantation involves the risk of loss of residual hearing, healing time of 1 to 4 weeks prior to activation, and extended habilitation of weeks to months before the user can experience significant improvements in word recognition. Implanting one ear at a time may allow for an easier acclimation period where she can still utilize residual hearing in her contralateral ear with a HA.

- For adults, the recipient's insurance may preclude them from obtaining a second CI; however, it should be considered for a few reasons. When deciding on adding a second CI or a contralateral HA, the following considerations should be made:
  - □ Both bimodal and bilateral CI users have better performance on speech-in-noise compared to recipients who only utilize one CI.
  - □ Bilateral CI users experience better localization compared to unilateral CI and bimodal users.
  - □ Bimodal users may have better music perception and sound quality due to improved fine temporal structure provided by the low frequencies from the HA.
- Bilateral CI use is much more widely accepted and approved in pediatrics and is preferred to unilateral use for patients with bilateral profound SNHL. It has significant implications for language and educational outcomes.
  - □ Optimal performance is achieved when there are <2 years between implantation (Gordon et al., 2010).

Single-Sided Deafness

Since 2019, CIs have been FDA approved for single-sided deafness (SSD) and asymmetric hearing loss for patients 5 years of age and over for MED-EL and, more recently, Cochlear recipients. Before that, CIs were provided in an off-label capacity and for research purposes for recipients for whom more traditional interventions were not sufficient or for those who had incapacitating tinnitus.

- The only way to restore hearing in unilateral deafness is a CI.
- CIs for people with SSD can improve speech understanding in quiet and in noise, localization, music appreciation, quality of life, and potentially speech and language development for pediatrics as compared to more traditional interventions of CROS, BCHD, and proactive environmental management.

Bone-Conduction Devices

Introduction

Conductive hearing losses may be medically managed by an otologist/neurotologist, but not all are medically manageable and/or not all patients desire surgical intervention. Even with surgical management, there may be a residual hearing loss for which audiologic management is recommended.

- Traditional bone-conduction devices function similarly to air-conduction devices until the last stage, which is when the signal is transduced to the patient. Instead of an acoustic signal, it is a vibratory signal that directly stimulates the inner ear, bypassing the outer and middle ear.

Candidacy

Bone-conduction devices have two indications: conductive hearing losses and SSD as a transcranial routing of signal device. These are also divided into implanted and nonimplanted devices.

Candidacy Evaluations

Candidacy evaluations include a comprehensive audiologic evaluation with air- and bone-conduction thresholds, speech recognition thresholds, word recognition testing, and subjective measures. Considerations for candidacy will be made based on the patient's bone-conduction thresholds and lifestyle. To help the patient decide on a device (nonimplantable or implantable), the audiologist should consider completing aided testing with a clinical demo device on a hard headband. Aided measures of functional gain, including soundfield thresholds and aided word recognition in quiet and in noise, may be performed. The patient may also undergo an at-home trial and wear a nonsurgical device for 2 to 6 weeks.

CASE EXAMPLE

A 65-year-old patient presents with a moderately severe conductive hearing loss in his right ear secondary to a failed ossicular chain reconstruction. He has an otherwise normal ear canal and no history of significant cerumen occlusion or drainage. His left ear presents with normal hearing. This patient has significant complaints of hearing in background noise. He has been trialing an air-conduction HA for his right ear for 1 month and is dissatisfied with the sound quality. At this time, it may be more appropriate to recommend a trial with a bone-conduction device. Since this patient has an air-bone gap greater than 35 to 45 dB HL, he will likely achieve better aided outcomes and better satisfaction with a bone-conduction device. He can trial a nonsurgical option first with counseling regarding the possibility of improved sound quality and gain characteristics with a surgically implanted device.

Bone-conduction devices may be implanted or nonimplanted. Uses, advantages, and disadvantages are reviewed in Table 9–11.

- Nonimplanted coupling methods
  - Hard headband: this resembles the traditional headband used for bone-conduction audiometric testing.
  - Soft headband: an elastic band that surrounds the head
  - SoundArc™: a hard headband that sits behind the head
  - Sticker (ADHEAR™): an adhesive that can be placed on the mastoid by which to affix the sound processor to the head
- Implanted coupling methods
  - Transcutaneous: vibratory communication occurs across the skin via an internal magnet that is affixed to the skull.
  - Percutaneous: vibratory communication occurs via a screw affixed to the skull that protrudes the skin.
  - Active transcutaneous bone-conduction implants: a semi-implanted device with the vibratory component being surgically implanted and the sound processor serving as the external component, which communicates through radiofrequency code across the skin to the internal component.

TABLE 9–11. Implanted Versus Nonimplanted Bone-Conduction Devices

TYPE	USES	ADVANTAGES	DISADVANTAGES
Nonimplanted	People that cannot undergo surgery based on age or surgical risks factors	Temporary, may be used in interim scenarios	High cost of device compared to traditional amplification, may not be covered by insurance if not implanted
	Trial devices prior to deciding on surgery	Access to sound immediately, no osseointegration or surgical healing	Consistent pressure needed, can cause discomfort and/or headaches; if consistent pressure not achieved, gain is not optimal
	Those who do not want to undergo surgery	Easy to discontinue if hearing improves or management changes	Aesthetics—not optimal for any coupling method
	Interim use prior to medical management of hearing loss	No internal components	Higher incidence of feedback and distortion—higher gain used to accommodate for placement
			High frequencies not transmitted as effectively
Implanted	Adults and children over 5 years of age; other indications are device-specific	More likely to be covered by insurance than nonsurgical; no pressure from headband; less feedback and distortion, better high-frequency transmission depending on coupling method; stable position; can be more optimally programmed; surgery is reversible without affecting patient hearing	Limitations based on patient age; patient needs to undergo surgery; others (discussed in chapter)

Nonimplanted Bone-Conduction Devices

Nonimplanted devices are in the same regulatory class as HAs and can be fit according to audiologic need and recommendations from the audiologist. Guidelines may help the clinician decide whether to choose an air-conduction or bone-conduction device for a patient with a conductive or mixed hearing loss.

■ For patients with conductive or mixed hearing loss who have an intact ear canal, air-conduction HAs may be an option. The managing audiologist should consider the following:

 □ Available gain: as discussed in the first section of this chapter, when there is an air-bone gap, the patient requires more gain than with a SNHL (to overcome the attenuation caused by the conductive component) with the same air-conduction thresholds.

☐ Drainage that occurs in the ear canal

- Frequent or persistent drainage can cause numerous challenges with traditional HA use, including damage to the internal components of the device, possible reinfection, and increased incidence of drainage with an occluded ear.

☐ Comfort of the patient

- Some patients find air-conduction HAs to be uncomfortable and dislike having to wear a device in the ear canal.

☐ Size of air-bone gap (de Wolf et al., 2011)

- Patients perform better on audiometric tasks with a bone-conduction device compared to traditional amplification when their air-bone-gap is >35 dB HL. Patients report improvements in their performance on subjective ranking on the APHAB when the air-bone gap is >45 dB HL.

- Based on these data, a bone-conduction device should be recommended when the air-bone gap is 35 to 45 dB HL.

- Patients may be candidates for bone-conduction devices if the audiologist cannot occlude the ear canal, they have a congenital malformation of the external ear, or a large air-bone gap is present.

- Audiologic bone-conduction thresholds should be normal to near-normal if the patient is being chosen for a nonimplanted bone-conduction device for optimal performance. If the device is going to be implanted, they can have poorer bone-conduction thresholds as there will be more available gain. This is discussed in more detail below.

☐ Normal high-frequency bone-conduction thresholds are of primary importance. All nonimplanted bone-conduction devices have suboptimal transmission of high-frequency sounds due to the dampening of high frequencies by the skin. Reduced transmission and

---

Q & A

Question: A 6-month-old with bilateral microtia and ear canal stenosis arrives for a follow-up visit. The patient has received an ABR, which suggested maximum (moderate to moderately severe) conductive hearing loss in both ears. The family asks if a watch-and-wait approach can be utilized as they believe the ear canals are likely to grow. What is the most appropriate audiologic management and what counseling should be provided to the family?

Answer: Timely intervention, with management of hearing loss by age 6 months, is critical to maximal spoken language outcomes. A traditional HA is not appropriate for this patient due to infant ear canal stenosis. Various bone-conduction devices can be presented to the family as options. Bone-conduction devices should not be implanted for children younger than age 5 years due to skull thickness. Therefore, nonimplanted coupling methods should be discussed. Counseling should also include a discussion of frequent audiologic reevaluation and adjustment of the management strategy with age, ear canal growth, and changes in hearing status.

perception of high-frequency speech sounds will have an adverse effect on the perception of speech.

- Nonimplanted device coupling
    - ☐ Cochlear Baha™ processor can be used on a Soundarc™ or Softband™.
    - ☐ Oticon Medical Ponto™ processor can be used on a soft headband or a hard traditional headband for trial purposes.
    - ☐ MED-EL ADHEAR™ processor does have a soft headband option for certain situational needs but is designed specifically to be connected to an adhesive that is placed on the mastoid. There is no surgical version of the ADHEAR™.
        - While the Baha and Ponto can be used in a nonsurgical capacity with up to 45 dB HL bone conduction thresholds, the ADHEAR™ processor should only be utilized if bone-conduction thresholds are in the normal range.

Implanted Bone-Conduction Devices

Implanted devices undergo FDA approval in the same regulatory class as CIs (III). Typical candidacy evaluations involve the otologist/neurotologist and the audiologist. Candidacy requirements are based on bone-conduction thresholds, air-bone gaps, patient goals, and suitability for surgery. Devices may be chosen based on lifestyle factors considering the pros and cons mentioned in the description of the internal devices earlier in this chapter.

- Transcutaneous and percutaneous devices have similar candidacy profiles.
    - ☐ FDA indicates patients need to be ≥5 years of age.
    - ☐ Hearing loss can be conductive, mixed, or SSD.
        - For SSD, normal hearing is required in the contralateral ear.
    - ☐ For bilateral surgical placement, symmetrical bone-conduction thresholds (no more than 10-dB difference on average between ears) are required.
    - ☐ As with CIs, other FDA indications are manufacturer specific.
    - ☐ Cochlear offers both transcutaneous and percutaneous devices.
        - Baha Connect™—percutaneous
        - Baha Attract™—transcutaneous
        - Sound processors can accommodate bone-conduction thresholds of up to 65 dB HL, depending on the coupling.
    - ☐ Oticon Medical offers percutaneous devices.
        - Ponto™ sound processors can accommodate up to 65 dB HL bone-conduction thresholds.
    - ☐ Medtronic Sophono™ is a transcutaneous device and is technically a bone fixture device as it attaches to the skull without osseointegration. It is the only device on the market that does not require osseointegration but is a traditional vibratory external device.
- Active transcutaneous bone-conduction implants
    - ☐ FDA indications are age 12 and older with conductive, mixed, or SSD.
        - Individuals between the ages of 5 and 12 may undergo placement of these devices in an off-label capacity.

- □ MED-EL BONEBRIDGE™

  - For mixed or conductive hearing losses, the pure-tone average bone-conduction thresholds should be better than 55 dB HL.

  - For SSD, the implanted ear needs to have profound SNHL and the contralateral ear pure-tone average bone-conduction thresholds should be better than 20 dB HL.

  - Patient should have experience with air-conduction or bone-conduction HAs as a trial, with length of time not specified.

- □ Cochlear Osia™

  - For mixed or conductive hearing losses, the pure-tone average bone-conduction thresholds should be better than 55 dB HL.

  - For SSD, the implanted ear needs to have profound SNHL and the contralateral ear pure-tone average bone-conduction thresholds should be better than 20 dB HL.

  - Patient should have experience with air-conduction or bone-conduction HAs as a trial, with length of time not specified.

Surgery

Transcutaneous and percutaneous implanted devices, with the exception of the Sophono™ device, undergo osseointegration, which is the bonding of the implanted device to living tissue. This is a natural process that occurs when titanium is placed into bone.

Internal Devices

- ■ Percutaneous

  - □ The titanium screw protrudes through the skin, and the abutment (connection point of the bone-conduction device to the osseointegrated component) is directly connected to the screw.

  - □ Advantages

    - High signal fidelity as there is no dampening from the skin and it is directly transmitted to the bone and therefore the cochlea.

    - Because the only surgically implanted component is the titanium screw, this is beneficial for people who need to undergo MRIs as it is approved for up to 3.0 Tesla (3T) with minimal shadow caused by the screw.

    - Retention is optimal.

  - □ Disadvantages

    - Skin overgrowth, infection, loss due to head trauma, extrusion of device, granulation tissue

    - Cannot be activated until osseointegration takes place, which on average takes 3 months

  - □ Percutaneous devices should not be used in cases of psychiatric concerns, poor hygiene, or diseases that impact wound healing.

- ■ Transcutaneous

  - □ A titanium screw is still placed into skull with an additional magnetic plate placed under the skin.

- ☐ Bone-conduction device is attached to an internal magnet component.
- ☐ Vibration of internal magnet + screw component occurs through the connection of the internal and external magnets, across the skin.
- ☐ Advantages
  - Lower complications and less wound care required compared to percutaneous
  - More aesthetically pleasing
  - Can be activated before full osseointegration has taken place, as soon as 4 weeks after surgery
  - Less risk of damage secondary to head trauma
  - May be easier to place by recipients
- ☐ Disadvantages
  - Dampening of high-frequency sounds by the skin
  - May be more susceptible to feedback due to higher gain needed to provide stimulation across the skin
  - Can only undergo MRI up to 1.5 Tesla (1.5T) and may have greater shadow if MRI is of the head
  - Poorer retention if recipient has an active lifestyle
  - Skin aggravation secondary to pressure of magnet external component
- ■ Active transcutaneous bone-conduction implants
  - ☐ These devices are more similar to CIs in that the vibratory device is affixed to the skull and a receiver stimulator is underneath the skin. The external device communicates via an electromagnetic signal to the internal device. Vibration is not generated in the external component, unlike the abovementioned bone-conduction devices. The vibration occurs at the level of the internal fixation point.
  - ☐ MED-EL BONEBRIDGE™
    - Utilizes a bone-conduction floating mass transducer that is placed in a bone bed in the skull
  - ☐ Cochlear Osia™

 KNOWLEDGE CHECKPOINT

Bone-conduction devices may be surgical or nonsurgical. Patients of any age can obtain a nonsurgical bone-conduction device and only patients 5 years of age or older can receive transcutaneous and percutaneous devices, with patients 12 years of age being indicated for active transcutaneous bone-conduction implants. Some patients may choose to defer surgery and utilize a bone-conduction device in a nonsurgical capacity. These patients should be counseled regarding significant benefits to surgical placement, including comfort, consistent device placement, available gain before feedback, and transmission of high-frequency sounds.

- Utilizes the same internal B300™ implant used for the Connect™ and Attract™, which is screwed into the skull, but physical location of the implant will be different. The B300™ implant is affixed to a piezoelectric transducer.

  □ Both of these devices have the benefit of being transcutaneous but without the limitations of skin dampening. There is superior high-frequency output and more useable gain before feedback, as such, that it is comparable to a percutaneous device.

Post-Implantation and Device Management

Verification is a challenge with bone-conduction devices as there is a not a currently acceptable, standardized method for verification as there is with air-conduction devices. The Verifit® system offers an artificial mastoid with which verification of electroacoustic device can be completed; however, the only available prescriptive targets are DSL-BCD, which should only be used with percutaneous devices. Other considerations are skin thickness, skull shape, and individual cochlear differences. Depending on the coupling of the device, the patient's skin and hair thickness, and placement, the gain will vary from that which would be recommended by connection to an artificial mastoid.

- Nearly all bone-conduction devices are programmed with in-situ audiometric measures, meaning the clinician identifies the patient's threshold via direct stimulation of the processor. As of the time of this writing, the only device that does not allow for in-situ measurement is the MED-EL ADHEAR™.

- This device comes preprogrammed with the sole intention of converting the auditory signal into mechanical transduction. Minor adjustments can be made to overall gain, but it is not meant to be individually programmed to a recipient's bone-conduction thresholds.

- Validation can be completed via aided audiologic measures of threshold detection, speech-in-quiet, and speech-in-noise.

Auditory Brainstem Implants

Introduction

Certain individuals may not benefit from the implantable options discussed above. These individuals may benefit from an auditory brainstem implant (ABI). The primary goal of an ABI is sound awareness and potential assistance in speech reading (Wong et al., 2019).

An ABI uses the same external components as the CI. The internal components consist of a receiver-stimulator and a paddle electrode, which communicates directly with the cochlear nucleus, located in the brainstem, using electrical pulses.

Candidacy

The only current FDA indication for use of an ABI is for patients with neurofibromatosis type 2 (NF2) who are 12 years of age and older. These individuals do not receive benefit from a CI due to the site of lesion being at the level of the auditory nerve, and the success of a CI is dependent on the status of the auditory nerve. In the United States, there are a few centers that will implant ABIs off-label. Those who may be considered for off-label candidacy include cases of a temporal bone fracture that severs the auditory nerve, congenital cochlear nerve aplasia, cochlear aplasia, or complete cochlear ossification. Outside of the United States, there is a wider recipient base of ABI devices.

Children may also receive ABIs. They may be required to undergo and fail cochlear implantation prior to receiving an ABI, if they have an intact cochlea. Below is a list of conditions that would make a person a potential off-label candidate (Wolfe, 2020):

- Congenital cochlear nerve aplasia or cochlear aplasia
- Bilateral profound hearing loss
- Age 18 months to 5 years
- Realistic expectations and family dedication

ABI Team

The ABI team is more extensive than the CI team. An ABI team includes an otologist, a neurosurgeon, a neuroradiologist, an audiologist, an electrophysiologist, and a SLP. It is imperative that the potential candidate and/or family understand that a small percentage of recipients achieve open-set word understanding secondary to ABI (Colletti & Shannon, 2005). As a result, children who are possible ABI candidates should be exposed to signed/manual language to ensure language development.

Candidacy Evaluations

Candidacy evaluations include the traditional test battery for cochlear implantation, MRI imaging, possible CT imaging, and extensive counseling regarding risks of surgery and potential outcomes. Counseling may include:

- Many of the same outcome predictors for performance with a CI can be applied to performance with an ABI. Additional factors for consideration include if there has been neural degeneration within the brainstem and placement of the electrode array.
- Individuals with NF2 have been identified as the poorest performers with an ABI, and recipients who do not have NF2 typically perform better (Colletti & Shannon, 2005).
- A small subset of people achieves open-set word understanding. More often, "good" outcomes include the ability to detect environmental sounds and slightly improved performance on speech tasks with visual cues.

Surgery

- Insertion of the auditory brainstem implant is completed via a craniotomy and therefore requires a comprehensive team with more specialty providers than a CI surgery. These providers are present during the surgery and may also be involved in candidacy evaluation.
  - Due to the placement within the brainstem (at the cochlear nucleus), the surgical team also needs to ensure the integrity of the cranial nerves remains intact.
  - Patients are usually admitted to the hospital for multiple days after surgery to ensure adequate recovery.

Internal Devices

- Cochlear is the only ABI device in use in the United States at the time of this publication. Cochlear's ABI device utilizes the same external processor as their CI device. The primary difference is in the electrode array. It is often referred to as a "paddle" that contains multiple rows of 21 total platinum electrodes. The paddle should be placed directly on the cochlear nucleus.

☐ MED-EL has an ABI that is used in other parts of the world.

☐ Advanced Bionics had an ABI that is no longer available.

Post-Implantation and Device Management

Recipients typically do not achieve open-set word understanding with ABI devices. Expected performance is discussed under ABI Candidacy Evaluations, above.

Programming

■ While there is potential for nonauditory effects from a CI (i.e., facial stimulation), nonauditory effects are much more common with an ABI due to the location of the device on the cochlear nucleus and in close proximity to other neural structures. Common nonauditory effects can include facial nerve stimulation, a tingling sensation, dizziness, nystagmus, or a cardiac or respiratory response. Therefore, initial activation is completed with access to emergency medical services or a cardiac code team.

■ During initial stimulation, the audiologist will determine which electrodes produce audition, as not all electrodes will produce an auditory effect. Only those electrodes are utilized for stimulation and the programming of lower and upper stimulation levels to set the electrical dynamic range in the same manner of programming a CI.

■ A critically important feature of programming an ABI is determining pitch ordering of the electrodes. The cochlear nucleus is not tonotopically organized like the cochlea but does contain some degree of tonotopic organization. The audiologist will have to change the pitch relationship of the electrodes to match the patient's pitch identifications.

☐ This is a difficult skill for patients to master and therefore will likely be completed over multiple sessions and may span months to years to determine ideal pitch relationships, if ever.

■ Loudness balancing also has more importance in ABI programming than in a traditional CI. As with pitch order, loudness relationships at the level of the paddle electrode's connection with the cochlear nucleus are not 1:1. There will be more variation in the current level needed for equal loudness across channels for ABI users.

☐ There is potential to use EABR and ESRT with ABI recipients to set loudness levels.

Middle Ear Implants

Introduction

Each manufacturer of middle ear implants (MEIs) approaches the design and composition from a different philosophy, but at its core, all (MEIs) have a piece that is surgically placed in the middle ear space to optimize stimulation of the cochlea. Specifics of MEIs are outside the scope of this text, but advantages and disadvantages are discussed.

- MEIs were initially designed as an alternative to traditional amplification due to limitations in technology in the late 1990s and early 2000s (Wolfe, 2020). They provide:
  - Increases in gain compared to traditional amplification and more available gain before feedback.
  - Less occlusion effect unless the MEI utilizes a microphone in the ear canal, which some require.
  - Some devices are more comfortable than traditional amplification.
  - At the time they were designed, the sound quality was reported to be better than amplification that was available; however, there have been significant advances in DSP with conventional amplification.
  - Since most of the device is implanted, there is less or no visible component, which may be preferable for discreet use.
  - If the device is one that is fully implanted, the recipient does not have to worry about not having improved hearing while sleeping, water activities, and so on.
- There are some reasons why a MEI is less desirable, which are listed here:
  - The device is placed surgically under general anesthesia.
  - Typically, 8 to 10 weeks of healing is required before the device can be used.
  - The devices and surgery are costly and not regularly covered by insurance.
  - For device placement, the ossicular chain may need to be disconnected, which can then worsen recipient hearing during the healing process or when they are not actively using the device.
  - Most devices have a magnet component, which therefore limits the recipient from undergoing MRIs.
  - There is no evidence-based verification method comparable to real ear probe microphone measures that are used with conventional amplification.

Candidacy

Due to insurance limitations and advances in traditional amplification, MEIs are much less common in audiologic/otologic care.

FDA criteria vary by manufacturer, but general candidacy considerations are as follows:

- Over the age of 18 with bilateral SNHL. An ideal candidate has thresholds better than 75 dB HL and a word recognition score better than 60% in the ear to be implanted.
- Chronic middle ear disease contraindicates use of these devices.

Surgery

The device is placed surgically in the middle ear space under general anesthesia. The exact placement procedure varies by device. The most common placement is fixation to the incus, either at the body or long process. Alternate placement options include the head of the stapes or round window. The external device also varies and may be similar either to the CI or to an in-the-canal style hearing aid. One device, the Envoy Esteem™, is totally implantable with no external component.

Internal Devices

Within the middle ear space, there are three primary transduction mechanisms for middle ear implants, dependent on manufacturer.

- Piezoelectric
  - ☐ Piezoelectric materials are crystals that vibrate in response to an electric stimulus. These materials also emit electricity when they experience movement or vibration.
  - ☐ These materials may be used to respond to vibrations of the tympanic membrane or the ossicles to serve as replacement for a microphone or to mechanically deliver a converted electrical signal to the ossicles or cochlea (Wolfe, 2020).
- Electromagnetic
  - ☐ Electromagnetic systems use a magnet placed in the middle ear along with a wired coil. The wired coil emits an electrically generated signal, causing the magnet to move, thereby moving the ossicular chain (Wolfe, 2020).
- Electromechanical
  - ☐ Electromechanical is similar to electromagnetic except that the wired coil is physically attached to the magnet (Wolfe, 2020).

Post-Implantation and Device Management

The reader is encouraged to view resources from the individual companies as these devices and their programming and management are evolving as their use increases.

Recommended Readings

Auditory Potential. (2011). New Minimum Speech Test Battery (MSTB) for adult cochlear implant users. https://www.auditorypotential.com/MSTB-files/MSTBManual2011-06-20%20.pdf

Bentler, R., & Chiou, L. K. (2006). Digital noise reduction: An overview. *Trends in Amplification, 10*(2), 67–82. https://doi.org/10.1177/1084713806289514

Fuglholt, M. L. (2010). Electrophysiological threshold estimation and infant hearing instrument fitting. *Pediatric Whitepaper. Oticon Pediatrics.* https://wdh02.azureedge.net/-/media/oticon-us/main/download-center/white-papers/20440-electrophys iological-threshold-estimation-and-infant-hearing-instrument-fitting.pdf?rev=D917&la=en

Killion, M. C., & Mueller, H. G. (2010). Twenty years later: A new count-the-dots method. *The Hearing Journal, 63*(1), 10, 12–14, 16–17. https://doi.org/10.1097/01.HJ.0000366911.63043.16

Ricketts, T. A. (2005). Directional hearing aids: Then and now. *Journal of Rehabilitation Research and Development, 42*(4, Suppl. 2), 133–144.

Zhang, X. (2020). New technologies of directional microphones for hearing aids. *Journal of Electrical and Electronic Engineering, 8*(3), 81–91. https://doi.org/ 10.11648/j.jeee.20200803.12

References

Alexander, J. M. (2013). Individual variability in recognition of frequency-lowered speech. *Seminars in Hearing, 34*, 86–109. http://doi.org/10.1055/s-0033-1341346

American Academy of Audiology (AAA). (2013). *American Academy of Audiology Clinical Practice Guidelines on pediatric amplification.* http://www.audiology.org/resources/documentlibrary/Documents/PediatricAmplificationGuidelines.pdf

American National Standard Institute. (2014) *Specification of hearing aid characteristics.* https://.ansi.org/standards/asa/ansiasas3222014r2020

Anderson, K. L., & Goldstein, H. (2004). Speech perception benefits of FM and infrared devices to children with hearing aids in a typical classroom. *Language, Speech, and Hearing Services in Schools, 35*(2), 169–184. https://doi.org/10.1044/0161-1461(2004/017)

Anderson, K. L., Goldstein, H., Colodzin, L., & Iglehart, F. (2005). Benefit of S/N enhancing devices to speech perception of children listening in a typical classroom with hearing aids or a cochlear implant. *Journal of Educational Audiology, 12,* 14–28.

Audioscan. (2022). *Audioscan Verifit® User's Guide 4.30.* https://docs.audioscan.com/userguides/vf2manual.pdf

Buchman, C. A., Gifford, R. H., Haynes, D. S., Lenarz, T., O'Donoghue, G., Adunka, O., . . . Zwolan, T. (2020). Unilateral cochlear implants for severe, profound, or moderate sloping to profound bilateral sensorineural hearing loss: A systematic review and consensus statements. *JAMA Otolaryngology-Head & Neck Surgery, 146*(10), 942–953. https://doi.org/10.1001/jamaoto.2020.0998

Colletti, V., & Shannon, R. V. (2005). Open set speech perception with auditory brainstem implant. *Laryngoscope, 115*(11), 1974–1978. https://doi.org/10.1097/01.mlg.0000178327.42926.ec

Cox, R. M., & Xu, J. (2010). Short and long compression release times: Speech understanding, real-world preferences, and association with cognitive ability. *Journal of the American Academy of Audiology, 21*(2), 121–138. https://doi.org/10.3766/jaaa.21.2.6

de Wolf, M. J., Hendrix, S., Cremers, C. W., & Snik, A. F. (2011). Better performance with bone-anchored HA than acoustic devices in patients with severe air-bone gap. *The Laryngoscope, 121*(3), 613–616.

Dillon, M. T., Buss, E., O'Connell, B. P., Rooth, M. A., King, E. R., Bucker, A. L., . . . Brown, K. D. (2020). Low-frequency hearing preservation with long electrode arrays: Inclusion of unaided hearing threshold assessment in the postoperative test battery. *American Journal of Audiology, 29*(1), 1–5.

Finley, C. C., Holden, T. A., Holden, L. K., Whiting, B. R., Chole, R. A., Neely, G. J., . . . Skinner, M. W. (2008). Role of electrode placement as a contributor to variability in cochlear implant outcomes. *Otology & Neurotology, 29*(7), 920–928. https://doi.org/10.1097/MAO.0b013e318184f492

Glista, D., Scollie, S., Bagatto, M., Seewald, R., Parsa, V., & Johnson, A. (2009). Evaluation of nonlinear frequency compression: Clinical outcomes. *International Journal of Audiology, 48*(9), 632–644. https://doi.org/10.1080/14992020902971349

Gordon, K. A., Wong, D. D., & Papsin, B. C. (2010). Cortical function in children receiving bilateral cochlear implants simultaneously or after a period of interimplant delay. *Otology & Neurotology, 31*(8), 1293–1299. https://doi.org/10.1097/MAO.0b013e3181e8f965

Hänsel, T., Gauger, U., Bernhard, N., Behzadi, N., Romo Ventura, M. E., Hofmann, V., . . . Coordes, A. (2018). Meta-analysis of subjective complaints of vertigo and vestibular tests after cochlear implantation. *Laryngoscope, 128*(9), 2110–2123. https://doi.org/10.1002/lary.27071

Hornsby, B. W., & Mueller, G. (2004). The speech intelligibility index: What is it and what's it good for? *The Hearing Journal, 57*(10), 10–17.

Koyama, H., Kashio, A., Fujimoto, C., Uranaka, T., Matsumoto, Y., Kamogashira, T., . . . Yamasoba, T. (2021). Alteration of vestibular function in pediatric cochlear implant recipients. *Frontiers in Neurology, 12,* 661302. https://doi.org/10.3389/fneur.2021.661302

Kuk, F., & Ludvigsen, C. (2003). Reconsidering the concept of the aided threshold for nonlinear hearing aids. *Trends in Amplification, 7*(3), 77–97. https://doi.org/10.1177/108471380300700302

McCreery, R. W., Venediktov, R. A., Coleman, J. J., & Leech, H. M. (2012). An evidence-based systematic review of directional microphones and digital noise reduction hearing aids in school-age children with hearing loss. *American Journal of Audiology, 21*(2), 295–312. https://doi.org/10.1044/1059-0889(2012/12-0014)

McCreery, R. W., Walker, E. A., Stiles, D. J., Spratford, M., Oleson, J. J., & Lewis, D. E. (2020). Audibility-based hearing aid fitting criteria for children with mild bilateral hearing loss. *Language, Speech, and Hearing Services in Schools, 51*(1), 55–67. https://doi.org/10.1044/2019_LSHSS-OCHL-19-0021

McKay, S., Gravel, J. S., & Tharpe, A. M. (2008). Amplification considerations for children with minimal or mild bilateral hearing loss and unilateral hearing loss. *Trends in Amplification, 12*(1), 43–54. https://doi.org/10.1177/1084713807313570

Messersmith, J. J., Entwisle, L., Warren, S., & Scott, M. (2019). Clinical practice guidelines: Cochlear implants. *Journal of the American Academy of Audiology, 30*(10), 827–844. https://doi.org/10.3766/jaaa.19088

Moore, B. C. (2008). The choice of compression speed in hearing aids: Theoretical and practical considerations and the role of individual differences. *Trends in Amplification, 12*(2), 103–112. https://doi.org/10.1177/1084713808317819

Mussoi, B., & Bentler, R. (2017). Binaural interference and the effects of age and hearing loss. *Journal of the American Academy of Audiology, 28*(1), 5–13. https://doi.org/10.3766/jaaa.15011

Park, L. R., Gagnon, E. B., & Brown, K. D. (2021). The limitations of FDA criteria: Inconsistencies with clinical practice, findings, and adult criteria as a barrier to pediatric implantation. *Seminars in Hearing, 42*(4), 373–380. https://doi.org/10.1055/s-0041-1739370

Rabelo, A. T. V., Santos, J. N., Oliveira, R. C., & Magalhães, M. de C. (2014). Effect of classroom acoustics on the speech intelligibility of students. *CoDAS, 26*(5), 360–366. https://doi.org/10.1590/2317-1782/20142014026

Rasmussen, K., West, N., Tian, L., & Cayé-Thomasen, P. (2021). Long-term vestibular outcomes in cochlear implant recipients. *Frontiers in Neurology, 12*, 686–681. https://doi.org/10.3389/fneur.2021.686681

Schafer, E. C., Kirby, B., & Miller, S. (2020). Remote microphone technology for children with hearing loss or auditory processing issues. *Seminars in Hearing, 41*(4), 277–290. https://doi.org/10.1055/s-0040-1718713

Sharma, A., Dorman, M. F., & Kral, A. (2005). The influence of a sensitive period on central auditory development in children with unilateral and bilateral cochlear implants. *Hearing Research, 203*(1–2), 134–143. https://doi.org/10.1016/j.heares.2004.12.010

Slade, K., Plack, C. J., & Nuttall, H. E. (2020). The effects of age-related hearing loss on the brain and cognitive function. *Trends in Neurosciences, 43*(10), 810–821.

Souza, P. (2002) Effects of compression on speech acoustics, intelligibility, and sound quality. *Trends in Amplification, 6*(4),131–165. https://doi.org/10.1177/108471380200600402

Stelmachowicz, P. G., Pittman, A. L., Hoover, B. M., Lewis, D. E., & Moeller, M. P. (2004). The importance of high-frequency audibility in the speech and language development of children with hearing loss. *Archives of Otolaryngology-Head & Neck Surgery, 130*(5), 556–562. https://doi.org/10.1001/archotol.130.5.556

Stewart, E., & Woodward, J. (2021). Out of the (head) shadow: A systematic review of CROS/BiCROS literature. *The Hearing Review, 28*(8), 22–25.

Stiles, D., Bentler, R., & McGregor, K. (2012). The speech intelligibility index and the pure-tone average as predictors of lexical ability in children fit with hearing aids. *Journal of Speech, Language, and Hearing Research, 55*, 764–778.

Uhler, K., Warner-Czyz, A., Gifford, R., & Working Group, P. (2017). Pediatric minimum speech test battery. *Journal of the American Academy of Audiology, 28*(3), 232–247. https://doi.org/10.3766/jaaa.15123

Walker, E., McCreery, R., Spratford, M., & Roush, P. (2016). Children with auditory neuropathy spectrum disorder fitted with hearing aids applying the American Academy of Audiology pediatric amplification guideline: Current practice and outcomes. *Journal of the American Academy of Audiology, 27*(3), 204–218. https://doi.org/10.3766/jaaa.15050

Walkowiak, A., Lorens, A., Polak, M., Kostek, B., Skarzynski, H., Szkielkowska, A., & Skarzynski, P. H. (2011). Evoked stapedius reflex and compound action potential thresholds versus most comfortable loudness level: Assessment of their relation for charge-based fitting strategies in implant users. *ORL; Journal for Oto-Rhino-Laryngology and Its Related Specialties, 73*(4), 189–195. https://doi.org/10.1159/000326892

Wolfe, J. (2020). *Cochlear implants: Audiologic management and considerations for implantable hearing devices.* Plural Publishing.

Wong, K., Kozin, E. D., Kanumuri, V. V., Vachicouras, N., Miller, J., Lacour, S., . . . Lee, D. J. (2019). Auditory brainstem implants: Recent progress and future perspectives. *Frontiers in Neuroscience, 13*, 10. https://doi.org/10.3389/fnins.2019.00010

Yeo, B. S. Y., Song, H. J. J. M. D., Toh, E. M. S., Ng, L. S., Ho, C. S. H., Ho, R., . . . Loh, W. S. (2022).

Association of hearing aids and cochlear implants with cognitive decline and dementia: A systematic review and meta-analysis. *JAMA Neurology*. Advance online publication. https://doi.org/10.1001/jamaneurol.2022.4427

Yin, S., Njai, R., Barker, L., Siegel, P. Z., & Liao, Y. (2016). Summarizing health-related quality of life (HRQOL): Development and testing of a one-factor model. *Population Health Metrics*, *14*, 1–9. https://doi.org/10.31887/DCNS.2014.16.2/drevicki

Zimmerling, M. J., & Hochmair, E. S. (2002). EAP recordings in Ineraid patients—correlations with psychophysical measures and possible implications for patient fitting. *Ear and Hearing*, *23*(2), 81–91. https://doi.org/10.1097/00003446–200204000–00001

Zwolan, T. A., Schvartz-Leyzac, K. C., & Pleasant, T. (2020). Development of a 60/60 guideline for referring adults for a traditional cochlear implant candidacy evaluation. *Otology & Neurotology*, *41*(7), 895–900. https://doi.org/10.1097/MAO.0000000000002664

✎ Practice Questions

1. A patient with high-frequency SNHL related to presbycusis is fit with binaural amplification for the first time. After a few days of wearing her devices, she returns to your office complaining of bothersome noises including the refrigerator at home, the HVAC system at church, and her key chain rattling in her purse as she walks. What programming strategy may best help this patient?

   a. Implementing a looped system at church to pair to her T-coil

   b. Implementing expansion into her hearing aid programming

   c. Reducing overall gain for all input levels

   d. Creating an earmold with smaller venting

Explanation: The bothersome sounds this patient is reporting are soft sounds that she has not likely heard for many years. With her aids, she now has access to these soft sounds. Expansion can be used as a noise reduction strategy for low-level sounds. By implementing expansion into her device settings, we can help the patient experience perceived quiet in quiet environments. Therefore, b is the correct answer.

2. A 3-year-old with CHARGE syndrome is fit with binaural amplification in the form of traditional BTEs coupled with half shell silicone earmolds. His parents report persistent feedback from the devices after the first 10 to 15 minutes that the patient has them in each morning. The feedback stops when the earmolds are pushed into the ear. His earmolds are new and, when they are properly inserted, appear to fit appropriately. What steps can be taken to reduce feedback for the patient?

   a. Remake the earmolds with a larger vent.

   b. Purchase a different hearing aid style. Instead of a BTE, the patient could try a RIC.

   c. Remake the earmold to be a full shell with helix lock for better retention.

   d. The patient is a better candidate for a cochlear implant due to his diagnosis of CHARGE syndrome. He should be referred to the CI team.

Explanation: Based on the parents' report and troubleshooting descriptions, the feedback seems to result from a poor-fitting earmold. As the half-shell earmolds are new and look well fit when properly inserted, the audiologist should consider switching to a different earmold style. The audiologist could try remaking the earmold to be larger with an additional retention feature. A full-shell earmold with a helix lock may prevent feedback by creating a more secure coupling method. Therefore, c is the correct answer.

3. An adult patient has a moderate SNHL in her right ear and a severe SNHL in her left ear. Her word recognition score was 100% in the right ear and 12% in the left ear. What is the most appropriate amplification option for this patient based solely on the audiometric information provided?

   a. BICROS; CROS device on the left ear

   b. CROS; CROS device on the right ear

   c. BICROS; CROS device on the right ear

   d. CROS; CROS device on the left ear

Explanation: This patient may benefit from traditional amplification in their right ear. The patient has poor word recognition and may not be a good candidate for traditional amplification in her left ear. The patient may benefit from a BICROS system. The CROS device is worn on the poorer hearing ear. Therefore, a is the correct answer.

4. A 4-year-old patient with moderate conductive hearing loss is seen for a hearing aid evaluation. Which is the best air-conduction HA and coupling option based on the information provided?

   a. RIC with open-dome modular fitting

   b. BTE with open-dome modular fitting

   c. BTE with traditional tube and custom earmold

   d. BTE with slim tube and custom earmold

Explanation: Based on the patient's age and degree of hearing loss, the best HA option is a BTE with a traditional tube coupled with a custom earmold. This provides increased durability and more consistent access to appropriate gain. Therefore, c is the correct answer.

5. A 25-year-old patient is seen for an annual hearing aid check. She has a bilateral, mild to moderately severe, high-frequency SNHL. She is currently fit binaurally with BTEs, slim tubes, and custom earmolds. An electroacoustic check is completed using the Verifit2® real ear speech mapping. Results show that her current aids are not meeting targets for high frequencies. What change could initially be implemented to improve high-frequency audibility?

   a. Replace slim tubes with traditional diameter tubing

   b. Switch from custom earmold to closed dome

   c. Change HA style to IIC

   d. Change HA style to a CROS system

Explanation: Slim tubes can create significant high-frequency roll-off. Switching to regular tubing is one way to try and better meet high-frequency targets. Therefore, a is the correct answer.

6. An adult patient with bilateral moderate sloping to severe SNHL arrives at your office with HAs that they acquired from another audiologist's office. The HAs are less than 1 year old. The patient reports wearing the devices during all waking hours but still having difficulty hearing in all situations. You evaluate the patient's aids and find they are not adequately meeting prescriptive targets for their hearing levels. The patient insists that hearing aids do not work for them. What is the best **next** step for this patient:

   a. Recommend the patient purchase new HAs from your office.

   b. Recommend the patient for a cochlear implant evaluation.

   c. Attempt to adjust the gain on the patient's current devices. Charge your standard hearing aid adjustment fee.

   d. Refer the patient for a medical evaluation.

Explanation: First, you should try to meet the patient's needs with the device they have purchased. If you cannot adjust their devices, you could then consider counseling they return to their original audiologist for adjustments. If you cannot adjust the devices to adequately meet their gain needs, then you may counsel them into new devices with more appropriate gain and/or coupling methods. Therefore, c is the correct answer.

7. A cochlear implant recipient arrives for a visit with a chief complaint of increased difficulty in background noise. They were last seen in the office 1 year ago. What is the best next step to address the patient's concerns?

   a. Increase the patient's upper stimulation levels.

   b. Activate a fixed directional program and counsel them regarding environmental modifications.

   c. Recommend they utilize remote microphone technology.

   d. Reevaluate the patient's internal dynamic range.

Explanation: The first thing you should do is reevaluate the internal dynamic range. Optimization of mapping parameters is the key to successful performance. After these are optimized, you can talk about directionality and remote microphone technology. Therefore, d is the correct answer.

8. A cochlear implant recipient is experiencing facial stimulation with their device. Which of these is the best **next** step to eliminate their facial stimulation:

   a. Globally lower their upper stimulation levels.

   b. Increase the pulse width of the patient's map.

   c. Contact the manufacturer and order an integrity test.

   d. Identify the electrode or region that is causing the facial stimulation.

Explanation: You should identify the electrode or region that is causing the facial stimulation and try to correct it within that region only without making global changes to the MAP. Therefore, d is the correct answer.

9. A 24-month-old child with auditory neuropathy has been wearing appropriately fitted HAs since age 9 months. The child presents with a moderate SNHL when tested via behavioral threshold measures. They are currently nonverbal with no other diagnoses or syndromes. Which THREE options are appropriate next steps for the child (select all that apply):

   a. Refer the child for a speech-language evaluation.

   b. Refer the child to an otolaryngologist for further medical evaluation.

   c. Recommend the child undergo an audiologic cochlear implant evaluation.

   d. Contact the child's pediatrician and recommend an evaluation for autism spectrum disorder.

Explanation: This child should undergo evaluation by the pediatric cochlear implant team members. Regardless of behavioral thresholds, children with ANSD may not be able to adequately access speech and language with HAs and should be considered for cochlear implantation. Therefore, a, b, and c are the correct answers.

10. Which of the following is considered current best practice for programming upper stimulation levels that are equally loud for an adult that can participate in behavioral mapping techniques?

    a. Electrically evoked compound action potential

    b. Electrically evoked stapedial reflex threshold

    c. Psychophysical loudness scaling

    d. Creating a map based on the manufacturer-specified population mean

Explanation: Even when the patient can participate in psychophysical loudness scaling, they may not be skilled at listening to loudness differences through the electrode array, especially if they are a new user. ESRT is the best way to ensure equal loudness regardless of the patient's subjective scaling abilities. Therefore, b is the correct answer.

Appendix 9–A

Hearing Aid Styles/Types

STYLE OF HEARING AID	DESCRIPTION	TYPE/SEVERITY OF HEARING LOSS	ADVANTAGES	DISADVANTAGES
Completely in Canal (CIC)	HA fits entirely into external auditory canal.	Fits a range of hearing loss severity. Less power than RIC or BTE.	Discreet and cosmetically appealing. Less wind noise. Receiver closer to TM, so less gain needed.	Fewer technology options. Requires patient dexterity. Risk of occlusion.
In The Canal (ITC)	HA fits in external auditory canal, partially filling concha. Custom fit using impression of ear.	Can fit a range of hearing loss severities. Less power than RIC or BTE.	No tubing or earmold needed. Discreet. Receiver closer to TM, so less gain needed.	Fewer technology options. Requires good patient dexterity. Risk of occlusion and cerumen damage.
In the Ear (ITE)	HA fits into concha. Custom fit using an impression of the ear.	Can fit a range of hearing loss severity. Less power than RIC or BTE.	No tubing or earmold needed. Discreet. Receiver closer to TM, so less gain needed.	Technology options depend on ear size. Risk of occlusion and cerumen damage. Requires good patient dexterity.
Receiver in Canal (RIC)	HA rests behind the ear. Receiver wire connects HA to receiver sitting in outer portion of EAC. Coupled by soft dome or custom earmold.	Different receiver strengths available to fit range of hearing loss.	Includes directional mics. Can accommodate advanced signal processing and wireless/Bluetooth technology. Rechargeable options.	Receiver wire is fragile. Risk of cerumen damage.
Behind the Ear Hearing Aid (BTE)	HA rests behind the ear. Tubing connects HA to in-ear retention device (e.g., an earmold).	Can be used with a variety of hearing loss types and degrees of severity.	Less repairs needed. Can accommodate severe hearing loss. Tamperproof options. Directional mics.	Bulkier and less cosmetically appealing compared to other options.

Appendix 9–B

Cochlear Implant Programming Parameters

PARAMETER	SUB-PARAMETER	DEFINITION	CLINICAL IMPLICATION	RECOMMENDATION
Impedance	Normal Impedances	Telemetry measure; assesses resistance of cochlear fluids to electrical current flow; normal to fluctuate within a few kOhms	Direct implications on maximum power output of device (compliance); compliance changes relative to impedance; high impedances = lower compliance; impedances high at activation, lower and stabilize first few months Normal fluctuations: changes in the recipient's hormones, reduction in device use, and cases of reimplantation Abnormal fluctuations: middle ear disease or inflammation, cases of migrating electrode array, device malfunction	With fluctuating impedances, verify recipient's MAP. If impedances increase, patient may become out of compliance.
	Open Circuit	Impedances >manufacturer-recommended limits	Possible cause: air bubble or significant protein buildup around electrode; too much energy needed to obtain normal loudness	Deactivate electrode(s); may spontaneously resolve
	Short Circuit	Impedances <manufacturer-recommended limits; no resistance between two electrodes	Possible cause: bends in the electrode array, folded over on itself, damaged electrode array	Deactivate electrode(s); remains deactivated for lifetime of device

continues

APPENDIX 9–B. *continued*

PARAMETER	SUB-PARAMETER	DEFINITION	CLINICAL IMPLICATION	RECOMMENDATION
Directional Microphones		Microphone configuration. Optimizes signal in front of listener, reduction of signal behind listener; exact configuration delineated by the manufacturer.	Adaptive directionality: more effective and provide easier utilization	Give both omnidirectional and directional microphone configurations, automatic or manual. No default directional-only program for pediatrics. Use with other manufacturer-specific signal processing algorithms.
Electrical Dynamic Range (EDR)	Threshold, Upper Stimulation Level	Difference between lowest current level and highest current level presented to the patient	EDR too large or too small = poorer performance on detection, word recognition Ideal EDR value is different depending on the manufacturer	Manufacturer-specific: threshold audibility Equally loud upper stimulation levels = better sound quality and word recognition
Input Dynamic Range (IDR)		Difference between softest sound picked up by the microphones and loudest sound picked up by the microphones	Ideal IDR: access to soft and loud sounds with comfortable loudness percepts Range: 25 dB SPL to level determined by manufacturer	Children: low IDR for access to distant and low-level speech Adults: increase IDR to improve comfort in noise
Volume		Determines amount of current is presented prior to being outputted by the array	Higher volume: higher current level for input signal; constrained by patient compliance levels	Adults: give volume control, especially during activation period as alternate to progressive programs
Sensitivity		Affects signal picked up by microphones and amount of gain applied	Higher sensitivity: greater access to soft speech, negative impact on performance in noise Lower sensitivity: positive outcomes in noise	Provide savvy patients access to sensitivity

PARAMETER	SUB-PARAMETER	DEFINITION	CLINICAL IMPLICATION	RECOMMENDATION
Rate		Number of biphasic pulses per second is presented during electric stimulation; varies per manufacturer	Changing rate can impact performance by improving or reducing speech understanding. Inversely related to duration-increased rate, increased maximum pulse.	Remap, verify performance after changing rate
Pulse duration (width)		Number of seconds pulse is presented during electric stimulation	Increased pulse width: increased percept of loudness without changes in stimulation level	Increase when stim level limited by patient compliance levels or facial stimulation
Processing/Coding Strategy		Proprietary algorithm used to present stimulation to patient; comprises default stimulation settings	Set prior manipulating upper and lower stimulation levels	Start with the manufacturer-recommended/newest strategy; reassess based on performance
Stimulation mode	Monopolar stimulation	Method of completing electrical circuit; extracochlear electrode is ground	Monopolar: broader current spread between electrodes; allows measurement of a few channels and interpolation between them	Monopolar is U.S. recommendation
	Bipolar stimulation	Method of completing electrical circuit; intracochlear electrode is ground	Bipolar: cannot use interpolation, measure every channel	
	Common ground	Method of completing electrical circuit; all remaining intracochlear electrodes are ground	Common ground: diagnostic only, not for active stimulation; most sensitive to detecting shorts	

continues

PARAMETER	SUB-PARAMETER	DEFINITION	CLINICAL IMPLICATION	RECOMMENDATION
Channels/ Bands/ Frequency Allocation Tables (FAT)		Specific frequency composition of channels, range, and assignment	Greater range of and a higher number of frequencies are ideal, constrained by individual capacity and residual spiral ganglion nerve survival Adjusted for users with residual acoustic hearing	Virtual channels can increase intermediary pitch percept, improved sound quality
Channel Gain		Amount of amplification as a function of channel	Varies per manufacturer	Optimize programming before changing channel gain

Source: Key parameters identified via Messersmith et al. (2019).

Chapter 10

Treatment: Topics in Aural Rehabilitation

Laura N. Galloway

Introduction

Aural rehabilitation is a broad term that is used to describe any intervention that seeks to reduce the impact of hearing loss on communication and on the emotional, psychosocial, educational, and vocational functioning of people with hearing loss. In the field of communication disorders, it has been referred to by a variety of terms over the years, including AR, auditory rehabilitation, audiologic rehabilitation, hearing rehabilitation, aural habilitation, and rehabilitative audiology. While these terms are often used interchangeably, there are a few differences that should be pointed out.

- Aural rehabilitation is arguably the broadest term as it is used to describe therapeutic activities of an interdisciplinary nature that may be performed by different providers, typically speech-language pathologists (SLPs), to address the impact of hearing impairment on receptive and expressive communication. Because hearing disorders inherently impact speech and language development, audiologists, SLPs, educators, therapists, and other professionals commonly have overlapping or complementary roles.

- Audiologic or auditory rehabilitation has been gaining favor as a term to describe interventions provided specifically by audiologists that includes many of the traditional aural rehabilitation activities, as well as the provision of sensory management devices, like hearing aids (HAs) or cochlear implants (CIs).

- Aural habilitation is commonly used when providing services to children, as the term habilitation refers to development of skills as opposed to the term rehabilitation, which refers to restoring former functioning.

For the purposes of this chapter, the term AR will be used to describe traditional rehabilitation activities like those aimed to enhance speech perception and understanding as well as activities that aim to address the psychosocial impact of hearing impairment on the whole person and clarify any distinguishing characteristics when appropriate.

487

Defining AR

AR is at the heart of audiology's professional origins as soldiers returning from World War II with noise-induced hearing loss were provided a comprehensive hearing loss rehabilitation program that included HA provision, counseling, and various types of speech perception training (Alpiner & McCarthy, 2014). Over time, as the profession of audiology has shifted toward more diagnostic and device-centered applications, AR has been continually redefined to position itself in the context of treatment for the person with hearing loss.

- Erdman (1993) described the importance of including a counseling component to AR to address nonauditory components of hearing loss, such as emotional, psychosocial, and vocational impacts.

- Boothroyd (2007) added components related to sensory management through provision of devices like HAs when describing a four-pronged approach to AR as "the reduction of hearing loss–induced deficits of function, activity, participation, and quality of life through a combination of sensory management, instruction, perceptual training and counseling" (p. 63).

- A more recent definition of AR comes from Montano (2014) and states that "AR is a person-centered approach to assessment and management of hearing loss that encourages the creation of a therapeutic environment conducive to shared decision process, which is necessary to explore and reduce the impact of hearing loss on communication, activities, and participations" (p. 27).
  - □ This final definition is a reminder of the emphasis on person-centered care and shared decision-making to optimize the rehabilitation process.

- AR can be provided:
  - □ For the person with hearing loss and for their frequent communication partner (FCP)
  - □ For patients of any age with tinnitus, hearing loss, HAs, CIs, auditory processing, and vestibular disorders
  - □ With the provision of HAs or other assistive devices as auditory training, counseling, vocational assessment, family intervention, and more

Regardless of the disorder, the goal of AR is to provide tailored, person-centered services to adults with hearing loss supported by scientific evidence so the patient can make informed treatment decisions to improve clinical outcomes. Figure 10–1 summarizes the many components of AR, each of which will be described in more detail in the sections below.

AR Components

Assessment

Practicing AR often starts with an evaluation of the hearing loss and its impact on auditory and nonauditory functioning. This can include:

- A detailed case history and assessments of current levels of functioning through diagnostic testing and validated outcome measures. It is important to note if the hearing loss is pre- or

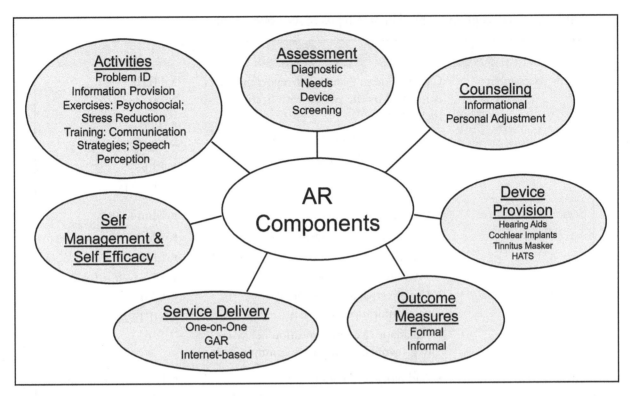

FIGURE 10–1. Summary of AR components.

postlingual and time factors related to prior interventions (e.g., how long have they worn HAs or CIs).

- Assessment for other auditory complaints, like tinnitus or vertigo, to determine the need for additional referrals

- Consideration of cultural and cognitive factors, not only for how they may impact the patient's daily functioning but for consideration of rehabilitative direction

- Gathering information on expectations and goals

- Formal and informal measures that may address educational, vocational, and social functioning

See Table 10–1 for a description of the different types of AR assessments.

Counseling

Counseling is used to shift the relationship between patient and audiologist into one that is therapeutic to facilitate the patient's adjustment to the hearing loss to promote proper management. Counseling can benefit patients by enhancing understanding of hearing loss and its impacts, increasing confidence, reducing stress, and improving motivation to seek and adhere to treatment plans. There are generally two types of counseling:

1. Informational counseling
    - Providing knowledge to the patient about their disorder, the associated symptoms, and the rationale for intervention and prevention

TABLE 10–1. Description of the Different Types of AR Assessments

MEASUREMENT	DETAILS	EXAMPLES
Needs Assessment	Can include subjective self-report measures completed by the person with hearing loss or their FCP on: • Functional impact of hearing loss • Psychological factors • Quality of life	• HHIE • HHIA • THI • CHILD • ELF • ITMAIS
Screening Measures	• Cognitive screening • Speech-language screening • Functional listening skills (e.g., everyday situations at work, school, etc.) • Use of verbal and nonverbal communication strategies • Maladaptive communication behaviors (e.g., avoidance of phone communication)	• Mini-Cog • ASQ • LDS • MacArthur-Bates CDI • SIFTER
Diagnostic Assessment	• Audiologic evaluation • (Central) auditory processing disorder ((C)APD) specific measures • Tinnitus-specific measures • Speech-language evaluation • Skills assessment: detection, discrimination, recognition, and comprehension • Speech recognition/comprehension at various presentation levels (e.g., words, sentences) with and without competing noise • Speechreading assessment at perceived, analytic, and synthetic levels	• Pure-tone hearing test • Classroom observation • Quick-SIN
Device Assessment	• Assessment of the person's current hearing device use (e.g., type, regularity of use, personal and family/significant other satisfaction with device) • Evaluation of differential listening abilities with various amplification options, including the use of hearing assistive technology systems • Determination of candidacy for hearing aid(s), cochlear implant(s), other implantable device(s), and/or hearing assistive technology systems	• APHAB • COSI • DOSO • ECHO • HASP

TABLE 10–1. *continued*

MEASUREMENT	DETAILS	EXAMPLES
Outcome Measures	• Used for tracking treatment progress and benefit	• Pre- and posttreatment comparisons that look at perceived benefit or limitations with the disorder (e.g., HHIE, COSI)

Note. Hearing Handicap Inventory for Adults (HHIA; Newman et al., 1990); Hearing Handicap Inventory for the Elderly (HHI-E; Ventry & Weinstein, 1982); Tinnitus Handicap Inventory (THI; Newman et al., 1996); Children's Home Inventory for Listening Difficulties (CHILD; Anderson & Smaldino, 2000); Early Listening Function (ELF; Anderson, 2002); Infant-Toddler Meaningful Auditory Integration Scale (IT-MAIS; Zimmerman-Phillips et al., 2001); Quick-Speech in Noise (Quick-SIN; Killion et al., 2004); Mini-Cog (Borson et al., 2000); Ages & Stages Questionnaire (ASQ; Squires et al., 2002) ; Language and Development Survey (LDS; Rescorla & Alley, 2001); Screening Instrument for Targeting Educational Risk (SIFTER; Anderson, 1989); Abbreviated Profile of Hearing Aid Benefit (APHAB; Cox & Alexander, 1995); Client Oriented Scale of Improvement (COSI; Dillon et al., 1999); Device Orientated Subjective Outcome scale (DOSO; Cox et al., 2014); Expected Consequences of Hearing Aid Ownership (ECHO; Cox & Alexander, 2000); Hearing Aid Selection Profile (HASP; Jacobson et al., 2001).

Source: Adapted from American Speech-Language-Hearing Association. (n.d.). Aural rehabilitation for adults. https://www.asha.org/practice-portal/professional-issues/aural-rehabilitation-for-adults/#collapse_1

■ Implemented routinely at the conclusion of a patient appointment when reviewing results and providing recommendations

■ As patients only retain about 15% of spoken information provided at medical appointments (Kessels, 2003), methods to improve retention, such as providing information in writing, keeping information brief and easily understandable, and repeating important information, are necessary.

2. Personal adjustment counseling

■ Addressing the psychosocial impacts of hearing loss, in other words the social, psychological, and emotional impact of the disorder

■ Often involves deep empathetic listening, reflection, and clarification to elicit patients' reactions and evaluate them for underlying meaning

■ Sometimes referred to as affective counseling

AR activities can involve both types of counseling and are often well suited to specifically address personal adjustment issues.

 AUDIOLOGY NUGGET

A recent study by Bennett et al. (2020) noted that two thirds of audiologists did not provide personal adjustment counseling for their patients with hearing loss, with over half of audiologists reporting that they lacked the skills to provide this

service for their patients. This highlights a gap in audiology training programs that could be addressed. With perceived threats to audiology service provision such as OTC HAs and third-party buying groups, AR, including personal adjustment counseling, is something that may set audiologists apart from other hearing care providers. Luckily, university programs are addressing this deficit in creative ways, including hands-on training with standardized patient labs and simulation software. The Ida Institute website (https://www.idainstitute.com) is a resource with free counseling tools to help audiologists better address the psychosocial impacts of hearing loss.

Self-Management and Self-Efficacy

The concepts of self-efficacy and self-management are both intertwined in patient-centered care.

- Self-management is used broadly to describe everything one knows and does to manage a problem. Hearing loss, like other chronic health conditions, requires patient action to engage in management of the condition. This can include managing the symptoms (e.g., by going to get a hearing test or choosing an amplification device). It can also include managing the psychosocial impacts by, for example, using good communication skills or stress reduction techniques. Patient participation is essential to the success of self-management. Many of the AR activities described below are self-management activities.

- Self-efficacy is used to describe how capable one is of managing a problem. Older adults with high self-efficacy are more likely to engage in self-management. Patients with low self-efficacy can be identified to engage them in targeted AR activities designed to increase self-efficacy and therefore increase the likelihood they take action to manage their hearing loss.

AR Service Delivery

AR is implemented in many forms, from one-on-one counseling during a routine appointment, to group sessions with other individuals with hearing impairment, to Internet-based designs like group-based message boards or computer-based programs that can be used in the home. As previously mentioned, AR can include services like HA provision, CI programming, and management of vestibular disorders or tinnitus, which are beyond the scope of this chapter. The following will focus primarily on activities related to addressing communication-related difficulties that do not include specific devices or relate to specific disorders.

Group AR

Using a group setting to deliver AR activities can be particularly beneficial as it helps address the concept of stigma.

- Stigma is a social construct whereby society attaches a label to a devalued trait. Hearing loss is considered a stigmatizing trait and often has negatively associated labels like "old" and "incapable" attached. Stigma constitutes a barrier for many people in the hearing loss rehabilitation process. An audiologist leading a group AR (GAR) session can address stigma by including activities that are designed to evoke the feelings, behaviors, and physical effects associated with hearing loss.

- GAR utilizes principles of social comparison theory (Suls et al., 2002), which promotes adjustment to hearing loss through comparisons with others. Those participating in GAR often believe they are managing well compared to others and find solace in realizing that others are living with some of the same issues.

A group setting for AR helps to reinstate the feeling of belonging as people with hearing loss benefit from sharing experiences and solutions to problems in an open environment.

 AUDIOLOGY NUGGET: STIGMA AND GAR

How does a group setting benefit individuals with hearing impairment during the rehabilitation process? Hétu (1996) described a two-step process for using a group setting to address hearing loss as a stigmatizing trait. In the first step, individuals with hearing loss interact with other individuals with hearing loss (i.e., other individuals that have the stigmatizing trait). As the trait of hearing loss is now shared and not deviant, members of the group can compare the difficulties they experienced and their solutions in a supportive environment. Individuals realize that the problems they are experiencing are due to hearing loss and not some personal deficit. The second step of Hétu's process involves interacting with normal-hearing individuals and using the skills and coping strategies learned in Step 1 with the ultimate goal of restoring former social identity. This two-step process of sharing and practicing is commonly employed in a GAR setting.

Internet-Based AR

Interned-based AR programs have gained popularity as access to technology and availability of new programs has increased exponentially over the last 10 to 20 years.

- More older adults than ever before are accessing the Internet for a variety of purposes, including for managing chronic conditions, like hearing loss (van Boekel et al., 2017).

- The inclusion of interactive, online curriculum helps connect older adults who may not be able to attend traditional AR activities with other older adults in similar settings, mimicking the impact of a traditional GAR setting.

- Internet- or computer-based programs are commonly used for speech perception training activities, especially for children or new CI users. The ability of a patient to complete the activities on their own frees up clinical time for other patient needs like programming devices or counseling.

- While technology helps increase the reach of AR services, it is important to remember that it will not be optimal for every patient.

Activities

AR practitioners have a variety of topics to choose from when implementing an AR plan for their patients.

- Treatment should be tailored to individual characteristics (e.g., age, hearing status), needs, and goals.

- Some activities are best suited for group settings, whereas others may be better suited for online or one-on-one meetings.

- It is important to first establish a set of guidelines or rules (expectations) for participants to abide by. This is especially important not only to improve adherence to treatment but in a group setting to keep participants on task.

  □ In a one-on-one or virtual setting, these guidelines can include expectations for the task, like how often and in what order tasks should be completed.

  □ In a group setting, these guidelines can include rules, like allowing only one person to speak at a time, or breaking into small groups for discussion and practice.

- Common AR activities include problem identification and solving, information provision, psychosocial exercises, communication strategies training, speech perception training, stress reduction exercises, and provision of hearing assistive technology systems (HATS). HATS are electronic devices that are designed to offer additional assistance to individuals with hearing impairment in specific listening environments (e.g., when there is a lot of noise in the room, when hearing from a distance, or in a highly reverberant environment). These devices can be used alone or in conjunction with HAs.

Problem Identification and Problem Solving

Problem identification (ID) is typically a good way to begin an AR activity as it can help determine follow-up activities that support solutions to these problems.

- Goal attainment scales can be used to identify problems, rank them, and implement and track appropriate strategies.

- Problem ID and problem solving in a group setting can promote adjustment to hearing loss through participation in the shared activity.

- In one-on-one or Internet-based programs, problems can be identified through formal measures like case history forms or questionnaires like the Client Oriented Scale of Improvement (COSI; Dillon et al., 1999) or through informal discussion. Formal measures offer a validated tool to identify treatment goals, but informal discussion may foster an environment where the patient is more open to discussing their difficulties. The "What's the worst thing about having a hearing loss?" described in this chapter is an example of an informal problem identification activity performed in a group. The group leader could choose future activities based on problems that are identified by multiple group members.

Information Provision

Informational lectures or handouts can be a useful way to increase the amount of knowledge that a patient gets outside of the face-to-face appointment time. It helps the patient avoid information overload and makes better use of clinical time. For example, in a group setting, audiologists can address a common HA patient complaint (e.g., Bluetooth connectivity) to multiple patients at once. Topics for informational content are best determined based on needs and can include:

- Getting the most out of HA features and functions
- HATS demonstrations

- Installing visual alerting systems
- Understanding your audiogram
- Tips for better communication

When holding informational group sessions, it is important to review suggestions for teaching adult learners, which can include planning interactive components that engage an audience.

Hearing Assistive Technology Systems (HATS)

Sometimes the problems identified by a patient can be solved with technology. HAs are often thought of as the first treatment option for older adults with hearing impairment, but HA benefit is limited in some environments. HATS offer additional assistance to hearing-impaired individuals in specific listening environments. HATS can include:

- Use of Bluetooth technology to improve the signal-to-noise ratio (SNR) for devices like the television or the telephone
- Use of remote microphones or frequency modulation (FM) systems to improve the SNR of the signal of interest, commonly speech
- Altering systems, for example, a smoke alarm with a flashing strobe light or an alarm clock that shakes the pillow
- Looped systems, which are useful for large, public venues like theaters, train stations, or churches. These use induction technology to transmit sound from the signal of interest to either a HA with a telecoil engaged or an individual headset.

See Table 10–2 for a comprehensive list of different types of HATS.

 AUDIOLOGY NUGGET: HATS

One of the often-cited limitations of well-fit HAs is the inability to hear the signal of interest in the presence of background noise. One of the only ways to overcome this limitation is by increasing the level of the signal so that it is louder than the level of the background noise in the room. This can be accomplished by using Bluetooth or FM technology to stream the signal of interest, picked up by a remote microphone, directly to the HAs. Research has shown that using HATS in this manner improves speech perception abilities in noise (Saunders et al., 2018; Thibodeau, 2014). Despite repeated studies showing the benefit of this technology, the adoption of HATS by adults with hearing impairment remains low; reasons for this are related to device malfunction, aesthetics, and stigma. Simply put, the situational benefit experienced by the users often did not outweigh the lifestyle cost of having another device to maintain, especially since use of these devices often requires cooperation from others (those who need to wear the remote microphone). For these reasons, practitioners may be selective in suggesting HATS for every patient. HATS are sometimes better suited as an alternative to HAs; for example, a standalone streaming device may be the best option for a person with hearing loss who only reports difficulty hearing on the television.

TABLE 10–2. Comprehensive List of HATS

TYPICAL PLACE OF USE	NAME OF DEVICE	DESCRIPTION
Classroom	FM system	• Sound is transmitted from a wireless microphone via FM radio waves to a receiver. • Can be a personal FM system or a soundfield FM system • For personal FM, receiver may be directly integrated into the hearing aid or may be an intermediary device, like a boot or neck loop. • For soundfield, receiver is a speaker placed near the person with hearing impairment (e.g., on classroom desktop).
	Classroom Audio Distribution System (CADS)	• Sound is transmitted from a microphone worn by the teacher as well as a pass-around microphone used by students in the classroom to speakers distributed evenly throughout the classroom. • All students in the class can benefit from the increase in SNR. • Decrease auditory fatigue and increase attention • Reduce vocal strain on the teacher
	Bluetooth wireless streaming	• Transmits signals wirelessly using 2.4 to 2.5 GHz radio waves • Higher-frequency range than FM, which allows for small antenna and multiple device connections at once • Limited range (10 m) • Multiple devices can use Bluetooth streaming, including remote microphones, cellphones, and computers, often without an intermediary device. • Many smartphones can use Bluetooth to act as a remote microphone and stream directly to hearing aids.
	Communication Access Realtime Translation (CART)	• Real-time, verbatim text of spoken presentations is typed onto a screen by a trained provider • Ideal for live events, like presentations, workshops or meetings • Can be accomplished remotely as long as there is a designated person on site to assist with setup and troubleshooting
Public Forums (e.g., theaters, places of worship)	Infrared streaming device	• Transmits the signal of interest to the receiver via infrared light waves • Receiver may be a standalone headset or use an intermediary device like a neck loop • Not appropriate for outdoor use (sunlight interferes with transmission) • Need a direct line of site between transmitter and receiver (does not work between walls) • Smartphone applications for live captioning of speech

TABLE 10–2. *continued*

TYPICAL PLACE OF USE	NAME OF DEVICE	DESCRIPTION
Public Forums (e.g., theaters, places of worship) *continued*	Induction Loop system	• Sound is picked up from the microphone and converted into an electric signal, which is transmitted via electromagnetic energy through a wired loop that surrounds the perimeter of the listening environment. • The sound can be picked up by hearing aid users with their telecoil setting engaged or through telecoil enabled headsets.
	Hardwired systems	• Sound is picked up by the microphone and transmitted directly to the listener via a cable that connects to the user's hearing aids or a headset.
Telephone	Amplified telephone	• Telephones that allow the user to adjust output volume to a preferred level.
	Captioned telephones	• A special telephone with a built-in screen that provides word-for-word captioning in nearly real time while the user simultaneously hears the speaker's voice
	Text telephones	• A telephone that also includes a keyboard and message display screen • Both parties must have a text telephone. • Parties communicate by typing their messages back and forth to each other. • Sometimes referred to as telecommunication devices for the Deaf (TDD)
	Relay systems	• A trained operator serves as an intermediary during a telephone conversation. • The person with hearing loss communicates with the operator by using a text telephone and the person with normal hearing communicates with the operator via voice.
Home/Hotels	Alerting systems	• Using sound, vibration, light, or a combination of the three to notify when a particular event is occurring • Sample devices include shaking pillow alarm clocks, flashing strobe lights for smoke detectors, or vibrating wristbands to alert when a baby is crying. • Apps and smartphone settings can provide alerts for specific environmental sounds.

Psychosocial Exercises

Psychosocial exercises are specifically designed to address how hearing loss impacts individuals in the psychological domain (e.g., self-image, stigma, stress) and the social domain (e.g., withdrawal, family relationships, work). It is especially important to address psychosocial outcomes due to the associations between hearing loss and negative health outcomes, like dementia and depression, and the proposed mechanism of social withdrawal (e.g., Pichora-Fuller et al., 2015).

- Psychosocial exercises involve asking individuals to share, discuss, and practice effective coping strategies, whether it be coping with a psychological or a social impact.
- Psychosocial support can be particularly beneficial when patients have a negative emotional response to their hearing loss or have withdrawn from their usual activities due to fear of communication breakdown.
- One example of a psychosocial exercise can be seen in the "What's the worst thing about having a hearing loss?" GAR activity described in the box below.
- When choosing psychosocial exercises, monitor the tone and phrasing of exercises to ensure a balance between positive and negative wording. For example, you could follow up "What's the worst thing about having a hearing loss?" activity with "What's the best thing about having a hearing loss?" The resulting humorous answers can lighten the mood and promote camaraderie among the group.

 ### CASE EXAMPLE: WHAT'S THE WORST THING ABOUT HAVING A HEARING LOSS?

During a recent GAR class, the group facilitator prompted the class with the question, "What's the worst thing about having a hearing loss?" One of the participants, Emmitt, a 68-year-old new HA user, responded, "I can't hear when my spouse whispers something to me." He was surprised when other members began to laugh, and almost all noted that none of them could hear whispered speech either. In this group, the stigma associated with hearing loss was lowered, allowing participants to share their experiences and feelings about living with hearing loss. At the end of the session, Emmitt reported that he felt better about his hearing problems when he realized that they were shared by others and not some personal deficit.

Additional problems identified by the group during this exercise included understanding on the telephone, strain on relationships with friends and family due to communication breakdown, and not being able to enjoy going to the movie theater. Once these problems were identified, the group facilitator decided to include a discussion on HATS, communication strategies, training exercises, stress reduction exercises, and a separate class for FCPs for future course agendas. This is an example of how problem identification exercises can be used to determine AR activities.

Communication Strategies Training

People with hearing impairment will have a primary complaint of difficulty communicating with others, which can be a source of anxiety. To facilitate communication, AR often involves talking with and teaching patients about communication strategies. These are tactics that patients can use to prevent a breakdown in communication from happening or to repair a breakdown after it occurs.

- Communication strategies training can occur in any setting. This type of training can be implemented during GAR by having participants role-play through different communication breakdown settings. Communication strategies can also be promoted by one-on-one counseling during a routine appointment or as a take-home printout.

- Anticipatory strategies: communication strategies that are designed to prevent a communication breakdown from occurring in the future

  - □ Example: 15 things activity (Trychin, 2003); participants work together to brainstorm 15 both common and creative solutions to a group-generated hearing loss-related problem (e.g., trouble hearing on the telephone).

  - □ Often involve exercises designed to promote self-advocacy, which may lead to a discussion of the Americans With Disabilities Act (ADA, 1990) and rights of people with hearing loss.

    - Example: an anticipatory strategy aimed at helping one hear better at a theater may also involve a self-advocacy activity describing and practicing steps needed to get ahold of HATS in a public theater.

- Repair strategies: designed to fix a communication breakdown that has already occurred

  - □ This often involves the person with hearing loss admitting to having a hearing loss, explaining the communication breakdown, and then offering a solution.

  - □ Some people with hearing loss would prefer to avoid this interaction due to stigma. Since the stigma of hearing loss is lowered in a GAR setting, this can be an ideal time to practice repair strategies.

Speech Perception Training

Speech perception training, like AR, has taken on a variety of meanings and terminology over the years. For adults with postlingual hearing impairment, speech perception training has been viewed as a means to address the inability of well-fit HAs to return spoken communication to preclinical abilities. For infants and children with prelingual hearing impairment, speech perception training may be viewed as a means to enhance access to the auditory signal to promote speech and language development. Speech perception training is often divided into three categories: lip reading training, speech reading training, and auditory training.

- Lip reading training—training based only on visual cues

  - □ Not typically an effective use of time and resources as lipreading abilities are highly variable among individuals (Hall et al., 2005)

- Speech reading training—training participants using auditory and visual stimuli

  - □ Has not been shown to improve speech understanding scores when implemented in a group setting (Preminger & Ziegler, 2008); however, participants did report benefit from the activity, likely from increased confidence and decreased perceptual effort when using visual cues to understand speech in a difficult listening environment.

- Auditory training—training with only auditory stimuli

  - □ The most widely used of the three methods; goal is to maximize residual hearing.

  - □ Often used with children with hearing loss, CI users, or even as part of a treatment plan for listeners with normal peripheral hearing (e.g., CAPD).

☐ Auditory training approaches can be analytic, synthetic, or a combination of both.

- Analytic auditory training—bottom-up processing approach to distinguish the smallest linguistic features in speech (e.g., phonemes, syllables); follows the auditory skills hierarchy of awareness, discrimination, identification, and comprehension to move from tasks that are easy to difficult.

- Synthetic auditory training—top-down processing that places an emphasis on larger segments of speech, like words, phrases, and sentences; advantage is that it uses ecologically valid tasks and trains the listener to use context to determine parts of the auditory signal that were missed.

■ Auditory training programs are generally available as computer-based programs with game-like activities designed to be completed over a specified time period and featuring adaptive exercises in different categories, like understanding degraded speech. Perhaps the most well-known computer-based auditory training program is the Listening and Communication Enhancement (LACE) program (Sweetow & Sabes, 2007). All three types of speech perception training can be done in conjunction with sensory aids or as a standalone alternative to sensory aids.

KNOWLEDGE CHECKPOINT

The primary goal of auditory training is to assist patients in recognizing and interpreting speech sounds based on the auditory signal. Auditory training activities are typically either analytic or synthetic. Analytic auditory training focuses on smaller units of speech, like phonemes and syllables, with the thought process being that these smaller units of speech must be detectable and differentiated before the whole word or phrase can be identified. An analytic activity may focus on differentiating the word "stop" from the word "chop." Synthetic training, on the other hand, focuses on understanding the meaning of an entire phrase or sentence, regardless of if every word is understood. The thought here is that understanding the whole idea and learning to use context is more important than understanding each word. An example of a synthetic training activity would involve reading a passage out loud and then having the patient answer questions based on the passage. Both types of activities should be employed in auditory training.

Stress Reduction Exercises

Individuals with hearing loss may experience stress not only from the impact of the hearing loss and subsequent communication breakdown but also from the increased listening effort and fatigue that comes from engaging in typical communication. For this reason, AR can include teaching patients stress management techniques, like breathing and relaxation exercises.

■ One example of a stress reduction exercise is the controlled breathing exercise for tinnitus patients from Henry et al. (2010). In this exercise, patients are instructed to lie on their back in a relaxed position and place one hand on their chest and one hand on their abdomen. Next, they are advised to notice the difference in hand movements when they take shallow breaths compared to when they take deep breaths. They are then instructed to focus on taking several deep breaths in a row until they are feeling calmer and more relaxed.

■ While the exercises themselves are designed to promote stress reduction, simply acknowledging the connection between hearing loss and stress can be a profound realization for some patients.

Measuring Outcomes

Success of treatment is influenced by patient adherence to treatment. Documenting outcomes is vital to professional accountability. AR outcomes can be measured in a variety of objective and subjective ways. One of the easiest ways to measure outcomes is with validated measures of benefit and quality of life. Commonly, researchers and clinicians compare pre- and postintervention scores on the Hearing Handicap Inventory for Adults (HHIA; Newman et al., 1990), the Hearing Handicap Inventory for the Elderly (HHIE; Ventry & Weinstein, 1982), or the International Outcome Inventory–Alternative Interventions (IOI-IA; Noble, 2002). All three of these measures have been shown to be sensitive to the impact of hearing loss–related interventions on activity limitations, participation restrictions, and psychosocial factors. A detailed list of common questionnaires and scales used in AR is outlined in Table 10–3. More informal measures can be used to track AR-related outcomes, for example, measuring the effectiveness of a GAR program for new HA users by making a comparison of the number of HA return rates among users who attended the GAR session and users who did not. The type of outcome measure chosen depends on the type of intervention and the goals of the treatment.

 KNOWLEDGE CHECKPOINT

It is clear that hearing loss can impact an individual on many levels, but hearing loss can have a measurable impact on the frequent communication partners (FCPs) of people with hearing loss as well. Scarinci et al. (2011) showed that spouses of adults with hearing loss encountered an increase in reported limitations and restrictions in activities and participation as a result of their partner's hearing loss. For example, FCPs, like spouses or adult children, may avoid joint activities they themselves enjoy if they think their loved one with hearing impairment will struggle to hear. They may report feeling fatigued and frustrated from always having to be the one who answers the phone or repeats things that are not understood. FCPs may not understand the limitations of HAs and wonder why their loved one still struggles despite consistent device usage. FCPs should always be encouraged to join in the rehabilitation process. This can be something as simple as calling them in from the waiting room before reviewing results to as complex as having a GAR class just for FCPs. FCPs can benefit from participation in the rehabilitation process by learning communication strategies to use with their partner and by gaining a better understanding of the difficulties their partner experiences. Additionally, perceived support from FCPs has been shown to improve outcomes, increase HA uptake, and improve satisfaction with devices (e.g., Singh et al., 2015).

TABLE 10–3. Common Questionnaires and Scales Used in AR

NAME	POPULATION	KEY FEATURES
Early Listening Function (ELF; Anderson, 2002)	Infants ≥5 months of age	• Teaches families to observe auditory behaviors and suggests activities to stimulate alerting responses in their young child • Validation measure of improvement in access to auditory signals and functional benefit of amplification system
LittlEars Auditory Questionnaire (Tsiakpini et al., 2004)	0–48 months (hearing age)	• Assessment of auditory skills of young children with hearing loss • Used to show need for hearing intervention and improvement in auditory skills during intervention
Children's Home Inventory Listening Difficulties (CHILD; Anderson & Smaldino, 2000)	3–12 years Caregiver completes if child is less than 7 years old	• Parents rate children's abilities for 15 different listening situations in the home/family environment • Assists in counseling regarding the communication difficulties a child with hearing loss can experience • Assesses need for assistive listening devices • Monitors auditory function with amplification and assistive devices over time
Infant-Toddler Meaningful Auditory Integration Scale (IT-MAIS; Zimmerman-Phillips et al., 2001)	1a: >age 5 1b: <age 5	• Structured interview schedule designed to assess the child's spontaneous responses to sound in his or her everyday environment • Must be completed in interview style
Ages and Stages Questionnaire (ASQ; Squires et al., 2002)	2–60 months	• Screening tool for caregiver to review child's development • Specific questionnaires for each age • Scores communication, gross motor, fine motor, problems solving, and personal-social development
Language Development Survey (LDS; Rescorla & Alley, 2001)	2 years	• Screening tool for identification of language delay in 2-year-old children • 10-minute completion time
MacArthur-Bates Communicative Development Inventories (CDI; Fenson et al., 2006)	Words and Gestures: 8–18 months Words and Sentences: 16 to 30 months	• Short- and long-form options • Spanish and English • Parent report instrument to capture information about a child's developing abilities in early language, including vocabulary comprehension, production, gestures, and grammar
Screening Instrument for Targeting Educational Risk (SIFTER; Anderson, 1989)	12–18 years	• Screening tool for area of educational risk as a result of hearing loss • Evaluates risk in academics, attention, communication, class participation, and social behavior

TABLE 10–3. *continued*

NAME	POPULATION	KEY FEATURES
Hearing Handicap Inventory for Adults (HHIA; Newman et al., 1990)	Preretirement age individuals with active lifestyles	• Measures perceived social and emotional handicap of hearing loss • Does not always correlate with degree of hearing loss
Hearing Handicap Inventory for the Elderly (HHIE; Ventry & Weinstein, 1982)	Retired individuals (typically 65 years and older)	• Measures perceived social and emotional handicap of hearing loss • Does not always correlate with degree of hearing loss
Tinnitus Handicap Inventory (THI; Newman et al., 1996)	Adults with tinnitus complaints	• Measures perceived social and emotional handicap of tinnitus
Abbreviated Profile of Hearing Aid Benefit (APHAB; Cox & Alexander, 1995)	Adults	• Predicts success from unaided scores, compares results with different hearing aids, evaluates fittings in an absolute sense, and measures benefit from the fitting • Evaluates ease of communication, reverberation, background noise, and aversiveness
Client Oriented Scale of Improvement (COSI; Dillon et al., 1999)	Adults	• Identifies three to five very specific listening goals/communication needs for amplification and measure expectations related to specific goals
Device Oriented Subjective Outcome (DOSO; Cox et al., 2014)	Adults	• Measures hearing aid outcomes focusing on the device itself in a manner that is relatively independent of wearer's personality • Evaluates speech cues, listening effort, pleasantness, quietness, convenience, and use • Short and long forms available
Hearing Aid Selection Profile (HASP; Jacobsen et al., 2001)	Adults	• Assesses eight patient factors related to the use of hearing aids, motivation, expectations, appearance, cost, technology, physical needs, communication needs, and lifestyle
Expected Consequences of Hearing Aid Ownership (ECHO; Cox & Alexander, 2000)	Adults	• Assessment of expectations to counsel patients on realistic expectations related to positive effects, service and cost, negative features, and personal image
Characteristics of Amplification Tool (COAT; Sandridge & Newman, 2006)	Adults	• Nine questions designed to determine the patient's communication needs, motivation expectations, cosmetics, and cost concerns
Satisfaction of Amplification in Daily Life (SADL; Cox & Alexander, 1999)	Adults	• Seventh-grade reading level with 10-minute completion time • Indirect measure of satisfaction

continues

TABLE 10–3. *continued*

NAME	POPULATION	KEY FEATURES
Significant Other Scale for Hearing Disability (SOS-HEAR; Scarinci et al., 2009)	FCP of adults with hearing loss	• Measures third-party disability experienced by spouses of older adults with hearing impairment • 27-item scale, with six subscales
International Outcomes Inventory for Hearing Aids (IOI-HA; Cox et al., 2003)	Adults with hearing aids	• 7-item questionnaire that evaluates the effectiveness of hearing aid treatments • Alternate version IOI-AI (Alternate Interventions) looks at impact of non–hearing aid interventions (e.g., GAR)
Hearing Impairment Impact–Significant Other Profile (HII-SOP; Preminger & Meeks, 2012)	FCP of adults with hearing loss	• Measures third-party disability experienced by spouses of adults with hearing impairment • 3 subscales: emotional impact, social impact, and communication strategies use
Self-Assessment of Communication (SAC; Schow & Nerbonne, 1982)	Adults	• 10-item scale that measures communication difficulties in a variety of settings • Includes questions related to disability, handicap, and perceptions of others' attitudes toward hearing loss
Significant Other Assessment of Communication (SOAC; Schow & Nerbonne, 1982)	FCP of adults with hearing loss	• 10-item scale that mimics the questions in the SAC but changes pronouns in order to reflect the FCP's point of view • Provides a proxy report of the person with hearing loss' perceived difficulties

Considerations for Older Adults and AR

Since hearing loss increases with age and older adults are the fastest-growing segment of the U.S. population, it makes sense to focus on considerations for older adults during the rehabilitation process. Increasingly, older adults are engaging with technology that can be beneficial not only for adopting sensory devices like HAs, but for engaging in Internet-based AR programs or social networks and discussion boards (Faverio, 2022). There are several factors that may need consideration when working with older adults:

- Multiple chronic health conditions: multiple providers will mandate an interdisciplinary approach to care.
- Cognitive impairment: rate is higher in this population and cognition can impact testing and rehabilitative direction; audiologists should feel comfortable screening for cognitive decline in both new and returning older patients.
- Case history: caregivers or family members may be relied upon to provide.
- Processing speed: may need to slow down approach to testing.
- Word recognition declines: requires additional counseling on device expectations and a greater need to determine and rely on effective communication strategies.

- Vision and dexterity declines: can impact rehabilitative choices (e.g., patients with vision or dexterity issues may need to be guided toward sensory management devices that are simple to use).

- Income: may be on a fixed income; it is important to explain lower cost options; they may end up choosing one amplification device instead of two or may choose to use a less expensive HATS like a TV amplifier. See Table 10–2 for more examples of HATS.

- Groups and programs: information about reputable and appropriate in-person and virtual social network groups and Internet-based auditory training programs for adults as rehabilitation options should be provided.

- Residence and service provision: may occur in nursing homes or other residential-type care facilities where patients are more likely to have multiple health concerns; high staff turnover may make it difficult for some facilities to keep track of and maintain any sensory devices or benefit from training on the impact of hearing loss and the unique needs of these patients.

KNOWLEDGE CHECKPOINT

With the increasing evidence linking untreated hearing loss and negative health outcomes, like dementia and depression, rehabilitation options for older adults with hearing impairment are more important than ever. One of the proposed mechanisms for these negative health outcomes is social isolation (Shukla et al., 2020). Older adults who cannot hear may stop engaging with others in social settings due to fear of communication breakdown. GAR may be an ideal setting for older adults, not only to increase social contacts but also to provide the extra time outside of an appointment that may be needed to discuss things like communication strategies or Bluetooth connectivity. Helping older adults connect with community or online groups like the Hearing Loss Association of America (HLAA) may be another way to combat social isolation in older adults with hearing impairment. HLAA is a nonprofit organization that promotes education, advocacy, and support for adults with hearing loss through regular meetings and events.

From assessments to measuring outcomes, AR is pervasive in all aspects of patient care. This can include counseling patients on the psychosocial aspects of having a hearing loss, providing information on the latest technology options, practicing communication strategies, or completing an online auditory training program. Special considerations are especially important when providing services to older adults. In the next section, we will discuss considerations for AR in the pediatric population.

Pediatric AR

AR is particularly important for children with hearing disorders, especially during the critical period for language development from birth to 3 years of age. AR can take a variety of forms, from counseling families during the initial diagnosis to implementing and monitoring sensory management and working with SLPs and other providers to ensure the child gets optimal access to sound in home, social, and educational environments.

Counseling

Counseling is often thought of as the first step in pediatric AR and one that will be needed at multiple time points during the professional relationship.

- When counseling families of newly diagnosed infants and children, providers should be prepared for a spectrum of emotional responses.

- After the initial diagnosis, some families will be ready to move forward quickly; others will need more time. Recognize that while an audiologist may be an expert on the disorder, that does not mean they understand what each family is going through.

- Utilize a family systems approach, which means always viewing the child within the context of the family and taking family-specific considerations into account during treatment planning.

- Connecting families with resources, including other families of children with hearing loss, is a great way to foster emotional adjustment to hearing loss as families can get reassurance and advice from others who are in the same circumstances as themselves.

- Not only do reactions and needs differ, but they will likely change over time, especially during times of transition, like when starting a new school.

Counseling can include both informational and personal adjustment techniques.

- The goal of informational counseling is to provide information that can empower families for informed decision-making by the family and eventually the child. Informed decision-making is associated with increased satisfaction with intervention and better compliance with recommendations (Margolis, 2004).

- Informational counseling should include techniques to improve retention of information. Clinicians should consider the role of the primacy effect, which states that memory is better

CASE EXAMPLE

When Aubrey was 5 weeks old, she was diagnosed with bilateral, moderate sensorineural hearing loss. One of her caregiver's first questions after the diagnosis was "Will she have to wear HAs all the time?" In this case, the practitioner's first instinct is to answer the informational content in the question. This could look like, "Yes, she should wear her HAs at all waking hours." A practitioner with training in personal adjustment counseling will be able to recognize that this may be an affective question in disguise, which would require a modified response. The caregiver may actually be concerned about HA visibility, stigma, and social acceptance. Therefore, a response that also acknowledges the emotions underlying the question may be more appropriate. For example, "It must be difficult not knowing how things will be in the future, but you are doing the right thing by taking steps to manage your child's hearing loss. With time and practice, the HAs should become a seamless part of your day-to-day routine, where they are placed first thing in the morning and worn all day." In this case, the clinician is still answering the informational request from the caregiver, but they are also responding to the unsaid emotional impact of the new diagnosis.

for information presented first. Clinicians should repeat the most important information and back up verbal information with written information in the family's preferred language.

- Personal adjustment counseling techniques will need to be modified as children grow. Affective listening to recognize and acknowledge emotionally charged statements may be more useful in the early days of a new diagnosis. As the child grows, personal adjustment techniques can be used to identify problems, set goals, and make, practice, and implement action plans.

Service Delivery

For families who choose listening and spoken language, AR activities should emphasize spoken language and include auditory training techniques. Pediatric AR service delivery can be home based, center based, or virtual. One of the primary techniques used in listening and spoken language therapy is a guide and coach technique. With this type of technique:

- Therapy is typically provided by a professional known as an auditory verbal therapist (AVT) or auditory verbal educator (AVE) with a specialty certification from the Alexander Graham Bell Academy in Listening and Spoken Language (LSLS) who has a background in audiology, speech pathology, or education of children who are deaf or hard of hearing.

- Therapy is often provided in the home setting, using toys or equipment that the family already has on hand, and therapy techniques are completed by the caregiver, while the therapist observes and coaches.

- Using this technique allows the caregiver to carry over what they learned during therapy sessions into their daily routine.

- Therapy can also be center based with the child attending therapy at a center, clinic, or school for a set number of hours per week. In this setting, caregiver participation is also encouraged.

Early intervention strategies should begin as soon as the child is diagnosed. From birth to age 3, services for infants and toddlers with hearing loss and their families are covered by Part C of the Individuals With Disabilities Education Act (IDEA, 2004). Specific services may be outlined in an individualized family service plan (IFSP), which considers family resources, goals, priorities, and the child's current level of development to determine the services needed. After the age of 3, AR service provision may be specifically outlined in an Individual Education Plan (IEP) or a 504 Plan, which is a written document that stipulates any special education programs or services, long-term goals, short-term objectives, accommodations, and related services that need to be provided for children with disabilities.

- Accommodation for the child with hearing loss could include provision of sensory devices, like HAs or HATS, interpreters, or classroom modifications, like acoustic treatment or preferential seating in the classroom.
- Related services could include:
  - Family instructions, counseling, and home visits
  - Sessions with an SLP, where students will focus on exercises aimed at improving receptive and expressive language
  - Occupational therapy
  - Case management
  - Medical services for diagnosis or evaluation
  - Transportation to and from services

AUDIOLOGY NUGGET

Both IEPs and 504 Plans are the product of legislative efforts designed to ensure that children with a disability identified under the law who are attending elementary or secondary schools have access to appropriate services for academic success. The IEP process is defined by the Individuals With Disabilities Education Act (IDEA) and is for students with disabilities who require specialized instruction. The process for receiving and implementing a 504 Plan is defined by Section 504 of the Rehabilitation Act and is designed for students with disabilities who do not require specialized instruction but may have specific accessibility requirements to receive equal access to public education. For this reason, 504 Plans are often available to children with hearing loss who may not qualify for an IEP but require additional support to access the learning environment within the general classroom. Both require documentation of measurable growth and should be updated annually.

Auditory habilitative therapy is one method of direct service provision for children with hearing loss. It is often performed by an SLP for children over the age of 3. By this age, children should be wearing technology during all waking hours and be stimulable (i.e., primed to respond to a particular auditory stimulus) for this kind of therapy. The clinician uses a stimulus-response paradigm (S-R paradigm) to reinforce appropriate responses to auditory stimuli. It is up to the clinician to evaluate inappropriate responses to determine the need for and type of activity to remediate the response. Activities can aim to address auditory awareness, perception, attention, inhibition, localization, discrimination, memory, sequencing, processing, and understanding. Activities can also focus on social competence factors, like turn taking, eye contact, and asking for help.

CASE EXAMPLE

Ana is a 6-year-old with Morquio syndrome, a rare genetic condition that impacts the body's ability to break down naturally occurring sugar chains in the body. She has a complex medical history, including multiple surgeries. Due to anatomical differences, Ana experiences chronic ear infections and fluid retention. At age 4, she was diagnosed with mild to moderate mixed hearing loss in both ears and fitted with bilateral HAs. She has an IEP and receives speech and language services at school. Recently, Ana's SLP has noted a lack of progress in fluency, and her teacher has reported increased trouble with spelling words. Following an IEP meeting, the SLP advised Ana's mother to schedule an appointment with the pediatric audiologist. An updated hearing evaluation showed that Ana's hearing loss had remained relatively stable. Aided speech perception testing was completed, and scores were calculated based on the number of correctly identified phonemes. This testing showed that Ana was consistently missing high-frequency consonants like /s/ and /th/. In coordination with Ana's AVT-LSLS, the pediatric audiologist reprogrammed Ana's HAs to allow for more high-frequency gain while the AVT worked specifically with Ana to detect and identify the high-pitched sounds that she was missing during aided speech perception testing. At the follow-up HA appointment, Ana's aided speech perception scores increased, and Ana's mother reported that she as well as Ana's teachers and other therapists had noticed an improvement in communication. This is an example of interprofessional practice where the audiologist, SLP, teacher, and family came together to identify and remediate the problem.

Activities

AR activities for infants and children fall under many of the same categories as adult activities, like communication strategies training and psychosocial exercises, but are modified for the intended audience.

- One activity that families are taught early on is to provide a language-rich environment by talking to their child as much as possible. For families who choose an LSL approach, this can include describing the surroundings, discussing past and future activities, reading books, and singing nursery rhymes or other songs.

- AR activities may also include the provision of HAs and instruction on use and care as well as strategies to foster consistent use. See Table 10–4 for self-management activities for children and families involving provision and instruction of HA and CI.

- Families who choose a different communication approach (e.g., sign language) also need instruction on providing a language-rich environment, which necessitates family members become proficient in the chosen communication method in a very short amount of time. It is essential that the family prepare to be ahead of their children's communication skills, so naturalistic learning can occur.

- Tracking outcomes and goal setting are vital during these appointments, so families understand the importance of their role in the rehabilitation process.

Psychosocial Exercises and Communication Strategies Training

As children with hearing loss are likely to be the only person they know with hearing impairment, psychosocial support should be a vital part of their AR services. Children with hearing loss are more likely to experience bullying from their peers. Like adults, children with hearing loss can develop maladaptive behaviors to cope with unresolved feelings brought about by the hearing loss.

- Teachers and other professionals need education regarding the connections between hearing loss, psychosocial outcomes, and cognitive load so they can better support children with hearing loss in their classrooms. Providing in-services to school professionals on these and other topics, like the importance of clear speech and limitations of sensory devices, is important for student success.

- Children with hearing loss have more mental health concerns than their peers with normal hearing. Issues can occur even in young children with hearing loss and can include attention problems and poor relationships with peers. As children grow, their mental health support needs change.

TABLE 10–4. Self-Management Activities for Children and Families Involving Provision and Instruction of HA and CI

AGE	USE AND CARE	SOCIAL ASPECTS
Toddlers	• Insert and remove devices as part of morning and bedtime routine • Help select device and earmold colors • Identifying names of device and some parts	• Read bedtime stories with characters who have hearing devices • Promote acceptance of devices and sense of ownership by linking up with other families of children with hearing impairment (e.g., join local chapter of Hands and Voices)
Preschool age	• Practice labeling the parts of the device • Introducing correct terms for parts/devices	• Learn to communicate when batteries need to be replaced or charged • Learn to communicate when additional support is needed (e.g., asking for a seat change in a difficult listening environment)
Elementary school age	• Help with cleaning and maintenance of devices • Be responsible for their device and accessories, especially when changing environments	• Practice answering questions from peers about the hearing loss and devices • Consider reading a book to the class about hearing loss and devices during show-and-tell • Educate peers to be proactive about social differences
Middle school age	• Watch for wear-time issues related to social pressure from peers and increased self-awareness • Identify barriers as they arise and consider creative solutions (e.g., adding volume control or switching to a RIC device) • Consider technology streaming for motivation and academic access	• Foster an environment where the child can express positive and negative feelings related to the hearing loss and device(s) • Role-play problem solving and resolution • Openly discuss frustrations with hearing aids
High school teenagers	• Work on autonomy with devices and appointments • Independently attend appointments • Role-play advocacy efforts around device use and other accommodations that may come up in postsecondary education or employment	• Identify barriers to use and consider problem-solving options for specific barriers • Begin to work on long-term planning for postgraduation • Educate on disability rights with job and college searching

- Practitioners are urged to focus on not only outcomes related to speech, language, and educational attainment but also emotional and social well-being outcomes.
- Adolescents with hearing loss have fewer close friendships and lower levels of self-perceived social acceptance than their normal-hearing peers.
- Strategies to support mental health in older children and adolescents can also include making connections with others with hearing impairment.

Psychosocial support and communication strategies training go hand in hand for children with hearing loss. These activities can focus on advocacy training techniques that will help the child improve communication by clarifying problems, setting goals, and developing action plans.

- Teaching family members effective communication strategies is vital to the child's success. Communication breakdowns can occur from limited speech production and perception abilities in the child with hearing loss. When this happens, parents should be encouraged to use receptive repair strategies, like asking the child to repeat, rephrase, or provide more information.
- As children age, they can be more involved in communication strategy training activities. Anticipatory role-playing exercises are a great way to do this. Helping children understand that communication breakdowns will occur and empowering them with repair strategies can go a long way toward improving communication for the child with hearing loss.

HATS

Like adults, children can benefit from the use of HATS in a variety of settings. The determination to fit a child with a HATS device depends on a number of things, including:

- Degree and configuration of hearing loss
- Current HA usage characteristics
- Listening environment (home, school, daycare)
- Additional concerns (attention or behavioral disorders, cognition, mobility, vision, fine motor, auditory processing difficulties)
- Technology compatibility
- Motivation of caregiver and child

Commonly, HATS are used in the classroom to increase the level of the teacher's voice relative to the noise in the classroom. HATS can take several forms:

- Personal FM system
- Remote microphone system that works with the child's HAs or CIs
- Classroom Auditory Distribution System (CADS): the teacher wears a microphone that amplifies their voice to one or more speakers positioned throughout the classroom
  - □ Additional microphones can be used by students for class discussion.
  - □ Extra boost in SNR that CADS provide can be beneficial for all students regardless of hearing status (Wolfe et al., 2013).

HATS may be included as part of the child's IEP or 504 Plan. All HATS should be appropriately verified through electroacoustic analysis or with behavioral testing. In addition, caregiver, child, and teacher questionnaires should be employed regularly as validation measures, and in fact, IDEA stipulates that any child using assistive technology receives a functional listening evaluation in their customary environment. Finally, training caregivers, teachers, and children on how to perform daily listening checks and troubleshoot issues is vital to a child's success with HATS.

Auditory Training

Auditory training for children with hearing loss closely follows the hierarchical continuum of skills.

1. Awareness: since children born with hearing loss cannot draw on previous memories of how speech sounds and what those sounds mean, auditory training typically begins with sound awareness activities. Once children can attend to the signal, they can begin to relate those sounds to their own vocabulary. Children with greater degrees of hearing loss may need to spend more time on sound awareness activities.

2. Discrimination: focus on the ability to distinguish that two sounds are different

3. Identification: attaching a label to an auditory stimulus

4. Comprehension: understanding the meaning of the auditory stimuli, the final level of auditory skill development

Activities can incorporate different levels of skills development and have various subfactors that affect difficulty level, including response set (open vs. closed), stimulus unit (phoneme, syllable, word, or phrase; analytic vs. synthetic), and listening conditions (quiet vs. noise). See Table 10–5 for sample auditory training activities for each of the four auditory skill development levels.

Conversational Fluency

Most people adhere to unwritten rules of conversation that may be based on cultural norms or conventions. This may include things like taking turns in a conversation in an organized manner or keeping the conversation related to a coherent topic. When these rules are adhered to, conversational fluency is high.

- When one or more of the individuals in a conversation have hearing loss, these rules may be broken. One example of this is disrupted turn taking by the person with hearing impairment, who may start talking over someone when they don't realize that person is talking. When this happens, conversational fluency is low and can result in increased stress, not just for the person with hearing loss but for all communication members and is a primary reason for maladaptive strategies, like bluffing or social withdrawal. Children with prelingual hearing loss will have more difficulty with conversational fluency as they may not be exposed to these conversational conventions as frequently during language development.

- Conversational fluency is typically measured with mean length turn (MLT) ratio or mean length utterance (MLU). Both of these terms are measures of language proficiency that can be used as a benchmark for rehabilitation.

  □ MLT is a ratio of the average number of words spoken by each participant in the conversation.

    • Calculated by counting the total number of words spoken by each individual and dividing by the number of turns in the conversation

TABLE 10–5. Auditory Training Activity Examples for the Four Different Types of Auditory Skill Development

AUDITORY SKILL	SAMPLE ACTIVITIES (all stimuli are presented in the auditory alone condition)	SPECIFIC EXAMPLES
1. Sound Awareness	Play a game where the child indicates that they have heard the sound by performing a task.	• Peek a boo • Musical chairs • Freeze dancing • Drop the toy in a bucket
2. Sound Discrimination	Play a game where the child has to match a sound with a picture.	• Select matching animal picture to animal sound heard • Children's Perception of Speech Test (NU-CHIPS) words recognition using picture pointing • Present similar words, then picture points to matching image • Jump when they hear one sound, sit when they hear another
3. Sound Identification	Play a game where the child has to listen and identify a word or phrase.	• Mr. Potato Head • Go Fish • Candyland
4. Sound Comprehension	Read aloud a story and answer questions. Play a game where the child must listen and comprehend directions.	• I spy • 20 questions • Simon Says • Make predictions from a story

☐ MLU is the average number of morphemes in a child's utterances or phrases.

  • Morphemes are the smallest meaningful level of speech and are used instead of words to account for the developing child's vocabulary.

  • A 2-year-old typically has MLUs that are 2 to 3 morphemes long, whereas a 4-year-old may have MLUs that have ≥6 morphemes. As children grow and develop language, these metrics should increase.

☐ MLT or MLUs can be used to monitor and track language intervention outcomes. Conversational fluency could also be assessed informally by observing the patient and their family during appointments.

■ There are many factors that can impact conversational fluency, including familiarity with the speaker and with the topic.

Cultural Responsiveness, Competence, and Humility

Cultural responsiveness, sometimes referred to as cultural competence or cultural humility, recognizes, affirms, and values people of all cultures, languages, classes, races, ethnic backgrounds, disabilities, religions, genders, and sexual orientations.

- ASHA describes its preferred term of "cultural responsiveness" as "understanding and appropriately including and responding to the combination of cultural variables and the full range of dimensions of diversity that an individual brings to interactions" (ASHA, 2022, Cultural Responsiveness section, para. 1).

- Cultural competence and cultural humility are generally related to personal knowledge, understanding, and growth.
  - □ Cultural competence involves continually learning about different cultural backgrounds and beliefs. Audiologists will come into contact with a diverse patient population during the rehabilitation process. The audiologist must be able to provide assessment and rehabilitation that is both relevant and purposeful to patients from these different backgrounds.
  - □ Cultural humility is accepting that the values system of others may conflict with one's own values system. By remaining open-minded about this conflict, one can engender trust in the provider-patient relationship, which will promote greater patient participation in the rehabilitation process and improve outcomes.

One of the best ways to practice cultural responsiveness is to adjust your interaction (verbiage, behaviors) to match the cultural expectations of the patient and their family. This can be done through language and communication style, representation, awareness, and information sharing.

- Language: every effort should be made to interact with the family in their natural or preferred language. Interpreters should be counseled beforehand on the intricacies of testing and the unique needs of the patient. Remember, family members, including children, should never be used as interpreters.

- Communication style: cultural backgrounds of patients and their families can vary and may include differences in eye contact and body language. Providers should follow the caregiver's lead and try to match communication styles. Learning about cultural backgrounds and communication styles prior to the appointment can help put the family at ease.

- Representation: posters, brochures, and other clinic materials should reflect a diverse array of cultures, ethnicities, and skin tones. This can show families that the practice values diversity by seeing patients that look like them.

- Awareness: bias can impact any cross-cultural interaction, often without one or both parties even being aware of the effect. Working to uncover your own bias is an important part of cultural responsiveness. The cultural competency check-ins from ASHA are a great place to begin engaging in cultural responsiveness (https://www.asha.org/practice/multicultural/self/).

- Information sharing: practitioners should also collaborate with families in order to increase knowledge. One way to practice this is by avoiding the use of yes or no questions to assess information retention. For example, if you ask the family, "do you understand" they may be reluctant to admit that they don't and simply answer, "yes." Instead, have them demonstrate understanding, either by repeating/rephrasing the information you provided or by using a hands-on activity, for example, changing a HA battery or doing a listening check.

Remember, engaging in cultural responsiveness should not be viewed as a standard that one becomes proficient in but rather as a lifelong commitment.

CASE EXAMPLE

Leo was identified at 18 months of age with bilateral moderate-to-severe SNHL. Records indicate that he passed his newborn hearing screening (NBHS) in one ear and failed in the other. His family reported that they did not follow up after the NBHS as they were unaware of his screening results. Leo's family speaks Spanish, so a Spanish language interpreter was used over the telephone for case history prior to testing and for delivering results at the end of testing. The pediatric audiologist was careful to speak in short, clear sentences and avoid technical jargon as she had been trained to do. After delivering the diagnosis, she paused to allow the family time to process the information, and Leo's mother burst into tears. It was clear that she had not anticipated the diagnosis at all, and the audiologist, despite all her training and experience, was at a loss. She found that acknowledging and affirming the emotional response to a new diagnosis was much more difficult when using a telephone interpreter to communicate. Luckily, she was able to connect Leo and his family with another Spanish-speaking family of a child with hearing loss who could provide support based on the shared experience, and she located an in-person interpreting service to use for his future visits. Now this pediatric audiologist spends more time with families during the case history to learn about their cultural and normative beliefs surrounding hearing loss and HAs. She has found that this helps establish rapport, which promotes trust in the provider-patient relationship. As her community has a large Spanish-speaking population, she found a local community group and spent time learning about their culture and customs. She started to arrange for in-person interpreters when possible and worked to spend time before appointments making sure the interpreter understood the testing process and some of the more technical terms. Additionally, she maintains a list of resources and information in multiple languages to provide to newly diagnosed families. Most importantly, this particular audiologist recognized that despite a license and a degree, learning and growth do not stop, especially when it comes to cultural responsiveness.

Interprofessional Approach to AR

AR is one area where audiology and speech-language pathology truly coexist; these roles can be complementary and cooperative. Despite clear delineations in knowledge and skill criteria for each profession, at this time, only SLPs can be reimbursed for AR activities as audiology is deemed to be exclusively a diagnostic profession. Other disciplines that may participate in AR can vary based on the service delivery setting.

- School setting: educators, psychologists, teachers of the deaf, special education teachers, occupational therapists, and more may play a role in AR provision.

- Assisted living facility: nurses, physicians, and other healthcare providers will be part of the team.

For some specific interventions, a team approach is also mandated. For example, a CI patient's interdisciplinary team may include an otologist, an audiologist, a psychologist, an SLP, and a social worker. An interprofessional approach is one where each member of the team can share their expertise to achieve the end goal of lessening the impact of the disorder.

Summary

AR provision and the role audiologists play in it has continued to progress, especially with advancements in healthcare delivery, technology, and the impact of hearing loss on patients of all ages. With AR encompassing such a broad scope of paramount clinical activities, it is more important than ever that audiologists use their knowledge to provide evidence-based, comprehensive care for all patients. Whether AR is practiced by giving informational handouts, holding GAR sessions, recognizing affective statements, or offering Internet-based auditory training, outcomes should be tracked, and adjustments should be made according to a patient's care plans. Keep in mind that the definition and provision of AR services is likely going to continue to shift as the field continues to grow and change.

Recommended Readings

AG Bell Academy, The AG Bell Academy for Listening and Spoken Language. (2023, February 9). AG Bell Academy | the AG Bell Academy for Listening and Spoken Language—Home to Listening and Spoken Language Professionals. https://agbellacademy.org/

American Academy of Audiology. (2011) *Clinical practice guidelines for fitting HATS birth–21 years.* https://www.audiology.org/practice-guideline/clinical-practice-guidelines-remote-microphone-hearing-assistance-technologies-for-children-and-youth-from-birth-to-21-years/

American Speech-Language-Hearing Association. (n.d.). *Cultural responsiveness* [Practice portal]. https://www.asha.org/Practice-Portal/Professional-Issues/Cultural-Responsiveness/

American Speech-Language-Hearing Association. (n.d.-a). *Hearing loss in adults.* https://www.asha.org/practice-portal/clinical-topics/hearing-loss/#collapse_6

American Speech-Language-Hearing Association. (2008). *Guidelines for audiologists providing informational and adjustment counseling to families of infants and young children with hearing loss birth to 5 years of age* [Guidelines]. https://www.asha.org/policy

Basura, G., Cienkowski, K., Hamlin, L., Ray, C., Rutherford, C., . . . Ambrose, J. (2023). American Speech-Language-Hearing Association clinical practice guideline on aural rehabilitation for adults with hearing loss. *American Journal of Audiology, 32*(1), 1–51. https://doi.org/10.1044/2022_AJA-21-00252

Boothroyd, A. (2007). Adult aural rehabilitation: What is it and does it work? *Trends in Amplification, 11*(2), 63–71. https://doi.org/10.1177/1084713807301073

Idainstitute.com. (n.d.). *Ida Institute.* https://idainstitute.com/

Montano, J. J., & Spitzer, J. B. (2019). *Adult audiologic rehabilitation.* Van Haren Publishing.

Tye-Murray, N. (2022). *Foundations of aural rehabilitation: Children, adults, and their family members.* Plural Publishing.

References

Alpiner, J., & McCarthy, P. (2014). History of adult audiologic rehabilitation: The past as a prologue. In J. Montano & J. Spitzer (Eds.), *Adult audiologic rehabilitation* (2nd ed., pp. 3–21). Plural Publishing.

American Speech-Language-Hearing Association. (n.d.). *Cultural responsiveness* [Practice portal]. https://www.asha.org/Practice-Portal/Professional-Issues/Cultural-Responsiveness/

Americans With Disabilities Act of 1990. 42 U.S.C. § 12101 et seq. (1990).

Anderson, K. L. (2002). *ELF-Early listening function.* https://successforkidswithhearingloss.com/wpcontent/uploads/2017/09/ELF_Questionnaire.pdf

Anderson, K. L., & Matkin, N. (1996). *Screening Instrument for Targeting Educational Risk in Preschool Children (Age 3Kindergarten) (Preschool SIFTER).* https://successforkidswithhearingloss.com/wpcontent/uploads/2017/09/Preschool_SIFTER.pdf

Anderson, K. L., & Smaldino, J. J. (2000). *Children's home inventory of listening difficulties.* https://successforkidswithhearingloss.com/wpcontent/uploads/2011/08/CHILD_pgs3-4.pdf

Anderson, K.L., & Matkin, N. (1989). S.I.F.T.E.R.—Screening instrument for targeting educational risk. *Success for Kids with Hearing Loss.* https://successforkidswithhearingloss.com/uploads/SIFTER.pdf

Bennett, R. J., Meyer, C. J., Ryan, B., Barr, C., Laird, E., & Eikelboom, R. H. (2020). Knowledge, beliefs, and practices of Australian audiologists in addressing the mental health needs of adults with hearing loss. *American Journal of Audiology, 29*(2), 129–142. https://doi.org/10.1044/2019_aja–19–00087

Boothroyd, A. (2007). Adult aural rehabilitation: What is it and does it work? *Trends in Amplification, 11*(2), 63–71.

Borson, S., Scanlan, J., Brush, M., Vitaliano, P. P., & Dokmak, A. M. (2000). The Mini-Cog: A cognitive vital signs measure for dementia screening in multi-lingual elderly. *International Journal of Geriatric Psychiatry, 15*(11), 1021–1027.

Cox, R. M., & Alexander, G. C. (1995). The abbreviated profile of hearing aid benefit. *Ear and Hearing, 16*(2), 176–186. https://doi.org/10.1097/00003446-199504000-00005

Cox, R. M., & Alexander, G. C. (1999). Measuring Satisfaction with Amplification in Daily Life: The SADL scale. *Ear and Hearing, 20*(4), 306–320. https://doi.org/10.1097/00003446-199908000-00004

Cox, R. M., & Alexander, G. C. (2000). Expectations about hearing aids and their relationship to fitting outcome. *Journal of the American Academy of Audiology, 11*(7), 368–382. https://doi.org/10.1055/s-0042-1748124

Cox, R. M., Alexander, G. C., & Beyer, C. M. (2003). Norms for the international outcome inventory for hearing aids. *Journal of the American Academy of Audiology, 14*(8), 403–413.

Cox, R. M., Alexander, G. C., & Xu, J. (2014). Development of the device-oriented subjective outcome (DOSO) scale. *Journal of the American Academy of Audiology, 25*(8), 727–736. https://doi.org/10.3766/jaaa.25.8.3

Dillon, H., Birtles, G., & Lovegrove, R. (1999). Measuring the outcomes of a national rehabilitation program: Normative data for the Client Oriented Scale of Improvement (COSI) and the HA User's Questionnaire (HAUQ). *Journal of the American Academy of Audiology, 10*(2), 67–79.

Erdman, S. (1993). Counseling adults with hearing impairment. In J. Alpiner & P. McCarthy (Eds.), *Rehabilitative audiology: Children & adults* (2nd ed., pp. 374–413). Williams & Wilkins.

Faverio, M. (2022, January 13). *Share of those 65 and older who are tech users has grown in the past decade.* Pew Research Center. https://www.pewresearch.org/fact-tank/2022/01/13/share-of-those-65-and-older-who-are-tech-users-has-grown-in-the-past-decade/

Fenson, L., Marchman, V. A., Thal, D. J., Dale, P. S., Reznick, J. S., & Bates, E. (2006). *MacArthur-Bates Communicative Development Inventories, Second Edition (CDIs)* [Database record]. APA PsycTests. https://doi.org/10.1037/t11538-000

Hall, D. A., Fussell, C., & Summerfield, A. Q. (2005). Reading fluent speech from talking faces: Typical brain networks and individual differences. *Journal of Cognitive Neuroscience, 17*(6), 939–953. https://doi.org/10.1162/0898929054021175

Henry, P. J., Zaugg, A. T., Myers, P. P., & Kendall, P. C. (2010). *How to manage your tinnitus: A step-by-step workbook.* Plural Publishing.

Hétu, R. (1996). The stigma attached to hearing impairment. *Scandinavian Audiology. Supplementum, 43,* 12–24.

Individuals With Disabilities Education Act, 20 U.S.C. § 1400 (2004).

Jacobson, G. P., Newman, C. W., Fabry, D. A., & Sandridge, S. A. (2001). Development of the Three-Clinic Hearing Aid Selection Profile (HASP). *Journal of the American Academy of Audiology, 12*(3), 128–166.

Kessels, R. P. C. (2003). Patients' memory for medical information. *JRSM, 96*(5), 219–222. https://doi.org/10.1258/jrsm.96.5.219

Killion, M. C., Niquette, P. A., Gudmundsen, G. I., Revit, L. J., & Banerjee, S. (2004). Development of a quick speech-in-noise test for measuring signal-to-noise ratio loss in normal-hearing and hearing-impaired listeners. *Journal of the Acoustical Society of America, 116*(4), 2395–2405. https://doi.org/10.1121/1.1784440

Margolis, R. (2004). Audiology information counseling. *Audiology Today, 16*(2), 14–15.

Montano, J. (2014). Defining audiologic rehabilitation. In J. Montano & J. Spitzer (Eds.), *Adult audiologic rehabilitation* (2nd ed., pp. 23–35). Plural Publishing.

Newman, C. W., Weinstein, B. E., Jacobson, G. P., & Hug, G. A. (1990). The Hearing Handicap Inventory for Adults: Psychometric adequacy and audiometric correlates. *Ear and Hearing, 11*(6), 430–433.

Newman, C. W., Jacobson, G. P., & Spitzer, J. B. (1996). Development of the tinnitus handicap inventory. *Archives of Otolaryngology-Head & Neck Surgery, 122*(2), 143–148. https://doi.org/10.1001/archotol.1996.01890140029007

Noble, W. (2002). Extending the IOI to significant others and to non-hearing-aid-based interventions. *International Journal of Audiology, 41*(1), 27–29.

Pichora-Fuller, M.K., Mick, P., & Reed, M. (2015). Hearing, cognition, and healthy aging: Social and public health implications of the links between age-related declines in hearing and cognition. *Seminars in Hearing, 36*, 122–139. https://doi.org/10.1055/s-0035-1555116

Preminger, J. E. & Ziegler, C. (2008). Can auditory and visual speech perception be trained within a group setting? *American Journal of Audiology, 17*(1), 80–97. https://doi.org/10.1044/1059-0889(2008/009

Preminger, J. E., & Meeks, S. (2012). The Hearing Impairment Impact-Significant Other Profile (HII-SOP): A tool to measure hearing loss-related quality of life in spouses of people with hearing loss. *Journal of the American Academy of Audiology, 23*(10), 807–823. https://doi.org/10.3766/jaaa.23.10.6

Rescorla, L., & Alley, A. C. (2001). Validation of the language development survey (LDS). *Journal of Speech Language and Hearing Research, 44*(2), 434–445.

Sandridge, S.A., & Newman, C.W. (2006). Improving the efficiency and accountability of the hearing aid selection process—Use of the COAT. *Audiology Online.* https://www.audiologyonline.com/articles/improving-efficiency-and-accountability-hearing-995

Saunders, G. H., Frederick, M. T., Arnold, M. L., Silverman, S. C., Chisolm, T. H., & Myers, P. J. (2018). A randomized controlled trial to evaluate approaches to auditory rehabilitation for blast-exposed veterans with normal or near-normal hearing who report hearing problems in difficult listening situations. *Journal of the American Academy of Audiology, 29*(1), 44–62. https://doi.org/10.3766/jaaa.16143

Scarinci, N., Worrall, L., & Hickson, L. (2009). The effect of hearing impairment in older people on the spouse: development and psychometric testing of the significant other scale for hearing disability (SOS-HEAR). *International Journal of Audiology, 48*(10), 671–683. https://doi.org/10.1080/14992020902998409

Scarinci, N. A., Hickson, L. M., & Worrall, L. E. (2011). Third-party disability in spouses of older people with hearing impairment. *Perspectives on Aural Rehabilitation and Its Instrumentation, 18*(1), 3–12.

Schow, R. L., & Nerbonne, M. A. (1982). Communication screening profile: Use with elderly clients. *Ear and Hearing, 3*(3), 135–147.

Shukla, A., Harper, M., Pedersen, E., Goman, A., Suen, J. J., Price, C., . . . Reed, N. S. (2020). Hearing loss, loneliness, and social isolation: A systematic review. *Otolaryngology–Head and Neck Surgery, 162*(5), 622–633. https://doi.org/10.1177/0194599820910377

Singh, G., Lau, S. T., & Pichora-Fuller, M. K. (2015). Social support predicts hearing aid satisfaction. *Ear and Hearing, 36*(6), 664–676. https://doi.org/10.1097/AUD.0000000000000182

Squires, J., Bricker, D., Heo, K., & Twombly, E. (2002). *Ages & stages questionnaires: Social-emotional: A parent-completed, child-monitoring system for social-emotional behaviors.* Paul H. Brookes.

Suls, J., Martin, R., & Wheeler, L. (2002). Social comparison: Why, with whom, and with what effect? *Current Directions in Psychological Science, 11*(5), 159–163. https://doi.org/10.1111/1467–8721.00191

Sweetow, R. W., & Sabes, J. H. (2007). Listening and communication enhancement (LACE). *Seminars in Hearing, 28*(2), 133–141.

Thibodeau, L. (2014). Comparison of speech recognition with adaptive digital and FM remote microphone hearing assistance technology by listeners who use hearing aids. *American Journal of Audiology, 23*(2), 201–210. https://doi.org/10.1044/2014_AJA-13-0065

Trychin, S. (2003). *Problem solving in families: Suggestions and procedures for negotiating behavior changes related to hearing loss.* Self-published.

Tsiakpini, L., Weichbold, V., Kuehn-Inacker, H., Coninx, F., D'haese, P., & Almadin, S. (2004). *LittlEARS auditory questionnaire.* MED-EL.

van Boekel, L. C., Peek, S. T., & Luijkx, K. G. (2017). Diversity in older adults' use of the internet: Identifying subgroups through latent class analysis. *Journal of Medical Internet Research, 19*(5), e180. https://doi.org/10.2196/jmir.6853

Ventry, I. M., & Weinstein, B. E. (1982). The hearing handicap inventory for the elderly. *Ear and Hearing, 3*(3), 128–134. https://doi.org/10.1097/00003446–198205000–00006

Wolfe, J., Morais, M., Neumann, S., Schafer, E., Mülder, H. E., Wells, N., . . . Hudson, M. (2013). Evaluation of speech recognition with personal FM and classroom audio distribution systems. *Journal of Educational Audiology, 19*, 65–79.

Zimmerman-Phillips, S., Osberger, M. J., & Robbins, A. M. (2001). *Infant-Toddler Meaningful Auditory Integration Scale.* Advanced Bionics Corporation.

✎ Practice Questions

Mr. Kellogg is a 68-year-old male who was recently fit with his first set of HAs. HA output was verified using real ear measures. Datalogging shows a consistent 10 hours of use per day, and postfitting scores on the HHIE showed a significant reduction compared to prefitting scores. He reported satisfaction with the devices, specifically in quiet environments, but noted that he still struggles to hear when there is background noise present. He specifically expressed frustration with communication with his wife when they go out to dinner.

1. Which of the following AR activities would be most appropriate for Mr. Kellogg?
   a. Problem identification exercises
   b. Psychosocial exercises
   c. Internet-based auditory training program
   d. Communication strategies training

Explanation: As Mr. Kellogg is a new HA user, it is important to discuss communication strategies, especially in the context of HA limitations. Mr. Kellogg and his wife should be counseled on strategies they can use in situations where the HA benefit is limited such as preferential seating, sitting with your back to the noise (when noise reduction strategies, like directional microphones are in use), and strategies for communication repair. Therefore, d is the correct answer.

2. After 3 years of successful use and perceived benefit, Mr. Kellogg starts to notice that he is more tired at the end of the day and feels like he is not hearing as well as he used to, despite updated diagnostic testing and objective measures showing appropriate HA output. He is also struggling to understand his wife more and is frustrated and embarrassed with how often he has to ask for repetition. What AR activities could you suggest to him now?
   a. Addition of a TV streamer
   b. Participation in a GAR program with FCPs
   c. Speech perception exercise worksheet
   d. Advocacy/self-management training

Explanation: Mr. Kellogg is reporting more than one issue related to his hearing impairment, suggesting the need for multiple activities. Since his complaints pertain more to the psychosocial impacts of hearing loss, a GAR program might help connect him with others experiencing the same issues. In a GAR setting, the impact of stigma is reduced, and participants can share solutions to problems in a more supportive environment. Specific GAR activities could also provide him with communication strategy tips to use with his FCPs, stress reduction exercises to help him cope with frustration, and informational content about HATS. Therefore, b is the correct answer.

3. Mr. Kellogg was planning to attend a play at the downtown center for the arts. Before going, he wanted to make sure he knew how to procure and use the loop system installed in the facility. What type of activity would this be called?

   a. Repair strategy

   b. Self-efficacy activity

   c. Anticipatory strategy

   d. Synthetic strategy

Explanation: Mr. Kellogg is doing "homework" ahead of time to prevent or reduce the occurrence of communication breakdown. Since he is making this effort as a proactive measure, it is an anticipatory strategy. Therefore, c is the correct answer.

4. What type of activity would be best suited for a patient who states, "HAs will make me look old"?

   a. Informational counseling

   b. Personal adjustment counseling

   c. Analytic counseling

   d. Advocacy counseling

Explanation: This patient is demonstrating self-stigma, that is, applying labels that are negatively associated with hearing loss (in this case "old") to himself as a person with hearing loss. We know that stigma can impact acceptance of hearing loss and serve as a barrier to successful intervention; therefore, personal adjustment counseling would be appropriate to promote adjustment to the hearing loss. Therefore, b is the correct answer.

5. Mr. Maxwell is an 82-year-old, long-term bilateral HA user. His current BTE HAs are 2 years old, and prior to today's appointment, he expressed satisfaction and demonstrated benefit on objective outcome measures with the devices. At today's appointment, Mr. Maxwell expressed frustration that his HAs are not working, noting that he is struggling to understand others. You retested his pure-tone hearing thresholds and noticed no significant change since his last evaluation. You also performed a listening check and verified gain using real ear measures to match HA output to the appropriate targets. What would be an appropriate next step for you as the clinician?

   a. Perform a cognitive screening to rule out age-related cognitive decline as a source of the problem

   b. Retest word recognition scores to look for age-related declines in speech perception

   c. Recommend a HAT, like a Bluetooth remote microphone, to help the patient understand speech better

   d. Advise the patient to attend HLAA meetings to better manage the psychosocial impact of the reported problem

Explanation: While you could argue that all of these options may help the patient, the next logical step would be to assess the patient for age-related changes in word recognition scores. As we age, our ability to understand speech can decline. If this testing did demonstrate a significant decline in word recognition abilities, then you could counsel the patient on these changes and recommend some options, including a HAT or psychosocial exercises. Therefore, b is the correct answer.

6. Baby J was identified at 5 weeks of age with bilateral moderate to severe sensorineural hearing loss. Her caregivers decided to use an LSL approach for communication and recently had impressions made for her first pair of earmolds. Which of the following would not be an appropriate AR activity for this family at this time?

   a. Written information on communication strategies for infants and young children

   b. Referral to a local program where parents of children with hearing loss serve as mentors to families of newly diagnosed children

   c. Referral for an Individualized Education Plan (IEP) to outline necessary AR services

   d. Referral to a certified LSLS specialist for AVT

Explanation: An IEP is only for children aged 3 or older who need specialized school instruction. All of the other answers would be appropriate activities for a newly diagnosed family who chooses LSL. Therefore, c is the correct answer.

7. A patient-centered AR program is one that:

   a. Considers background, current status, needs, and wants to develop a custom treatment plan

   b. Has an ultimate goal of persuading a patient to take up and maintain services offered in the treatment plan

   c. Covers as many activities as possible in the shortest amount of time

   d. Includes informational counseling and personal adjustment counseling

Explanation: Patient-centered care occurs when a practitioner takes into account all of the individual patient factors to provide information about all available treatment options so that the patient can make an informed choice. Therefore, a is the correct answer.

8. Elena is a 4-year-old with bilateral hearing loss and has a 504 Plan that stipulates that she attend therapy with an SLP at her school three times per week. One of the activities she has been working on targets sound identification through playing the game Candyland. The SLP notices that Elena has steadily improved and is now responding correctly during game play at least 90% of the time. What should the SLP do next?

   a. Seek to terminate the 504 Plan on the grounds that therapy is no longer needed

   b. Change to a comprehension task, like 20 questions

   c. Change to a closed-set task that works on sound discrimination

   d. Change to a communication strategies task

Explanation: Auditory skills training is typically done on a continuum. Since the child is doing well with an identification task, the next step would be to move to a harder task on the continuum, in this case a comprehension task. Therefore, b is the correct answer.

9. During therapy, Elena's SLP notes that her conversational fluency has improved since her last evaluation. How could the SLP measure this?

    a. Informally through talking with Elena and observing interactions with her classmates

    b. By recording a structured conversation and then using the recording to calculate mean length turn (MLT) ratio

    c. By asking her teachers to rate Elena's fluency on a scale of 1 to 10

    d. Both a and b

Explanation: Conversational fluency can be measured formally by calculating the MLT ratio or informally by a trained professional (in this case the SLP). While Elena's teacher may be able to provide some input, evaluating conversational fluency is beyond her area of expertise so a subjective rating from the teacher would not be of much value. Therefore, d is the correct answer.

10. Which of these would not be considered an effort to improve cultural responsiveness at your practice?

    a. Recruit and retain minority staff

    b. Attend a cultural competence workshop

    c. Use family members as interpreters

    d. Engage in introspection to discover any implicit biases

Explanation: Using family members as interpreters is strongly discouraged in a healthcare setting. Family members are not likely to be neutral when relaying information, and any emotional impact that the information may contain could result in it not being correctly relayed. It is recommended to always retain a qualified medical interpreter to ensure that the patient is getting all the information they need. The rest of the responses are all appropriate examples. Therefore, c is the correct answer.

Chapter 11

Counseling and Audiological Documentation

Alex Meibos

Importance of Audiological Counseling and Documentation

Patients and families affected by audiological disorders are impacted in diverse ways. To effectively meet the informational and adjustment needs of patients, effective communication and health/medical recordkeeping skills are essential. Although these subjects may be covered separately in graduate audiology curricula, the topics are combined in this chapter to better help students study and review introductory characteristics of professional audiological communication knowledge and skills for their major exams.

- Audiological counseling: intentional communication with patients and families impacted by hearing loss and other ear-related conditions, including the provision of emotional, rehabilitative, and educational support throughout a patient's audiological journey from diagnosis to treatment and through the rehabilitation process.

- Audiological documentation: the recording of medical and health-related results of audiological testing and details of patient encounters.

Audiological Counseling

To best help patients through audiological counseling, audiologists and patients need to develop a therapeutic relationship. A therapeutic relationship includes:

- Having mutual trust
- Respect for differing perspectives
- Assessment of and responsiveness to patient interests
- Shared decision-making
- Aptly addressing patient emotions

To effectively develop therapeutic relationships, audiologists should become familiar with:

- Basic theories of counseling
- Approaches to audiological counseling
- The dynamic impacts that hearing loss and other ear-related disorders can have on individuals and families across the lifespan
- Cultural and linguistic diversity (CLD) of patients

Basic Theories of Counseling

A counseling *theory* is "an intellectual model that purports certain ideas about underlying factors that affect behavior, thoughts, emotions, interpersonal interactions, or interpersonal interpretations" (Cottone, 2017, p. 4). Numerous counseling theories and therapy approaches exist in healthcare; however, some are more useful as applied to audiologic practice, including:

- Person-centered counseling theory: psychologist Carl Rogers developed this theory rooted in humanistic counseling theory, where patients focus on identifying their own answers to problems or barriers, looking at current aspirations rather than past experiences, and the belief that everyone has the capacity to recover, learn, and grow. Clinicians applying this theory in practice focus on three key qualities: unconditional positive regard, genuineness, and empathetic understanding. The therapist must accept the client for who they are, feel comfortable sharing their feelings with the client, and express empathy to the client to form a trusting relationship.

- Behavioral theory: a theory emphasizing that all behavior is learned and that that which can be learned can also be unlearned (Wolpe, 1990). Behavioral approaches focus on assisting individuals in extinguishing unwanted behaviors and relearning new or desirable behaviors.

- Cognitive theory: a theory and therapy approach developed by psychiatrist Aaron Beck (1979), describing how people's thinking can change feelings and behaviors. Oriented toward problem solving, cognitive therapy approaches focus more on the client's present situation and distorted thinking than on their past. Cognitive and behavioral therapy are often combined as one form of theory practiced by counselors and therapists.

- Family-systems theory: this theory describes the relationship system the family exhibits as the interlocking concepts of familial development and behavior are carefully analyzed (Devlin, 2018). Psychiatrist Murray Bowen developed this theory, purporting that behavioral patterns can lead to either balance or dysfunction of the system or both. Even for seemingly disconnected families, Bowen suggested that one's family unit, family of origin, or family center can still have a profound impact on individual emotions and actions.

Audiological Counseling Approaches

Counseling in audiology has long been defined as addressing two broad aspects of individual patient/family needs for information and adjustment support (Clark & English, 2019; Sanders, 1975). The balancing of these two aspects is achieved through careful observation and active listening to patients/families across the continuum of audiological care and services.

- Informational counseling: educating a patient regarding the nature and impact hearing or vestibular health challenges may be affecting their daily function, quality of life, and well-being, and how different interventions help mitigate impacts of their disorder(s).

- Adjustment audiological counseling: helping patients/families accurately identify and address internal barriers (e.g., denial, stress, anxiety) and external barriers (e.g., logistical, financial, learning new information) associated with their ear-related disorder(s), and support the personal development and implementation of new skills to help manage daily living with their disorder(s).

Other types of counseling approaches in audiology are provided below.

- Diagnostic counseling: evaluating a patient in audiology includes gathering sufficient information from a patient through a variety of means to answer specific questions regarding the status of hearing, communication, or vestibular function related health to drive an individualized audiological treatment plan. Diagnostic counseling in audiology includes the skills of taking a thorough case history about why a patient is seeking services, ensuring the instructions for diagnostic procedures are understood and adhered to through effective communication, and maintaining a shared agenda throughout diagnostic encounters. The use of patient demographic forms, special questionnaires, and other subjective tools and instruments can be used in audiology to help in this process. A critical aspect of diagnostic counseling includes being prepared to share results of diagnostic procedures in culturally, linguistically, and socially sensitive ways.

 CASE EXAMPLE

Consider the case of Mr. Jones, who underwent a hearing evaluation and is sitting down to discuss the results with his audiologist. Note how the audiologist opens the clinician-patient dialogue with questions to gauge what may be most important/useful to Mr. Jones instead of jumping straight into information sharing.

Audiologist: *We are now done with the evaluation, Mr. Jones, and ready to discuss the results. Would you like to have a detailed explanation of the results or more of the big picture?*

Mr. Jones: *I think I'd like the big picture.*

Audiologist: *I understand. Per our testing today, Mr. Jones, you have moderate hearing loss in both ears, which is consistent with your reporting having a hard time hearing and understanding others speaking, especially noisy situations. The likely cause of your hearing loss is due to a combination of aging as well as your occupational and recreational exposure to noise.*

Mr. Jones: *So, I do have a hearing loss, huh?*

Audiologist: *Yes; however, we also saw that when speech is loud enough, you can hear and understand very well in both quiet and background noise test situations, meaning you are a candidate for hearing aids in both ears. Right now, I would like to discuss technology options that may work to meet your*

> *communication needs, but, before I move on, do you have any other questions about the testing we completed today?*
>
> **Mr. Jones:** *Well, I suppose this was going to happen to me sooner or later. I don't think I have any other questions, so, let's go ahead and talk about my options.*

- Intervention counseling: developing an audiologic treatment plan is dependent on both the comprehensive diagnostic work of a clinician and the readiness of a patient or family member to participate in a health behavior change process. Treatment for hearing and vestibular-related disorders can take many forms and will differ based on an individual's diagnosis and perceived challenges. Some aspects of audiologic intervention may even be delayed pending referrals and results from outside evaluations, including medical and surgical treatments. Readjusting plans is common with patients and usually requires effective intervention counseling skills when an abrupt change may catch a patient or family off-guard.

CASE EXAMPLE

Consider the case of the following patient who is overwhelmed about using amplification following a trial period with hearing aids. The patient had a recent knee surgery and is being seen for regular physical therapy and outside follow-up. The patient works as a store manager and is surrounded by a large family, including eight grandchildren.

Audiologist: *Can we spend some time now talking about how you have been doing at home as I know you are balancing recovering from knee surgery as well as to these new hearing devices?*

Patient: *Well, I suppose I've not been the poster child when it comes to hearing aid use.*

Audiologist: *It sounds like maybe you would like to be using your hearing aids more frequently than you are. Is that the case?*

Patient: *Well, I feel like . . . look, it's just not a good time to try these things out right now. I know my wife thinks I could really benefit from them, but I'm hearing in most situations without them, and I'm just having a hard enough time learning how to walk on this new knee that remembering to put these things in my head every day is just frustrating.*

Audiologist: *Would it be fair to say that, although your wife is noticing benefit, for you, having hearing aids at the same time as going through your knee recovery right now is too much, and that you have different priorities?*

Patient: *I've really got to get back to work or I could lose my job, and the things I do at work require my knee to work, not so much my hearing.*

> **Audiologist:** *So, your top priority is getting your knee working well enough to get back to work so you do not lose your job?*
>
> **Patient:** *Yes, I think I'd really like my therapy out of the way and to get back to work before I start anything else new like hearing aids.*
>
> **Audiologist:** *I see. It's important to notice when you feel overwhelmed, and it sounds like there may be too much going on in your personal life for us to be working with hearing aids right now. If getting back to work and physical therapy is the higher priority, it may be best for us to put this hearing aid trial on hold, so you are not feeling overwhelmed. Does that sound like something you would like to do?*
>
> **Patient:** *Yes, please. Don't get me wrong, I appreciate the time you've taken with me, and I do really notice some improvement with the hearing aids, especially when the family is over and being able to hear my grandkids is much easier. But I just don't think right now is the right time to invest in them.*
>
> **Audiologist:** *I understand. If you decide that after physical therapy and getting back to work that you would like to pursue hearing aids again, we can certainly revisit this process when you're ready.*
>
> **Patient:** *Sure, fine. I understand I can return these at the front desk today, so I'll do that on my way out. I appreciate your understanding and do really think I will come back when I'm done with therapy and back to working.*

- Individual counseling: most patients seeking audiology services may not need robust personal adjustment support; however, a small percentage may experience emotional or adjustment challenges that are best met by the knowledge and skills of audiologists. The following counseling approaches developed in the fields of professional counseling and psychotherapy have shown benefit in with audiology populations (Aazh, 2016; Molander et al., 2018) and continue to be studied.

  □ Motivational interviewing (MI) (Rollnick et al., 2008) is a counseling approach described as a comprehensive guiding style to behavior change, used most with those who may be ambivalent or weighing the pros and cons of making a change, as opposed to taking a persuasive approach. MI conversations are designed to strengthen a person's motivation and movement to achieving behavior change by eliciting and exploring their motivation within a context of acceptance and compassion.

  □ Cognitive-behavioral therapy (CBT) is an intervention approach that aims to alleviate anxiety by helping patients to modify unhelpful, erroneous cognitions (distorted thinking) and safety-seeking behaviors. Audiologist-delivered CBT is most often focused on managing hyperacusis/tinnitus-related distress (Fuller et al., 2020).

  □ Acceptance and commitment therapy (ACT) (Hayes et al., 1999), rooted in CBT, can also help to assist a patient in better aligning their hearing/vestibular health choices and behaviors to their personal beliefs and values. ACT is an empirically developed psychological intervention that uses strategies of acceptance and mindfulness to increase psychological flexibility and reduce ineffective control and avoidance strategies, helping individuals to live a fulfilling and valued life despite experiencing negative evaluated feelings, thoughts, and physical sensations.

CASE EXAMPLE

Sammy arrives for a hearing aid consultation appointment. She and the audiologist walk back to the consult room and talk briefly about the weather and busy downtown traffic, and the audiologist begins to detect some ambivalence in Sammy's being in the office as their dialogue continues into the consult room.

Audiologist: *What brings you in to see me today?*

Sammy: *I'm here for a hearing test and hearing aids.*

Audiologist: *Very good. Were you referred to our center by anyone?*

Sammy: *My daughter Mallory.*

Audiologist: *Tell me a little about your daughter.*

Sammy: *Well, she's been pestering me to get hearing aids for years.*

Audiologist: *I see. Is there anyone else who may be concerned about your hearing?*

Sammy: *My son Joe and his wife, Julia.*

Audiologist: *Of the three of them—Mallory, Joe, or Julia—who do you feel is the most interested in you getting hearing aids today?*

Sammy: *Well, I guess that would have to be Mal. Joe and Julia are more understanding that it's my decision, my money, and my health.*

Audiologist: *I see. And what would each of them do if you didn't get hearing aids?*

Sammy: *Mal would get upset and continue pestering me. Joe would defend me, and then he and Mal would most likely get in a fight. Julia I'm not sure, but she may be indifferent as my daughter-in-law.*

Audiologist: *And how would all this affect you?*

Sammy: *Well, Mal should be the one in here to buy her own hearing aids and . . . and frankly, ever since my husband passed away, I feel like I'm not going to live much longer myself, so what's the point.*

Audiologist: [providing space with a short pause]. *I'm sorry for your loss. It seems like this situation seems very dire to you. There are a lot of emotions and multiple people involved.*

Sammy: [nods her head]

Audiologist: *It is not my interest to force anyone into buying or wearing hearing aids. Would it be okay today if we talk about your concerns and test your hearing, but hold off on discussing hearing aids or other treatment options until I understand more how it would fit into your life and family issues?*

> **Sammy:** *Yes, I would appreciate that very much.*
>
> The audiologist completed a thorough patient history, tested Sammy's hearing, and a bilateral mild sloping to moderately severe sensorineural hearing loss was diagnosed. Having a sense of the family dynamics prior to testing and now the evaluation results, they can now move on to assessing Sammy's level of motivation for hearing aids.

- Group counseling: for some patients and caregivers, the support of peers, family, and significant others in group settings may help them make gains in intervention that are not always feasible in a clinical setting. For audiologists acting as facilitators, group counseling can be a valuable tool to augment many of the direct clinical services they provide. A variety of group options for enrolling members are available to patients depending on the specific needs they may have. Examples include parent groups, mother groups, father groups, sibling groups, adults new to technology, patients with tinnitus and other ear-related disorders, aural rehabilitation groups, and many more.

Patient Reactions to Nonsupportive Communication

Recent qualitative studies in audiology have illustrated instances of nonsupportive communication observed among audiologists and patients, including not empathically responding to emotional concerns of patients, audiologists dominating conversations, using excessive complex language or technical jargon, and exhibiting multitasking behaviors during appointment conversations. Such counseling behaviors may dissuade patients from trusting their audiologists. While informational counseling is important and greatly emphasized in graduate training programs, limited experiences in adjustment counseling training and targeted feedback are primary reasons why audiologists may fall short of patient and family expectations.

 AUDIOLOGY NUGGET

Developing effective interviewing skills is a process that requires practice. Observing oneself through video recordings and asking someone with counseling expertise to critique and provide feedback about how communication skills are being conveyed/perceived can be very helpful to reveal things that are working well and where to improve.

Interviewing Patients

Interviewing patients and families in audiology is the basic process for gathering and sharing information, providing advice, and suggesting alternative working solutions to perceived challenges and concerns. Specific skills related to interviewing patients and why these areas are important skills to develop are described below, adapted from professional counseling texts (Ivey et al., 2017; Rollnick et al., 2008).

Asking Questions

When interviewing and counseling patients, the appropriate use of questions can really enhance communicating with and understanding patients and their families. An audiologist can use questions to gather relevant information related to hearing and vestibular health history, but they should avoid using interrogative-style questioning or overwhelming a patient with too many questions. Common question types include:

- Closed: used to facilitate obtaining specific information that is usually important to the clinician (typically beginning with the words *is, are,* or *do*) and can be answered in a few words

- Open-ended: used to facilitate deeper exploration of issues that are usually important to the patient/family (typically beginning with the words *what, how,* or *why*) and often are not answered in a few words

- Clarifying: if the audiologist feels they are understanding what is being said, questions such as "So what you are saying is _____. Is that right?" or "If I understand, you are feeling that _____, is that correct?" convey a sincere interest in understanding. If the audiologist is not sure they understand, asking the patient for clarification with these types of questions can also help avoid communication breakdowns.

 Q & A

Question: What are some examples of these questions as applied in an audiology appointment?

Answer: The following are some examples of questions that may be used during a dialogue when performing an intake case history with a patient.

- Closed questions

  "Was your change in hearing sudden or progressive?"

  "Are you currently taking any medications?"

  "Have you been taking your medication as prescribed?"

  "How long have you been feeling dizzy?"

  "Does your tinnitus seem worse in the morning or in the evening?"

- Open-ended

  "Tell me more about how conversing in a restaurant is difficult for you."

  "How are you hearing today?"

  "How do you fit meditation in your daily routine for managing your tinnitus?"

- Clarifying

  "So, you are saying you only hear the ringing in your left ear, correct?"

  "If I understand correctly, you were told you have normal hearing, but you still feel like you're having challenges hearing and understanding speech in background noise?"

- Funnel/circular: questions like these involve starting with general questions and then drilling down to a more specific point in each. Usually asking for more and more detail at each level. Generally interrogative in nature, these questions are often used by detectives taking a statement from a witness.

- Leading: these questions tend to be closed-ended and are used to lead the respondent to a preferred perspective or way of thinking with an assumption, personal appeal to agree, phrasing the wording so that the "easiest" response is "yes," and/or giving someone a choice between two options or preferences.

Responding to Patients

There are times in audiological care when the most important and most healing thing that an audiologist can do is simply be there with their patient(s) and take the time to listen and understand. What patients communicate, including their intention, needs, meanings, and emotions, can be communicated both nonverbally and verbally. Listening and responding empathically takes practice and the following are specific counseling skills that can help convey sincere and intentional listening:

Nonverbal Communication Skills

- Nonverbal skills that can have a positive impact include using appropriate facial expressions, eye contact, gestures, motioning, tone of voice, speaking rate, posture, body positions, comfortable spacing/distance between patient and clinician, setting up a welcoming clinical environment, and strategic placement of furniture and other objects (e.g., computer, cell phone, or hearing technologies). Sitting forward in one's chair toward the patient, facing the patient directly, and head and face movements such as head nods and appropriate facial expressions are also some specific nonverbal ways to convey listening.

- Nonverbal skills that can have a negative impact include nervous habits (e.g., continually tapping a pen, wringing/fidgeting with hands, bouncing leg), which can be distracting or perceived adversely by a patient (whether intentional or not).

Verbal Communication Skills

- Encouragers
  - Patients are usually reluctant to share personal thoughts without prompts, encouragement, and intentional guiding by audiologists to uncover issues currently being experienced. Patients need to know that their audiologist hears what they say, sees what they see (their point of view), and can empathize with or appreciate their experience and demonstrate understanding.
  - Verbal encouragers can be used to help with this process, including the use of "door openers" such as "tell me what brings you into the clinic today," or "tell me more about . . . ," essentially leaving the communication door open to all clinically relevant information. Other verbal encouragers include listening to the responses of the patient and using minimal encouragers, such as saying "uh-huh," "what else about . . . ," "is there anything else . . . ," and so on.

- Reflective listening
  - Another effective way to demonstrate active listening in counseling is through the skill of reflecting communication back to the patient, including restating, paraphrasing, and

summarizing the content of what has been said, avoiding the use/creation of your own words, except when needing to clarify.

☐ Reflective listening is helpful in reducing the clinical knee-jerk reactions to solve, right, or fix someone's problem(s), concern(s), or issue(s) that may arise during a clinical encounter. Reflecting content allows the clinician to let the patient say what they want to say and feel heard, without any judgment, criticism, or blame for what has been shared.

☐ It is not uncommon for a patient/family to experience strong emotions during the news of a diagnosis or recommendations they were not expecting or wanting. Reflecting what feelings or emotions the clinician may be observing (both positive and negative) is as equally important as reflecting content and information. For example, based on nonverbal cues, you might say something to a patient experiencing strong emotions, such as: "It seems like you may be confused, or upset, etc., about. . . . Is this what you are feeling/experiencing right now?" Reflecting back what the clinicians observe about the emotional state of the patient can give clarity to the quality of the communication and help the clinician readjust as needed.

■ Validation

☐ The psychosocial impact of auditory and vestibular disorders can vary widely among patients. Validation in counseling involves communicating an understanding and acceptance of a patients' feelings, thoughts, reactions, and fears (whatever they are) without judgment.

☐ Validating statements are like those used in reflective listening, such as: "I hear what you are saying," "I understand," "This must be difficult for you," "It sounds like you did your best," "You are not alone," "I can see you are trying," and "I can see you are _____ (sad, upset, frightened, etc.)."

Q & A

Question: What are the differences between patient values and patient goals?

Answer: Understanding a patient's/family's values that drive decisions can aid in understanding how the intervention process relates to what is important. Goals are often things a patient can work for and achieve, whereas values are always present and seldom change (e.g., striving for consistency is a value, being on time for an appointment is a goal). Values often refer to chosen life directions that motivate actions. Distinguishing between values and goals is an important skill that can help audiologists know how to best support patients and families to feel motivated to make desired changes in their lives.

Addressing the Functional and Social Impacts of Auditory and Vestibular Disorders

The World Health Organization's (WHO) International Classification of Functioning, Disability and Health (ICF) theoretical framework provides standard language for describing individual functioning and health, while also promoting patient-centered practices in healthcare (WHO, 2001). The

ICF framework is used within a wide range of disability and health professions and is organized into two parts: (a) functioning and disability (body functions/structures and activity/participation) and (b) contextual factors (environmental and personal factors). A paradigm shift toward this framework has been advocated for in audiology (Erdman, 2019), moving away from a medical model (or site-of-lesion) approach. Experts agree that individuals affected by ear-related disorders are impacted in diverse ways because of the "types of activities they do, [the] societal roles they have, who they are, and the [environments] in which they participate" (Meyer et al., 2016, p. 163).

AUDIOLOGY NUGGET

Individuals who do not participate in social activities/events such as attending movies, musicals, plays, music concerts, or theatrical productions because of their hearing loss are often limited by their hearing challenges because of their having trouble understanding speech in those settings. Under the ICF framework, these would be considered "participation restrictions" in activities that require them to understand speech.

Examples of Audiological Counseling Across the Lifespan

This section is designed to illustrate portions of scripted clinical encounters or vignettes of audiologist-patient interactions at different stages of life. At the end of each example are some review questions and brief explanations or answers to support the reader in their review and identifying basic counseling skills present within each vignette.

- Pediatric diagnosis example
  - □ Shaun, age 2 months, was referred for a pediatric auditory brainstem response evaluation after referring from his universal newborn hearing screening. The case history obtained by the audiologist was unremarkable in terms of the child and maternal overall health and hearing-related health history reported. Following the evaluation, the audiologist had the following discussion with the mother, Mrs. Smith:

    Audiologist: *Mrs. Smith, what was your initial reaction when Shaun referred from his hearing screening at the hospital?*

    Mrs. Smith: *I was quite surprised. I never suspected my first child wouldn't be able to hear. No one in my family is deaf. How were the results of your test today?*

    Audiologist: *Well, according to our testing today, it does appear that Shaun does have hearing loss in his left ear.*

    Mrs. Smith: *Really, why would that be?*

    Audiologist: *I cannot say for certain, but additional medical and genetic information may help to pinpoint exactly what may be the cause for this difference in hearing between his ears. Would it be important to you to be able to have this kind of information?*

    Mrs. Smith: *I don't really know. Maybe. I'll have to talk to my husband about that. When you say he has hearing loss in just the left ear, does that mean he cannot hear anything in that ear?*

Audiologist: *Great question. The results indicate that Shaun's auditory system responded to sounds at elevated volume levels in his left ear, but not typical volume levels, meaning if sounds are loud enough in the left ear, he can hear them. With this being the case, Shaun may be a candidate for using a hearing aid in the left ear to bring sounds back into a typical hearing range in that ear.*

Mrs. Smith: *A hearing aid? I thought only old people wore hearing aids. Do they make hearing aids for babies, and does he need to wear it now?*

Audiologist: *It sounds like you would like to learn more about pediatric hearing aids and the timing of when Shaun would be eligible for technology. In short, yes, there are hearing aids that are made for infants and we can start the process of acquiring hearing technology today if you feel ready; however, I want to make sure that you and your husband have time to let this sink in, it's a lot, I know. Would some more time and information be helpful to you before discussing anything more about a hearing aid?*

Mrs. Smith: *Thank you for your consideration. This is new and unexpected, and I think I would like some more time to talk about this with my husband and have him come with me to talk about the hearing aid before we proceed.*

Audiologist: *Certainly. I understand and would be more than happy to visit with you and your husband to discuss the next steps. How soon do you think you and your husband may be able to return to our office?*

☐ Should the audiologist have used more technical information to describe the test results to Shaun's mother?

☐ Did the audiologist use active listening skills such as reflective listening or validating statements to help Mrs. Smith feel heard and understood?

☐ Answers: In this example, the audiologist addressed Mrs. Smith's questions immediately and followed her lead. Although there is urgency to early intervention improving outcomes, if audiologists push their agenda too much and too fast, it may dissuade families from proceeding with intervention. The audiologist in this case did use active listening responses and addressed the underlying concerns of the mother, who was surprised at the news and was not wanting to decide next steps without her husband's input. He followed through on this response also by inviting Mrs. Smith to set up a time for the family to return soon with her husband.

■ School-age classroom participation example

☐ Eric, age 9 years, was referred for a hearing evaluation by his third-grade teacher, who feels like he is not paying attention and missing instructions in class. The case history obtained by the audiologist was unremarkable in terms of the child and family health and otologic history. Following the evaluation, the audiologist had a teacher assistant escort Eric back to his classroom, and the educational audiologist had the following discussion with Eric's father, Mr. Brown:

Audiologist: *Mr. Brown, thank you for coming in to support Eric today. I believe you are aware of his teacher's recent concerns in class.*

Mr. Brown: *Yes, his teacher sent a letter regarding why she thought this test was needed, but I honestly haven't seen or suspected anything wrong with his hearing.*

> **Audiologist:** *I would agree based on today's results as he does appear to have normal hearing by our measures. For some reason, it did take a little longer for me to get through testing and for Eric to respond to instructions.*
>
> **Mr. Brown:** *Interesting. Sounds kind of like what the teacher's been reporting.*
>
> **Audiologist:** *Right. I couldn't say from my observation why this might be, but I do see a lot of kids Eric's age and know them to make some creative decisions when other things in life aren't going as well. Sometimes children Eric's age seek attention without asking for it. Could you tell me if there's anything going on in Eric's life that might be bothering him?*
>
> **Mr. Brown:** *Well, to be frank, both of his maternal grandparents recently passed away in a tragic accident, and he was quite close to them. Eric's mother has also been taking it quite hard and has been receiving professional counseling support. I've been encouraging him to just kind of move on and take it like a man—I didn't have grandparents and lost both of my parents at a pretty young age myself and was raised by an uncle. Do you think perhaps this may be contributing to Eric's recent classroom behaviors?*

- ☐ Did the audiologist assert the longer/challenging test time to Eric being a mischievous or noncooperative child?

- ☐ How did the father, Mr. Brown, respond to the audiologist's questions about other reasons outside of school that may be contributing to Eric's behavior?

- ☐ Answers: In this example, the audiologist focused on the positive side of Eric's behaviors. Mr. Brown additionally responded with a willingness to disclose some crucial information, which may be the real source of the classroom challenges that the audiologist could confidently then share with Eric's teacher and others in the school who could work to consider other ways of supporting Eric in class.

- ■ Young adult college needs example

  - ☐ Emery, a 19-year-old female, has recently started her second year in a premedical biology program, and the material is becoming increasingly difficult to master in classes. She comes to her first audiology appointment after nearly 4 years since she last saw an audiologist while still in high school:

    > **Audiologist:** *Emery, I see you wrote a note on your intake history form that you frequently feeling lost and frustrated in class because of your hearing loss and that it is interfering with your academic performance. This sounds stressful.*
    >
    > **Emery:** *It really is. As you know, I'm a college student studying premed biology, and as I've gotten into my more advanced sophomore biology classes, the subject material is becoming harder to hear and understand in classes and I do feel like I'm not understanding my professors who are from other countries and whose accents are really hard to understand.*
    >
    > **Audiologist:** *How have you been managing with these classes so far?*
    >
    > **Emery:** *Very badly. I pretend I know what they're saying, nod my head, or claim that I understand something when they ask me questions, but when it comes to a direct question about specific concepts in class, I am extremely anxious about answering, I've gotten a couple questions right because of good luck, but have even gone as far as excusing myself from class to go to the bathroom one time because I really had no idea what they were asking me about.*

- What kinds of questions or statements did the audiologist use to gain a better understanding of Emery's recent concerns related to her hearing?
- Answer: In this brief example, the audiologist used open-ended statements and questions to give Emery time to explain how her hearing loss is impacting her functioning in school.

■ Working adult resistant to hearing aids example

- Mr. Johnson, a 40-year-old male, has been referred from multiple occupational hearing screenings and has a known noise-induced hearing loss but has been reluctant to obtain hearing aids since his work requires him to always wear hearing protection, and he only seems to have trouble outside of work when conversing in small and large groups or when there is background noise. He is beginning to consider hearing aids to help in these situations but is skeptical/doubtful they will provide any benefit.

> **Audiologist:** *Mr. Johnson, tell me a little more about the difficulty you experience conversing in groups.*
>
> **Mr. Johnson:** *I'm not sure. I can hear that everyone is talking, I just can't make out any one voice over another.*
>
> **Audiologist:** *I imagine that must be frustrating for you. What have you done in those situations?*
>
> **Mr. Johnson:** *What do I do? Well, recently I don't do anything because I try to avoid talking groups whenever I can. I know I probably shouldn't, but when I miss things, all I can do is fake it or pretend I heard what was said.*
>
> **Audiologist:** *So, because you don't want to feign understanding in groups, you find yourself avoiding those kinds of listening situations?*
>
> **Mr. Johnson:** *Yeah, it can be really embarrassing, especially at breaks on work, or if my wife tells me we're going out to eat with friends or family. Mostly I just leave my hearing protection in all the time at work now unless my boss or a supervisor needs to talk to me . . . and I guess I just make excuses not to go out, which means my wife ends up cancelling and we stay home a lot more from outings.*
>
> **Audiologist:** *It sounds like your challenges conversing in groups are starting to have a significant impact on your relationships with coworkers and now even with your wife, friends, and family.*
>
> **Mr. Johnson:** *I suppose you're right, but, like I said, most of the time, I can hear, I just don't understand everything.*
>
> **Audiologist:** *Would you like to be able to understand everything better in these situations?*
>
> **Mr. Johnson:** *Sure.*
>
> **Audiologist:** *If there were something we could do together to make conversing in groups more successful for you, would that be a good thing?*
>
> **Mr. Johnson:** *It would be good for my wife perhaps.*
>
> **Audiologist:** *While that may be true, and I hope your wife can join us in the future to see what she can do to help, I assume you'd agree that we can't hold your wife responsible to fix all the challenges you are experiencing because of the changes you've experienced with your hearing.*

> **Mr. Johnson:** *Right, she can't do it all, but I'm still not all that sure about getting hearing aids.*
>
> **Audiologist:** *On a scale of 0 to 10, with 0 being not motivated and 10 being highly motivated, how motivated do you feel it might be to follow my recommendations to make conversing in groups easier if part of what we did included using hearing aids?*
>
> **Mr. Johnson:** *On that scale, maybe a 5.*
>
> **Audiologist:** *Any thoughts on what would shift your rating to a 7 or 8?*

☐ Did the audiologist in this case jump straight to solutions as to how hearing aids could help Mr. Johnson hear better in group settings?

☐ How does the audiologist show acceptance of Mr. Johnson's skepticism regarding hearing aids?

☐ Answers: In this example, it could have been very easy for the audiologist to just jump straight to reasons why hearing aids could improve Mr. Johnson's listening challenges, but this is a scenario where Mr. Johnson doesn't need all the information about hearing aids, but rather, encouragement to see what a hearing health behavior change can do to enhance his quality of life and relationships. The audiologist recognized and accepted Mr. Johnson's skepticism and opened the door for a more supportive counseling dialogue based on using a question about exploring Mr. Johnson's thoughts related to the potential for future change.

■ Older adult strained relationship concerns example

☐ Cecilia, an 88-year-old female, recently lost her husband of 62 years, moved into an assisted living center, and was dropped off for her first hearing evaluation by her adult daughter because of concerns they have with her hearing and memory:

> **Audiologist:** *Good day, Ms. Cecilia. What brings you to our clinic today?*
>
> **Ms. Cecilia:** *My daughter made me come. She is always complaining that I set my TV volume too loud and that I'm not understanding what my grandkids are saying. If they wouldn't talk so fast, I wouldn't have any trouble understanding them.*
>
> **Audiologist:** *I see. It sounds like your daughter is wondering if there may be changes in your hearing, is that correct?*
>
> **Ms. Cecilia:** *Yes.*
>
> **Audiologist:** *It also sounds like communication may be causing some tension. . . .*
>
> **Ms. Cecilia:** *I would say there is a lot of contention in our family lately.*
>
> **Audiologist:** *That must be hard. Can you tell me what you are noticing?*
>
> **Ms. Cecilia:** *I notice . . . well, nothing really that bad. I occasionally cannot hear the preacher on the broadcast I watch on my TV, even with the volume louder, but if other people would just speak slower and clearer, things wouldn't be so hard.*
>
> **Audiologist:** *So, you feel like you are noticing some hearing difficulties you didn't before, and maybe you're unsure of the reasons. Although your daughter dropped you off for today's appointment, what are you hoping to get out of your visit? Would you like to find out if your hearing is changing?*
>
> **Ms. Cecilia:** *Yes, I suppose I would like to find out.*

- ☐ Did the audiologist move through a standard check list of case history questions to interview Ms. Cecilia at the outset of meeting this patient?

- ☐ Did the audiologist define Ms. Cecilia's challenges for her?

- ☐ Answers: At the outset of this dialogue, the audiologist could have easily gone through the motions of using a standard checklist of intake history questions. Instead, they chose to use open-ended statements, acknowledging and listening to the patient without labeling any hearing or listening challenges for the patient. It can be helpful to let the patient define in their own words what their situation is and what they would like to do about it. The dialogue in this example was productive because it resulted in forward movement.

Cultural and Linguistic Diversity (CLD)

Cultures, languages, and dimensions of diversity throughout the world are constantly in change. Culture can be defined as the learned, shared, inherited, or taught set of shared values, beliefs, norms, behaviors, communication, and roles among a group (Rosal et al., 2014). It is estimated that 95% of audiologists in the United States identify with Western (North and South America, Europe, Australia, and New Zealand) cultural values (Clark & English, 2019). If audiologists and patients are unfamiliar with other cultures or backgrounds than their own, it can create issues through the continuum of clinical care. The following are important culture-related definitions and approaches to consider for addressing the audiological counseling needs of culturally and linguistically diverse patients.

- ■ Cultural influence
  - ☐ Cultural influence is the extent to which the values, beliefs, traditions, and norms of a group influence their behaviors within the group (Rosal et al., 2014). A model illustrating a broad range of values that may influence patient behaviors in an audiological practice setting is provided in Figure 11–1.
  - ☐ Time: cultural perceptions of time can influence attitudes toward punctuality and timeliness, or the lack thereof.
  - ☐ Autonomy: cultural perceptions of individualism can influence how patients may make decisions regarding their hearing health. Some may be comfortable making choices on their own, whereas others depend or rely on the opinions and decisions of those they are socially connected to such as family or other trusted individuals.
  - ☐ Gender: cultural perceptions of gender can influence what patients expect from audiological services. Some may not feel comfortable relating to, sharing personal health information with, taking direction from, or refuse services altogether from an audiologist of the opposite sex.
  - ☐ Health beliefs: cultural perceptions of health can influence expectations about the value of audiological care. In some cultures, even the decision to seek healthcare is made by considering the monetary, time, and psychological costs to the patient themselves, their family, possible caregivers, and society. Mainstream expectations of advanced and optimal healthcare solutions such as modern hearing technology may be perceived in some cultures as unnecessary when weighing the cost of their personal health against the needs of others of their community and culture.

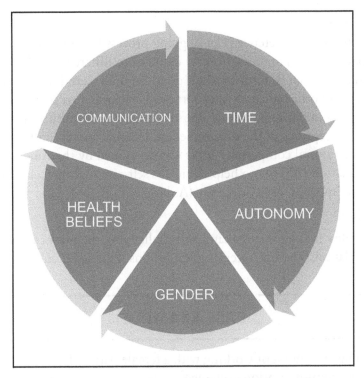

FIGURE 11–1. Broad values that differ between cultures.

□ Communication: cultural perceptions of communication norms vary widely across cultures. There are both nonverbal communication cues (e.g., eye contact, amount of personal space when conversing, professional dress, and appearance) and verbal communication cues (e.g., appropriate language and vocabulary use, linguistically code-switching) that should be considered when a patient/family is from a different culture. There may be different cultural norms about how audiologists may be expected to speak differently to adults, older adults, and children from various backgrounds. Some patients additionally may base their decision to communicate with audiologists who are only of a certain age, sex, occupation, or who hold a higher position of rank or status within the clinical setting. As an example, a patient may choose to accept the recommendations from a more senior or seasoned audiologist but not from a younger one.

■ Deaf culture considerations

□ A specific culture of interest to audiologists includes individuals from Deaf culture and Deaf populations. A small percentage of individuals in the United States who have severe to profound hearing loss are described as culturally D/deaf. The capital "D" refers to a cultural identification with the Deaf community, whereas the lowercase "d" deaf relates to individuals who may not wholly identify as being a part of the Deaf community exclusively. Some within this community prefer verbal communication, but most rely on visual, manual, or signed communication such as American Sign Language (ASL). Hearing loss in Deaf culture is not viewed as a disability or in any way a detriment to function; rather, deafness is seen from a social model of disability, that of it being society's reluctance to accommodate to their needs as what is disabling (Dobie & Van Hemel, 2004).

■ Cultural competence

  ☐ Developing cultural competence is an ongoing process for clinicians who interact with individual patients and families who may come from different culturally and linguistically diverse populations that differ from their own. An understanding of one's own worldview and sensitivities to other cultures is important. Developing cultural competence comes through a process of self-reflection of one's own biases and culture and developing positive attitudes and perceptions of the diverse beliefs, feelings, values, and experiences of others. A collection of cultural competency tools was developed by the American Speech-Language-Hearing Association (ASHA) to help clinicians self-rate their perceived levels of cultural competence to improve service delivery (ASHA, n.d.-a).

■ Cultural humility

  ☐ Cultural humility is about recognizing and challenging the power imbalances in clinician and patient relationships and accepting limitations. Practicing cultural humility is a lifelong

---

CASE EXAMPLE

Consider a male audiologist working with a female patient from Saudi Arabia in the following communication exchange:

Audiologist: *Mrs. Ahmed, please look at my face as I am talking with you. You will understand what I'm saying better if you look at my lips, expressions, and my eyes as I talk. The habit of looking down all the time will not help you understand what I'm saying.*

Mrs. Ahmed: [looks briefly at the audiologist's face, but then quickly returns her gaze to the floor, followed by darting her gaze back and forth toward the door, ensuring others in the hall can see her and the audiologist in the room].

When patients are from a culture that has customs that vary from those of the audiologist, the potential for problems increases. In Anglo-American culture, eye contact is often seen as a sign of direct and honest communication, and thus the avoidance of eye contact may be seen as disrespectful or distrustful. Such interpretations of avoiding eye contact would likely be incorrect for patients from an Asian, a Middle Eastern, a Native American, or possibly a Hispanic/Latin cultural background. Among many Middle Eastern cultures, such as Mrs. Ahmed's cultural background, eye contact is avoided between men and women out of propriety. Direct eye contact may be seen as sexually suggestive, and thus care should be taken to avoid such inferences. Mrs. Ahmed's audiologist demonstrated a lack of cultural competence and humility regarding her cultural background, causing her to feel uncomfortable with the services being provided. The audiologist in this scenario should have acknowledged Mrs. Ahmed's lack of eye contact more empathically using appropriate questions to ask why she was not making eye contact. Doing so could've helped the audiologist understand the underlying cultural reasons behind her nonverbal behaviors while also creating a more comfortable healthcare environment for Mrs. Ahmed's appointment.

self-reflection process that includes learning to put aside personal biases and perceptions and having an interest in learning from others about their biases and perceptions.

- Using interpreters
  - When working with patients who speak different languages, using an interpreter can help overcome linguistic barriers. In counseling patients with the help of an interpreter, it is important that audiologists should avoid talking to the interpreter as if the patient were absent. Instead, they should direct all communication as if the patient spoke the same language, including actively facing the patient, using appropriate eye contact, and addressing the patient in the first person. Word-for-word translations of what patients say may also be needed with the help of the interpreter to check for understanding or clarify points that may have been unclear or misunderstood by the patient.

What audiologists choose to say and communicate to patients and families is important for the success of audiological services to meet the needs of patients. We have spent the first section of this chapter reviewing important and foundational counseling skills that can be used in practice. In addition to what is said, audiological documentation can also affect patient care, and the next section of this chapter will help with the review of important concepts related to documentation in practice.

Audiological Documentation

Audiologists work in a variety of healthcare and educational settings. As a result of the needs that vary in each setting, there are no universal formats or time frames that are set for documenting health records in audiology. Key principles are outlined in detail by ASHA (n.d.-b) that are helpful to guide documentation of audiological records.

The use of the acronym ACUTE can be used to recall five of these principles in proper documentation: Accurate, Code-able, Understanding, Timely, Error-free. These principles are further delineated in how they include demonstrating medical necessity, based on if services are reasonable (appropriate amount, frequency, and duration of services), necessary (contribute to patient's diagnosis and functioning), specific, effective (expected improvement in a reasonable time), and that services are provided by, or referrals made to, skilled and competent providers.

Another commonly used structure for audiologic and other medical reporting includes the use of the acronym SOAP: subjective, objective, assessment, and plan. Routinely used in healthcare documentation, it is a helpful format to organize both thinking about a patient's situation and the recording of this information in a logical manner that is linked often with the summary of how an appointment was carried out (Figure 11–2). The SOAP format for documenting patient encounters is designed to expand the problem list of challenges a patient may be experiencing and seeking the provider out for and summarizing this list into a simplified list of vital information regarding the key problems and what was being done about them (Ramachandran & Stach, 2013).

Demonstrating medical necessity is crucial for audiology services, and effective documentation can help to accomplish this. Reimbursement or payment by medical insurance or self-paying patients requires documentation of medical/behavioral history, diagnosis, date of onset, physician referral, initial evaluation/date, evaluation procedures, individualized plan of care, and intervention/progress notes. Details are generally specific to appointment types (e.g., diagnostic, evaluation, treatment, follow-up) and depend on the types of services rendered. Annual or routine audiological evaluations are not considered medically necessary by Medicare.

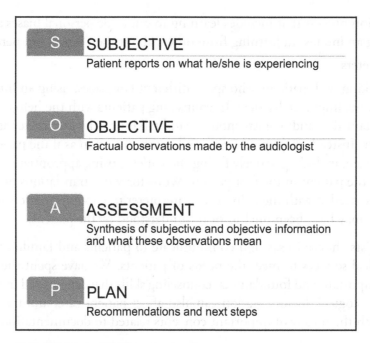

FIGURE 11–2. SOAP note structure.

 KNOWLEDGE CHECKPOINT

An example of an abbreviated SOAP note in audiology:

Patient reports recent hearing loss in the right ear (S) and audiologist finds deep and occluding cerumen (O), which coincides with the complaint. Audiologist's state licensure does not permit removal of wax beyond the cartilaginous portion and removal is needed prior to continuing with hearing evaluation (A). Audiologist refers patient to otolaryngologist for cerumen removal in the right ear (P) and recommends that the patient return for hearing evaluation post medical clearance.

- Clinical encounters
  - Documentation of all clinical interactions should include date of encounter, procedures performed, patient and family/caregiver participation, subjective and objective data, clinical interpretations, recommendations, accommodations and modifications to clinical procedure(s), patient and family counseling, patient consent forms, provider signature(s), and credentials of clinician.
  - Types of documentation may include evaluation reports (summary of evaluation, diagnosis, and plan for service/discharge), intervention notes (documentation of patient encounter postdiagnosis), progress notes (for patients who receive regular services with long- or short-term goals), or discharge summaries (reasons for stopping services and patient status at that time).

- Equipment/protocols
  - □ Having a documentation of records to verify regulations were met for clinical equipment (e.g., ANSI standards) and protocols followed regarding calibration, equipment function, and test environment can help to ensure the operations of a practice are working smoothly and also help prevent medical errors in administrative oversight, clinical use of equipment/ protocols, and treatment procedures.
- Referring patients
  - □ When encountering patient problems that are beyond the professional scope of practice of audiology or competence level of the clinician, audiologists are ethically obligated to refer patients to professionals better suited to meet their needs.
  - □ If providing services after receiving a referral from a physician, a referral back or written report to the physician is common.
  - □ Medical referrals are common for red-flag indications to rule out ear-related medical pathologies/disorders, as well as when medical clearance is needed prior to the start of audiologic intervention (e.g., pediatric amplification). Providers commonly referred to from audiology include otolaryngologists (ear, nose, and throat physicians), pediatricians, primary care physicians (PCPs), and other allied health professionals.
  - □ A subset of patients who experience mental health challenges because of or in addition to their hearing loss, balance loss, or other auditory/ear-related disorders may need to be referred to mental health professionals (e.g., psychologists, psychiatrists, licensed professional counselors) for specialized services related to their mental health needs (e.g., depression, anxiety, stress); specific concerns can be collected and shared with these professionals using both behavioral observations and self-report instruments (e.g., Patient Health Questionnaire–9 [PHQ-9] [Kroenke & Spitzer, 2002]; Depression, Anxiety and Stress Scale–21 [DASS-21] [Antony et al., 1998]).
- Institutional guidelines for documentation
  - □ Medicare
    - Evaluation: includes diagnosis, results of ASHA National Outcomes Measures (NOMs) or functional assessment scores and measurable benchmarks/progress; ONE TIME SERVICE may be implied in the diagnosis.
    - Plan of care: reported separately or together with the evaluation; includes long-term treatment goals and type/duration/frequency of therapies.
    - Progress reports: to justify medical necessity, completed once every treatment day or once each certification interval; includes assessment of progress/improvement, plans to continue treatment, or changes to goals.
    - Treatment notes: to record encounters and intervention, required for every date of service.
    - Discharge note: includes all treatment since last progress report in the form of a handover document explaining to patient or any other healthcare professional why the patient was admitted or enrolled in treatment, what happened to them during treatment, and all information that they may be needed in the future for another provider to pick up the care of the patient efficiently and effectively.
  - □ Medicaid: documentation required for all services

- Considerations include prior authorization, PCP referral, evaluation report, diagnosis, reevaluation, and claim form requirements.
- Private practice guidelines for documentation
  - □ In private practice, documentation can be variable but typically includes reason for patient visit, services provided, diagnosis, and recommendations (aligned with procedure codes).
- Electronic medical records (EMRs)
  - □ The use of EMRs provides substantial flexibility to the clinician to easily locate documentation and reports for a particular patient about reasons for referrals or any relevant patient history.
  - □ "Medicare requires electronic submission of billing information if the practice employs more than 10 full-time employees" (ASHA, n.d.-b); this may be more stringent for large healthcare facilities.
  - □ Documentation templates must include individualized patient information options, including needs, goals, and recommendations.
- Communication with patients, professionals, and interpreters
  - □ Most health interactions in audiology may occur face-to-face and important information can be shared with patients via handouts, pamphlets, brochures, and other paper materials. Increasingly, however, patients have appreciated the ability to communicate electronically, via methods such as e-mail or systems that may exist through their hearing technology mobile applications or EMR software.
  - □ The option to use telecommunications (phone communication) is also a support to families who may not have the ability to visit an office but just need a quick question answered over the phone.
  - □ For electronic and telecommunications that require a significant amount of the provider's time to address, there may be systems in place to bill for that time that they take to address patient concerns in these formats.
- Telehealth applications: also called telepractice or teleaudiology or telerehabilitation
  - □ Teleaudiology is the provision of audiology services that encompass the audiology scope of practice.
  - □ To provide these services, providers must comply with ASHA code of ethics and state/federal laws; requires consideration for technological training, understanding, and troubleshooting.
  - □ ASHA guidelines recommend having the requisite licensure for the location of both provider and patient to provide teleaudiology services. The Audiology and Speech-Language Pathology Interstate Compact (ASLP-IC) is under development to allow professionals to practice in multiple states without multiple licenses.
  - □ The Veteran's Health Administration (VHA) might have different requirements for teleaudiology (ASHA, n.d.-c).
  - □ Services in teleaudiology can be synchronous, asynchronous, or hybrid.
    - Synchronous: live, two-way flow of information and communication encounter between audiologist and patient

- Asynchronous: information stored at the patient site and later forwarded to the audiologist via telecommunications or other technology means

  - Hybrid: a combination of synchronous and asynchronous modalities

  □ Reimbursement for teleaudiology depends on federal and state regulations.

  □ Documentation of teleaudiology encounters should demonstrate services and procedures were provided or accomplished to the same extent and benefit as to what a patient would have received in person (face-to-face).

- Legal and ethical considerations

  □ Confidentiality and security of records and documentation of services in audiology is extremely important, and each state may have unique record retention laws that vary by setting or type of record.

  □ Federal laws, such as the Health Insurance Portability and Accountability Act (HIPAA) and the Family Educational Rights and Privacy Act (FERPA), must be considered in the creation and granting of access to identifiable medical, health, or educational records, and unless required under other laws, these records cannot be released to anyone other than the patient without written permission.

  □ All forms of medical records are legal documents, and any changes or edits to records should be dated and initialed by the original documenter.

  □ Payers, insurers (both private and public), and regulatory or accrediting agencies may set forth regulations governing record retention, and it is the duty of audiologists to learn applicable regulations to their setting, facility, or type(s) of record(s) and abide by the most stringent policy(s) as warranted.

Recommended Readings

Blonna, R., & Watter, D. (2005). *Health counseling: A microskills approach*. Jones & Bartlett.

Dilollo, A., & Neimeyer, R.A. (2022). *Counseling in speech-language pathology and audiology: Reconstructing personal narratives* (2nd ed.). Plural Publishing.

Flasher, L. V., & Fogle, P. (2012). *Counseling skills for speech-language pathologists and audiologists* (2nd ed.). Delmar.

Holland, A. L., & Nelson, R. L. (2020). *Counseling in communication disorders: A wellness perspective* (3rd ed.). Plural Publishing.

Meier, S. T., & Davis, S. R. (2019). *The elements of counseling* (8th ed.). Waveland Press.

Moreno, N. J. (2020). *Patient-centered communication: The seven keys to connecting with patients*. Thieme Publishing.

References

Aazh, H. (2016). Feasibility of conducting a randomized controlled trial to evaluate the effect of motivational interviewing on hearing-aid use. *International Journal of Audiology, 55*(3), 149–156. https://doi.org/10.3109/14992027.2015.1074733

American Speech-Language-Hearing Association. (n.d.-a). *Cultural competence check-ins* [Practice management]. https://www.asha.org/practice/multicultural/self/

American Speech-Language-Hearing Association. (n.d.-b). *Documentation of audiology services* [Practice portal]. https://www.asha.org/Practice-Portal/Professional-Issues/Documentation-of-Audiology-Services/

American Speech-Language-Hearing Association. (n.d.-c). *Telepractice* [Practice portal]. https://www.asha.org/Practice-Portal/Professional-Issues/Telepractice/

Antony, M. M., Bieling, P. J., Cox, B. J., Enns, M. W., & Swinson, R. P. (1998). Psychometric properties of the 42-item and 21-item versions of the Depression Anxiety Stress Scales in clinical groups and a community sample. *Psychological Assessment, 10*(2), 176. https://doi.org/10.1037/1040-3590.10.2.176

Beck, A. T. (Ed.). (1979). *Cognitive therapy of depression.* Guilford.

Clark, J. G., & English, K. M. (2019). *Counseling-infused audiologic care* (3rd ed.). Inkus Press.

Cottone, R. R. (2017). *Theories of counseling and psychotherapy: Individual and relational approaches.* Springer. https://connect.springerpub.com/content/book/978-0-8261-6866-5

Devlin, K. (2018, June 13). *Family systems theory definition & what is it?* https://www.regain.us/advice/family/family-systems-theory-definition-what-is-it/

Dobie, R. A., & Van Hemel, S. (2004). *Hearing loss: Determining eligibility for social security benefits.* National Academies Press.

Erdman, S. A. (2019). Biopsychosocial approaches to audiologic counseling. In J. J. Montano & J. B. Spitzer (Eds.), *Adult audiologic rehabilitation* (3rd ed., pp. 199–247). Plural Publishing.

Fuller, T., Cima, R., Langguth, B., Mazurek, B., Vlaeyen, J. W., & Hoare, D. J. (2020). Cognitive behavioural therapy for tinnitus. *Cochrane Database of Systematic Reviews, 1*(1), CD012614. https://doi.org/10.1002/14651858.CD012614.pub2

Hayes, S. C., Strosahl, K. D., & Wilson, K. G. (1999). *Acceptance and commitment therapy an experiential approach to behavior change.* Guilford.

Ivey, A. E., Ivey, M. B., & Zalaquett, C. P. (2017). *Intentional interviewing and counseling: Facilitating client development in a multicultural society* (9th ed.). Cengage.

Kroenke, K., & Spitzer, R. L. (2002). The PHQ-9: A new depression diagnostic and severity measure. *Psychiatric Annals, 32*(9), 509–515. https://doi.org/10.3928/0048-5713-20020901-06

Meyer, C., Grenness, C., Scarinci, N., & Hickson, L. (2016). What is the international classification of functioning, disability and health and why is it relevant to audiology? *Seminars in Hearing, 37*(3), 163–186. https://doi.org/10.1055/s-0036-1584412

Molander, P., Hesser, H., Weineland, S., Bergwall, K., Buck, S., Jäder Malmlöf, J., . . . Andersson, G. (2018). Internet-based acceptance and commitment therapy for psychological distress experienced by people with hearing problems: A pilot randomized controlled trial. *Cognitive Behaviour Therapy, 47*(2), 169–184. https://doi.org/10.1080/16506073.2017.1365929

Ramachandran, V., & Stach, B. A. (2013). *Professional communication in audiology.* Plural Publishing.

Rollnick, S., Miller, W. R., & Butler, C. C. (2008). *Motivational interviewing in health care: Helping patients change behavior.* Guilford.

Rosal, M. C., Wang, M. L., & Bodenlos, J. S. (2014). Culture, behavior, and health. In K. A. Riekert, J. K. Ockene, & L. Pbert (Eds.), *The handbook of health behavior change* (pp. 109–136). Springer.

Sanders, D. A. (1975). Hearing aid orientation and counseling. In M. C. Pollack (Ed.), *Amplification for the hearing-impaired* (pp. 323–372). Grune & Stratton.

Wolpe, J. (1990). *The practice of behavior therapy* (4th ed.). Pergamon Press.

World Health Organization. (2001). *International classification of functioning, disability and health: ICF.* http://www.who.int/classifications/icf/en/

✎ Practice Questions

1. Counseling in audiology is defined as intentional communication with patients and families impacted by audiological conditions. Which of the following types of counseling is intended to the educational needs of a patient/family?

   a. Informational counseling

   b. Adjustment counseling

   c. Diagnostic counseling

   d. Intervention counseling

Explanation: In this question, educational needs of a patient/family are best addressed through informational counseling. Therefore, a is the correct answer.

2. Which of the following questions is the best example of a *closed* question?

   a. Tell me more about the music you've been hearing in your head?

   b. Other than your husband, son, and daughter-in-law, is there anyone else who would like you to get hearing aids?

   c. Are you taking any medications?

   d. Is there anyone else who you would like to better communicate with at home?

Explanation: Closed questions often lead a patient to respond with a short or sometimes yes/no type of answer. Therefore, c is the correct answer.

3. Sally, an 18-year-old female with bilateral cochlear implants, has been working with the same cochlear implant audiologist since she was a toddler. There were times she got along well during mapping sessions and others she would've rather been someplace else. She is nearly ready to graduate from high school. Which of the following is an example of a patient goal that Sally, her parents, and her audiologist could work together on setting?

   a. Being reliable and decisive

   b. Scheduling her own appointments

   c. Showing respect and dignity

   d. Being courteous and civil

Explanation: Only one goal is provided: "showing up on time." Values are attitudinal characteristics that drive and motivate actions, including being reliable, respectful, or courteous. Therefore, b is the correct answer.

4. Which of the following statements best demonstrates an example of a patient who is resistant to changing their hearing health behavior?

   a. My wife thinks I am having trouble hearing at home and I have noticed similar things.

   b. I need to hear and understand people better at work, or I may lose my job.

   c. My wife is nagging me to get hearing aids, I don't think I have enough hearing loss yet.

   d. I would like to get the best hearing aids to meet my communication needs possible.

Explanation: All listed answers are examples of a desire to change, except for the one that presents a statement of denial. Therefore, c is the correct answer.

5. Mr. Echohawk, a 55-year-old male from a Native American background, was diagnosed with a bilateral flat moderately severe sensorineural hearing loss. When discussing options after his hearing test, he is having a hard time understanding the audiologist's words and does not make eye contact. The audiologist notices this and offers Mr. Echohawk a handheld personal sound amplifying device (e.g., a Pocket Talker) to use for the remainder of the appointment. Mr. Echohawk is relieved that he can now hear the audiologist's voice better without having to rely on visual or lip cues. What cultural counseling principle did the audiologist apply in this encounter?

   a. Cultural humility
   b. Cultural humiliation
   c. Cultural adaptation
   d. Cultural disrespect

Explanation: In this question, the audiologist was culturally familiar with Native Americans not making direct eye contact out of respect and demonstrated cultural humility by offering an alternative solution to help them communicate better. Therefore, a is the correct answer.

6. Ms. Hampton, an 88-year-old female, who lives on limited Social Security income and has no Medicare hearing aid benefits was recently diagnosed with a mild steeply sloping to severe sensorineural hearing loss in both ears and is greatly interested in purchasing hearing aids. Which of the following is the best example of an external barrier that may be present to Ms. Hampton in reaching her hearing health goal of acquiring hearing technology?

   a. Emotional
   b. Financial
   c. Cognitive
   d. Stress

Explanation: In this question, the only external variable listed is "financial" due to Ms. Hampton's limited income. All other answers are example of internal barriers to patient goals (i.e., emotional, cognitive, stress). Therefore, b is the correct answer.

7. Consider the following audiological encounter:

   Audiologist: "How long were you exposed to this loud music at the concert?"
   Patient: "About 2 hours."
   Audiologist: "Were you wearing any hearing protection?"
   Patient: "I had some foam plugs, but I don't think I had them deep enough."
   Audiologist: "What sort of foam plugs were they?"
   Patient: "Ones I got at a local drug store."
   Audiologist: "Did you take them out at any point during the concert?"
   Patient: "Yes, they were getting sore after about an hour in, so I just went the rest of the concert without them."

Audiologist: "Can you remember if the music got any louder toward the end of the concert?"

Patient: "Now that you mention it, yes, I do remember the band getting really loud during the closing number and seeing a bunch of kids around me starting to plug their fingers into their ears when a guitar amp burst."

Which of the following types of questions best describes the types of questions used by the audiologist to gather more and more detail in developing levels?

a. Funnel questions

b. Closed questions

c. Leading questions

d. Clarifying questions

Explanation: General questions that drill down to a more specific point in each, asking for more and more detail at each level that are interrogative in nature act like a funnel, and are thus called funnel questions. Therefore, a is the correct answer.

8. Jimmy, a 2-year-old male, was recently fit with a pair of wireless rechargeable BTE hearing aids with custom earmolds compatible with direct streaming to mobile technologies like smartphones and tablets. He and his family live a 2.5-hour drive from the children's hospital where his pediatric audiologist works. Jimmy's parents own a tablet device with videoconferencing abilities and the pediatric audiologist expressed that due to their state's licensure laws permitting, they would like to set up some intermittent follow-up teleaudiology appointments to see how Jimmy is doing at 1 week and 3 weeks postfitting to reduce the travel burden on the family. What type of service category would these types of appointments fall under?

a. Synchronous

b. Asynchronous

c. Hybrid

d. None of the listed options

Explanation: For videoconferencing appointments, synchronous sessions would provide for the best setup in this case; therefore, a is the correct answer.

9. Which of the following best describes what a discharge note for a Medicare patient should include?

a. Assessment of progress/improvement and/or changes to goals

b. Diagnosis and functional assessment scores from earliest encounters

c. All information a future provider may need to pick up patient care

d. The most recent encounter and notes on intervention

Explanation: Medicare suggests a discharge note should include documentation of all treatment since last progress report in the form of a handover document explaining to a patient or any other healthcare professional why the patient was admitted or enrolled in treatment, what happened to them during treatment, and all information that they may be needed in the future for another provider to pick up the care of the patient efficiently and effectively. Therefore, c is the correct answer.

10. Which of the following statements is true of electronic medical record (EMR) systems?

    a. There are no Medicare requirements for electronic submission of billing information when using an EMR.

    b. They offer substantial flexibility to locate any available relevant patient history.

    c. It is not possible to use documentation templates in an EMR system.

    d. They are not as secure as paper charts.

Explanation: EMR systems offer substantial flexibility to providers, including from multiple professions, to locate any relevant patient history when working easily and conveniently in a setting such as a hospital network. Therefore, b is the correct answer.

Section V

Research and Professional Topics

Chapter 12

Research Applications and Evidence-Based Practice

Katharine Fitzharris, Jenna Cramer, and Jeremy J. Donai

Research Principles

Research is a process of systematic inquiry. Typically, this involves asking a question and subsequently engaging in a process to derive the answer. Often referred to as the scientific method, this process includes a series of steps that begins with identifying an issue or problem, formulating a question, collecting data, and ultimately uncovering possible answers to the question.

- Research involves many types of activities that healthcare professionals already participate in during clinical practice. It is through evidence resulting from the research process that healthcare professions develop, norm, and implement clinical protocols and procedures. This is commonly referred to evidence-based practice or EBP. Other components of EBP include clinical expertise and patient values, which help guide clinical decision-making. Clinicians should constantly seek to ask and answer questions about issues relating to evaluation, diagnosis, and treatment and practice as consumers of research.

Variable Levels

Variables are the elements or characteristics that are being investigated or measured; they are usually expected to change attributes depending upon the experimental question or procedures. They can be categorized in a number of ways, as described in the next section.

- Nominal: mutually exclusive (i.e., a data point cannot be categorized/grouped into multiple areas) categories or named groupings (e.g., yes/no response, type of hearing loss, biological sex)
  - ☐ Commonly referred to as a classification or categorical variable, the nominal level is the most basic level of measurement or naming of objects, response types, or events.
- Ordinal: mutually exclusive categories or named groupings with ranked or ordered levels (e.g., hearing loss severity: mild, moderate, moderately severe, severe, profound)

- ☐ The ordinal level accounts for the identity of the members of a category, as well as the magnitude of the attributes by ranking from least to most.

- ■ Interval: mutually exclusive categories or named groupings, ordered levels, with a constant distance between adjacent intervals (e.g., standard scores on behavioral tests like the SCAN-3, temperature in degrees Fahrenheit or Celsius, sound intensity in dB HL, Likert-scale ratings)

  - ☐ The interval level includes category and magnitude and specifies the equality of intervals between adjacent values of the attribute measured.

- ■ Ratio: mutually exclusive categories or named groupings, ranks or ordered levels, with a constant distance between adjacent intervals, equivalence of ratios among values, and a true zero point (e.g., frequency of sound in Hz word recognition score in percent correct)

  - ☐ The ratio level requires the establishment of an absolute zero and the determination of the equality of the ratios between the attribute measured.

Variable Types

- ■ Independent variable (IV): the presumed cause of the dependent variable (the presumed effect). This is conceptualized as conditions that can cause or change behavior and is typically controlled or manipulated by the researcher (variables that **I** control). IVs are also referred to as predictor variables.

- ■ Dependent variable (DV): this can be viewed as the behavior that is changed or the outcome (variables or tasks that subjects **do**). This is also referred to as a criterion or response variable. The formula (DV = f(IV)) highlights the fact that the DV is dependent upon a "function" or effect of the IV.

- ■ Confounding variable: a variable that influences both the dependent variable and independent variable. These can be known or unknown to the researcher. If known, efforts to control for this type of variable should be undertaken.

- ■ Moderating variable: a variable that can strengthen, diminish, or negate the association between an IV and a DV.

 AUDIOLOGY NUGGET

A researcher is studying the effects of age and sex on the degree of hearing loss, pure-tone average in dB HL, and word recognition score in a group of younger adults and a group of older adults. In this example, sex is a nominal variable. Degree of hearing loss and age group (young and old) are ordinal variables, pure-tone average is an interval variable, and word recognition score is a ratio variable. Additionally, this study has IVs of age groups and sex and the DVs are the measurements being made (degree of loss, pure-tone average, and word recognition score).

- Discrete variable: a quantitative variable whose value can be calculated by counting (e.g., number of people with hearing loss within a specified population at a given time).

- Continuous variable: a quantitative variable whose value can be measured to an infinite degree (e.g., a person's age in years, months, days, hours, minutes, seconds, centiseconds, milliseconds, microseconds, nanoseconds, and so on). These can be made into discrete variables by placing specific constraints (e.g., age calculated in months) on the data being measured.

Study Design

Study design can be separated into categories based on the means by which the outcomes are derived (quantitative or qualitative), if the variables or conditions are manipulated (experimental or nonexperimental), if subjects are randomly assigned (experimental or quasi-experimental), and how the results are reported (group or single subject) (Nelson & Gilbert, 2021).

- Experimental studies: in an experimental design, researchers identify one or more factors that they will manipulate or control during the experiment. In this design, it is assumed that the effects of the experimental manipulation (independent variables) influence (or cause) changes in the participants' behavior (dependent variables).

- Quasi-experimental studies: these studies are also common. True experiments require that subjects are randomly assigned to experimental groups where quasi-experimental designs do not have such a requirement. It is generally accepted that "cause-effect" relationships require some degree of experimental manipulation.

- Nonexperimental/descriptive studies: these types of studies are typically used to describe patterns of disease, public opinion, or some characteristic of a particular group. These studies may be qualitative or quantitative in nature, depending on the goal of the study. It is important to note that no experimental manipulation occurs during these types of studies, and due to this, a cause-effect relationship may not be drawn from the results.

- Between-subjects studies: these studies can be experimental or nonexperimental and involve two or more groups of subjects who are divided by some characteristic (e.g., men vs. women, musicians vs. nonmusicians, normal hearing vs. hearing impaired). These typically examine the same dependent variables (outcomes) in two or more groups of subjects. Consider the case where a researcher wanted to answer the question: What are the effects of musical training on speech perception in noise abilities? The IV is the presence or absence of musical training (musician group vs. nonmusician group) and the DV is the score on the speech-in-noise measure.

- Within-subjects studies: these can be experimental or nonexperimental with one group of participants. The IVs are the various conditions or test measures completed by the participant and the DVs are the outcomes of the measures. Similar to between-subjects designs, within-subjects designs evaluate the effects of the IVs on the DVs. These are often completed when examining outcomes of different products (e.g., hearing aids) or characteristics of the independent variable (e.g., signal-to-noise ratio [SNR]). Consider a researcher who wants to evaluate the effects of SNR on a particular speech-processing strategy currently implemented in hearing aids. The researcher uses four SNRs, including −10, −5, 0, and +5 dB (IVs), and measures sentence recognition abilities (DV) among 30 subjects with mild-to-moderate sensorineural hearing loss. In this example, all 30 subjects will be tested in each of the four SNRs. One advantage of this study design is the fact that each subject acts as his or her own control, so any effects of subject selection are present and distributed among all DVs (outcomes).

■ Mixed studies: these studies possess aspects of both within- and between-subjects designs and utilize multiple groups of subjects tested in multiple conditions with comparisons made both between and within each group of subjects.

■ Prospective studies: these studies collect and analyze data that have not yet been acquired. These studies can be experimental or nonexperimental.

■ Retrospective studies: these studies analyze data that have already been acquired (e.g., chart reviews). These studies are nonexperimental as there are no variables being manipulated by the researcher.

■ Correlational studies: the purpose of correlational studies is to examine the relationship between IVs of interest. These studies are nonexperimental in nature in that no experimental manipulation to the IV occurs. This is commonly evaluated via the Pearson product-moment correlation coefficient and often noted as r. The r value can range from −1.0 to +1.0 (perfect correlations), with the strength of the relationship getting stronger toward ±1.0 and weaker as it approaches 0.0 (no correlation). Correlation data are usually displayed on a scatterplot with one variable on the x-axis and the other on the y-axis. As shown in Figure 12–1, the closer r gets to ±1.0, the closer the data approximate a straight line, which is typically called the line of best fit (see Figure 12–1 for specific and detailed examples).

  □ The relationship between the two variables can be positive (e.g., direct) or negative (e.g., inverse) based on the direction of the relationship. Positive r values indicate a direct

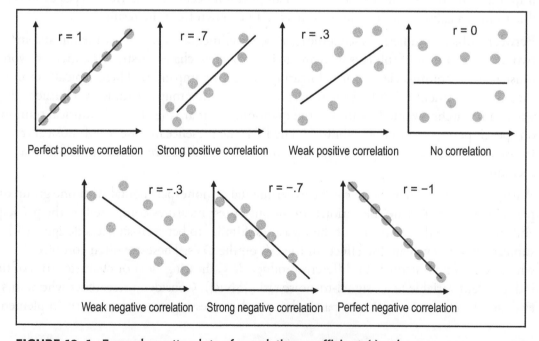

FIGURE 12–1. Example scatterplots of correlation coefficient (*r*) values.

relationship (as one variable increases in value, so does the other variable). An example of this relationship is degree of hearing loss and the amount of hearing aid gain required to achieve signal audibility. Negative *r* values indicate an inverse relationship (as one variable increases in value, the other variable decreases). An example of a negative relationship is audiometric thresholds (in dB HL) and word recognition scores.

☐ Other study types are outlined in Table 12–1. Note: this is not an exhaustive list but some of the commonly used ones from the current literature.

Hypothesis Testing

The purpose of hypothesis testing is to reject or fail to reject (never "prove" or "accept") a null hypothesis. This is accomplished through statistical testing, which will be discussed later in the chapter.

- Null hypothesis (H_0): a null hypothesis is stated in the negative and assumes that no significant differences between groups and/or no significant relationships among variables exist.

  ☐ Example: no difference in speech recognition scores exists for individuals with hearing loss and individuals with normal hearing.

- Alternative hypothesis (H_1): an alternative hypothesis is contradictory to the null hypothesis and is generally a statement that the study is testing.

  ☐ Example: differences in speech perception scores exist for individuals with and without hearing loss.

- In research studies, one can reject the null hypothesis in favor of the alternative hypothesis. However, individuals cannot "prove" the null is true. Researchers test a hypothesis by determining whether there is enough statistical evidence to "reject" the null in favor of the alternative hypothesis.

Statistical Analyses

- Statistical tests are used to evaluate and determine the statistical probability of the null hypothesis or alternative hypothesis (Oleson et al., 2019). This is accomplished via probability testing, which will be discussed later.

- Statistical significance is a concept that relates to making decisions about the existence versus the absence of differences between groups or relationships among variables. It should be noted that statistical and clinical significance are different measures.

Types of Statistics

Descriptive statistics put quantitative data into numerical form to summarize and present salient information, while inferential statistics are a tool to assist researchers in evaluating the representative nature of their findings (i.e., how the findings from a sample relate to the findings for a population). One role of inferential statistics is to provide information about the probability that study outcomes are a result of their experimental manipulation or groupings and not due to random chance.

TABLE 12–1. Study Design Table

STUDY DESIGN	DESCRIPTION	EXAMPLE
Case control	Compares two groups (one with the disease/condition [case] and one without [control]); can be quantitative or qualitative or mixed; nonexperimental	Experiment comparing auditory skills between a group of children with cochlear implants and those with normal hearing
Case series	Observations of an individual or a group with a disorder/undergoing an intervention to establish possible outcomes; quantitative, qualitative, or mixed; nonexperimental	Retrospective study describing test outcomes of a group of children with auditory processing disorder undergoing music training
Randomized control trials	Experimental study comparing outcomes for two or more randomly assigned groups undergoing different interventions; quantitative, qualitative, or mixed	Prospective study examining different hearing aid settings for two groups of subjects on speech-in-noise outcome measures
Cross-sectional	Observational study that collects and analyzes data collected from a group/subset of a population at one particular time; quantitative, qualitative, or mixed; nonexperimental	Retrospective study reporting on the data gathered from a Special Olympics Healthy Hearing event
Crossover	Compare subjects' responses to the multiple treatments delivered at different points of time on the same outcome measures to determine the most effective option; quantitative, qualitative, or mixed; experimental or nonexperimental	Prospective study examining effects of multiple different hearing aid settings for one group of subjects on speech-in-noise outcome measures, changing the settings every 6 weeks
Single-subject	Examine a participant's actions or behaviors over time, usually on some repeated measure, to evaluate effects of different treatments or interventions; quantitative, qualitative, or mixed; nonexperimental	Measuring auditory discrimination skills on a child with a cochlear implant as they age
Cohort	Longitudinal study reporting on data collected over time for a group of subjects that share a common characteristic; quantitative, qualitative, or mixed; nonexperimental	Prospective study examining veterans with blast exposure performance on auditory processing measures every year after the blast exposure for 15 years
Normative	Prospective or retrospective data collection to establish normative values for some measure; quantitative; experimental or nonexperimental	Establishing the latency cutoffs for expected normal-hearing thresholds via ABR on a new piece of electrophysiological equipment

Descriptive Statistics

If data values are plotted on a figure with the value of the data on the *x*-axis and the frequency (count) of data points on the *y*-axis, it yields something like is shown in Figure 12–2. Researchers can use many aspects of the data set to describe its trends and shape, as described in the following points.

- Mean, median, mode: mean is a common measure of central tendency, often referred to as the "average" of a set of numbers. The median is a number that occurs at the midpoint in a series of scores after ordering them (usually from high to low). Mode is based on frequency information (how often a value occurs) and is the category, response, or score that occurs most often.

- Standard deviation: standard deviation (SD) is the most used measure of variability for a level of measurement. The SD reflects the dispersion of scores around the mean; 1 SD represents approximately 68% and 2 SD represents approximately 95% of the data falling within the specified range. Some consider it the most important statistic for organizing data of a study, one that should always be reported with the mean to provide a complete picture of the data.

- *z*-score: A *z*-score is a standardized numerical measurement that describes a value's relationship to the mean of a group of values when measured in standard deviation units. The formula for *z*-scores is: $z = X$ (obtained score) – Mean (population)/SD. A *z*-score equal to 0 equates to the mean value, while $z = -1$ refers to 1 SD below the mean and $z = 1$ refers to 1 SD above the mean.

- Confidence interval (CI): a measure of the probability that a value will fall within a specific range of numbers around the mean. The CI is affected by its value (usually 95% or 99%), the sample's variance, and the sample size (number of collected values) in the data set.

- Variance: variance refers to how far each number in a data set is from the mean (average) or the spread of the data.

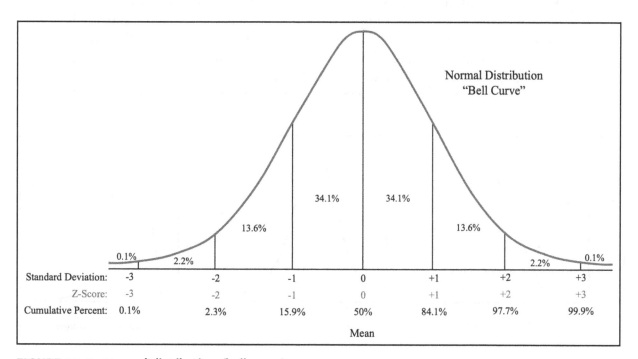

FIGURE 12–2. Normal distribution (bell curve).

- Skewness: skewness refers to the symmetry or asymmetry of a distribution. A distribution is said to be skewed if the majority of scores fall at the extremes (high or low scores). For example, if 100 subjects were evaluated and 90 of them scored between 90% and 100% on the measure, the data would be skewed toward the upper limit of performance (negative skew). Distributions are described as having a symmetrical, positive, or negative skew (Figure 12–3) and are categorized according to the tail. The tail is the portion opposite of the peaked portion of the distribution. Note that distributions of scores on a given measure can also be qualified as having ceiling (negative skew; mostly high scores) or floor (positive skew; mostly low scores) effects.

- Kurtosis: kurtosis is a descriptor of the general concentration of scores around the center of the distribution, which can be seen on the graph by looking at the center to see if it is broad or peaked.

AUDIOLOGY NUGGET

When describing a data set, a researcher wants to represent as much of the data as they can, but in terms that are straightforward to illustrate. An overall value, such as the mean, is one level of descriptor, but it does not account for a great deal of the data. Adding the standard deviation (SD) to the descriptors can help further explain the spread of the data—how large a range the data fall. Data with a small SD can be interpreted as that the data collected are clustered around the mean, that is, the mean number is a strong descriptor of the data set as a whole. For instance, if a mean pure-tone average in a study of adults is 17 dB HL with a standard deviation of 4, a reader can safely assume that the vast majority of the subjects in the study had normal hearing (or at least a pure-tone average ≤25 dB HL with 95% of the data [2 SD] falling between 9 and 25 dB HL). However, if the SD is large, say 12 dB for the previous example, a reader cannot necessarily assume normal hearing for everyone in the study. In fact, it would be difficult to estimate the degree of hearing loss for the sample as a whole since the range of 95% of the data would fall between –7 and 41 dB HL.

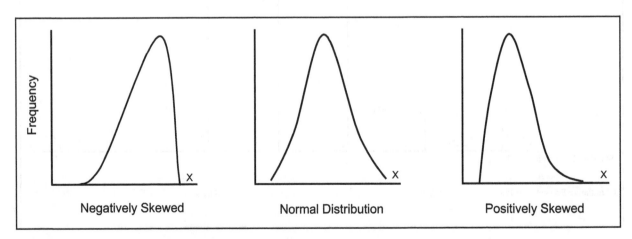

FIGURE 12–3. Examples of skewed and normal distribution.

Inferential Statistics

Inferential statistics allow researchers to make inferences or draw conclusions about the results of a study that extend beyond simply describing the data using descriptive statistics. Inferential statistics can be divided into qualitative and quantitative statistics. Both are important as they provide different outcomes and thus are often used together to provide a "full picture" of what is being studied.

- Qualitative statistics: these describe data in terms of features, trends, themes, or characteristics. Qualitative statistics can be converted to quantitative statistics by calculating the mean (or other values) of qualitative responses (e.g., determining what percentage a particular theme arises during qualitative analysis). Tests for qualitative data (nominal or ordinal variables) include those like the chi-squared test.

  - Chi-squared test: the chi-squared test (χ^2 test) is a way to examine categorical variables, specifically to compare the obtained frequencies of the defined variables to the expected frequencies of those same variables. These tests are performed on data in a contingency table, wherein the variables are distributed along the columns and rows, and the frequency of occurrence for each combination of variables is put into the corresponding cells.

- Quantitative statistics: quantitative statistics describe data in terms of discrete, measurable values (i.e., discrete variables and continuous variables). There are numerous quantitative statistics that can be used depending upon the assumptions about the population from which the data were derived (parametric or nonparametric), type of outcome and predictor variables (continuous or discrete), the number of predictor variables, and the study design (between or within subjects). Some of the possible tests are included in Figures 12–4, 12–5, and 12–6. Several common tests are described below.

KNOWLEDGE CHECKPOINT

When choosing a statistical test, it is important to decide between parametric and nonparametric measures. Parametric tests are used when the following assumptions can be made about the data:

1. The data are normally distributed.

2. The data were sampled randomly and independently.

3. There are no outliers in the data (points that are at the extremes from the majority of the data).

4. The different groups of data have similar variances (i.e., how much the data varies from the mean).

   If these assumptions are not met, then nonparametric tests should be used. Nonparametric tests are appropriate for data with small numbers of subjects or observations, outliers, and all data types (nominal, ordinal, and continuous). Examples of parametric and nonparametric tests are included in Figures 12–4 and 12–5.

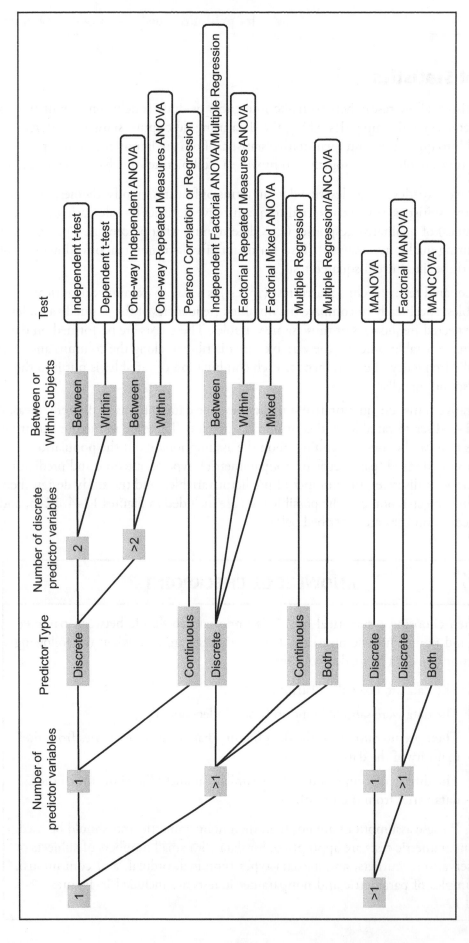

FIGURE 12–4. Characteristics of different statistical tests for studies with parametric data that use continuous outcome variables.

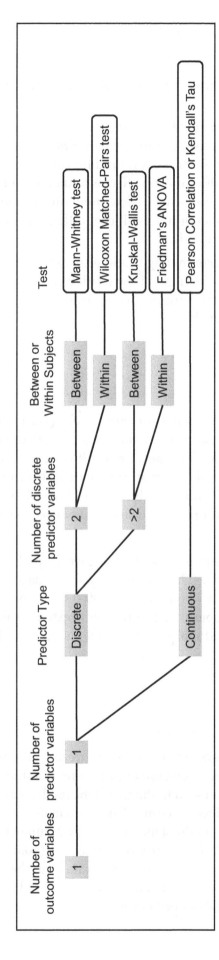

FIGURE 12–5. Characteristics of different statistical tests for studies with nonparametric data that use continuous outcome variables.

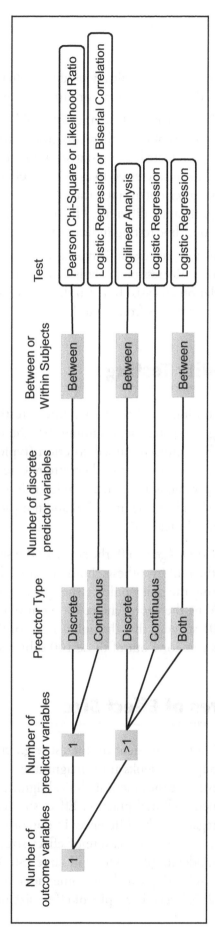

FIGURE 12–6. Characteristics of different statistical tests for studies with data that use discrete outcome variables.

- *t*-tests: *t*-tests are typically used to evaluate for statistically significant differences between two sets of data with interval- or ratio-level measures.

- ANOVA: analysis of variance (ANOVA) is commonly used in instances where there are comparisons of more than two groups and more than two conditions under which each group is being evaluated. It is a statistical procedure that presents as a test for differences among several means, referred to as a "main effect." If a significant main effect is found, post hoc testing (after initial statistical evaluation) should be conducted to determine which conditions are significantly different. The main effect tells whether or not significant differences exist, while post hoc testing indicates where these differences exist.

- Regression: regression is typically performed when determining relationships among multiple variables. Regression analysis determines not only the strength of the relationship (similar to correlation analysis) but also the variables that have the most predictive power for determining future outcomes from an independent (predictor) variable.

Probability Testing

Probability testing is utilized in hypothesis testing where the p value (or alpha level) is the probability of observing a test statistic, assuming that the null hypothesis is true (typically at $p = .05$ or greater). If results meet a predetermined criterion (typically $p < .05$), it is considered sufficient evidence that the null is likely not true and therefore rejected in favor of the alternative hypothesis (Oleson et al., 2019). The p value is a measure in reference to the Type I error rate (the chance of rejecting the null hypothesis when it is true in reality) and not the Type II error rate (the chance of not rejecting the null when it is false in reality).

- The closer p gets to 0, the stronger the statistical significance, and the higher the probability that the null hypothesis should be confidently rejected. This means that $p < .05$ suggests that rejecting the null would be the appropriate choice for 95 out of every 100 subjects, but it would be the wrong choice for 5 out of every 100 subjects. Taken to a more extreme value, $p < .01$ suggests that the null is false for 99 out of 100 subjects (and should be rejected) but holds true for 1 out of those 100 subjects.

Measures of Effect Size

Effect size is a measurement of interest (e.g., change in outcome in response to treatment, difference between groups) that looks at the magnitude of difference between outcome measures in a study. It can be used to estimate the practical/clinical significance of a statistical finding, or if the results of the study should influence clinical practice. Effect sizes can be qualified in terms of their strength—calculated using data regarding the differences in outcome measures and the standard error (SD/number of data points). For a common measure of effect size, Cohen's d, these categories are trivial (<0.02), small (0.2–0.5), moderate (0.5–0.8), and large (>0.08) effect sizes. Note that these values can be positive or negative, indicating which outcome measure (e.g., control vs. experimental group, Condition 1 vs. Condition 2) is larger. Examples of effect size measures are described below.

Examples of effect sizes:

- r^2: referred to as the coefficient of determination and is the proportion of the variation in the dependent variable predictable from the independent variable
- R^2: similar to r^2, but relates to multivariate regression, with a range from 0 to 1, with 0 indicating no relationship and 1 a perfect relationship
- eta-squared (η^2): measures the proportion of variance associated with each main effect and interaction effect in the ANOVA model
- omega-squared (ω^2): estimation of how much variance in the response variables is accounted for by explanatory variables in the ANOVA model
- Cohen's d: based on R^2 and is used to indicate the standardized difference between two means, it is an alternate indicator of effect size for multiple linear regression (MLR)
- Odds ratio (OR): likelihood of an event occurring in one group (experimental group) compared to the likelihood of the same event occurring in another group (control group). OR values less than 1 (OR < 1) suggest the outcome is more likely to occur in the control group, with OR > 1 suggesting an outcome more likely to occur in the experimental group.

Statistical Significance Versus Clinical Significance (Effect Sizes)

Statistical significance refers to the probability that your result is due to chance. Effect size refers to the strength of relationships or importance of the findings (Sullivan & Feinn, 2012). As previously discussed, it is possible to obtain statistically significant results with a small effect size. This can occur when data are collected from a large number of subjects or a measure with high precision.

- Consider an example where a 3% difference in mean word recognition score is obtained when these scores are obtained using two different models of hearing aids. Based on probability statistics, these results are found to be significant (null hypothesis is rejected in favor of the alternative).
- Once the researcher determines if their results are significant, it is important to review the effect size. In this example, the effect size is found to be .08 or 8%. This value is interpreted as a small effect size, suggesting that while statistically significant, the effect of hearing aid type on word recognition score among participants in this study is limited.

Sensitivity and Specificity

Sensitivity and specificity are measures used to evaluate relationships between outcomes on some measure, typically screening measures for the presence of a disease or disorder. These are important to clinicians because they are used on a regular basis (e.g., universal newborn hearing screening via automated auditory brainstem response or otoacoustic emission testing, school hearing screenings with different presentation levels) to determine what constitutes best clinical practice in terms of EBP. Data used to calculate sensitivity and specificity are collected and analyzed as part of research protocols. These calculations are shown in Figure 12–7.

	Number with Disease	Number with No Disease	Total
Positive test result	A *True Positive*	B *False Positive*	All with Positive Test
Negative test result	C *False Negative*	D *True Negative*	All with Negative Test
	All with Disease	All with No Disease	Total
	Sensitivity: A/(A+C)	Specificity: D/(D+B)	

FIGURE 12–7. Sensitivity and specificity information.

- Sensitivity: sensitivity refers to the relationship between a true positive (i.e., hit) and a false negative (i.e., miss) when the condition is positive. This describes how well a condition is detected when it is present.

- Specificity: specificity refers to the relationship between false positives (i.e., false alarms) and true negatives (i.e., correct rejections) when the condition is negative. This describes how well a condition is rejected when it is absent.

- Predictive value: predictive value is the likelihood that the observed results are true. These can be described in terms of positive predictive value (among individuals with positive results, the probability of individuals having the disorder) or a negative predictive value (among individuals with negative results, the probability of individuals not having the disorder).

Ceiling and Floor Effects

When designing a new outcome measure or evaluating measures to use either for clinical or research purposes, ceiling and floor effects must be considered as they will skew the data that are collected. This can make interpretation and application of findings difficult or distorted.

- Ceiling effect: if a measure is too easy, scores will cluster at the maximum end of the scale, for example, around 100%. Here, a bell curve (see Figure 12–2 for a normal "bell curve") would have an abnormally high mean, skewing the data to the left (i.e., the peak of the curve would be at the right of the figure, a negative skew).

- Floor effect: if a measure is too difficult, scores will cluster toward the minimum end of the scale, closer to 0%. On a bell curve, the mean would be extremely low, leading to a rightward-skewing curve (i.e., the peak of the curve would be at the left side of the figure, a positive skew).

Norm- Versus Criterion-Referenced Tests

In audiology practice and education, it is common to use test measures that are both norm- and criterion-referenced. The difference between the two is as follows: Norm-referenced tests compare the test taker's outcome to a normative group of test takers' scores, whereas criterion-referenced tests do

Q & A

Question: Can the results of a study be statistically significant but have a low effect size, and if so, what does this mean?

Answer: Yes, this can and does occur. Statistical significance provides information related to whether results are due to experimental manipulation or grouped conditions or simply random chance; however, it does not provide information regarding how important or strong they are in terms of the population. For example, let's say a researcher wanted to examine the relationship between AuD students' grade point average (GPA) and the number of hours slept per night. Results of a statistical test show that a statistical significance exist between these two factors, and the effect size (r^2) is .15 $(r^2 = .15)$. This suggests that, although statistically significant, the strength of the relationship between these two variables is 15%. In other words, only 15% of GPA values is accounted for or predicted by the number of hours slept per night. The moral of the fictitious story: Sleeping well does not guarantee a high GPA during graduate studies, so go out and enjoy yourself!

not take the performance of others into consideration. Norm-referenced measures are often reported in terms of percentile rankings; a score of 90% would mean that the individual performed better than 90 out of 100 peers that took the same test. A criterion-referenced test would be something like the Praxis or other exams—an earned score must meet a certain cutoff to pass, but this score was not determined by testing others. Tests can use both norm- and criterion-referenced cutoffs, such as the SCAN-3:C and SCAN-3:A. Here, absolute scores are converted into standard scores, which are criterion-referenced, and also yield percentile rankings, which are norm-referenced.

Systematic Reviews and Meta-Analyses

Systematic reviews and meta-analyses are two mechanisms involved in determining the best available evidence to assist in the clinical decision-making process. Universally considered the highest level or strongest research evidence, these techniques involve the accumulation of research studies in a systematic fashion, including only articles that meet certain, stringent, inclusion criteria. The following information represents commonly utilized methods and issues for conducting a systematic review with a meta-analysis and information related to the interpretation of these techniques.

1. Formulate question: define the review question and formulate hypotheses.
2. Define inclusion and exclusion criteria: develop PICO(T) question and details about studies to be included or excluded from the analyses.
    - PICO(T) is an acronym standing for Population/Patient, Intervention, Comparison, Outcome, and Time. These terms are defined further on in the chapter.
3. Define search strategy and locate relevant studies: develop a comprehensive list of search terms and databases.

4. Select studies to include: review abstracts and retain studies meeting inclusion criteria for full review. Commonly, two reviewers judge articles to establish interrater reliability.

5. Extract data and assess study quality: extract data and create a table or form to organize information from each study. Review each study for quality of research design, methods, and outcomes.

6. Analyze and interpret findings: calculate effect sizes and create visuals to display the data (e.g., summary table with forest plot).

7. Disseminate findings: submit for publication in academic journal or Cochrane Database of Systematic Reviews.

- Results of systematic reviews and meta-analyses are typically provided in table format (refer to Figure 12–8). Shown in the far-right potion of the table is a forest plot. A forest plot is a graphic display of estimated effect measures from scientific studies included in a meta-analysis. Take note of the x-axis (often arranged in terms of the odds ratio or OR) ranging from –2 to +2, with a central value of 0. In this example, effect measures below 0 (to the left) favor the control, while values to the right (above 0) favor the treatment.

- A summary effect measure (indicated by the diamond-shaped figure) provides information regarding the cumulative outcome from studies included in the analysis. For a more exhaustive review, refer to Haidich (2010).

- Meta-analyses are not without limitations, however. These analyses are subject to publication bias. Publication bias occurs because studies failing to produce significant findings are less likely to be published in peer-reviewed outlets than those with significant outcomes. Because of this, it is likely that studies without significant findings are excluded from meta-analyses. This can skew the outcome of the analysis and should be evaluated and accounted for through statistical tests that adjust the summary effect measure.

EBP

Evidence-based practice (EBP) is a process for decision-making that incorporates external scientific evidence with practitioner expertise and client perspectives to improve clinical outcomes (Figure 12–9). Providing services in an evidence-based way allows practitioners to evaluate and recognize the needs of the individuals to which we are providing services. EBP also assists in making clinical decisions based on evolving knowledge.

- Commonly referred to as a process of clinical problem solving, providing evidence-based care involves four steps: (1) framing the clinical question (ask), (2) searching the evidence (access), (3) evaluating the evidence (appraise), and (4) making a clinical decision (apply).

PICO(T) Questions

Framing a clinical question involves determining characteristics related to PICO(T). In framing the question using the PICO(T) framework, the researcher/clinician is creating what is referred to as a foreground question (a question with specific details about the patient). Information regarding each of these areas is provided below.

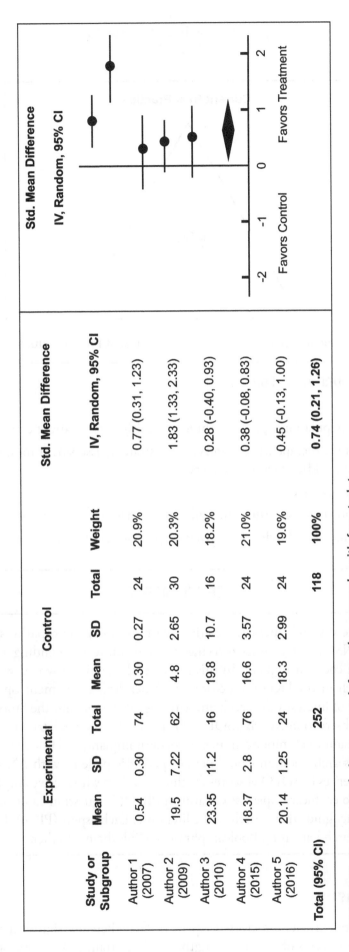

Study or Subgroup	Experimental			Control			Weight	Std. Mean Difference IV, Random, 95% CI
	Mean	SD	Total	Mean	SD	Total		
Author 1 (2007)	0.54	0.30	74	0.30	0.27	24	20.9%	0.77 (0.31, 1.23)
Author 2 (2009)	19.5	7.22	62	4.8	2.65	30	20.3%	1.83 (1.33, 2.33)
Author 3 (2010)	23.35	11.2	16	19.8	10.7	16	18.2%	0.28 (−0.40, 0.93)
Author 4 (2015)	18.37	2.8	76	16.6	3.57	24	21.0%	0.38 (−0.08, 0.83)
Author 5 (2016)	20.14	1.25	24	18.3	2.99	24	19.6%	0.45 (−0.13, 1.00)
Total (95% CI)			252			118	100%	0.74 (0.21, 1.26)

FIGURE 12–8. Meta-analysis summary information example with forest plot.

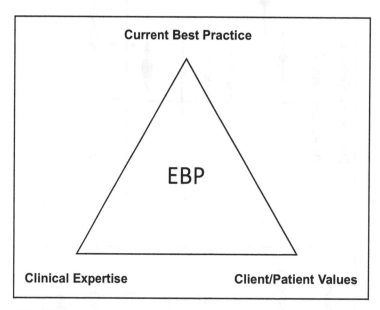

FIGURE 12–9. EBP triangle.

- P: patient/client population: age, sex, ethnicity, health status, patient category
- I: intervention issue: therapeutic or intervention strategy, assessment tool, therapeutic tool or device (e.g., hearing aid), or service delivery
- C: comparison/alternative
- O: outcome: short- or long-term goal, skill, ability, mastery, or accuracy
- T: time: time frame of evaluation (not always a part of the question)

 CASE EXAMPLE

Consider the case of a pediatric patient with auditory neuropathy spectrum disorder (ANSD) and a clinician trying to decide on recommending amplification versus a cochlear implant. In this instance, the clinician would want to do some research in the literature before recommending a treatment option. Say the outcome of interest was speech and language development, the Student Oral Language Observation Matrix (SOLOM). Here, P = the pediatric patient with ANSD, I = traditional amplification, C = cochlear implant, and O = the SOLOM. Thus, the research question would be: For pediatric patients with ANSD, what are the differences in SOLOM scores for those children who receive amplification as opposed to cochlear implants? Creating a PICO(T) question can help a clinician/researcher guide their search of the literature: Each aspect (PICO(T)) can be entered in search bars using Boolean phrases to link them together.

Levels of Evidence

Not all published research articles are created equal. In fact, there are significant differences among the published literature in terms of quality, strength, and importance. Assessing each article individually based on established guidelines affords clinicians and researchers to make these determinations. Table 12–2 contains information related to the type of published study and its relative strength and level (increasing from Level VI to Level I). It should be noted that there are numerous formats for evidence tables; however, they all contain a general structure that should be applied when evaluating the quality of and reporting research evidence. In other words, the highest level of evidence (Level I) takes the form of well-designed systematic reviews and/or meta-analyses of randomized controlled trials. Due to the amassing and analysis of multiple sources of evidence regarding a similar topic, these scholarly analyses contain less bias and increased statistical power (due to combining subjects from multiple studies) than studies reviewed individually. However, as previously discussed, publication bias does occur.

 AUDIOLOGY NUGGET

Recall the buzz within the hearing health professions regarding research documenting the association between hearing loss, hearing aid use, and the slowing or decrease in the incidence of dementia. A recent retrospective cohort study by Chern et al. (2022) found a strong association of dementia among elderly individuals with hearing loss compared to those without hearing loss (incidence was twice as high for those with hearing loss). The authors of the study note the correlational relationship (noncausal) found in their study and suggest that randomized controlled trials (one of the strongest levels of evidence) are needed to determine if treating hearing loss (through hearing aids) reduces incident dementia. They go on to suggest "although hearing aids have been shown to be associated with decreased incident dementia and cognitive decline, this does not imply that hearing aid use prevents dementia or cognitive decline, as association does not imply causation" (p. 40). This highlights the need for experimental manipulation to imply cause-effect relationships.

TABLE 12–2. Level of Evidence Table

LEVEL	STRENGTH OF EVIDENCE	DESCRIPTION
I	Strongest	Systematic reviews and well-designed meta-analyses of several randomized controlled clinical studies
II	Strong	Well-designed randomized control clinical studies
III	Moderate	Well-designed nonrandomized quasi-experimental studies
IV	Limited	Controlled noninterventional descriptive studies, correlational and case-control studies
V	Weak	Uncontrolled noninterventional studies, including case reports
VI	Weakest	Expert opinion of authorities

Source: Adapted from Orlikoff et al. (2015).

Institutional Review Board (IRB)

Research activities are overseen by the IRB at various institutions to ensure scientific integrity and safety for participants who take part in research studies. All research, whether prospective or retrospective, is expected to be examined and approved by the IRB prior to data collection.

- Purpose: the IRB reviews research proposals and works to ensure that respect, beneficence, and justice are maintained for all participants prior to their involvement in research activities. The IRB considers the risk-to-benefit ratio of the studies that are submitted prior to approval and monitors the study during its duration for any events (i.e., adverse events) that may endanger the participants/subjects.

- Protection for human subjects includes the requirement that participation is voluntary, that individuals are safe from harm, and that they have information about the purpose of the research before they are asked to participate, which is referred to as informed consent.

- Assent refers to when individuals (adults or children) are considered a minor or otherwise unable to sign for informed consent but are old enough to understand the purpose of the study. In this case, the possible best possible explanation of study procedures is provided to the subject and guardian. The participant must sign the assent form prior to participating in the study, with the guardian being required to sign the consent form.

 KNOWLEDGE CHECKPOINT

In speech-in-noise measures with fixed signal-to-noise ratios (SNR), such as the Auditory Figure-Ground subtest of the SCAN-3, the specific SNR being tested (0, +8, +12 on the SCAN-3) is calculated to avoid ceiling or floor effects. This allows for a broad range of scores to be elicited, which leads to better delineation between normal and abnormal findings. Looked at another way, most academic exams are designed to have scores distributed in a normal bell-shaped curve. If an exam had a floor effect, most students would do poorly, which would not be the optimal outcome. If an exam had a ceiling effect, students would be understandably happy since their scores would be on the higher side of the distribution.

Types of IRB Review

- Expedited review: where certain kinds of research can be reviewed and approved without a meeting of the full IRB, requiring that the study meets the categories of research that involve no more than minimal risk.

- Full-board review: involves research that is greater than minimal risk but also includes minimal risk research that does not meet the requirements of the expedited review categories.

- Exempt review: a project may be "exempt" from higher review if it presents no more than minimal risk and all of the research procedures fall within one or more of the exemption categories specified in the federal IRB regulations. Examples include, but are not limited to, surveys, education research, benign behavioral interventions, and taste and food evaluations.

Ethics in Research

Research ethics have been shaped by a long history of documentation and events, which readers are encouraged to review (e.g., Belmont Report, Tuskegee syphilis study, Willowbrook hepatitis study). There are three basic principles governing the use of human participants in research: respect for persons, beneficence, and justice.

- Respect for persons is the recognition of potential participants' abilities to make their own decisions as to whether they participate in a study. The informed consent process plays a vital role in ensuring respect for persons.

- Beneficence is the protection of the well-being of those who choose to participate in research. Study review by the IRB ensures this concept is maintained throughout the study.

- Justice is the assurance of equitable recruitment and involvement of participants in research and is also maintained by the IRB.

Protections

- The IRB requires that participants' personal information be kept private and that the research records remain confidential and secure. Most often, records must be deidentified prior to data entry to maintain confidentiality.

- Vulnerable populations, such as children, prisoners, pregnant women and fetuses, individuals with developmental disabilities, and students, have special protections. These are in place to prevent undue harm to these populations who may be coerced (intentionally or unintentionally) into participating in a study.

- There are special protections for these groups since they may be under additional influences to participate in a study or at a greater risk for negative effects of a study. There must be a strong rationale, as determined by the IRB, for the inclusion of vulnerable groups.
    - Informed consent or assent (if the participant is a child or otherwise unable to give consent on their own behalf without another responsible party) must be obtained from all participants prior to their involvement in a research study unless otherwise determined by the IRB.

    - All individuals must give voluntary informed consent to participate in a research study. To do so, the participant needs to be made aware of the nature, purpose, and expectations of the study. Special considerations and procedures are made for vulnerable populations listed above. Even when informed consent is provided by an appropriate legal representative, the research participant must still be willing and able to participate after receiving the appropriate explanation of the study (often referred to as assent). Regardless, additional justification and safeguards are necessary in these vulnerable populations.

Research Integrity

Research must be conducted in a responsible manner and include the protection of human and nonhuman subjects, avoidance/acknowledgment of potential conflicts of interest, care when collecting or handling data, and publication of accurate findings with appropriate attribution of concepts and researcher contribution. Research with nonhuman animals is generally managed by a separate office than human subject research, titled the Institutional Animal Care and Use Committee (IACUC).

- Conflicts of interest can arise when an individual or group is performing multiple roles with different types of responsibilities. It is important to avoid these as much as possible, especially in the researcher/clinician role, but if they cannot be avoided, conflicts must be acknowledged and disclosed to the parties involved.

- It is also important to establish relationships between mentors and mentees, collaborating authors, and others involved in research. Expectations should be set regarding roles and responsibilities, as well as authorship guidelines for the research team contributors.

Researchers must not intentionally misrepresent the data and/or findings. Further, publications should include appropriate citations and acknowledgments of the work of others who contributed to the paper (ASHA, 2016).

Recommended Readings

American Speech-Language-Hearing Association. (n.d.-a). *Evidence-based practice (EBP)*. https://www.asha.org/research/ebp/

American Speech-Language-Hearing Association. (n.d.-b). *Statistics refresher*. https://www.asha.org/research/ebp/statistics-refresher/

CITI Program. (n.d.). *Research, ethics, and compliance training*. https://about.citiprogram.org/

Haidich, A. B. (2010). Meta-analysis in medical research. *Hippokratia, 14*, 2937.

Oleson, J. J., Brown, G. D., & McCreery, R. (2019). Essential statistical concepts for research in speech, language, and hearing sciences. *Journal of Speech, Language, and Hearing Research, 62*(3), 489–497.

Sullivan, G. M., & Feinn, R. (2012). Using effect size—or why the P value is not enough. *Journal of Graduate Medical Education*, 279–282.

References

American Speech-Language-Hearing Association. (2016). *Code of ethics*. https://www.asha.org/policy/ET2016-00342/

Chern, A., Sharma, R. K., & Golub, J. S. (2022). Hearing loss and incident dementia: Claims data from the New York SPARCS database. *Otology & Neurotology, 43*, 36–41.

Haidich, A. B. (2010). Meta-analysis in medical research. *Hippokratia, 14*, 2937.

Nelson, L. K., & Gilbert, J. L. (2021). *Research in communication sciences and disorders: Methods for systematic inquiry*. Plural Publishing.

Oleson, J. J., Brown, G. D., & McCreery, R. (2019). Essential statistical concepts for research in speech, language, and hearing sciences. *Journal of Speech, Language, and Hearing Research, 62*(3), 489–497.

Orlikoff, R. F., Schiavetti, N., & Metz, D. E. (2015). *Evaluating research in communication disorders* (7th ed.). Pearson.

Sullivan, G. M. & Feinn, R. (2012). Using effect size—or why the P value is not enough. *Journal of Graduate Medical Education, 4*(3), 279-282.

Practice Questions

Use the passage below to answer Questions 1–4.

Researchers conducted an experiment to examine how pediatric patients with unilateral hearing loss (anacusic ear) performed on speech-in-noise measures with a CROS device versus a bone-conduction device on a headband. Fifteen children between the ages of 10 and 12 years participated in a laboratory setting with speakers set up at 30° angles surrounding the test chair. The task was twofold: a CRM (coordinate response measure; a measure of button-press reaction time to identifying which speaker the target talker as noted by a call sign was originating) and speech recognition measure (repeating the word from the target talker) with the signal coming from speakers at 0°, 90°, 180°, and 270° azimuth; 12-talker speech babble was presented at 90° and 270° azimuth. Performance was measured to stimuli presented at a +3 dB signal-to-noise ratio (SNR) at 65 dB SPL.

Results indicated that the best speech recognition in noise was when the signal was directed to the normal-hearing ear regardless of device. The poorest performance was when the target and noise were co-located with the bone-conduction device. Performance on the CRM reaction time metric was best for the CROS condition and poorest for the unaided condition. These findings support an advantage for the CROS device over the bone-conduction device for speech-in-noise tasks in children with unilateral hearing loss.

1. What kind of study design was used in the study described?

    a. Crossover

    b. Between-subjects

    c. Within-subjects

    d. Mixed

Explanation: In this example, one group of 15 subjects with unilateral hearing loss completed all of the experimental conditions. Thus, there are only within-subject comparisons. Therefore, c is the correct answer.

2. What type of variable was the devices (CROS, bone conduction) used?

    a. Dependent

    b. Independent

    c. Nominal

    d. Ordinal

Explanation: Remember that the independent variable, by definition, is the presumed cause of the dependent variable (the presumed effect). In this example, the devices serve as the independent variable, and the performance measures are the dependent variable. The devices are controlled by the researcher, and the measures are the change observed. Therefore, b is the correct answer.

3. What type of research was used in the described experiment?
   a. Experimental
   b. Nonexperimental
   c. Quasi-experimental
   d. Normative

Explanation: In the example, we know it is experimental in nature because we have independent and dependent variables that we are controlling. However, the example does not specify if the groups are randomized, which is a requirement of true experimental designs. The study fits the quasi-experimental design best. Therefore, c is the correct answer.

4. Suppose the study above used 24 participants with normal hearing, plugged one ear with a foam hearing protection device, and used the two devices in two randomly assigned groups. What would the type of research be in this case?
   a. Experimental
   b. Nonexperimental
   c. Quasi-experimental
   d. Normative

Explanation: The study is similar to the one we just discussed, but now it includes the randomly assigned groups, which satisfies the requirements of a true experimental design. Therefore, a is the correct answer.

5. The ability of a screening measure to correctly identify individuals who do not have a disorder is referred to as:
   a. Sensitivity
   b. Specificity
   c. False positive
   d. False negative

Explanation: The definition of specificity refers to when the condition is negative. Or in other words, describes how well a condition is rejected when it is **absent**. In this example, we are looking to correctly identify those who do NOT have a disorder, or reject the condition because it is absent. Thus, b is the correct answer.

6. An experiment is conducted to explore the mean length of utterance (MLU) in 20 young children (aged 18–41 months; divided into groups) with mild to moderately severe sensorineural hearing loss who received amplification as compared to their age-matched peers with normal hearing. The MLUs across age groups were subjected to t-tests for statistical analysis with the following results:

Age group (months)	df	t	p
18–23	4	2.25	.049
24–29	4	0.56	.890
30–35	4	1.23	.420
36–41	4	1.50	.085

Which age group had significantly different MLUs between those children with and without hearing loss?

a. 18–23

b. 24–29

c. 30–35

d. 36–41

Explanation: In order to determine which group has significantly different results, we need to look at the p value that was provided in the chart. Remember, the p value is the probability of observing a test statistic, assuming that the null hypothesis is true (typically at $p = .05$ or greater). In this example, we want to determine which age group has a p value of $<.05$. The only one that satisfies this is the 18–23 group at .049. All other values are $>.05$ (i.e., 0.890, 0.420, 0.085), and therefore are not the right answer. If results meet a predetermined criterion (typically $p < .05$), it is considered sufficient evidence that the null is likely not true and therefore rejected in favor of the alternative hypothesis. Therefore, a is the correct answer.

7. A clinician is trying to decide whether to pursue mild gain amplification for a pediatric patient diagnosed with auditory processing disorder. They search the literature and are determining the level of evidence for eight recently published articles (in the last 10 years). Which study would provide the strongest level of evidence upon which to base the clinician's decision?

a. Randomized control trial

b. Meta-analysis

c. Cohort study

d. Expert opinion

Explanation: Recall the level of evidence figure earlier in the chapter; expert opinion is the weakest level of evidence. Randomized control trials are strong, but meta-analyses are the strongest level of evidence and would be considered correct given the answer choices. Therefore, b is the correct answer.

8. A researcher performs informed consent on all human participants in a trial of tinnitus treatments before beginning testing procedures. What research principle(s) does informed consent represent?

    a. Beneficence

    b. Justice

    c. Respect for persons

    d. All of the above

Explanation: Informed consent ensures that participants are able to make their own decisions as to their participation in the study. This relates to the principle of respect for persons. Therefore, c is the correct answer.

9. An experiment is conducted to evaluate the presence of elevated pure-tone thresholds with severity of perceived tinnitus handicap. A correlational analysis is completed. What is the expected result if the two dependent variables are not related to one another?

    a. Negative r

    b. Positive r

    c. p approaching 1

    d. r approaching 0

Explanation: In this example, an r (correlation coefficient) value approaching 0 suggests no correlation (no relationship between the two variables). Therefore, d is the correct answer.

10. Which of the following represents the most complete PICO question?

    a. In adults with sensorineural hearing loss, does frequency-lowering technology affect speech recognition scores in noise?

    b. Does frequency-lowering technology improve speech recognition scores in noise?

    c. In adults with mild sensorineural hearing loss, does frequency-lowering technology lead to better speech recognition scores in noise than extended bandwidth technology?

    d. Does extended bandwidth technology improve speech recognition scores in noise more than frequency-lowering technology?

Explanation: In this question, each of the answers contains some elements of the PICO question. Answer c, however, contains all of the categories needed to formulate a complete PICO question.

Chapter 13

Audiology Professional Topics

Renee Zimmerman and Jeremy J. Donai

Professionalism

Audiologists are bound to practice within both legal and ethical guidelines. It is the individual's responsibility to maintain knowledge of this information, which is readily available and provided by professional organizations, continuing education opportunities, and state licensing entities. Professional organizations, including the American Academy of Audiology (AAA) and the American Speech-Language-Hearing Association (ASHA), publish a Code of Ethics under which members should practice. Codes of Ethics and rules of practice are also published by licensing bodies (e.g., state licensure boards) and state-level professional organizations. Professionalism, the conduct, aims, or qualities that characterize an individual professional and their practice, should be guided by the information contained in these documents.

Moral, Legal, and Ethical Issues

There are specific legal and ethical issues relevant to the profession of audiology. It is important to disassociate ethics from law but also realize that the two areas influence one another. Figure 13–1 provides information related to laws and ethics. One can think of ethical principles as information to help guide actions and decision-making, whereas laws are intended to direct, restrict, or modify behavior in some way. Typically, punishment for violating legal statutes is more severe than ethical violations, which often results in education or training to assist in remedying the unethical behavior. Liang (2006) provides a comprehensive review of legal considerations relevant to the profession of audiology. Morality is similar to ethics but is typically considered applicable to personal rather than professional situations and decisions.

The Anti-Kickback Statute

The Anti-Kickback Statute prohibits payment for referrals for anyone participating in a federally funded healthcare program. According to Liang (2006), "this law prohibits any knowing and willful conduct involving: (1) the solicitation, receipt, offer, or payment of any kind of remuneration, (2) in return for referring an individual for services or recommending or arranging the purchase, lease, or ordering of any item, (3) that may be wholly or partly paid for by a federal healthcare program" (p. 51).

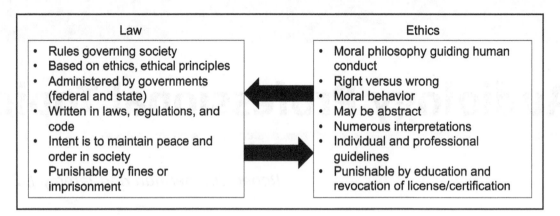

Law	Ethics
• Rules governing society • Based on ethics, ethical principles • Administered by governments (federal and state) • Written in laws, regulations, and code • Intent is to maintain peace and order in society • Punishable by fines or imprisonment	• Moral philosophy guiding human conduct • Right versus wrong • Moral behavior • May be abstract • Numerous interpretations • Individual and professional guidelines • Punishable by education and revocation of license/certification

FIGURE 13–1. Differences between law and ethics.

- Example violation: Dr. S owns a private practice and is discussing a referral system with a local ENT physician. Dr. S is offered $25.00 per patient referred to the ENT practice for otologic evaluation. The ENT physician offered to send Dr. S a quarterly check based on the number of referrals provided by his audiology practice. Dr. S's practice participates with most private insurance companies common to the geographic area (e.g., Blue Cross/Blue Shield, AETNA) but also participates with Medicare and Medicaid. Because Dr. S participates in Medicare (federal) and Medicaid (federal and state) and is receiving remuneration for referrals to the ENT practice, she is in violation of the Anti-Kickback Statute.

- Penalties: both civil and criminal providers may be held liable for both civil and criminal penalties for the same offense.

   □ Criminal penalties are felonies and must be proven to the standard of "beyond a reasonable doubt" as with all other crimes.

   □ Criminal: fines up to $25,000 and imprisonment up to 5 years for each offense; provider is subject to program exclusion (exclusion from health insurance plans)

   □ Civil penalties up to $50,000 and damage to the government for each violation

Stark Self-Referral

The Stark Self-Referral statute (sometimes referred to as the Stark law) prohibits referrals by physicians to entities in which they or an immediate family member maintains a financial interest. Under this law, the word "physician" is inclusive of only traditional allopathic physicians and does not explicitly include audiologists. However, subsequent interpretations have established the statute to be applicable to the profession of audiology.

- According to Liang (2006), "if a physician or immediate family member maintains a financial relationship with an entity, then: (1) the physician may not make a referral to the entity to furnish health services, (2) for which payment would otherwise be made by a federal healthcare program, (3) and the entity may not present a claim to a federal healthcare program, or bill any individual, third-party payer, or other entity for the service" (p. 52).

- Example violation: Dr. B is a private practice audiologist who creates a separate company (Company X) with a physical therapist who performs vestibular rehabilitation for the purpose of referring his vestibular patients. Dr. B refers all of his patients who are candidates for vestibular rehabilitation to Company X, in which he is part owner. Dr. B participates in most insurances, including Medicare and Medicaid. Because Dr. B participates in federally funded insurance programs and has financial interest in Company X, he is in violation of the Stark Self-Referral statute.

- Penalties: Civil

  - Civil: denial of payment for designated healthcare services provided; refunds of the amounts that were paid for these services; civil monetary penalties of up to $15,000 for individuals; civil monetary penalties of up to $100,000 per scheme

False Claims Act

The False Claims Act prohibits the submission of false claims (including healthcare claims) and fraudulent billing to the federal government. According to Liang (2006), no false claim may be submitted or fraudulent billing made under any federal healthcare program for any item or service provided by a person who knowingly and willfully has made any false statement or representation in application for payment. This includes claims for uncovered services or services or supplies that are determined to be substantially in excess of those needed or are so lacking as to be considered useless.

- Example: Dr. M has a large pediatric patient base and routinely performs OAE screenings using equipment limited to testing only three frequencies (2, 3, and 4 kHz). The practice is a provider for both private and federal health insurances. Dr. M's office manager informs her that the diagnostic OAE Current Procedural Terminology (CPT) code (92588) reimburses at a higher rate than the screening (limited) code (92587). Dr. M requests the office manager use the diagnostic code to improve reimbursement for the OAEs performed at her office (commonly referred to as "upcoding"). Because the practice participates with federal health insurances, knowingly filing a fraudulent claim with the federal health insurance plans is a violation of the False Claims Act.

  - Penalties: criminal and civil

 Q & A

Question: An audiologist performs air-conduction screenings for patients of a residential facility for individuals with developmental delays. The practice accepts both private and governmental insurance, including Medicare and Medicaid. Because the code used for air-conduction screening is consistently denied by Medicare, the audiologist decides to use a comprehensive evaluation code (92557) because he knows it is a reimbursable code. Is the audiologist violating a federal statute, and if so, which statute?

Answer: Yes, the audiologist is violating the False Claims Act, which prohibits filing a false claim against the government. In this instance, the audiologist is knowingly using a form of "upcoding" by filing the claim using a code for a more extensive diagnostic service than that being performed.

- Criminal: felonies and fines up to $25,000 and up to 5 years of imprisonment (same as Anti-Kickback)
- Civil: penalties up to $11,000

☐ No proof of damage is required to prove a violation

☐ Insurance program exclusion

Malpractice

According to Bal (2009), medical malpractice is defined as any act or omission by a physician during treatment of a patient that deviates from accepted norms of practice in the medical community and causes injury to the patient.

- According to Liang (2006), medical malpractice is often adjudicated at the state level in civil court between private parties (e.g., the patient and the audiologist) using the negligence rule.
- Negligence rule contains four parts: duty, breach of duty, causation, and damages.

☐ To demonstrate medical malpractice, the patient must show that the audiologist had a duty to provide nonnegligent care, the audiologist breached that duty, and that breach caused the patient harm or some form of damage.

- Audiologists will typically purchase malpractice insurance to cover themselves in these cases. Alternately, individual audiologists may fall under the malpractice insurance of their larger organization, like a hospital or university.

Licensure Versus Certification

Certifications and professional licenses are time-limited (typically 1 or 2 years) credentials intended to ensure a level of skill or knowledge required to perform a specific occupation. The fundamental difference between the two is the issuer of the credential. Certifications are issued by nongovernmental certification bodies (ASHA or AAA in audiology), whereas licenses are awarded by federal, state, or local government agencies. As such, licenses provide a legal authority to work in an occupation, while certifications on their own do not.

- In most instances, both credentials require completion of continuing education for maintenance and renewal.
- Certifications are typically optional for practitioners, whereas licensure (state licensure) is required for practice.
- Optional specialty certifications in areas of audiological practice (e.g., vestibular evaluation/treatment, cochlear implants, pediatrics) are also offered by independent professional organizations.

Code of Ethics Review

Codes of Ethics are provided by the AAA and ASHA (as well as other organizations) and are intended to help guide professional behavior. The following are five general ethical concepts upon which most Codes are established.

- Beneficence: doing good for others
- Autonomy: protects and defends informed choices of capable patients
- Nonmaleficence: obligation not to inflict harm on others
- Justice: moral obligation to act based on fair adjudication between competing claims
- Fidelity: personal responsibility to be honest and truthful in relationships

ASHA Code of Ethics

ASHA describe four general ethical principles, under which specific rules are provided. Please review the entire Code of Ethics document for each rule relating to the four principles (https://www.asha.org/policy/et2016-00342/).

- Principle 1: Individuals shall honor their responsibility to hold paramount the welfare of persons they serve professionally or who are participants in research and scholarly activities, and they shall treat animals involved in research in a humane manner.
- Principle 2: Individuals shall honor their responsibility to achieve and maintain the highest level of professional competence and performance.
- Principle 3: In their professional role, individuals shall act with honesty and integrity when engaging with the public and shall provide accurate information involving any aspect of the professions.
- Principle 4: Individuals shall uphold the dignity and autonomy of the professions, maintain collaborative and harmonious interprofessional and intraprofessional relationships, and accept the professions' self-imposed standards.

ASHA Terminology

ASHA provides definitions for salient terminology related to their published Code of Ethics. Knowledge of this terminology should assist in reading and understanding the Code and are provided in Table 13–1.

AAA Code of Ethics

Similar to the ASHA Code of Ethics, the AAA Code contains eight general principles (provided below), with specific rules related to each principle. Please review the original Code of Ethics document for individual rules (https://www.audiology.org/clinical-resources/code-of-ethics/). Additionally, the Code provides procedures for potential violations or noncompliance (provided in Part II).

Part I: Statement of Principles and Rules

- Principle 1: Members shall provide professional services and conduct research with honesty and compassion, and shall respect the dignity, worth, and rights of those served.
- Principle 2: Members shall maintain the highest standards of professional competence in rendering services.
- Principle 3: Members shall maintain the confidentiality of the information and records of those receiving services or involved in research.

TABLE 13–1. Code of Ethics Definitions (ASHA)

TERM	DEFINITION
Advertising	Any form of communication with the public about services, therapies, products, or publications
Conflict of interest	An opposition between the private interests and the official or professional responsibilities of a person in a position of trust, power, and/or authority
Crime	Any felony; or any misdemeanor involving dishonesty, physical harm to the person or property or another, or a threat of physical harm to the person or property of another
Diminished decision-making ability	Any condition that renders a person unable to for the specific intent necessary to determine a reasonable course of action
Fraud	Any act, expression, omission, or concealment—the intent of which is either actual or constructive—calculated to deceive others to their disadvantage
Impaired practitioner	An individual whose professional practice is adversely affected by addiction, substance abuse, or health-related and/or mental health–related conditions
Individuals	Members and/or certificate holders, including applicants for certification
Informed consent	May be verbal, unless written consent is required; constitutes consent by persons served, research participants engaged, or parents and/or guardians of persons served to a proposed course of action after the communication of adequate information regarding expected outcomes and potential risks
Jurisdiction	The "personal jurisdiction" and authority of the ASHA Board of Ethics over an individual holding ASHA certification and/or membership, regardless of the individual's geographic location
Know, known, or knowingly	Having or reflection knowledge
May vs. shall	*May* denotes an allowance for discretion; *shall* denotes no discretion
Misrepresentation	Any statement by words or other conduct that, under the circumstances, amounts to an assertion that is false or erroneous (i.e., not in accordance with the facts); any statement made with conscious ignorance or a reckless disregard for the truth
Negligence	Breaching of a duty owed to another, which occurs because of a failure to conform to a requirement, and this failure has caused harm to another individual, which led to damages to this person(s); failure to exercise the care toward others that a reasonable or prudent person would take in the circumstances, or taking actions that such a reasonable person would not
Nolo contendere	No contest
Plagiarism	False representation of another person's idea, research, presentation, result, or product as one's own through irresponsible citation, attribution, or paraphrasing; ethical misconduct does not include honest error or differences of opinion
Publicly sanctioned	A formal disciplinary action of public record, excluding actions due to insufficient continuing education, checks returned for insufficient funds, or late payment of fees not resulting in unlicensed practice

TABLE 13–1. *continued*

TERM	DEFINITION
Reasonable or reasonably	Supported or justified by fact or circumstance and being in accordance with reason, fairness, duty, or prudence
Shall vs. may	*Shall* denotes no discretion; *may* denotes an allowance for discretion
Support personnel	Those providing support to audiologists, speech-language pathologists, or speech, language, and hearing scientists (e.g., technician, paraprofessional, aide, or assistant in audiology, speech-language pathology, or communication sciences and disorders)
Telepractice, teletherapy	Application of telecommunications technology to the delivery of audiology and speech-language pathology professional services at a distance by linking clinician to client/patient or clinical to clinical for assessment, intervention, and/or consultation. The quality of the service should be equivalent to in-person service.
Written	Encompasses both electronic and hard-copy writings or communications

Source: Information taken from American Speech-Language-Hearing Association. (n.d.). *Code of Ethics.* https://inte.asha.org/Code-of-Ethics#Terminology

- Principle 4: Members shall provide only services and products that are in the best interest of those served.
- Principle 5: Members shall provide accurate information about the nature and management of communicative disorders and about the services and products offered.
- Principle 6: Members shall comply with the ethical standards of the Academy with regard to public statements or publication.
- Principle 7: Members shall honor their responsibilities to the public and to professional colleagues.
- Principle 8: Members shall uphold the dignity of the profession and freely accept the Academy's self-imposed standards.

Part II: Procedures for the Management of Alleged Noncompliance

- Part II of the AAA Code of Ethics details the processes and procedures involved in cases of potential noncompliance such as reporting alleged cases of noncompliance and the role of the Ethical Practices Committee (the committee responsible for final decision-making on ethical misconduct). Outcomes of misconduct can include education (educative letter or mandatory continuing education) or revocation of membership (maximum penalty for blatant disregard for ethical conduct). Members have the right to appeal the Ethical Practices Committee decision.

Ethical Dilemmas

Professionals may find themselves in situations where they question the ethical nature of an action, decision, or behavior of a colleague or supervisor. Sometimes, this takes the form of being asked to do something potentially unethical in the work environment. A few ethical dilemmas common to the profession of audiology are the misrepresentation of credentials (e.g., audiology student or practice misrepresenting an audiology student as an audiologist), issues related to billing compliance (e.g., billing for unnecessary services or services not beneficial to the patient), and patient confidentiality (e.g., posting patient information, often innocuous information, on social media platforms). In these instances, the individual should refer to the relevant ethical guidelines and/or consult with the relevant professional organization or licensure board if concerns persist.

CASE EXAMPLE

An audiologist evaluates a 20-year-old patient who shows a severe-to-profound sensorineural hearing loss with 12% word recognition bilaterally. The audiologist believes strongly that the patient would benefit from a cochlear implant and recommends he be scheduled for an evaluation. The patient states a lack of interest in pursuing a cochlear implant, yet the audiologist persists in trying to convince him to schedule the evaluation. In this example, the ethical concept of autonomy is relevant. While the audiologist may have the best interest of the patient in mind, it is important to allow patients to have control over the decision-making process (autonomy) and respect their decision.

Patient Abandonment

Patient abandonment occurs when a provider unilaterally terminates the provider-patient relationship without providing adequate notice for the patient to obtain replacement care. Some consider patient abandonment as a form of medical malpractice. While there is a lack of universal agreement about what precisely constitutes patient abandonment, a few examples are provided.

- A private audiology practice closes without notifying patients and providing them with information regarding alternative locations where care is offered.
- An audiologist who is the sole audiology provider for an ENT practice quits her job without notice due to a disagreement with the ENT at the practice.
- An audiologist is scheduled to see patients at a satellite clinic but does not attend clinic/work that day due to a dispute over being paid for travel.

Examples that do not constitute patient abandonment:

- Leaving a position prior to a replacement being found after giving sufficient notice
- Leaving a position immediately after giving notice if instructed to do so by the employer
  - If this is the case, make a record of the employer's termination request.
- Taking a vacation as the sole audiology provider in a practice as long as patients have been given sufficient notice or a replacement provider is identified for patients to receive services
- Closing an audiology practice after providing current patients with alternative locations where care can be obtained

For additional information, please refer to the following information: https://www.asha.org/practice/ethics/client-abandonment/

Health Insurance Portability and Accountability Act

The Health Insurance Portability and Accountability Act (HIPAA) of 1996 (PL 104-191) was intended to (1) improve efficiency in healthcare and (2) enhance the privacy and security of health information.

- HIPAA regulations apply to covered entities and business associates (e.g., healthcare plans [insurance companies], hearing aid companies, and other organizations involved [directly or indirectly] with patient care).
- Created term protected health information (PHI)
- Example violations:
  - Accessing files without meeting the "need to know" criterion
    - Example: accessing the records of a family member or a coworker
  - Speaking about a patient's condition and/or care in a public space in a way that allows them to be identified
  - Posting identifiable patient information on social media without patient permission
  - Sending documentation with PHI to a noncovered entity in error (e.g., a misdirected fax)
    - Misdirected faxes are a common problem in healthcare due to physicians changing practices, clinics not keeping updated lists of faxes for referring providers, and fax/phone databases in EMRs not being kept up to date. To protect against the unintended disclosure of PHI, clinics should make every effort to verify the correct fax number before sending patient information and use an HIPAA-compliant coversheet whenever sending PHI over fax.
- Penalties: monetary penalties can range from $100 per violation with a yearly maximum fine of $25,000 to $50,000 per violation and yearly maximum of $1.5 million.
- HIPAA regulations require administrative, physical, and technical safeguards to protect PHI.
  - Administrative safeguards include staff training on compliance with policies and procedures, planning for emergencies or to restore lost data, and management of access to PHI.
  - Physical safeguards include access controls (locks and alarms) to ensure only authorized personnel have access, workstation security measures such as cable locks and computer monitory privacy filters designed to restrict access for unauthorized users.
  - Technical safeguards include hardware, software, and other technology that limits access to PHI. Audit controls to restrict access to PHI for unauthorized users and transmission security measures for PHI when transmitted over an electronic network.
- For additional information, please review the following website: https://www.asha.org/practice/reimbursement/hipaa/

 AUDIOLOGY NUGGET

While accessing one's personal health information in an electronic medical record (EMR) system is not a violation of HIPAA, most healthcare organizations have a policy against doing so. Accessing one's own health record may result disciplinary action according to the employer's policy up to and including termination.

Family Educational Rights and Privacy Act (FERPA)

FERPA is federal legislation that allows parents the right to access their child's educational records, amend those records as needed, and control the disclosure of information. Once a student turns 18 years of age or enters a postsecondary institution prior that age, the rights are transferred to the student. In general, schools must have permission from a parent or eligible student to release information except in the following conditions:

- School officials with legitimate need for the information
- Schools to which students are transferring
- Auditory or evaluation purposes
- Accrediting organizations
- Compliance with judicial orders or lawfully issued subpoenas
- State and local authorities pursuant to state law

FERPA is relevant for students, as well as audiologists working in schools or institutes of higher learning.

Advocacy

Advocacy is how professional organizations support and advance their respective professions (as well as services/benefits for patients) in areas related to public policy, reimbursement, political action, and public opinion. This process is intended to educate and persuade relevant stakeholders, including consumers, politicians, and reimbursement entities (e.g., insurance companies). It is important to obtain "buy-in" for advocacy efforts from members of the profession. State and national professional organizations promote advocacy through lobbying efforts, providing expert testimony, writing sample legislation, as well as other activities. However, all members of a profession have a role to play in advocacy. Professionals make up the organizations of which they are a member, and therefore, any advocacy effort undertaken by a professional organization is only as effective as the amount of support it receives from membership.

ADA and Accessibility Legislation

The Americans With Disabilities Act (ADA) was passed and signed into law in 1990. It protects individuals against discrimination based on disability, in similar way that the Civil Rights Act of 1964 protected individuals against discrimination based on race, religion, sex, national origin, and other identified characteristics. The ADA has five sections.

- Title I—Employment: prevents employers from discriminating against individuals with both mental and physical medical condition. It also requires employers to provide reasonable accommodations to employees in order to be able to do their job.
  - Example: an employee with hearing loss may request captioning for all meetings held via teleconference to aid in understanding.
- Title II—Public entities/transportation: Ensures that individuals with disabilities will be able to access benefits, programs, services, and other activities offered by state and local governments. Title II also provides for equal access to public transportation.

- □ Example: providing hearing loops in government buildings to ensure hearing aid compatibility and improved speech understanding

- ■ Title III—Places of public accommodation: prevents discrimination against individuals with disabilities in places of public accommodation (e.g., restaurants, theaters, hotels, hospitals, medical offices) and ensure equal access to goods and services provided. Title III also explicitly covers guidelines related to service animals and the provision of auxiliary aids.

  - □ Examples:
    - • Installing wheelchair accessible entrances and clearances throughout the facility
    - • Providing a sign language interpreter at no charge to the patient for scheduled visits at medical practices

- ■ Title IV—Telecommunications: requires that all telecommunications companies provide functionally equivalent services for consumers with disabilities, specifically those with disabilities for those that are deaf and hard of hearing

  - □ Example: requirement for television programming to include closed captioning

- ■ Title V—Miscellaneous provisions: includes technical provisions as well as provisions to prevent retaliation or coercion; it also specifies that ADA does not override or cancel any provisions in Section 504 of the Rehabilitation Act of 1973.

In addition to the Americans With Disabilities Act, audiologists should also be aware of relevant state laws regarding accessibility and discrimination. While state laws cannot nullify federal requirements, they can place additional requirements on an entity to which they must adhere.

CASE EXAMPLE

An audiologist at a private practice has an appointment for an audiological evaluation scheduled with a patient that communicates via American Sign Language (ASL). The patient has notified the practice that they will require a sign language interpreter for the appointment. The practice is required to provide a certified ASL interpreter for the patient at no cost to the patient. In addition, the practice may not bill the patient's health insurance for the cost of the interpreter. As a place of public accommodation, the practice is required to provide access to their services for any individual with a disability at no additional cost above what others would pay to access their services.

Interprofessional Education (IPE) and Interprofessional Practice (IPP)

IPE occurs when students from two or more disciplines learn from each other in a collaborative manner, with the goal of improving health outcomes through effective collaboration. IPP is the deliberate collaboration of multiple professions in providing healthcare services.

- ■ IPE example: pharmacy students working with audiology and physical therapy students learning about the auditory and vestibular effects of various medications

- IPP example: physical therapist working with an audiologist on gait training following a vestibular assessment

- For additional information on topics related to IPE and IPP, please see the following websites: https://www.asha.org/practice/ipe-ipp/what-is-ipe/ and https://www.asha.org/practice/ipe-ipp/what-is-ipp/

Supervision Principles

Clinical supervision of students is the mechanism by which the profession of audiology educates and trains future generations of practitioners. As such, it is important for audiologists to have a general understanding of concepts related to effective supervision. Professionals participating in the clinical education component of an audiology program may be referred to by different terms such as clinical educator, clinical preceptor, or clinical supervisor. While the term clinical supervisor is the traditional term, the word supervision broadly refers to overseeing and directing work. Professionals involved in the clinical education process do far more than simply oversee a student in their clinical education. Therefore, many in the field prefer the term clinical preceptor because it more accurately reflects the role of a professional working with a student to develop and practice new clinical skills and provide feedback during a clinical practicum.

A traditional model of clinical education assumes that those who are competent to provide clinical services are also competent to provide clinical supervision. However, the skills required to effectively serve as a clinical educator/preceptor are distinct from those of a competent clinician.

For clinical preceptors, it is important to have knowledge and skills related to the hierarchy of cognition and learning, adult learning styles, the continuum of supervision, and conflict resolution, among others. To emphasize the importance of clinical preceptors being specifically trained to provide supervision under the 2020 standards, ASHA introduced a requirement that professionals holding the Certificate of Clinical Competence in Audiology (CCC-A) complete a specific amount of continuing education (currently 2 hours) on the topic of clinical supervision prior to serving as a clinical preceptor/educator.

 AUDIOLOGY NUGGET

Anderson's Continuum of Supervision (Anderson, 1988)

- Understanding the supervisory process—discussing the process, understanding respective roles, and sharing expectations and objectives

- Planning—joint planning for the clinical process (client and clinician) and the supervisory process (supervisee and supervisor)

- Observing—collecting and recording objective data by both supervisor and supervisee

- Analyzing—examining and interpreting data in relation to changes in clinician and client

- Integrating—integrating content from all components at various points throughout the experience

- For additional details regarding topics relevant to the clinical supervision process, please refer to the following website: https://www.asha.org/practice-portal/professional-issues/clinical-education-and-supervision/

Practice Management

Audiologists should have a basic understanding of practice management topics. Topic areas of interest are types of insurance, insurance models, billing and coding for audiological services, and concepts related to financial management of audiology practices.

Medicare Versus Medicaid

Medicare is a federally administered health insurance program for individuals over the age of 65 and some individuals with disabilities. Medicaid is a jointly funded (federal and state) health insurance program for individuals with limited income and their children. Both insurances have specific guidelines to which audiologists must comply.

Medicare

- Medicare comprises Part A (hospital insurance), Part B (outpatient insurance), Part C (Medicare Advantage plans), and Part D (prescription coverage). Most often, Part B is billed for audiological services performed outside of the inpatient setting.

- Typically requires physician referral, but changes announced in 2023 allow for claims to be amended with a modifier without physician referral.

- Audiological service can only be provided in cases of medical necessity and not for routine screening, annual evaluations without medical necessity, or hearing aid purposes.

- There are six generally accepted components of adequate documentation including: (1) signature, (2) date of service, (3) case history sufficiently describing chief complaints, symptoms, and medical/familial history, to justify medical necessity, (4) procedures performed and outcome of each, (5) assessment/interpretation of results, and (6) recommendations.

Medicaid

- Medicaid is a means-tested (income-driven) health insurance program jointly funded by the state and federal government.
  - Funding from the federal government varies by state and is calculated using a specific formula. States determine mechanisms to administer the Medicaid program within guidelines specified by the federal government.

- Federal funding of Medicaid programs requires states cover specific individuals, including pregnant women, children, individuals with disabilities, and senior citizens with low income or who are blind or disabled.

- Audiological diagnostic and intervention services are covered in varying degrees across states at this time under Medicaid.

Insurance Models

In the United States, various models of health insurance exist. Each type maintains specific advantages and disadvantages, primarily related to costs (premiums and out-of-pocket requirements) and choice of providers. The most common models include health maintenance organizations (HMOs), point of service (POS), and preferred provider organizations (PPOs).

- HMO
  - Low premiums, low deductibles, fixed copays
  - Primary care physician (PCP) required; acts as "gatekeeper" to care
  - PCP referral required for specialist visits
  - Limited network of providers
- POS
  - PCP referrals are required.
  - Higher premiums compared to HMO
  - Greater flexibility in selecting provider
  - Covers out-of-network doctors
- PPO
  - Higher premiums
  - Access to out-of-network without referrals
  - Greater access to providers
  - Low copays for in-network doctors

A general rule regarding health insurance is the more access to and choice in provider, the higher the out-of-pocket expense (premiums and co-pays).

 AUDIOLOGY NUGGET

In 1992, Medicare adopted a resource-based relative value scale (RBRVS) payment system that is based on the principle that payments for clinical services vary depending on the resources required to provide specific services. Three considerations in determining reimbursement rates for each service include (1) the work involved, (2) expenses to the practice, and (3) cost of professional liability insurance. Reimbursement rates are periodically updated based on the recommendation of a committee, often referred to as the RUC (RVS Update Committee), which comprises professionals from multiple specialties, including audiologists, otolaryngologists, and other related professions. The RUC committee makes recommendations to Medicare, which ultimately makes the final decision on reimbursement rates.

Billing and Coding in Audiology

Efficient and accurate billing and coding for audiological services provided are vital facets of practice operation. Inaccurate or inefficient billing can lead to increased denials of claims (reduced revenue/cash flow and increased workload for billing personnel), increased likelihood of issues resulting from insurance audits, and potential legal actions taken against the practice. This section provides an overview into the complex and ever-changing area of billing and coding for audiological services.

- In 2007, the federal government began requiring all healthcare providers obtain a National Provider Identification (NPI) number in order to bill Medicare for services provided.

- Codes for audiological services (and other medical services) and supplies are contained in the Current Procedural Terminology (CPT) and Healthcare Common Procedure Coding System (HCPCS). CPT codes are primarily for diagnostic and therapeutic services, while HCPCS codes are for supplies and products such as hearing aids and related services.

  - Common CPT and HCPCS codes are provided in Tables 13–2 and 13–3.

- International Classification of Diseases, Tenth Revision (ICD-10) codes are used to specify the diagnosis associated with a healthcare encounter. Appropriate codes to use are determined by the signs and symptoms that prompted the evaluation and/or by the results obtained (e.g., type of hearing loss).

  - Common ICD-10 codes relevant to audiologic service provision are provided in Table 13–4.

- Additional details can be found by reviewing the practice management sites of the AAA and ASHA.

AUDIOLOGY NUGGET

In the past, there was discussion within the profession of audiology regarding the usefulness of conducting speech reception threshold (SRT) testing. Some suggested SRT measures provided little in the form of clinical utility (which can be debated); however, it was correctly pointed out that in order to charge insurance for a comprehensive audiological evaluation (92557), air conduction, bone conduction, SRT, and word recognition scores must be completed. So, whether one supports obtaining the SRT or not, the measure must be completed in order to charge for the standard comprehensive audiological test battery.

Time-Based Coding

Most CPT/HPCPS codes reported by audiologists are untimed and do not include time designations in the code descriptor. These codes represent the majority of services provided by audiologists and can be billed once per day. Timed codes include a time designation in the descriptor. Timed codes should only be used when face-to-face time spent in an evaluation is at least 51% of the time designated in the code's descriptor.

TABLE 13–2. Common Current Procedural Terminology (CPT) Codes for Audiology

92537	Caloric vestibular test, with recoding, bilateral, bithermal
92540	Basic vestibular evaluation
92546	Sinusoidal vertical axis rotational testing
92557	Comprehensive audiometry threshold evaluation and speech recognition
92565	Stenger test, pure tone
92567	Tympanometry (impedance testing)
92568	Acoustic reflex testing, threshold
92570	Acoustic immittance testing, includes tympanometry (impedance testing), acoustic reflex threshold testing, and acoustic reflex decay testing
92579	Visual reinforcement audiometry (VRA)
92582	Conditioning play audiometry
92587	Distortion product evoked otoacoustic emissions; **limited evaluation**
92588	Distortion product evoked otoacoustic emissions; **comprehensive diagnostic evaluation**
92601	Diagnostic analysis of cochlear implant, patient under 7 years of age; **with programming**
92602	Diagnostic analysis of cochlear implant, patient under 7 years of age; **subsequent reprogramming**
92603	Diagnostic analysis of cochlear implant, age 7 years or older; **with programming**
92604	Diagnostic analysis of cochlear implant, age 7 years or older; **subsequent reprogramming**
92620	Evaluation of central auditory processing, with report; **initial 60 minutes**
92625	Tinnitus assessment (includes pitch, loudness, matching, and masking)
92626	Evaluation of auditory function for surgically implanted device(s) candidacy or postoperative status of a surgically implanted device(s); **first hour**
92651	Auditory evoked potentials; **for hearing status determination, broadband stimuli**, with interpretation and report
92652	Auditory evoked potentials; **for threshold estimation at multiple frequencies**, with interpretation and report
92653	Auditory evoked potentials; **neurodiagnostic**, with interpretation and report
92591	Hearing aid examination and selection; **binaural**
92593	Hearing aid check; **binaural**

TABLE 13–3. Common Healthcare Common Procedure Coding System (HCPCS) Codes for Audiology

V5011	Fitting/orientation/checking of hearing aid
V5014	Repair/modification of a hearing aid
V5110	Dispensing fee, bilateral
V5211	Hearing aid, contralateral routing system, binaural, ITE/ITE
V5221	Hearing aid, contralateral routing system, binaural, BTE/BTE
V5241	Dispensing fee, monaural hearing aid, any type
V5254	Hearing aid, digital, monaural, CIC
V5255	Hearing aid, digital, monaural, ITC
V5256	Hearing aid, digital, monaural, ITE
V5257	Hearing aid, digital, monaural, BTE
V5258	Hearing aid, digital, binaural, CIC
V5259	Hearing aid, digital, binaural, ITC
V5260	Hearing aid, digital, binaural, ITE
V5261	Hearing aid, digital, binaural, BTE
V5264	Ear mold/insert, not disposable, any type
V5270	Assistive listening device, television amplifier, any type
V5274	Assistive listening device, not otherwise specified
V5275	Ear impression, each

- The primary time-based audiology codes are 92620 (Evaluation of central auditory processing, with report; initial 60 minutes) and 92626 (Evaluation of auditory function for surgically implanted device(s) candidacy or postoperative status of a surgically implanted device(s); first hour).

- In addition, 92621 (Evaluation of central auditory processing, with report; each additional 15 minutes) and 92627 (Evaluation of auditory function for surgically implanted device(s) candidacy or postoperative status of a surgically implanted device(s); each additional 15 minutes).

- It is important to document the start and finish times of testing when billing time-based codes. And, although time-based codes may be billed multiple times to reflect the time spent performing an assessment, payers may limit the number of units of a code they will reimburse in a single day.

TABLE 13–4. Common International Classification of Disease, 10th Revision (ICD-10) Codes for Audiology

H90.0	Conductive hearing loss, bilateral
H90.11	Conductive hearing loss, unilateral, right ear, with unrestricted hearing on the contralateral side
H90.12	Conductive hearing loss, unilateral, left ear, with unrestricted hearing on the contralateral side
H90.3	Sensorineural hearing loss, bilateral
H90.41	Sensorineural hearing loss, unilateral, right ear, with unrestricted hearing on the contralateral side
H90.42	Sensorineural hearing loss, unilateral, left ear, with unrestricted hearing on the contralateral side
H90.6	Mixed conductive and sensorineural hearing loss, bilateral
H90.71	Mixed conductive and sensorineural hearing loss, unilateral, right ear, with unrestricted hearing on the contralateral side
H90.72	Mixed conductive and sensorineural hearing loss, unilateral, left ear, with unrestricted hearing on the contralateral side
H91.90	Unspecified hearing loss, unspecified ear
H93.25	Central auditory processing disorder
H93.29	Other abnormal auditory perception
H93.3	Disorders of the acoustic nerve
Signs/Symptoms Codes	
F03	Unspecified dementia
F79	Unspecified intellectual disabilities
F80.4	Speech and language delay due to hearing loss
F80.9	Speech and language delay, unspecified
H55.0	Nystagmus
H61.2	Impacted cerumen
H83.3X3	Noise effects on inner ear, bilateral
H92.0	Otalgia
H92.1	Otorrhea
H93.13	Tinnitus, bilateral
H93.233	Hyperacusis, bilateral

AUDIOLOGY NUGGET

In cases where the type/nature of hearing loss differs between the left and right ears, each ear should be coded separately. For example, if a patient was found to have a sensorineural hearing loss in the right ear and a mixed hearing loss in the left ear, the following diagnosis codes are used:

- H90.A21 Sensorineural hearing loss, unilateral, right ear, with restricted hearing on the contralateral side
- H90.A32 Mixed conductive and sensorineural hearing loss, unilateral, left ear with restricted hearing on the contralateral side

Modifiers

Modifiers are used to add information or change the description of a procedure to the insurance payer. These are denoted by a dash (-) followed by two numbers (in some cases, two letters). For significantly atypical procedures, a -22 modifier can be used to indicate that the work is substantially greater than typically required, and a -52 modifier is used for an abbreviated procedure, such as testing only one ear. Claims with the -22 modifier require an additional description of the need for extended services. Modifiers -22 and -52 may not be used in conjunction with timed codes. Modifier -59 is used to establish one procedure as distinct from another procedure billed on the same day but typically should only be used with instruction from the payer. For additional details on modifiers please refer to the following website: https://www.asha.org/practice/reimbursement/medicare/aud_coding_rules/

CASE EXAMPLE

When performing an ABR, it is assumed that both ears will be tested. If testing is discontinued after testing the right ear due to patient movement or physiological state resulting in excessive artifact, a -52 modifier can be used with documentation explaining why testing was discontinued.

Basics of Teleaudiology/Telehealth

Telehealth (teleaudiology in the case of audiologic care) is becoming increasingly commonplace as a means of providing healthcare in the United States. Teleaudiology occurs when audiologic services are provided in cases where the audiologist and patient are in separate locations. The location (state) in which the services are provided is called the originating site and all applicable laws and regulations apply to the encounter.

- Audiologists must be licensed in the state in which the patient encounter occurs (where the patient is physically located).

- State law determines scope of practice for teleaudiology (and all audiology) services and terms of telepractice service provision for audiologists, support staff (audiology assistants), and audiology students.

- For a comprehensive review, please see Jilla, Arnold, and Miller (2021).

Healthcare Finance Concepts

It is important for audiologists to be aware of financial concepts involved in the provision of healthcare services. Familiarity with concepts related to audiology practice operation enhances one's marketability as a leader in the hearing healthcare job market. The information provided in this section is a cursory review of these concepts. For a more detailed discussion, please refer to Donai (2014a, 2014b) and Restrepo and Prentiss (2022).

- Revenue: income resulting from the provision of goods and services (total revenues from patient services, investments, and merchandise sales)

- Expenses: costs associated with doing business

  □ Fixed expenses: costs that remain constant in a given period of time (e.g., rent)

  □ Variable expenses: costs that fluctuate (e.g., costs of supplies, costs of goods to sell—hearing aids, assistive listening devices, batteries)

- Assets: any resource with current or future economic value owned or controlled by a business economic entity

- Liabilities: legally binding obligation payable to another person or entity

- Cost of goods sold (COGS): direct costs of goods (e.g., hearing aids, batteries, assistive listening devices) sold by the practice

- Profit margin: a measure of business profit

  □ Gross profit margin: money left over from sales after subtracting COGS, often expressed as a percentage of sales

    - Gross Profit Margin = (Net Sales – COGS)/Net Sales

  □ Net profit margin: measure of how much net income (profit) is generated as a percentage of total revenues

    - Net profit margin = (Net Income/Total Revenue) × 100

    - Strong indicator of practice's overall financial health

- Breakeven analysis: process used to determine the number of services or the amount of sales it will take to recoup the expense on a given expenditure. Breakeven point occurs when revenue and expenses are equal.

  □ Prior to that point, expenses exceed revenues (negative). Following that point, revenues exceed expenses (profit). See Figure 13–2 for a visual example.

- Return on investment (ROI): provides an indication of a practice's profitability relative to its total assets—specifies how well practice assets are being used to generate profits

- Average selling price (related to hearing aids): average cost of hearing aids sold

  □ Often used as a measure of sales performance

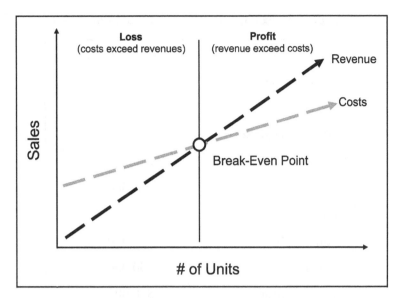

FIGURE 13–2. Breakeven analysis visual.

- Cash flow statement: describes the movement of cash from operations, investing, and financing activities in and out of the organization
  - Measure of how well a company generates cash to pay its debts and fund operating expenses
- Balance sheet: a financial statement that describes a company's assets, liabilities, and shareholder equity
- Profit and Loss (P&L) statement: financial statement that summarizes costs, revenues, and expenses incurred during a specified period of time, typically monthly or quarterly
  - Table 13–5 provides a hypothetical P&L statement (please review the individual components contained therein)
  - Provides information regarding a company's ability (or inability) to generate profit and determine the financial health of a company
  - Helpful when used in conjunction with cash flow statement and balance sheet for determining financial health
- Accounts receivable: amount of money owed to a practice for a good or service that has already been provided
- Days in accounts receivable (Days in AR): provides objective information on how effectively patient accounts receivable are collected
- Accounts payable: money owed to suppliers of goods or services
- Key performance indicators (KPIs): a set of metrics used to evaluate the activity, behaviors, and performance of individual employees and practices
  - Many of the concepts described in this section are used as KPIs from which practice performance is evaluated
  - For additional details, please review Taylor (2016).

TABLE 13–5. Example Profit & Loss (P&L) Statement

Total revenue	$100,000
Cost of goods sold	$20,000
Gross profit	$80,000
Operating expenses	
Salaries	$10,000
Rent	$10,000
Utilities	$5,000
Depreciation	$5,000
Total operating expenses	$30,000
Operating profit	$50,000
Interest expense	$10,000
Income before taxes	$40,000
Taxes	$10,000
Net income	$30,000

KNOWLEDGE CHECKPOINT

Most insurance companies will not reimburse for audiological services when provided with codes specifying results within normal limits. In these cases, it is important to provide an ICD-10 code related to the signs or symptoms that prompted the evaluation rather than coding normal findings. For example, if a patient reports experiencing persistent bilateral tinnitus during the case history (a symptom that prompted the referral and appointment) but testing yields normal (peripheral) hearing. In this case, a code of H93.13 (tinnitus, bilateral) is appropriate to use. This code reflects the symptom of tinnitus reported during the case history and reason for the appointment.

Bundled Versus Unbundled Models of Service Delivery

Traditionally, audiologists provide hearing aid services using a bundled method where many of the costs associated with obtaining the hearing device are paid upon receipt. These costs include fees associated with fitting and dispensing and follow-up (e.g., programming adjustments, appointments related to fitting concerns, verification/validation), routine checks (typically while under warranty), and repairs under warranty. Conversely, the unbundled method involves itemizing (i.e., separating products and services for billing purposes) costs for products and services related to hearing aid fittings. For example, in a bundled model, a patient purchases a pair of hearing aids for $3,000.00, which includes the hearing aids, fitting/dispensing, all follow-up appointments for 2 years (while in warranty), routine checks (while in warranty), and probe-microphone measures for verification as needed. In an unbundled model, the patient might pay $1,500.00 for the same hearing aids but be charged separately for the fitting/dispensing, initial follow-up appointments, and other services previously mentioned. While there are a host of opinions about each of these models, the following provides general advantages and disadvantages without preference for a particular model.

Bundled method

- Advantages: easy to explain and manage; fees paid up front; good for cash flow; patients who consistently utilize services may benefit

- Disadvantages: patient may be paying for services not utilized; less price transparency

Unbundled method

- Advantages: potentially lower short- and long-term cost for patients; increased price transparency; can help compete for patients with third-party coverage

- Disadvantages: potential reductions in cash flow for practice in the short term; potential difficulty transitioning established patients from bundled method

Risk Management in Audiology

Risk management is a process that identifies current and future risk in the areas of financial transactions, safety, infection control, and patient satisfaction. Risk management falls under the area of quality improvement (QI). QI measures are typically required by accreditation or certification bodies such as the Joint Commission (which typically certifies hospitals and rehabilitation centers) and/or part of a company's strategic plan. The employee handbook, which should be reviewed annually with employees, provides information regarding policies (including infection control, safety, and administrative) and other pertinent information. Increases in scope of practice and complexity of audiological services currently provided have created increased risk and the need for risk management and quality improvement programs.

- Internal controls: refers to mechanisms, policies, and procedures used to ensure fidelity in financial transactions and accounting procedures, with the goal of preventing fraud
  - Internal controls can improve operational efficiency by improving accuracy and timeliness of financial reporting.
- Patient satisfaction reporting is an area of QI that solicits perceptions related to the patient experience.
  - Areas typically assessed in measures of patient satisfaction include, but are not limited to, ease of appointment making and interactions with front office staff, punctuality of the appointment, interactions with clinical staff, provision of information by clinical staff (counseling), satisfaction with completeness of answers to patient questions, and patient outcomes.
  - Satisfaction data should be analyzed and used for QI purposes to improve satisfaction and alert administration to any issues (clerical or clinical) related to audiological service provision.

Infection Control

Patient safety is paramount to the provision of healthcare–related services. As such, infection control should be at the core of any QI program, with eliminating (or minimizing) the spread of infectious disease through contact transmission (transmission of disease through direct contact with patient or objects) as a primary goal. When providing audiological services, patients and clinicians encounter a number of pieces of equipment and have direct contact with patients by which infectious diseases can be transmitted. Clark et al. (2003) provide important information regarding environmental infection control and differentiate between common terms used to describe infection control measures: cleaning, disinfection, and sterilization. A review of the information is provided here.

- Cleaning: removing gross contamination from equipment or surface without concern for eliminating germs, which acts as an important precursor to disinfection and sterilization. For the process of disinfection and sterilization to be effective, an initial cleaning is required.
- Disinfection: killing a specific amount of germs, which is determined by the level of disinfectant used in the process.
  - ☐ Audiology practices should use a hospital-grade disinfectant that may come in the form of a spray, towelette, or soaking in ultrasonic tray.
  - ☐ Disinfection is acceptable for items that do not come into contact with blood or other potentially infectious substances or when it is unlikely that a break in the skin will occur. Surfaces and equipment in an audiological practice should be disinfected routinely, daily if possible.
    - Examples: earmolds, headphones, otoscope specula, probe tips (immittance and OAE), ABR electrodes
- Sterilization: involves killing 100% of vegetative microorganisms 100% of the time and is required when an object is in contact with a potentially infectious substance such as blood, mucous, or other bodily fluid
  - ☐ Objects capable of breaking the skin barrier such as curettes or other cerumen management tools should be sterilized after use regardless of contact with potentially infectious substances.
  - ☐ Sterilization options
    - Autoclave: preferred technique that provides heat under extreme pressure to sterilize
    - Cold sterilization: accomplished via soaking materials in specific substances (e.g., glutaraldehyde, hydrogen peroxide) for a period of time.
    - Glutaraldehyde is effective for use and reuse for 14 to 28 days depending on the brand.

Single-Use Versus Reusable Tips

Audiologists use many different probe tips and instruments during an evaluation. While disinfecting and reusing tips is cost-effective, it is important to know which tips can be disinfected/sterilized and which are designed for single use. Some items such as insert ear tips are designed for single use. Others, such as tympanometry probe tips, may seem reusable but are designed for single use. Before choosing to disinfect/sterilize an item for reuse, audiologists should consult the packaging for proper cleaning instructions.

Other Definitions Related to Infection Control

- Standard precautions
  - ☐ Formally known as universal precautions
  - ☐ Includes the following: hand hygiene/hand washing, sterilization and disinfection of reusable equipment as appropriate, utilizing personal protective equipment (PPE), following needle safety and sharp disposable procedures, and appropriately disposing of medical waste
  - ☐ Various procedures will require different levels of standard precautions depending on the level of contact and the risk for infection.

- Hand hygiene
  - ☐ Hand hygiene is the most effective way to prevent infection and is important for the safety of both patients and the healthcare workers that treat them. It is the most basic component of any infection control plan. Hand hygiene can be accomplished by alcohol-based hand rubs and soap and water.
  - ☐ Additional information about proper hand hygiene protocols can be found from the CDC: https://www.cdc.gov/handhygiene/providers/guideline.html

- Environmental surface/patient care equipment infection control
  - ☐ Office furniture and equipment should undergo periodic disinfection and sterilization (depending on the level of potential exposure). Make sure to follow instructions specific to any disinfecting or sterilization agent in regards to use (i.e., wait time, appropriate surface).
  - ☐ Important information can be found at: Methods for Sterilizing and Disinfecting Patient-Care Items and Environment Surfaces from the CDC: https://www.cdc.gov/infection control/guidelines/disinfection/index.html

- Isolation precautions
  - ☐ Isolation precautions are taken in healthcare settings to prevent the spread of an infectious agent from an infected or colonized patient to others. Isolation precautions are frequently used in hospital settings for patients with known infectious disease and require specific PPE.

- Personal protective equipment (PPE)
  - ☐ PPE is worn to minimize exposure to illnesses or hazardous chemicals. Common PPE consists of gloves, masks, gowns, and head and shoe coverings.
  - ☐ Employers should provide employees with adequate protection for all patient contact that is consistent with the CDC-recommended guidelines for PPE.
  - ☐ Employees should be familiar with PPE policies of the facility at which they are employed.

- Vaccinations
  - ☐ Vaccinations are one way to protect clinicians and patients from infectious diseases.
  - ☐ Employment or student placements at certain healthcare facilities may require certain vaccinations or proof of the disease through titers.

For additional information, please review Clark et al. (2003) and the following websites: (1) https://www.audiology.org/practice-guideline/infection-control-in-audiological-practice/ and (2) https://www.asha.org/practice/infection-control/

Recommended Readings

American Speech-Language-Hearing Association. (n.d.). *Practice management portal.* https://www.asha.org/practice/

American Speech-Language-Hearing Association. (n.d.). *Question and answer: Self referral/stark law and anti-kickback regulations.* https://www.asha.org/practice/reimbursement/medicare/qas/

ASHA Code of Ethics link: https://www.asha.org/policy/et2016-00342/#:~:text=The%20ASHA%20Code%20of%20Ethics,and%20integrity%20of%20the%20professions

AAA Code of Ethics link: https://www.audiology.org/clinical-resources/code-of-ethics/

Glaser, R., & Traynor, R. M. (2019). *Strategic practice management: Business considerations for audiologists and other health care professionals.* Plural Publishing.

Jilla, A. M., Arnold, M. L., & Miller, E. (2021). U.S. policy consideration for telehealth provision in audiology. *Seminars in Hearing, 42*(2), 165–174. https://doi.org/10.1055/s-0041-1731697

References

Anderson, J. (1988). *The supervisory process in speech-language pathology and audiology.* College-Hill.

Bal, S. B. (2009). An introduction to medical malpractice in the United States. *Clinical Orthopaedics and Related Research, 467*(2), 339–347.

Clark, J. G., Kemp, R. J., & Bankaitis, A. U. (2003). Infection control in audiological practice. *Audiology Today, 15*(5), 12–19.

Donai, J. J. (2014a). Practice management: Look to financial statements before you leap. *The Hearing Journal, 67*(2), 26–28.

Donai, J. J. (2014b). Putting the financial 'health' in hearing healthcare. *The Hearing Journal, 76*(4), 40, 42.

Liang, B. A. (2006). Law and audiology practice: Understanding malpractice and conflict of interest rules. *Seminars in Hearing, 27*(1), 48–56. https://doi.org/10.1055/s-2006-932122

Restrepo, A. M., & Prentiss, S. (2022). Business 101 for audiology: Business principles and clinical productivity. *The Hearing Journal, 75*(8), 18–21.

Taylor, B. T. (2016). Using key performance indicators to do more with less in your practice. *Seminars in Hearing, 37*(4), 301–315. https://doi.org/10.1055/s-0036-1594000

Practice Questions

1. An audiology practice provides hearing care services for employees of a large multinational company whose health benefits include full coverage for hearing aids. The practice also participates with governmental insurance, including Medicare and Medicaid. The audiologist routinely encourages individuals with normal hearing who are close to retirement to obtain hearing aids while they still have insurance since that benefit is not available in retirement. The audiologist uses the diagnosis code for bilateral sensorineural hearing loss (H90.3) for these patients. In this situation, which legal statute is the audiologist violating?

    a. Anti-Kickback Statute

    b. False Claims Act

    c. Stark Self-Referral

    d. Autonomy act

Explanation: The patient does not have a sensorineural hearing loss. The audiologist is selecting an inaccurate code for the purposes of insurance coverage and violating the False Claims Act. Therefore, the answer is b.

2. Which of the following is the ethical principle that requires audiologists to be faithful and honest in professional relationships?

    a. Autonomy

    b. Beneficence

    c. Nonmaleficence

    d. Fidelity

Explanation: Fidelity is defined as personal responsibility to be honest and truthful in relationships. Therefore, the answer is d.

3. An adult patient with developmental disabilities is being seen for a comprehensive audiological exam. The audiologist must end the appointment after obtaining results only for the right ear. Which of the following modifiers would be the best for the audiologist to use?

    a. -52

    b. -59

    c. -72

    d. -99

Explanation: The billing CPT code 92557 assumes testing of pure-tone air and bone conduction, speech threshold testing, and speech recognition testing bilaterally. If the appointment was ended without obtaining all of the required results for both ears, the audiologist should use the -52 modifier to indicate to the payer that the testing was incomplete. Therefore, the answer is a.

4. The parent of your 18-year-old patient is seeking to obtain the educational records (to share with you) from the local university that the student attended during the previous year. Which of the following legal statutes applies to this situation?

   a. Family Educational Rights and Privacy Act (FERPA)

   b. Health Insurance Portability and Accountability Act (HIPAA)

   c. Public Law 94-142

   d. Individuals With Disabilities Education Act (IDEA)

Explanation: FERPA is a federal privacy law that protects the privacy of student educational records and restricts access and disclosure of those records. Therefore, the answer is a.

5. The owner and audiologist of a single-provider private practice retires and closes his practice. Prior to the closure, he fails to notify patients and provide information regarding alternative providers from which they could receive services. Which of the following concepts is relevant in this instance?

   a. Patient abandonment

   b. Patient abuse

   c. Patient mismanagement

   d. Patient separation

Explanation: Because the patients were not provided notice or information regarding how to obtain services from another provider once the audiologist retires, patient abandonment was committed. Therefore, the answer is a.

6. Which of the following insurance types is typically characterized as having the lowest premium, requires a "gatekeeper" for specialty care, and is often more limited in the choice of providers?

   a. Health maintenance organization (HMO)

   b. Point of service (POS)

   c. Preferred provider organization (PPO)

   d. Health savings account (HSA)

Explanation: PCPs are the "gatekeeper" for HMO plans because a PCP referral is typically needed for access to specialty provides. HMOs also try to keep costs down by offering limited provider that are in-network providers. Therefore, the answer is a.

7. An audiologist is considering the purchase of a piece of vestibular equipment but notes a decline in the number of vestibular evaluations provided by the practice. There is concern that if new equipment is purchased, it will become nonfunctional prior to generating revenue for the practice. Which of the following calculations would be most helpful to the audiologist in deciding whether to purchase the equipment?

   a. Gross profit margin

   b. Costs of goods sold

   c. Breakeven analysis

   d. Key performance indicators

Explanation: The breakeven analysis is the process used to determine the number of services it will take to recoup the expense of a given expenditure. In this case, the breakeven analysis would calculate the number of vestibular tests that are likely to be performed over the expected lifespan of the equipment and compare the reimbursement for the tests compared to the cost of purchasing the equipment. This will allow the audiologist to determine what the breakeven point for the equipment is and if they are likely to perform enough vestibular tests to make a profit from the purchase of the equipment. Therefore, the answer is c.

8. The provision of outpatient audiological services in a private practice setting should be billed to which component of Medicare insurance?

   a. Part A

   b. Part B

   c. Part C

   d. Part D

Explanation: Medicare Part B covers medical services obtained on an outpatient basis. Audiology services are typically provided at outpatient clinics. Therefore, the answer is b.

9. An audiology practice bills an insurance company for a comprehensive audiological evaluation (92557) and tympanometry (92567) completed on a patient. Until the insurance company reimburses the practice for these services, the amount due is placed in which of the following accounts?

   a. Accounts receivable

   b. Accounts payable

   c. Cost of goods sold

   d. Diagnostic revenue

Explanation: Once a service is provided but yet to be reimbursed, the amount owed the practice is placed in accounts receivable until payment is received. Therefore, the answer is a.

10. Which of the following allows an audiologist to legally provide clinical services in a given state?

    a. American Board of Audiology (ABA) certification

    b. Malpractice insurance

    c. Licensure

    d. Certificate of Clinical Competence (CCC) '

Explanation: Licenses to practice in a healthcare field are awarded by federal, state, or local government agencies and are a requirement to practice. Certifications are awarded by nongovernmental organizations and are optional. Malpractice insurance is highly recommended but not required unless by state law. Therefore, the answer is c.

11. A patient is seen for an auditory processing disorder evaluation. The portion of the assessment specific to evaluating areas of auditory processing lasted 1 hour and 20 minutes. Which CPT code(s) should the audiologist select based on the testing?

    a. 92627

    b. 92620

    c. 92620 & 1 unit of 92621

    d. 92620 & 2 units of 92621

Explanation: The total evaluation time is 80 minutes. 92620 is the CPT code for the first 60 minutes of an evaluation of central auditory processing, with report. The additional 20 minutes meets the criteria to bill one unit of 92621 (each additional 15 minutes) but not 2 units since the assessment time did not meet the criteria of at least 51% of the next 15-minute time increment. Therefore, the answer is c.